ANTISEPSIS, DISINFECTION, AND STERILIZATION

TYPES, ACTION, AND RESISTANCE

ANTISEPSIS, DISINFECTION, AND STERILIZATION

TYPES, ACTION, AND RESISTANCE

GERALD E. McDONNELL, B.Sc., Ph.D.
Vice President of Research and EMEA Affairs
STERIS Limited
Basingstoke, Hampshire, United Kingdom

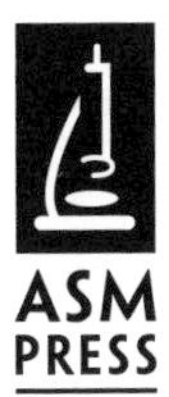

ASM PRESS WASHINGTON, D.C.

Address editorial correspondence to ASM Press, 1752 N St. NW, Washington, DC 20036-2904, USA

Send orders to ASM Press, P.O. Box 605, Herndon, VA 20172, USA
Phone: (800) 546-2416 or (703) 661-1593
Fax: (703) 661-1501
E-mail: books@asmusa.org
Online: estore.asm.org

Library of Congress Cataloging-in-Publication Data

McDonnell, Gerald E.
Antisepsis, disinfection, and sterilization : types, action, and resistance / Gerald E. McDonnell.
p. ; cm.
Includes bibliographical references and index.
ISBN-13: 978-1-55581-392-5 (hardcover)
ISBN-10: 1-55581-392-5 (hardcover)
1. Sterilization. 2. Asepsis and antisepsis. 3. Disinfection and disinfectants. I. Title.
[DNLM: 1. Antisepsis. 2. Disinfection. 3. Sterilization. WA 240 M478a 2007]

QR69.S75M33 2007
614.4′8—dc22 2006031854

10 9 8 7 6 5 4 3 2 1

Printed in the United States of America

Cover photo: Scanning electron micrograph of a mixed biofilm of yeast and bacteria on an indwelling silicone rubber voice prosthesis after 3 to 4 months in a laryngectomized patient. Courtesy of Henny C. van der Mei and Henk J. Busscher (Department of Biomedical Engineering, University Medical Center Groningen and University of Groningen, Groningen, The Netherlands).

Dedicated to the memory of Professor A. Denver Russell

CONTENTS

Chapter 8

MECHANISMS OF MICROBIAL RESISTANCE / 253

PREFACE

The control of microorganisms and microbial growth is an important consideration in medical, veterinary, dental, industrial, pharmaceutical, environmental, and food processing settings. This book has been developed to provide a basic understanding of the various chemical and physical antisepsis, disinfection, and sterilization methods used for infection prevention and contamination control. Disinfection and sterilization technologies are used for the control of microorganisms on surfaces, in products, or in air, while antisepsis is particularly associated with microbial reduction on the skin or mucous membranes. These varied applications play important roles in our daily lives, including the provision of safe drinking water, production and preservation of products, sterilization of medical devices, and decontamination of surfaces. The benefits of microbial control have been appreciated since ancient times—for example, in the use of heating, salts, and metals for preservation and wound treatment—despite the absence of any pure understanding of microbiology. Over the last 200 years, we have gained a greater appreciation of microorganisms and their roles in contamination and infection. In parallel, various chemical (referred to as "biocidal") and physical antisepsis, disinfection, and sterilization methods have been developed and are widely used to render surfaces and products safe for use. Despite these advancements, microbial control issues continue to challenge us. Recent examples include the aftermath of the bioterrorism attacks in the United States; the alarming spread of viral and reemerging bacterial infections such as influenza viruses and tuberculosis, respectively; the more recent identification of newer infectious agents (notably prions and viroids); and the continuing concern of anti-infective (including antibiotic)-resistant microorganisms in hospitals and the general community.

As a background to this subject, an introduction to microbiology is provided, including a discussion of the spectrum of action, determination of efficacy, and common variables that affect the performance of antisepsis, disinfection, and sterilization methods. Disinfection and sterilization are considered as either chemical (biocide) or physical technologies. Chemical biocides include aldehydes, halogens, and phenolics, while physical processes include the use of heat, filtration, and radiation. For each biocide class or process, the various types are discussed, along with their applications, spectrum of activity, advantages, and disadvantages and a brief description of their modes of action. A wider range of methods is used for disinfection and antisepsis applications. Many of these are required to reduce the number of microorganisms, or even the number of certain types of microorganisms, to an acceptable level. In contrast, only a limited number of technologies are utilized for sterilization, which has the ultimate goal of rendering a surface, area, or substance free of all viable microbial contamination. For this reason, disinfection and sterilization methods are considered separately, with a specific chapter dedicated to the various biocides used as antiseptics and in antisepsis applications.

The current understanding of the mechanisms of biocidal action on microorganisms is considered. In most cases, the modes of action of biocides are quite distinct from the more specific mechanisms of action described for anti-infective agents such as antibiotics and antiviral agents. Most biocides demonstrate a wider range of antimicrobial activity, generally corresponding to nonspecific and varied modes of action. The mechanisms of action of biocides are considered in four general categories: oxidizing agents, cross-linking agents, agents that act by transfer of energy, and other structure-disrupting agents. Despite these general mechanisms, some biocides have been shown to have primary targets similar to those of certain antibiotics, and a better understanding of their mechanisms of action is of interest in the development of the next generation of anti-infectives.

Microorganisms demonstrate various natural (intrinsic) and acquired mechanisms to resist the biocidal effects of chemical and physical processes. These mechanisms are also discussed and are important to consider in order to ensure the safe and effective use of biocides and biocidal processes. This topic has been particularly highlighted with the development of resistance to widely used anti-infectives (notably antibiotic-resistant bacteria), but similar mechanisms in microbial resistance to biocides and biocidal processes have been described. Biocide resistance in bacteria has been studied in some detail, with many examples of intrinsic and acquired mechanisms of resistance. Intrinsic mechanisms include biofilm formation and the development of dormant endospores. Acquired resistance mechanisms due to mutations and the acquisition of plasmids, not unlike those described for antibiotics, have also been described. Although many of these mechanisms allow for tolerance in the presence of biocides only at normally inhibitory levels, other mechanisms have been shown to dramatically change the response of a microorganism to biocides and to enable it to survive highly toxic conditions. Although less studied, specific mechanisms of resistance in viruses, prions, and fungi and other eukaryotes are also described.

Overall, it is intended that this book will give a basic understanding of and reference for the various types, modes of action, and mechanisms of resistance of antiseptics, disinfectants, and sterilants for students of microbiology, chemistry, infection control, contamination control, public health, and manufacturing. A greater understanding and appreciation of these technologies will ensure their long-term safe and effective use in contamination and infection prevention.

Acknowledgments

I greatly appreciate the many colleagues and friends who reviewed selected chapters of this book, as well as my wife, Lesley, for her encouragement.

GERALD E. McDONNELL
Basingstoke, Hampshire,
United Kingdom

ABOUT THE AUTHOR

Gerald E. McDonnell received a B.Sc. degree in medical laboratory sciences from the University of Ulster (1989) and a Ph.D. in microbial genetics at the Department of Genetics, Trinity College, University of Dublin (1992). His graduate work involved studies on the control of gene expression in *Bacillus subtilis*. He spent 3 years at the Mycobacterial Research Laboratories, Colorado State University, investigating the mechanisms of antibiotic resistance and cell wall biosynthesis in mycobacteria. In 1995 he joined the St. Louis, Mo., operations of ConvaTec, a division of Bristol-Myers Squibb, as a group leader in microbiology in the research and development of skin care, hard surface disinfection, and cleaning chemistries. He then joined STERIS Corporation and has worked for STERIS for more than 10 years in the United States and in the company's European, Middle East, and Africa (EMEA) region on the development, research, and support of infection and contamination prevention products and services, including cleaning, antisepsis, disinfection, and sterilization. Dr. McDonnell is currently the vice president of research and EMEA affairs for STERIS, based at its facility in Basingstoke, United Kingdom. He is responsible for the development and support of decontamination processes and services, and he provides training on various aspects of decontamination and contamination control. His basic research interests include infection prevention, decontamination microbiology, emerging pathogens, and modes of action and resistance to biocides. His work also includes the development and implementation of international and national guidance and standards in decontamination. He has published widely in peer-reviewed journals and books, has been granted patents in decontamination technologies, and frequently gives presentations on various aspects of his work at scientific meetings around the world.

IMPORTANT NOTICE

INTRODUCTION

1

1.1 GENERAL INTRODUCTION

Microbiology is the study of microscopic organisms (microorganisms). Microorganisms play important roles in our lives, for our benefit as well as to our detriment. Of primary interest are those microorganisms that cause diseases under a variety of circumstances. Other issues include the economic aspects associated with microbial contamination, such as food spoilage, plant infections, and surface damage. The control of microorganisms is therefore an important concern in preventing contamination, as well as removing or reducing it when it occurs. A variety of physical and chemical methods are used for these purposes in antisepsis, disinfection, and sterilization applications. Disinfection and sterilization are used for the control of microorganisms on surfaces, in liquids, or in areas, while antisepsis is particularly associated with microbial reduction on the skin or mucous membranes. These biocidal applications are varied and include skin washing, wound treatment, product preservation, food and water disinfection, surgical-device decontamination, and product sterilization. Many of these processes have been used historically and are described in many ancient texts and writings. Despite this, it is only in the last 150 years, as our knowledge and understanding of microbiology has expanded, that the impact of antiseptics, disinfectants, and sterilants has been truly appreciated. Their utilization has played and continues to play an important role in significantly reducing the incidence of infectious diseases, such as gastroenteritis and pneumonia. Today, microorganisms are still a significant cause of morbidity, mortality, and economic loss, and we continue to be challenged with the identification of "newer" microorganisms, like *Legionella*, antibiotic-resistant bacteria, human immunodeficiency virus (HIV), Ebola virus, viroids, and prions.

Biocidal processes include many physical and chemical methods. Physical processes include heat (e.g., steam) and radiation (e.g., UV radiation). A wide range of chemicals, such as aldehydes, halogens, and phenolics, are also used due to their antimicrobial activities. The choice and use of a biocide will depend on the required application. For example, many aggressive chemicals or high-temperature processes can be used on various hard surfaces, like medical devices, but would not be acceptable for use as antiseptics on the skin. Therefore, there are three primary considerations in the choice of a biocide: antimicrobial efficacy, safety, and compatibility. There is no perfect biocide for any application, but the desired attributes include the following:

- Activity against a wide range of (if not all) microorganisms
- Rapid activity
- Efficacy in the presence of contaminating organic and inorganic materials, which can inhibit the activity of the biocide
- Low or no toxicity, irritancy, mutagenicity (causing genetic mutations), or carcinogenicity (causing cancer)
- Safe use
- Lack of damage to surfaces or areas (compatibility)
- Lack of unwanted or toxic residues
- Stability, yet ability to be readily broken down in the environment
- Environmental friendliness

It is clear that the advantages and disadvantages of each biocide should be considered in deciding its suitability in a given application.

This book describes the major antiseptic, disinfectant, and sterilization practices that are used. For the purpose of introduction, this chapter gives a brief description of the various types of target microorganisms, as well as a discussion of some key considerations for biocidal applications, including the evaluation of efficacy, formulation effects, and the importance of cleaning. Chapters 2 and 3 describe the various types of physical and chemical biocides and biocidal processes, including filtration, which is not a true biocidal process but is widely used in the disinfection and sterilization of liquids and gases. For each biocide group, the various types, applications, spectra of antimicrobial activities, advantages, and disadvantages and a brief discussion of the mode of action are given. Chapter 4 addresses the use of biocides as antiseptics and antiseptic applications. Chapters 5 and 6 discuss various types of physical and chemical sterilization methods, which are considered distinct from disinfection applications. Chapter 7 addresses the current understanding of the mechanisms of biocidal action on microorganisms. In most cases, the modes of action of biocides are quite distinct from the more specific anti-infective agents, like antibiotics. Biocide mechanisms are considered in four general groups with similar mechanisms of action, including oxidizing agents, cross-linking agents, action by transfer of energy, and other structure-disrupting agents. Finally, chapter 8 introduces the growing concern about microbial resistance to biocides. This topic has been particularly well studied in bacteria, and a discussion of the various intrinsic and acquired mechanisms of resistance is provided. Further, descriptions of specific mechanisms of resistance in viruses, prions, and fungi and other eukaryotes are also given.

1.2 DEFINITIONS

In considering biocidal applications, definitions can vary widely. The following terms and their definitions, where possible, are consistent with international consensus documents.

Aerobe (adj., *aerobic*): An organism that grows in the presence of oxygen. Can be obligate (requiring oxygen), facultative (able to grow in the presence or absence of oxygen), or microaerophilic (requiring a lower concentration of oxygen than is present in air).

Anaerobe (adj., *anaerobic*): An organism that grows in the absence of oxygen. Can be obligate (requiring the absence of oxygen) or facultative (able to grow in the presence or absence of oxygen).

Antibiotic: A substance (or drug) that kills or inhibits the growth of bacteria. This definition has also been applied to substances that affect other microorganisms, in particular, fungi. Originally, antibiotics were discovered as substances that were produced by one type of microorganism (in particular, fungi) which selectively inhibited the growth of other microorganisms (in particular, bacteria). Many antibiotics are now synthetically produced.

Anti-infective: A substance (or drug) capable of killing microorganisms or inhibiting their growth, in particular, pathogenic microorganisms. This term is used to encompass drugs that specifically act on certain microbial types, including antibacterials (antibiotics), antifungals, antivirals, and antiprotozoal agents. For the purpose of discussion, the term anti-infectives will be used to described drugs that are used to treat specific infections within animals, plants, and humans. This is in contrast to biocides or biocidal processes, which are considered to be broad-spectrum antimicrobials that are used on inanimate surfaces or the skin and mucous membranes. The differentiation between anti-infectives and biocides is considered further in section 7.1.

Antimicrobial: A process or product that is effective at killing microorganisms. This can vary, depending on the process or product and the target microorganism (e.g., antibacterial or antifungal). Antimicrobial agents include physical and chemical methods.

Antisepsis (noun and adj., *antiseptic*): Destruction or inhibition of microorganisms in or on living tissue, e.g., on the skin. An antiseptic is a biocidal product used on the skin.

Aseptic (noun, *asepsis*): Free of, or using methods to keep free of, microorganisms.

Aseptic processing: The act of handling materials in a controlled environment in which the air supply, materials, equipment, and personnel are regulated to control microbial and particulate contamination within acceptable levels.

Bioburden: The microbial load, or numbers and types of microorganisms, with which an item (surface or product) is contaminated.

Biocide: A chemical or physical agent, usually with a broad spectrum of activity, that inactivates microorganisms. Chemical biocides include hydrogen peroxide and phenols, while physical biocides include heat and radiation. Biocides are generally broad spectrum, in contrast to anti-infectives, which have a narrower range of antimicrobial activity (see section 7.1).

Biofilm: A community of microorganisms (either single or multiple species) developed on or associated with a surface.

-Cidal: Suffix indicating lethal activity against a group of microorganisms (e.g., sporicidal means having activity to kill bacterial spores, and bactericidal means having the ability to kill bacteria). Compare to *-static*.

Cleaning: Removal of contamination (often referred to as "soil") from a surface to the extent necessary for further processing or for the intended use.

Decontamination: Physical and/or chemical means to render a surface or item safe for handling, use, or disposal. Decontamination can refer to either chemical and biological removal or inactivation, with emphasis on biological decontamination. Decontamination is generally a combination of cleaning and disinfection or sterilization.

Deinfestation: Removal or destruction of macroorganisms (e.g., insects).

Disinfection (noun, *disinfectant*): The antimicrobial reduction of the number of viable microorganisms, or bioburden, on or in a product or surface to a level previously specified as appropriate for its intended further handling or use. In general, disinfection is used to describe a product (a disinfectant) or process that is effective against most pathogens, with the exception of bacterial spores, which are considered the organisms most resistant to disinfection and sterilization. Disinfectants are often subdivided into high level, intermediate, and low level (depending on the product claims and registrations). High-level disinfectants are considered effective against most microbial pathogens, with the exception of large numbers of bacterial spores. These products are usually sporicidal over longer exposure times. Intermediate-level disinfectants are effective against mycobacteria, vegetative bacteria, most viruses, and fungi, but not necessarily bacterial or some fungal spores. Low-level disinfectants are generally effective against most bacteria, some (in particular, enveloped) viruses, and some fungi, but not mycobacteria and bacterial spores.

Depyrogenation: The inactivation or removal of pyrogens.

Detergent: A surface-active agent (surfactant) that can emulsify oils and hold dirt in suspension; generally related to cleaning, where "detergents" can refer to cleaning mixtures that contain surfactants.

D value: The time required to achieve inactivation of 90% (or 1 log unit) of a population of a given test microorganism under stated conditions.

Endotoxin: Any of a class of toxins (or pyrogens) present in a microorganism but released only on cell disintegration. Specifically, a major component (lipopolysaccharide [LPS]) of the outer membrane in gram-negative bacteria.

Exotoxin: Any of a class of toxins produced by and secreted from a microorganism.

Formulation: Combination of ingredients, including active (biocide) and inert ingredients, into a biocidal product for its intended use (e.g., cosmetics, antiseptics, and disinfectants).

Fumigation: Delivery of an antimicrobial process (gas or liquid) indirectly to the internal surfaces of an enclosed area. An example is fogging, which is the indirect application of a biocidal liquid to a given area.

Germ: A general term referring to a microorganism.

Germicidal (noun, *germicide*): Able to kill microorganisms. In some countries, this specifically refers to bactericidal activity only.

Germination: The initiation of growth in a dormant spore.

Hydrophilic (*polar*): Able to attract and absorb water ("water loving"). Similar to lipophobic ("lipid hating"; avoiding lipid).

Hydrophobic (*nonpolar*): Having the properties of repelling and not absorbing water ("water hating"). Similar to lipophilic ("lipid loving"; having an affinity for lipid).

Parasite: An organism able to live on and cause damage to another organism.

Pathogen: A disease-causing organism.

Pasteurization: The antimicrobial reduction, usually by heat, of microorganisms that can be harmful or cause product spoilage.

Preservation: The prevention of the multiplication of microorganisms in products.

Pyrogen: A substance that can cause a rise in body temperature; for example, some exotoxins and endotoxins.

Resistance: The inability of an anti-infective or biocide to be effective against a target microorganism. See *Tolerance*.

Sanitization: The removal or inactivation of microorganisms that pose a threat to public health.

Secondary metabolites: Various products produced by microorganisms at the end of exponential growth or during stationary phase.

Sporulation: The process of spore development in microorganisms.

-Static: Suffix indicating the ability to inhibit the growth of a group of microorganisms (e.g., bacteriostatic means having activity to inhibit the growth of vegetative bacteria, and fungistatic means having activity to inhibit the growth of fungi). Compare to *-cidal*.

Sterile (noun, *sterility*): Free from viable organisms.

Sterilization: A defined process used to render a surface or product free from viable organisms, including bacterial spores.

Sterilizing agent: A physical or chemical agent (or combination of agents) that has sufficient microbicidal activity to achieve sterility under defined conditions.

Tolerance: A decreased effect of an anti-infective or biocide against a target microorganism, requiring an increased concentration or other modifications for it to be effective. Compare to *Resistance*.

Validation: A documented procedure for obtaining, recording, and interpreting the results required to establish that a process will consistently yield a product complying with predetermined specifications.

Viable: Alive and able to reproduce.

1.3 GENERAL MICROBIOLOGY

1.3.1 Introduction

Microbiology is the study of microscopic organisms, which include multicellular forms (helminths), unicellular forms (classified as eukaryotes and prokaryotes), and noncellular forms (e.g., viruses) (Table 1.1).

Microorganisms play a large part in our daily lives, both for our benefit and to our detriment (Table 1.2). The use of antiseptics, disinfectants, and sterilization methods is essential for control of the growth, multiplication, and transfer of microorganisms. Of particular concern are pathogenic, or disease-causing, organisms that can cause a variety of infections and stresses in humans, plants, and animals. A further consideration is the control of product contamination or spoilage, including that of foodstuffs and pharmaceutical drugs, which can have significant commercial consequences.

1.3.2 Eukaryotes and Prokaryotes

Eukaryotes and prokaryotes in their basic structure consist of single discrete cells. Cells are the basic units of life for these microorganisms, as well as the building blocks for multicellular organisms—plants and animals. Eukaryotes and prokaryotes are distinguished based on their microscopic structures; prokaryotes are considered much smaller and simpler in structure, while eukaryotes are larger and more organized (Table 1.3). Eukaryotic cells include fungi, protozoa, algae, and human and plant cells. Prokaryotes include a diverse variety of eubacteria and archaea. Viruses are distinct and are considered separately, because they do not possess mechanisms for self-replication and depend on cells, in which they grow and multiply, for survival.

1.3.3 Eukaryotes

1.3.3.1 MULTICELLULAR EUKARYOTES

Multicellular eukaryotes include microscopic (or, indeed, macroscopic) arthropods and helminths (or worms). These are higher forms of life, composed of eukaryotic cells that are specialized into organs and structures. Arthropods are not considered further here, but some introduction is given to the helminths. Helminths are a diverse group of multicellular parasites and can be further classified as nematodes (roundworms) and platyhelminthes (flatworms). Over 20,000 species of nematodes have been defined, although it is estimated that 10 to 100 times this number possibly exist. The flatworms can be further separated into trematodes (flukes) and cestodes (tapeworms). Many helminths can be free-living in water environments (in particular, the roundworms), but most are parasitic in nature. Some of the key diseases caused by helminths are summarized in Table 1.4. Helminths reproduce sexually and have a typical associated life cycle (Fig. 1.1).

Externally, the adult forms (including worms and flukes) are protected by a rigid proteinaceous (collagen) cuticle, which can resist the effects of biocidal processes; however, parasitic forms will not survive in the environment without their respective hosts (including, in some cases, intermediate hosts). Further, during their respective life cycles they produce dormant forms (including ova [eggs] or cysts) that can survive under harsh environmental conditions. Little work has been published on the structure of these eggs and their relative resist-

TABLE 1.1 Examples of various types of microorganisms

Microorganism	Typical structures[a]	Size (μm)	Nucleic acid	Cell wall
Prions	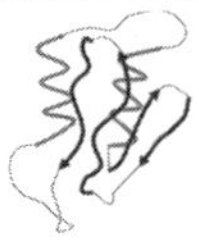	<0.01	None	No
Viruses	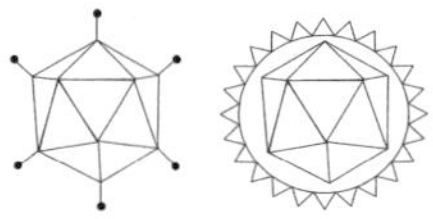	0.01–0.4	DNA or RNA	No Envelope may be present
Chlamydias, rickettsias	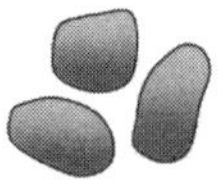	0.3	DNA	Minimal or simple cell wall
Mycoplasmas	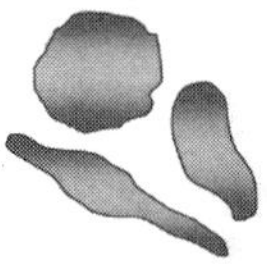	0.1–0.3	DNA	No
Bacteria	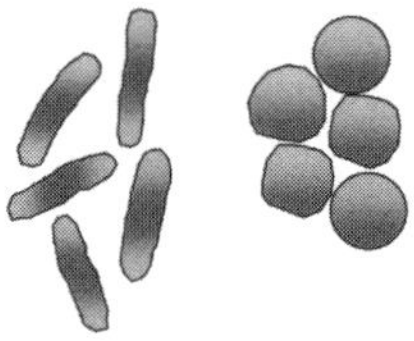	0.3–0.8	DNA	Yes
Fungi	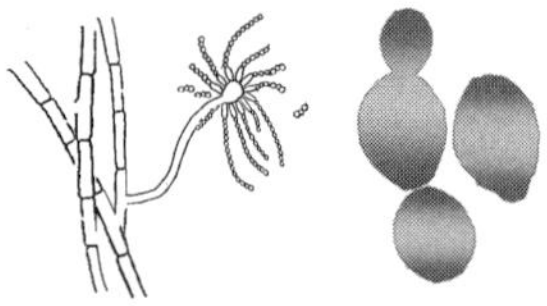	Yeast, 8–10 Fungi, >0.5 (wide), >5 (long)	DNA	Yes
Algae	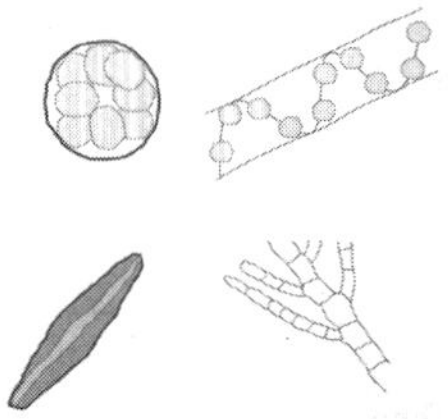	1 – >1,000	DNA	Yes/no (some)
Protozoa	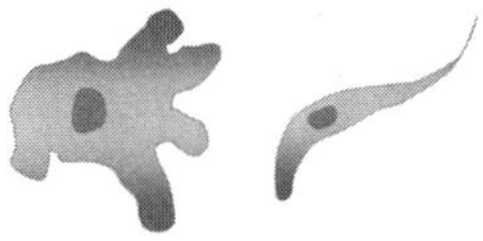	10–200	DNA	No
Helminths	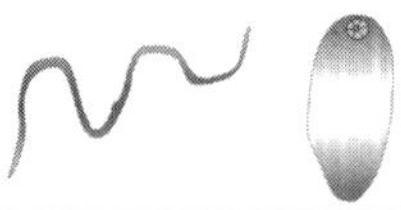	>1,000	DNA	NA[b]

[a]Not to scale; simplified structures are shown. In addition, the basic structures of microorganisms can vary considerably based on their type, environmental conditions, and growth (or life cycle) phase.

[b]NA, not applicable.

TABLE 1.2 Some advantages and disadvantages of microorganisms

Advantage or disadvantage	Example(s)
Advantages	
Food and beverage production	*Saccharomyces cerevisiae*: bread and beer production *Saccharomyces ellipsoideus*: wine fermentation
Antibiotic production	*Bacillus licheniformis*: bacitracin *Penicillium chrysogenum*: penicillin
Vitamin metabolism	*Pseudomonas* spp.: vitamin B_{12} production *Escherichia* spp.: vitamin K synthesis in the gut
Genetic engineering	*Agrobacterium tumefaciens*: plasmids used for generating transgenic plants (e.g., herbicide or pathogen resistance)
Disease prevention	*Bacteroides*, *Enterococcus* spp.: prevention of pathogen colonization of the intestinal tract
Bioremediation	*Desulfotomaculum* spp.: arsenic detoxification
Disadvantages	
Animal/human diseases	*Mycobacterium* spp.: tuberculosis HIV: AIDS *Plasmodium* spp.: malaria
Plant diseases	*Phytophthora*: potato blight *Corynebacterium*: vegetable infections
Surface damage	*Pseudomonas* spp.: biofilm development and surface corrosion
Food spoilage	*Rhizopus*: bread mold *Streptococcus*: milk souring
Allergic reactions	Fungal spores, including *Aspergillus* spp.
General product contamination	Bacterial and fungal spores, including *Bacillus* spp.

ances to biocides, but microscopically they are diverse, consisting of various proteins and carbohydrates and having a variety of thicknesses (see section 8.11).

1.3.3.2 FUNGI

Fungi are eukaryotic cells, many of which can reproduce asexually (by cell division) or sexually (by the production of spores). A limited number of fungi have been implicated in plant and animal diseases (mycoses), but fungi are also widely used for bioremediation and biodegradation, product fermentation (e.g., beer, wine, and bread), and the production of biochemical products (e.g., antibiotics, enzymes, and vitamins). Due to their ubiquitous nature, they are often implicated in spoilage and as general contaminants. They are chemoheterotrophs (requiring organic nutrition), and many are saprophytes (living off dead organic matter), acquiring their food by absorption. They are generally classified as filamentous (molds) or unicellular (Fig. 1.2).

Filamentous fungi multiply by cell division, but the cells do not separate and form long tubular structures known as hyphae (singular, hypha). The further development and branching of hyphae leads to the development of a mass of fungal growth on a surface known as a mycelium (plural, mycelia). Mycelia can often grow to such an extent that they are clearly visible to the naked eye on a surface (e.g., mold growth on bread). Fragments of hyphae can break off and allow the development of further mycelia. As the mycelia develop, a variety of fruiting bodies or other structures, which contain spores, are formed. Fungal spores can be present in a variety of shapes and sizes and can be asexual and/or sexual. The various molecular structures of fungal spores have not been studied in detail, but most are surrounded by a rigid wall distinguished by its low

TABLE 1.3 Comparison of general prokaryotic and eukaryotic structures[a]

Structure	Prokaryotes	Eukaryotes
Basic structure	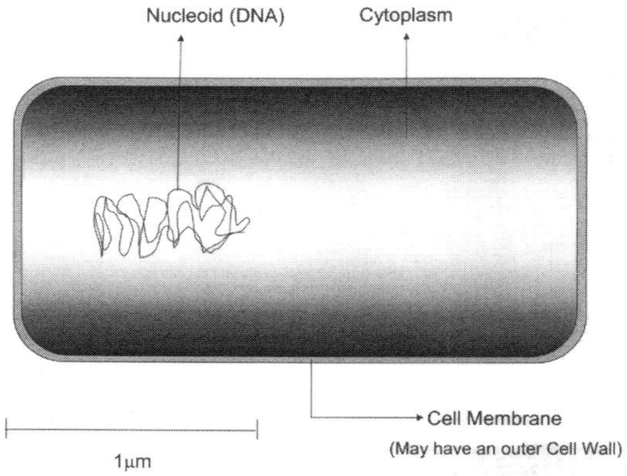 Nucleoid (DNA) Cytoplasm Cell Membrane (May have an outer Cell Wall) 1µm	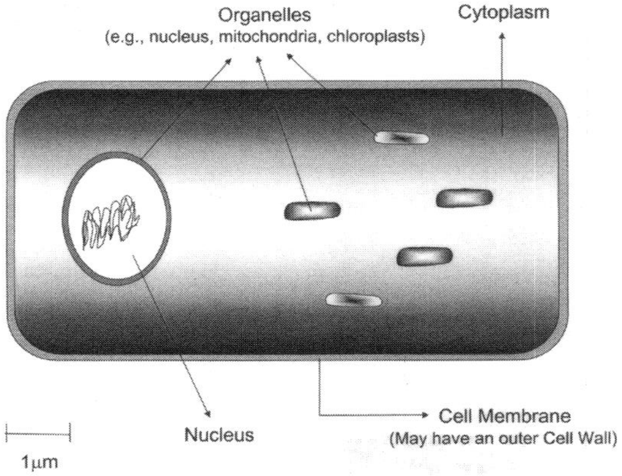 Organelles (e.g., nucleus, mitochondria, chloroplasts) Cytoplasm Nucleus Cell Membrane (May have an outer Cell Wall) 1µm
Cytoplasmic membrane	+	+
Organelles, e.g., chloroplasts, mitochondria	–	+
Nucleus defined by a membrane	–	+
Ribosomes	70S	80S
Cell wall	+/–	+/–

[a]Prokaryotic cells are simple, smaller structures, while eukaryotic cells are larger and more organized. Structural differences will vary, depending on the microorganism. For example, some prokaryotes (e.g., mycoplasmas) and eukaryotes (animal cells) do not have a cell wall.

TABLE 1.4 Helminths associated with disease

Species	Disease	Comments
Nematodes (roundworms)		
Wuchereria bancrofti	Elephantiasis (blood or lymphatic system blockage)	Transferred via mosquitoes; can grow up to 10 cm long
Onchocerca volvulus	River blindness	Transferred via blackflies
Ascaris lumbricoides	Generally asymptomatic, but can develop into ascariasis (pneumonitis and intestinal obstruction)	From contaminated water, food, or direct surface contact; worms can grow up to 30 cm long
Enterobius vermicularis	"Pinworms"; dysentery, intestinal blockage	From contaminated water, food, or direct surface contact; worms ~1 cm long
Cestodes (tapeworms)		
Taenia saginata	Generally asymptomatic, but can cause mild intestinal complications (including abdominal pain and diarrhea)	Contaminated meat; worms can be very long (>100 cm)
Trematodes (flukes)		
Fasciola hepatica	Can be asymptomatic, with complications including liver abscesses	Contaminated grasses; snails are intermediate hosts
Schistosoma spp.	Schistomiasis; can cause many complications due to growth in the bloodstream and body tissues	Water contamination; snails are intermediate hosts

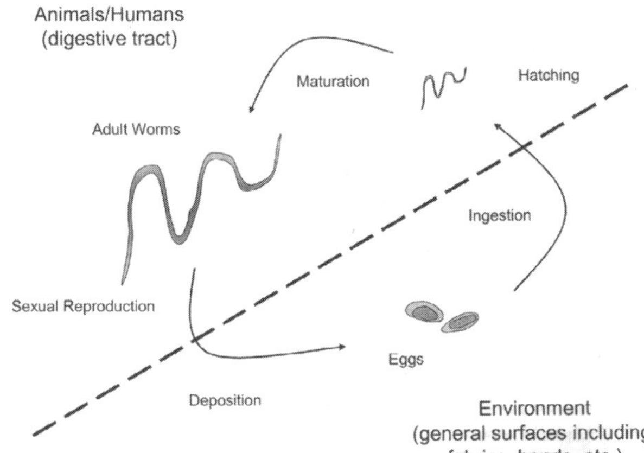

FIGURE 1.1 A typical helminth life cycle (example: *Enterobius vermicularis*).

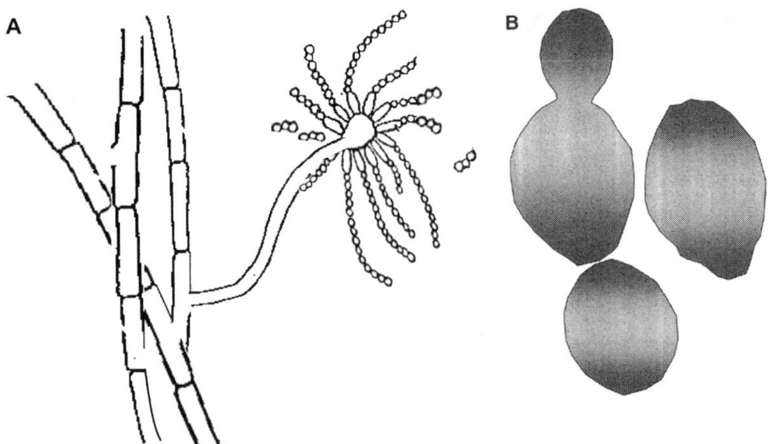

FIGURE 1.2 Typical fungal structures. (A) Filamentous fungus (mold). Hyphae are shown as long lines of unseparated cells, with the development of a fruiting body with attached spores. (B) Typical unicellular fungal (yeast) cells. The cells are generally polymorphic. In one case, a budding cell is shown.

water content and low metabolic activity and which can contain lipids and pigments, as well as nutrient reserves; these are discussed further in section 8.10.

Unicellular fungi (yeasts) do not generally form hyphae and produce growth that appears similar to bacteria (see section 1.3.4.1). Asexual reproduction of yeasts can occur by binary fission (e.g., in *Schizosaccharomyces*), similar to bacterial fission, or by budding directly from the parent cell (e.g., in *Saccharomyces* [Fig. 1.2]). In addition, some fungi are dimorphic, growing as either unicellular or hyphal (or pseudohyphal) forms. Common fungi are listed in Table 1.5.

The fungal protoplasm is surrounded by a rigid cell envelope consisting of the plasma membrane, periplasmic space, and outer cell wall (Fig. 1.3).

Many studies have investigated the structure and function of the yeast cell envelopes of *Saccharomyces cerevisiae* and *Candida albicans*, but much less is known about the range of various fungal structures. The plasma membrane is a lipid bilayer, similar to bacterial membranes (see section 1.3.4.1), but also includes some unique sterols, such as ergosterol and zymosterol. The membrane contains many integral proteins that are involved in various processes, such as cell wall synthesis and solute and/or molecule transport. Examples include various chitin and glucan synthases. Between the membrane and the outer cell wall is a narrow periplasm that can contain various mannoproteins, including enzymes such as invertase and acid phosphatase, which play a role in substrate uptake by the cell. The cell wall is a cross-linked, modular structure that varies between different molds and yeasts. It is a major component of the cell, typically comprising 15 to 25% of the cell and consisting of ~80 to 90% polysaccharide. The basic structure consists of chitin (~5% of the cell wall) or, in some cases, cellulose fibrils within an amorphous matrix of various polysaccharide glucans with associated proteins and lipids. Chitin is a polysaccharide of acetylglucosamine and gives the cell wall rigidity. In yeasts, the chitin fibrils are normally located toward the inner surface of the cell membrane, associated with various mannans and the cell membrane; however, only some species, such as *C. albicans*, have chitin, while others do not. The outer layers of the cell wall are primarily composed of β-1,3- and β-1,6-glucan fibrils,

TABLE 1.5 Examples of common fungi

Type	Example	Comments
Filamentous	*Trichophyton* (e.g., *T. mentagrophytes*)	Dermatophytes causing superficial infections on the outer layers of skin, hair, and nails, e.g., ringworm (tinea) or athlete's foot
	Aspergillus (e.g., *A. niger*, *A. fumigatus*)	Ubiquitous in nature and often isolated as microbial contaminants; rare cause of ear infections (otitis) and pulmonary disease (aspergillosis) in immunocompromised individuals; also used in the bioremediation of tannins and for the bioproduction of citric acid
	Phytophthora (e.g., *P. infestans*)	Causes potato blight, a plant disease
	Penicillium (e.g., *P. chrysogenum*, *P. roqueforti*)	Ubiquitous in nature and often isolated as microbial contaminants (e.g., as a bread mold); rarely identified as pathogenic; some strains used for the production of penicillin and cheese
Unicellular	*Cryptococcus* (e.g., *C. neoformans*)	Ubiquitous, but can cause meningitis or pulmonary infections (cryptococcosis; valley fever)
	Saccharomyces (e.g., *S. cerevisiae*)	Used for wine and beer production
Dimorphic	*Candida* (e.g., *C. albicans*)	Widely found as a commensal, including as part of normal human flora, but can cause candidiasis in immunocompromised patients (e.g., thrush and, in some cases, septicemia)
	Histoplasma (e.g., *H. capsulatum*)	Causes histoplasmosis, a pulmonary disease similar to tuberculosis

with various associated proteins, mannoproteins, and lipids. In some cases, like that of the ascomycetes, a defined protein layer has been described between the outer glucans and the inner chitin fibrils. Overall, fungal cell walls are predominantly (80 to 90%) composed of polysaccharides. The various mold cell walls have a similar, but overall more rigid, structure than those of yeasts.

The cell wall acts as a barrier for the action of biocides, and for this reason, fungi are considered relatively resistant to many antimicrobial processes in comparison to most bacteria. Some fungi (e.g., *Cryptococcus*) also produce a capsule structure external to the cell wall, which can act as an additional barrier. Further, fungal spores are generally more resistant than vegetative cells to biocides and heat, but not

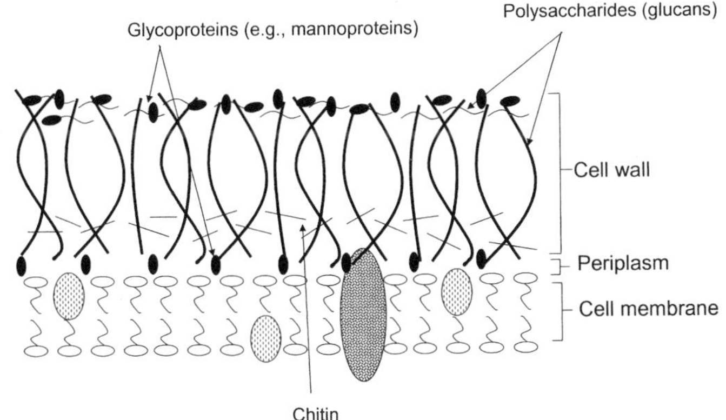

FIGURE 1.3 Simplified fungal cell envelope. The cross-linked cell wall is linked to the cell membrane. The cell wall usually consists of innermost fibrils of chitin or cellulose, with outer layers of amorphous, cross-linked glucans.

to the same extent as bacterial spores; fungal spores can be more resistant to radiation methods, as is observed when they are exposed to UV light.

1.3.3.3 ALGAE

Algae are a diverse group that can be found as single, free-living cells, but also as colonies, including multicellular filaments. Algae are phototrophs and therefore derive their energy by photosynthesis (light-mediated energy biosynthesis). Photosynthesis is conducted within special cytoplasmic organelles (chloroplasts), which contain light-sensitive pigments known as chlorophylls. Some bacteria and plants also use photosynthesis. The major habitats of algae are in water (marine or freshwater), and they are commonly encountered as colorful slimes on the water surface and, in particular, on polluted water. Examples are chlorophyta ("green algae," e.g., *Chlamydomonas*), rhodophyta ("red algae"), and dinoflagellata (e.g., *Gonyaulax*). Some species produce toxins, which can be lethal to fish and other marine life, as well as causing mild effects (headaches and respiratory problems) in humans. Structurally, algae are typical eukaryotes. Their cell wall structures vary considerably, including cellulose-, chitin-, and silica-based structures modified by polysaccharides and peptides.

1.3.3.4 PROTOZOA

Protozoa represent one of the most abundant groups of life in the world. Over 60,000 species have been described, but estimates of the total variety that exist are much higher. They are single-celled eukaryotes, but unlike fungi, they lack a cell wall. They can be found in a variety of ecosystems, including water, soil, and as parasites in animals and plants. They are generally mobile and can be classified based on their respective modes of movement and microscopic morphologies (Table 1.6).

Similar to helminths, protozoa produce multiple forms during their respective life cycles, including oocysts and cysts that can survive for extended periods in the environment (Fig. 1.4). The amebas and flagellates mostly reproduce asexually, while the human-parasitic sporozoans are capable of both asexual and sexual reproduction.

1.3.4 Prokaryotes

Prokaryotes are a diverse group that show some similarities in their basic structures but are also very distinct. They are generally single celled, range in size from ~0.1 to 10 μm, and unlike eukaryotes, their nucleic acid is free in the cytoplasm (Table 1.3). They can be considered as two general groups, the archaea and eubacteria.

1.3.4.1 EUBACTERIA

Eubacteria (or bacteria) can be subdivided into those that have cell walls and those that do not. The cell wall-free types are known as the mycoplasmas (or mollicutes). Mycoplasmas are a distinct group of prokaryotes containing a small genome and surrounded by a unique cell membrane. The surface structure of a typical mycoplasma cell is shown in Fig. 1.5.

The cytoplasm is surrounded by a lipid bilayer consisting of phospholipids. Phospholipids are molecules made up of fatty acids linked to glycerol and then, via a phosphate group, to an alcohol. Essentially, these molecules form the basic structure of the cell membranes of most bacteria (with the exception of archaea [see section 1.3.4.2]). They contain a hydrophilic (alcohol) end and a hydrophobic (fatty acid) end, which associate to form two layers (known as a bilayer) consisting of an inner hydrophobic core and an outer hydrophilic surface. Mycoplasmas are unique among prokaryotes, as they can also contain other lipids (sterols, such as cholesterol) associated in the lipid core of the membrane; sterols are usually present only in eukaryotes and add rigidity to the cell membrane, which confers greater resistance to extracellular factors than typical bacterial cell membranes do. Proteins may also be present, spanning the membrane or associated with the membrane surface. Glycolipids (polysaccharides linked to surface lipids) have

TABLE 1.6 Classification of protozoa, based on their motility mechanisms and microscopic morphologies

Classification and organism	Disease(s)	Comments
Flagellates (motility by flagella)	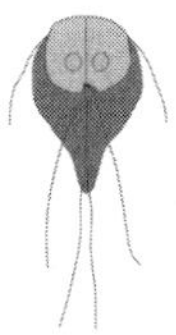	
Giardia lamblia	Giardiasis, including dysentery	Trophozoites (~20 μm; shown above) produce cysts, which can survive water chlorination
Trypanosoma gambiense	Sleeping sickness	Transferred in tsetse flies
Leishmania donovani	Leishmaniasis (kala-azar)	Transferred in sand flies
Amebas (motility by flowing cytoplasm, "pseudopodia")	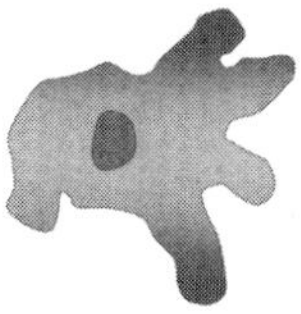	
Entamoeba histolytica	Amebiasis, including dysentery and liver abscesses	The trophozoites reproduce asexually by binary division and can produce cysts, which can be transferred in contaminated food or water (surviving for up to 5 weeks at room temperature)
Acanthamoeba castellanii	Eye infections; associated with contaminated contact lenses	Commonly found free living in water, with two stages in life cycle (trophozoites and cysts)
Ciliates (motility using cilia)	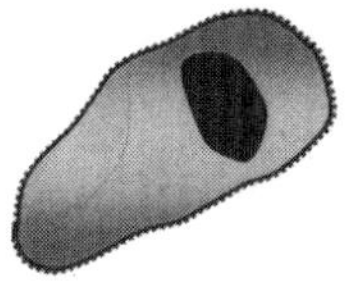	
Paramecium spp.	Dysentery	The trophozoite has two types of nuclei and can be up to 60 μm in length
Balantidium coli	Dysentery	Trophozoites can measure up to 150 μm, with transmission via cyst-contaminated meat
Sporozoans, apicomplexans (no specific motility extensions used)	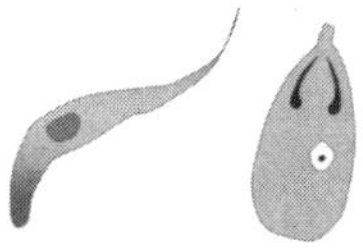	
Plasmodium falciparum	Malaria	Complicated life cycle; sporozoites transferred to humans by female mosquitoes
Cryptosporidium parvum	Severe diarrhea	Oocysts have marked resistance to biocides, surviving in water. When ingested, they hatch to release sporozoites. These forms invade cells of the intestine; they can reproduce asexually through two generations and then produce oocysts by sexual reproduction.
Toxoplasma gondii	Toxoplasmosis	The oocysts are formed in the cat intestine and transferred to other animals

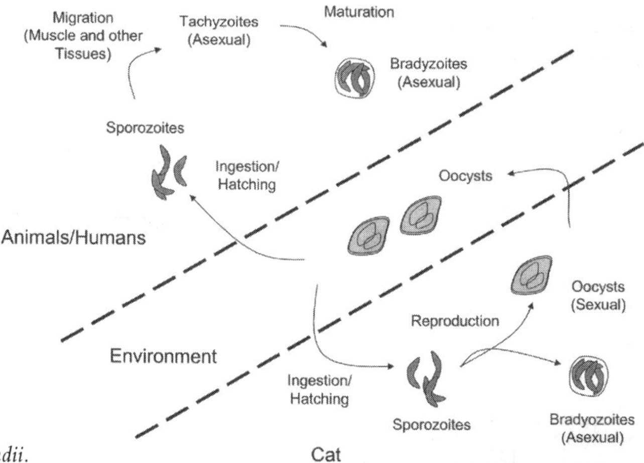

FIGURE 1.4 Life cycle of *Toxoplasma gondii*.

also been reported on cell surfaces, and they are believed to be involved in cell attachment. The reduced genome size is presumably linked to the lack of cell wall metabolism and other biosynthetic pathways (e.g., purine metabolism) that are required in other bacteria. Overall, as mycoplasmas have no cell wall, they are pleomorphic (many shaped) (Table 1.1). They can be commensals or pathogens of plants, humans, and animals (Table 1.7). Mycoplasmas are common contaminants of cell cultures and are also implicated in chronic diseases, such as chronic fatigue syndrome and rheumatoid arthritis. The lack of a protective cell wall may make mycoplasmas more sensitive to drying, heat, and some biocides. Other bacteria (as discussed below) that normally have a cell wall can also be present in a cell wall-free form and are referred to as L or cell wall-deficient forms. These forms have been found in artificial culture media and in infected tissues. They may be stationary forms that can circumvent host defense mechanisms. Examples of described cell wall-deficient forms of bacteria are *Helicobacter*, *Mycobacterium*, *Pseudomonas*, and *Brucella*. Some are suspected of being involved in autoimmune diseases, such as rheumatoid arthritis (*Propionibacterium acnes*) and multiple sclerosis (*Borrelia mylophora*).

Bacteria that contain cell walls can be simply classified based on their cell morphology and general reaction to a staining method known as the Gram stain. The Gram stain is used to differentiate between two types of cell wall structures: gram positive and gram negative. Microscopic examination of stained preparations allows further differentiation based on their shape (Table 1.8). However, this is an oversimplification, as bacteria vary widely in their morphologies and staining characteristics; many other methods are used for further differentiation, including assays of oxygen requirements, growth characteristics, and lipid composition; immunoassays; and molecular biological procedures.

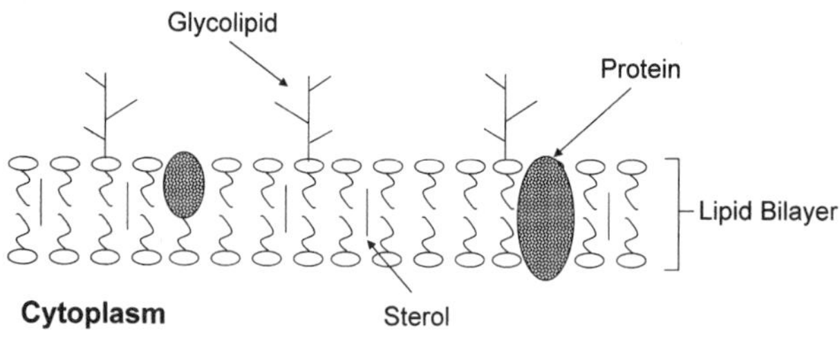

FIGURE 1.5 Simple representation of a mycoplasma cell surface structure.

TABLE 1.7 Examples of pathogenic mycoplasmas

Type	Example(s)	Significance
Spiroplasma	*S. citri*	Plant pathogens, insect parasites
Ureaplasma	*U. urealyticum*	Human parasites, genital tract diseases
Mycoplasma	*M. genitalium*, *M. pneumoniae*	Urethritis, atypical pneumonia

The basic structure of cell wall-containing bacteria consists of an outer cell wall and an inner cell membrane surrounding the internal cytoplasm (Fig. 1.6). The cell surface can also contain additional structures, such as pili, flagella, and capsules, depending on the bacterial species and its growth conditions.

The cell membrane is similar to that in mycoplasmas and consists of a phospholipid bilayer (without sterols) and associated proteins. Membrane proteins can be at the interface with the cytoplasm, embedded within the membrane, and/or associated with the external wall of the cell. Examples are some lipoproteins (proteins with lipid groups attached), in which the lipid component allows anchoring to the membrane. The overall structure is fluid but serves as a barrier to contain the cytoplasm and to restrict the passage of nutrients and ions into and out of the cell. Membrane proteins play vital roles in many cellular activities, including transport mechanisms, enzymatic reactions, cell signaling, energy generation, and cell wall syn-

TABLE 1.8 General differentiation of types of bacteria based on their microscopic morphologies and reactions to Gram staining

Bacterial structure	Shape	Example(s)
Cocci		Gram positive: *Staphylococcus*, *Streptococcus* Gram negative: *Neisseria*, *Veillonella*
Bacilli (rods)		Gram positive: *Bacillus*, *Listeria* Gram negative: *Escherichia*, *Pseudomonas*
Spirals		Gram negative: *Treponema*, *Borrelia*
Pleomorphic		Gram negative: *Bacteroides* Cell-wall-free bacteria, e.g., *Mycoplasma*

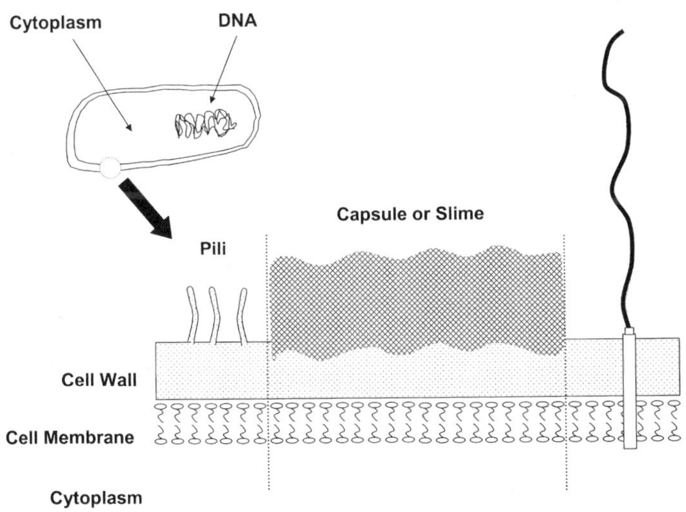

FIGURE 1.6 Basic structure of a bacterial cell, showing the cell surface in greater detail.

thesis. For this reason, damage to the cell membrane can render bacteria nonviable. The cell wall structures are less similar and can be considered as three basic types: gram-positive, gram-negative, and mycobacterial cell walls (Fig. 1.7). Mycobacteria (not to be confused with the cell wall-free mycoplasmas) are considered separately due to their unique cell wall structure. The cell wall can play an important role in the resistance of bacteria to disinfection (see chapter 8).

A key component of all bacterial cell walls is peptidoglycan, which is a polysaccharide (a polymer of sugar units) of two repeating sugars, *N*-acetylglucosamine and *N*-acetylmuramic acid, linked by β-1,4 glycosidic (sugar-sugar) bonds (Fig. 1.8). The *N*-acetylmuramic acids have attached tetrapeptides (peptides of four amino acids), which are composed of amino acids such as L-alanine, D-alanine, D-glutamic acid, and lysine (usually in gram-positive bacteria) or diaminopimelic acid (DAP) (usually in gram-negative bacteria). These tetrapeptides cross-link the polysaccharide layers. The exact structure, extent of cross-linking, and thickness of the peptidoglycan vary among bacteria. For example, *Escherichia coli* (a gram-negative bacterium) tetrapeptides consist of L-alanine, D-glutamic acid, DAP, and D-alanine, and the peptidoglycan is only a minor component of the cell wall (~10%), which is loosely cross-linked. In contrast, the *Staphylococcus aureus* peptidoglycan has lysine instead of DAP in the tetrapeptide but is also indirectly linked to an adjacent tetrapeptide by a five-amino-acid (glycine) bridge. The peptidoglycan makes up ~90% of the staphylococcal cell wall and is highly cross linked. It is the dense nature of peptidoglycan in the gram-positive cell walls that allows differentiation in the Gram stain. Some archaea have been found to have a similar but distinct peptidoglycan structure present in their cell walls (see section 1.3.4.2).

Overall, the basic structure of a gram-positive bacterium's cell wall consists of peptidoglycan; however, other proteins and polysaccharides have been described and can be specific to different bacterial species. These include polysaccharides (e.g., the A, B, and C streptococcal polysaccharides), teichoic acids, and teichuronic acids. The teichoic acids are found in the cell walls of many gram-positive bacteria, including those of *Bacillus*, *Staphylococcus*, and *Lactobacillus*. They are polysaccharides based on ribitol or glycerol, with attached sugars and amino acids, and are covalently linked to peptidoglycan. Some may also be bound to the cell membrane and are known as lipoteichoic acids. Other polysaccharides include the teichuronic acids (e.g., in *Bacillus*), which are also linked to peptidoglycan. Proteins and enzymes are also found attached to the peptidoglycan or otherwise associated with the cell wall; they may be involved in interaction with host tissues, peptidoglycan turnover, cell division, and nutrient acquisition. Finally, the actinomycetes typically stain gram positive, but with a different cell wall structure. Structurally, they resemble fungi, can form hyphae, and produce spores (sporophores) by filament fragmentation; however, the nucleic acid is free in the cytoplasm and the filaments and cell sizes are much smaller than in eukaryotic fungi (see section 1.3.2). *Nocardia*, as an example, has a tripartite cell wall structure similar to that of mycobacteria (see below), while *Streptomyces* has a more typical gram-positive cell wall structure consisting of an external peptidoglycan but also contains a major portion of fatty acids. Table 1.9 gives some common examples of gram-positive bacteria.

In general, the cell wall in gram-negative bacteria has a minor peptidoglycan layer directly bound to an external outer membrane by lipoproteins (Fig. 1.7). The area between the inner and outer membranes is known as the periplasm. The periplasm can contain a variety of proteins involved in cellular metabolism or in interactions with the extracellular environment. The outer membrane is essentially similar to the inner, cytoplasmic membrane but, in addition to phospholipids and integral proteins, also contains LPSs. LPS contains a lipid portion (known as lipid A) that forms part of the external surface of the outer membrane, linked to a polysaccharide (containing a core and an O-

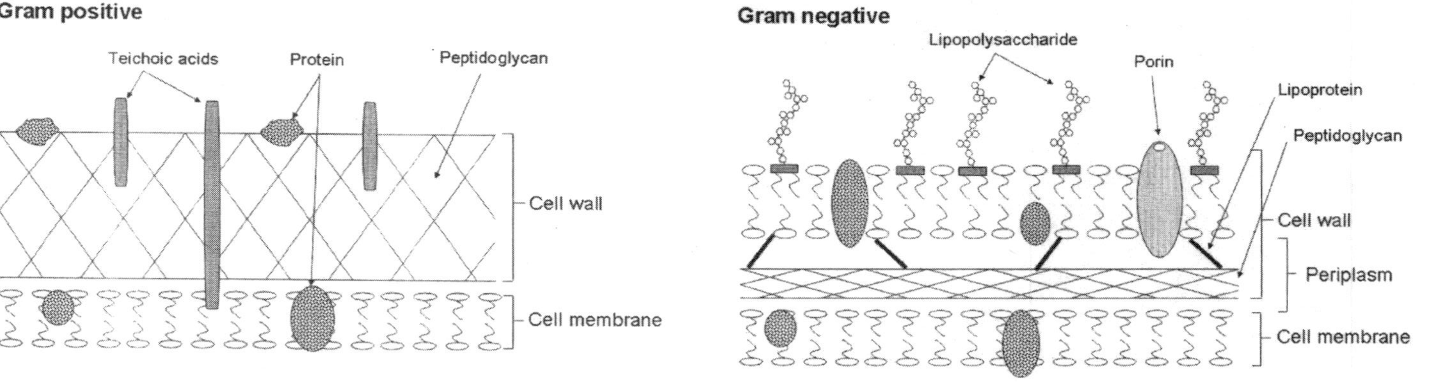

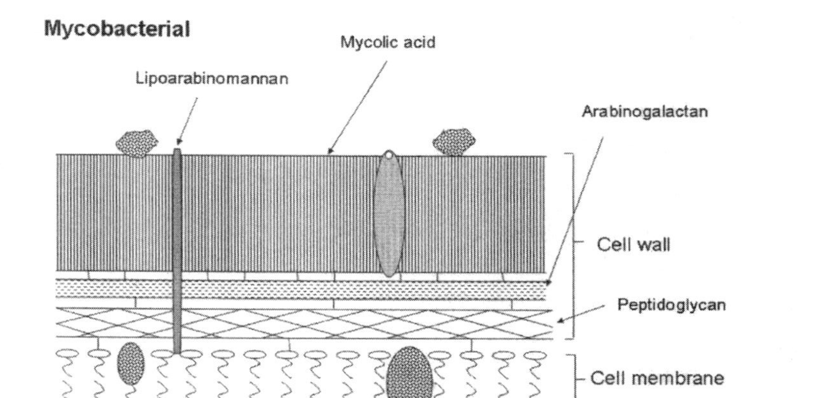

FIGURE 1.7 Bacterial cell wall structures. The cell membranes are similar structures in all types. Gram-positive bacteria have a large peptidoglycan layer (shown as crossed lines) with associated polysaccharides and proteins. Gram-negative bacteria have a smaller peptidoglycan layer linked to an outer membrane. The mycobacterial cell has a series of covalently linked layers, including the peptidoglycan-, arabinogalactan-, and mycolic acid-containing sections.

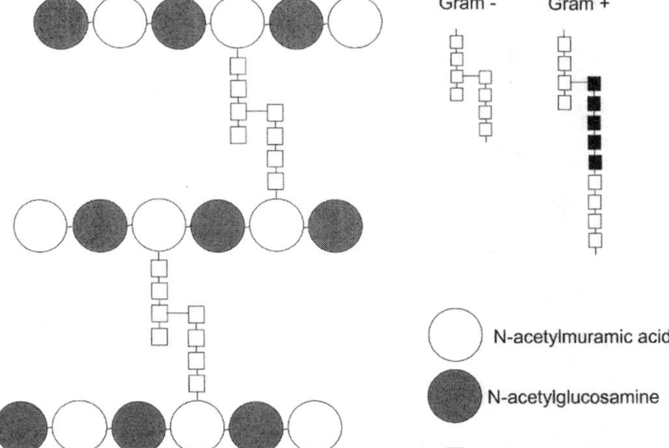

FIGURE 1.8 Basic structure of peptidoglycan. Polysaccharides of repeating sugars are cross-linked by peptide bridges. Two different types of peptide bridges, which have been described in gram-positive and gram-negative bacterial cell walls, are shown.

TABLE 1.9 Examples of gram-positive bacteria

General type	Key characteristics	Example(s)	Significance
Gram-positive cocci	Diverse group of gram-positive cocci; nonspore-formers	*Enterococcus* (e.g., *E. faecalis*, *E. faecium*)	Widely distributed in soil, water, and animals; normal flora in lower gastrointestinal tract; often identified as causing urinary tract diseases and wound infections. Vancomycin-resistant strains (VRE) are a concern in hospital-acquired infections.
		Lactococcus	Found in plant and dairy products; can cause food spoilage
		Staphylococcus (e.g., *S. epidermidis*, *S. aureus*)	Common human and animal parasites. *S. epidermidis* is usually found on the skin and mucous membranes. *S. aureus* is commonly identified as a pathogen, including in skin, wound, gastrointestinal, and lower respiratory tract diseases. Methicillin-resistant *S. aureus* (MRSA) strains are a leading cause of hospital-acquired wound infections.
		Streptococcus (e.g., *S. pyogenes*, *S. pneumoniae*)	Common human and animal pathogens. *S. pyogenes* and *S. pneumoniae* are both associated with upper and lower respiratory tract diseases, including pharyngitis (sore throat), pneumonia, and scarlet fever. *S. pyogenes* can also cause a wide variety of other diseases, including skin and soft tissue infections (e.g., cellulitis).
Endospore-forming rods/cocci	Rods or cocci that form dormant, heat-resistant endospores; can be aerobic or anaerobic	*Geobacillus*	*G. stearothermophilus* spores are widely regarded as the most resistant to heat and other sterilization methods; used as biological indicators of sterilization efficacy.
		Bacillus	Aerobic, rod-shaped bacteria; various strains also used as biological indicators for chemical sterilization processes (e.g., *B. atrophaeus*, formally known as *B. subtilis*, for ethylene oxide sterilization); some strains also pathogenic, including *B. cereus* (food poisoning) and *B. anthracis* (anthrax in animals/humans); widely distributed and often identified as environmental contaminants

TABLE 1.9 *(continued)*

General type	Key characteristics	Example(s)	Significance
		Clostridium	Anaerobic, rod-shaped bacteria; widely distributed, including in soil and water. Some species form part of the normal flora of the human intestine (e.g., *C. difficile*, which is also a leading cause of hospital-acquired diarrhea). Others can cause wound infections (including *C. perfringens* and *C. tetani*, the cause of tetanus) and food poisoning (e.g., *C. botulinum*).
Regular, non-sporulating rods	Rods, but also other regular forms	*Lactobacillus, Listeria*	Used in the preparation of fermented dairy products, such as yogurt; widely distributed. *L. monocytogenes* is a leading cause of food-borne illness, which can cause meningitis and septicemia.
Irregular, non-sporulating rods	Rods, but form irregular shapes	*Corynebacterium*	Often isolated as human/animal pathogens, in particular, on skin and mucous membranes; *C. diphtheriae* causes an upper respiratory tract infection with systemic effects (diphtheria) (see Table 1.11).
		Propionibacterium	*P. acnes* is a leading cause of skin acne. Some strains can be found as contaminants in dairy products.
Other gram-positive bacteria	Mycobacteria: rods	*Mycobacterium*	See Table 1.11
	Actinomycetes: pleomorphic, including the production of hyphae similar in appearance to those of fungi	*Nocardia, Streptomyces*	Widely distributed; some are opportunistic pathogens (see Table 1.11) Some strains produce antibiotics (e.g., streptomycin) and form spores; widely distributed; some pathogenic, including plant pathogens

polymer of sugars); the types of fatty acids and sugars that make up LPS structure vary among gram-negative species. LPSs, in particular the lipid A portions, are also known as endotoxins, which are pyrogenic and play a role in bacterial infections (see section 1.3.7). Similar to the inner membrane, proteins can be found associated through or at the periplasmic or external surface of the outer membrane. An important group of integral proteins are the porins, which form channels to allow the transport of molecules through the outer membrane. Some common examples of gram-negative bacteria are given in Table 1.10.

Some unique gram-negative-staining, obligate intracellular bacteria that were previously thought to be viral in nature have been identified, including the chlamydias and rickettsias. Rickettsias are small bacteria with a simple cell wall structure, similar to gram-negative bacteria, and are pleomorphic in shape (ranging from rods to cocci). Most are transferred to humans by arthropods (ticks and lice). Typical diseases caused by rickettsias include typhus (*Rickettsia prowazekii* and *Rickettsia typhi*) and Q fever (*Coxiella burnetii*). The chlamydias are also small obligate parasites. They are therefore difficult to isolate in vitro, requiring cell culturing, and typically stain as gram-negative coccoid bacteria. They are a serious cause of urogenital infections (*Chlamydia trachomatis*) and pneumonia (*Chlamydophila pneumoniae* and *Chlamydophila psittaci*). Chlamydia cell wall structure is unique; similar to the gram-negative cell wall, it contains an inner and outer membrane and LPS, but it does not appear to have a peptidoglycan layer. As obligate parasites, the cells are very sensitive to heat, drying, and biocides.

Figure 1.6 also shows that other structures can be present on the surfaces of bacteria. Of particular interest in the consideration of biocidal processes are external barriers that can

TABLE 1.10 Examples of gram-negative bacteria

General type	Key characteristics	Example(s)	Significance
Spirochetes	Thin; helical or spiral shaped	*Borrelia*	Cause what are often described as tick-borne diseases in animals, humans, and birds (e.g., *B. burgdorferi*, implicated in Lyme disease)
		Treponema	Cause human and animal diseases; *T. pallidum* causes syphilis, a persistent sexually transmitted disease
Helical, vibroid	Usually mobile; vibroid shaped	*Campylobacter*	*C. jejuni* causes gastroenteritis
		Helicobacter	*H. pylori* causes peptic ulcers due to gastritis
Aerobic or micro-aerophilic rods and cocci	Diverse group of rods or cocci that use oxygen for growth	*Acetobacter*	Cause food spoilage
		Bordetella	*B. pertussis* causes whooping cough, a respiratory disease
		Legionella	Associated with water or moist environments; *L. pneumophila* causes a form of pneumonia known as Legionnaires' disease
		Neisseria	Most strains are nonpathogenic and found on mucous membranes. *N. gonorrhoeae* causes the sexually transmitted disease gonorrhoea, and *N. meningitidis* can cause meningitis in young adults.
		Pseudomonas, Burkholderia	Common environmental contaminants in water and soil; some strains are plant pathogens. *P. aeruginosa* and *B. cepacia* are frequently implicated in hospital-acquired infections, usually associated with proliferation in moist environments and water lines. Pseudomonads can cause biofilm fouling in industrial water lines.
Facultative anaerobes	Rod-shaped; can grow in the presence or absence of oxygen	*Enterobacteriaceae*	
		Erwinia	Plant saprophytes and pathogens
		Escherichia	*E. coli* is the most prevalent microorganism in the lower intestinal tract and a common cause of intestinal and urinary tract infections. It is also widely used as a cloning host in molecular biology.
		Salmonella	Leading cause of gastroenteritis, mostly food or water borne; examples are *S. enterica* serovar Typhi (causing typhoid fever) and *S enterica* serovar Typhimurium (causing gastroenteritis and enteric fever)
		Yersinia	Zoonotic infections; *Y. pestis* causes plague
		Vibrionaceae	
		Vibrio	Gastrointestinal diseases, including cholera (*V. cholerae*) and food poisoning (*V. parahaemolyticus*)
		Pasteurellaceae	
		Haemophilus	Commonly found in the upper respiratory tracts of humans and some animals; *H. influenzae* is a leading cause of meningitis in children
		Pasteurella	Can cause septicemia in animals and humans
Other gram-negative bacteria	Various shapes and growth requirements	*Bacteroides*	Anaerobic rods; commonly found in the intestine and as opportunistic pathogens in wounds
		Veillonella	Anaerobic cocci; human and animal parasites
		Rickettsia, Chlamydia, Chlamydophila	Obligate intracellular pathogens
		Cyanobacteria	Free-living in water; photosynthetic; can be unicellular or filamentous
		Myxobacteria	Waterborne bacteria that are motile by a gliding mechanism
		Leptothrix	Sheathed, filamentous bacteria associated with polluted water

protect the cell from its environment. Many bacteria produce an external layer of high-molecular-weight polysaccharides, as well as associated lipids and proteins, which is referred to as a glycocalyx. This can be a simple, loosely associated slime layer or a more rigid, thicker, and firmly attached capsule structure. Capsules can range in structure and size, typically from one-half to five times the cell diameter in thickness. Glycocalyx production plays an important role in the development of bacterial biofilms, which are a further intrinsic resistance mechanism (see section 8.3.8). Glycocalyx structures are found in both gram-positive and gram-negative bacteria. Examples are *Streptococcus mutans* (in dental plaque), *Streptococcus pneumoniae* (in nasopharyngeal colonization), and *E. coli* (enteropathogenic strains that attach to epithelial cells in the intestine). In addition to direct cell protection, they can also play roles in pathogenesis, in bacterial attachment to surfaces, and in preventing drying of the cell. Other bacteria (including archaea) produce an S-layer, similar to polysaccharide capsules, which is composed of protein and glycoproteins to form an external crystalline structure; an example is the external surface of *Bacillus anthracis*, which produces an S-layer consisting of two protein types that is itself covered by a unique protein (poly-D-glutamic acid) capsule layer.

Bacteria can also have a variety of other proteinaceous cell surface appendages, including pili, fimbriae, and flagella (Fig. 1.6). For example, flagellar filaments are composed primarily of flagellin protein subunits and have other proteins that interact with the cell membrane and/or cell wall structure. Flagella are specifically involved in bacterial motility. Fimbriae and pili play important roles in surface, including cell surface, interactions.

A further cell wall structure that deserves separate consideration is the mycobacterial cell wall (Fig. 1.7). Mycobacteria are aerobic, slow-growing, rod-shaped bacteria (for example, *Mycobacterium tuberculosis* [Fig. 1.9]), which typically stain gram positive and can be further differentiated by acid-fast stain (staining with fuchsin, which resists acid and alcohol decolorization) due to their unique hydrophobic cell wall structure.

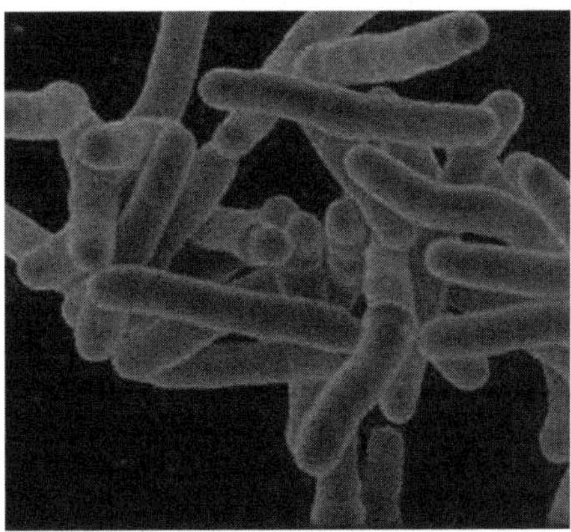

FIGURE 1.9 Cells of *Mycobacterium tuberculosis*. Courtesy of Clifton Barry, NIAID.

This mycobacterial cell wall structure presents a strong permeability barrier and is responsible for the higher level of resistance to antibiotics and biocides in comparison to other bacteria. The cell membrane is similar to that described in other bacteria, which can be linked to the cell wall by glycolipids. The cell wall has a three-layer structure, consisting of a peptidoglycan layer external to the cell membrane, which is covalently linked to a specific polysaccharide (known as arabinogalactan), and finally an external mycolic acid layer. The peptidoglycan is similar to that in other bacteria, but *N*-acetylmuramic acid is replaced with *N*-glycoylmuramic acid and cross-linked by three- and four-amino-acid peptides. Arabinogalactan is a polysaccharide of arabinose and galactose. The mycolic acids are attached to arabinose residues of the arabinogalactan and are some of the longest fatty acids known in nature. In mycobacteria, they typically range in carbon length from C_{60} to C_{90} and can make up $> 50\%$ of the cell weight. In addition, the mycobacterial cell wall can contain a variety of proteins (including enzymes), short-chain fatty acids, waxes, and LPSs. Examples are the LPS lipoarabinomannan, which plays a role in host interactions during *M. tuberculosis* infections, and porin proteins, with a function in molecule transport

TABLE 1.11 Cell wall structures in mycobacteria and related organisms

General type	Key characteristics	Example(s)	Significance
Mycobacteria	Slowly to very slowly growing; acid-fast; generally gram positive; aerobic; rod shaped but also pleomorphic or filamentous	*Mycobacterium* • Slowly growing (weeks to months)	
		M. tuberculosis, M. bovis	Cause tuberculosis, a respiratory tract disease, in humans and animals
		M. leprae	Causes leprosy, a skin and nerve disease
		M. avium	Ubiquitous in nature, including water, dust, and soil; can cause disease in poultry, swine, and immunocompromised humans
		• Rapidly growing (3 to 7 days)	
		M. chelonae, M. gordonae	Can be found as water contaminants and have been identified as pseudoinfections; some strains show high resistance to some biocides
		M. fortuitum	Identified in a variety of immunocompromised patient infections, including wound infections
Actinomycetes	Filamentous; gram negative; pleomorphic	*Nocardia*	Widely distributed, including in soil; some pathogenic, including *N. asteroides* in pulmonary and systemic infections in humans
Irregular rods	Irregular rods; gram positive	*Corynebacterium*	Obligate parasites on skin and mucous membranes; pathogenic strains include *C. diphtheriae*

similar to that seen in the outer membranes of gram-negative bacteria. In some disease-causing mycobacteria, these may also form an external capsule containing enzymes and adherence factors that play roles in mycobacterial pathogenesis. Similar basic cell wall structures have been identified in other bacteria, including actinomycetes (*Nocardia*) and gram-positive rods (*Corynebacterium*), with notably shorter-chained mycolic acids of C_{46} to C_{60} and C_{22} to C_{32}, respectively, and in some cases (*Amycolatopsis*) no mycolic acids. Examples of bacteria with mycobacterium-like cell wall structures are given in Table 1.11.

1.3.4.2 ARCHAEA

Archaea are prokaryotic but are phylogenetically distinct from eubacteria. They are a diverse group that has not been widely studied due to difficulties in culturing them from various environments. They are considered briefly, as many survive in severe environments that may be biocidal to other microorganisms and offer some interesting, if not rare, examples of microbial resistance mechanisms (see sections 8.3.9 and 8.3.10). It should be noted that bacteria and other microorganisms can survive and even multiply over a quite wide range of conditions, including temperature, pH, and the presence or absence of oxygen (aerobic or anaerobic). Those that grow under extremes of these conditions are referred to in combining form as "-philes"; for example, thermophiles (or thermophilic microorganisms) can survive at high temperatures, psychrophiles grow in cold environments, halophiles survive extreme salt conditions, and acidophiles or alkaliphiles are found in low- or high-pH environments (for further discussion, see section 8.3.10). In general, the archaea are found under extreme conditions within these ranges. For this reason, they are often referred to as extremophiles and can be considered to form four general groups: thermophiles (which survive in extreme high or low temperatures), halophiles (which survive in extreme high-salt concentrations), methanogens (which can survive under unique anaerobic conditions), and barophiles (which can survive high hydrostatic pressure). Examples are given in Table 1.12.

It should be noted that in many cases these extreme conditions are actually required for the growth of archaea. As an example, *Pyrococcus*

TABLE 1.12 Examples of extremophile archaea

Type	Description	Habitat example(s)	Typical conditions	Example(s)
Halophiles	Grow under high-saline conditions	Salt or soda lakes	9–32% NaCl	*Halobacterium, Natronobacterium*
Thermophiles	Grow at high temperatures, some under extreme acidic or basic conditions	Hydrothermal vents, hot springs	50–110°C	*Sulfolobus, Thermococcus, Pyrococcus*
Methanogens	Strict anerobes that produce methane (CH_4) gas from CO_2 and other substrates	Sediments, bovine rumens (anaerobic digesters)	Strictly anaerobic; H_2 and CO_2 used for CH_4 production	*Methanobacterium, Methanospirillium*
Barophiles (or piezophiles)	Grow optimally at high hydrostatic pressure	Deep sea	Low temperature (2–3°C) and high pressure (>100 kPa, e.g., 20–100 MPa)	*Methanococcus*

cells have an optimum temperature of 100°C but require at least 70°C for growth. Further, halobacteria, such as *Halobacterium*, require a minimum salt level of 1.5 M for growth.

Structurally, the archaea are similar to eubacteria (Table 1.3), but they present diverse cellular mechanisms that allow survival under extreme conditions. Overall, they have unique lipids (generally short-chain fatty acids) in their cell membranes, but also polysaccharides and/or proteins in their cell walls that differ from those of eubacteria. It is interesting that, similar to the mycoplasmas (see section 1.3.4.1), some archaea have no associated cell wall. Examples are *Thermoplasma* species, which contain a thick, unique cell membrane, which allows the growth and metabolism of the genus (see section 8.3.10). The cell membrane contains a unique LPS consisting of mannose-glucose polysaccharide attached to lipid molecules and glycoproteins that gives the membrane greater rigidity and temperature resistance. Some archaea have a surface structure similar to that of eubacteria, with a cell membrane bounded by a cell wall. The cell wall may contain a polysaccharide similar to peptidoglycan called pseudopeptidoglycan, with alternating *N*-acetylglucosamine and *N*-acetylalosaminuronic acid. Others do not have a peptidoglycan but a cell wall made up of proteins and polysaccharides. An example is the halophilic *Halobacterium*, which contains a salt-stabilized glycoprotein cell wall. Others species produce an external proteinaceous layer, similar to bacterial capsules (see section 8.3.7), which is known as an S-layer. In many methanogens, S-layers consisting of a crystalline structure of proteins may be found.

1.3.5 Viruses

Viruses are considered simple forms of life, consisting of a nucleic acid surrounded by protein. They are much smaller than bacteria (<0.5 μm) and are obligate intracellular parasites that depend on host cells, both prokaryotes and eukaryotes, for replication. They can be classified by a variety of methods, including size, structure, presence or absence of a lipid-containing envelope, type of nucleic acid, diseases they cause, and cell types they infect. In the consideration of biocides, viruses can be classified as being nonenveloped (or naked) or enveloped (Fig. 1.10).

Nonenveloped viruses consist of a nucleic acid surrounded by a protein-based capsid and are considered hydrophilic. Enveloped viruses also contain an external lipid bilayer envelope, which can include proteins (usually glycoproteins, or proteins with linked carbohydrate groups). Central to all viral structures is the nucleocapsid, consisting of the nucleic acid (which can be single- or double-stranded DNA or RNA) protected by a protein capsid. The capsid is made of individual capsomeres, which

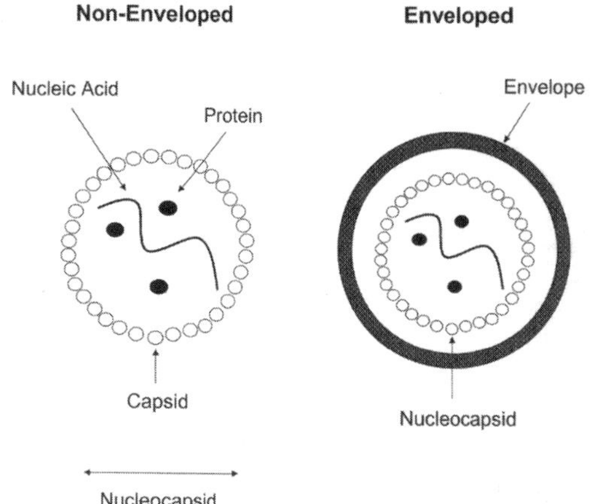

FIGURE 1.10 Basic viral structure.

consist of single or multiple protein types. Examples of nonenveloped viruses are the parvoviruses. Parvoviruses consist of 50% DNA and 50% protein, and the capsid is composed of three proteins that are responsible for their considerable resistance to disinfection. In addition, some viruses contain proteins, associated within the capsid or externally within an outer envelope, which play a role in the infection or replication of the virus particle in a susceptible host. An example is the adenoviruses, which are nonenveloped DNA viruses with a capsid containing 252 capsomeres of at least 10 different proteins, which are involved in viral structure, cell binding, and penetration; in addition, they have slender glycoproteins projecting from the capsid. Enveloped viruses are more complicated in their structure. Herpesviruses, for example, have an inner core consisting of DNA wound around a proteinaceous scaffold and surrounded by a capsid of 162 capsomeres, a protein-filled tegument, and finally an outer lipophilic envelope containing numerous glycoproteins and evenly dispersed surface spikes. Another group is the enveloped orthomyxoviruses, which contain two envelope-associated surface proteins that are involved in virus infectivity: hemagglutinins, which bind the virus to the recipient cell, and neuraminidases, which break down muramic acid in the protective mucopolysaccharide layer, which is found on the surfaces of target epithelial cells and allows contact with sensitive cellular receptor proteins. Additional proteins can be associated with the viral nucleic acid, including nucleic acid polymerases; for example, retroviruses are RNA viruses that contain reverse transcriptases that allow the generation of DNA from the viral RNA molecule, which is subsequently transcribed and translated to produce viral proteins in the host.

Based on these basic viral structures, a variety of virus families which vary in shape and composition have been described. Examples of virus families are given in Table 1.13, but this list is not complete. For example, at least 20 families of viruses that are of medical importance and that vary in size, shape, and chemical composition have been identified; additional virus families have been described for plants, fungi, protozoa, and bacteria.

Viruses are dependent on host cells for survival and multiplication. Despite the range of viruses described, viral infection occurs in a similar series of steps: attachment, penetration, synthesis of biomolecules, assembly, and release (Fig. 1.11). The first stage is attachment of the virus to the cell surface. This is mediated by specific proteins on the capsid or envelope surface that specifically interact with molecules on the cell surface known as receptors. Receptors can be cell membrane or cell wall proteins, lipids, carbohydrates, and even combinations of these. Therefore, the presence of specific receptors on the cell surface determines sensitivity or resistance to virus infection. Examples of receptors include the HIV receptor CD4 protein on the surfaces of human T cells and the binding of influenza virus to sialic acid, a carbohydrate linked to a cell membrane protein.

The next stage is penetration of the virus into the target cell, which can occur by different mechanisms. The nucleocapsid or nucleic acid, as the source genetic material that encodes the viral structure, can be injected or released into the cell. Similarly, the whole virus can be endocytosed into the cell or, in the case of enveloped viruses, by fusion with the cell membrane, which is subsequently uncoated to allow

TABLE 1.13 Viral families, with examples of classifications, including size, presence of a lipophilic envelope, and nucleic acid type

Viral family	Structure	Size (nm)	Envelope	Nucleic acid	Example(s)
Parvoviridae		18–26	No	DNA	Mouse parvovirus, parvovirus B19
Flaviviridae		40–50	Yes	RNA	Ebola virus, Marburg virus
Adenoviridae		70–90	No	DNA	Adenovirus serotypes
Retroviridae		90–120	Yes	RNA	HIV type 1
Herpesviridae		180–200	Yes	RNA	Epstein-Barr virus, herpes simplex virus
Poxviridae		250–400	Yes	DNA	Monkeypox virus, variola (smallpox) virus

nucleic acid release. Endocytosis is typical for penetration of many vertebrate viruses. As mentioned above, some enzymes that are associated with the virus capsid are required for viral multiplication (e.g., reverse transcriptase in retroviruses, such as HIV) and are released into the target cell. In some viruses, the nucleic acid is modified (e.g., by methylation) to protect it from damage (by nucleases) when it is free in the cell. Once the cell is infected, the virus uses

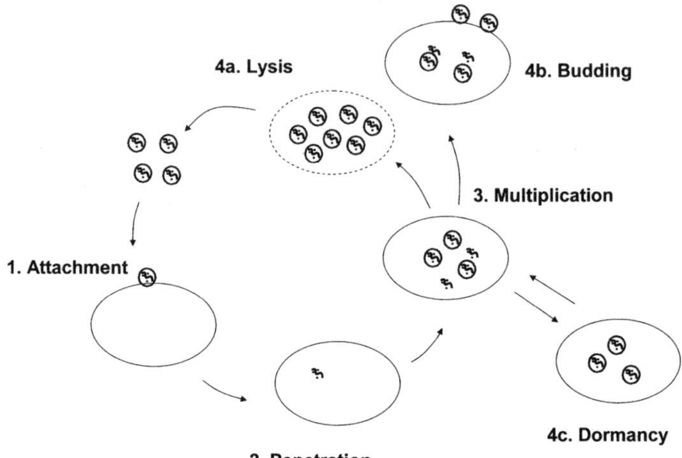

FIGURE 1.11 Typical viral life cycle. The stages include (1) attachment, (2) penetration into the cell, and (3) multiplication. Depending on the virus type, viral particles can be released by cell lysis (4a) or by budding (4b); alternatively, the virus can remain dormant in the cell (4c).

the available cell metabolic processes to replicate its nucleic acid and to allow the synthesis of specific viral proteins during the multiplication stage. Multiplication depends on the transcription and translation of viral mRNA. For DNA viruses, this can be achieved by the use of existing host enzymes, such as DNA-dependant RNA polymerases; in the case of RNA viruses, it may require specific viral proteins. An example already mentioned is the use of reverse transcriptase in retroviral multiplication, which generates DNA from a single-stranded RNA virus template. The viral proteins that are subsequently produced can be involved in the multiplication process (e.g., viral replication) or as structural parts of the virus. If viral multiplication continues, the cell will eventually burst or lyse to release the viral particles (Fig. 1.11, step 4a); an example is poliovirus. Lysing, however, does not occur with all viruses. A further mechanism of virus release is budding from the cell surface, which produces a persistent infection in a cell. Examples include influenza virus and HIV; it should be noted that both of these are enveloped viruses and that the viral envelope is actually formed around the viral nucleocapsid during the budding release from the cell surface. Some viruses can remain dormant in their host cells; these are referred to as latent infections, which can reactivate at a later stage to cause disease. During dormancy, the virus may not affect the normal cellular functions. An example of a virus causing latent infection is the varicella-zoster virus, which can remain dormant in neurons; varicella-zoster virus can cause chickenpox, commonly in children, and can reactivate to cause shingles, which is more prevalent in adults. In some cases, the presence of the virus may also trigger the uncontrolled growth of cells, leading to the development of cancers. Strong associations of viruses with cancers include papillomaviruses with skin and cervical cancers and some herpesviruses with lymphomas and carcinomas.

Viruses have been identified as the causes of a variety of plant, human, and animal diseases, including respiratory, sexually transmitted, neurological, and dermatological diseases (Table 1.14). The traditional difficulty of isolation and identification of viruses limits their study; however, it is thought that many more viruses remain to be identified and implicated in diseases by developing molecular biology and electron microscopy techniques.

Separate families of plant viruses have also been described, including tobamoviruses (nonenveloped RNA viruses; e.g., tomato-tobacco mosaic virus is a significant agricultural and horticultural concern, because it infects vegetables, flowers, and weeds, leading to leaf, flower, and fruit damage), *Comoviridae* (nonenveloped RNA viruses), and *Geminiviridae*

TABLE 1.14 Examples of viral diseases

Family and virus	Disease(s)
***Parvoviridae* (DNA, nonenveloped)**	
Human parvovirus B19	Erythema infectiosum (fifth disease)
Minute virus of mice	Cell line contamination, oncolysis
***Papovaviridae* (DNA, nonenveloped)**	
Human papillomavirus	Cervical cancer, genital warts
***Picornaviridae* (RNA, nonenveloped)**	
Poliovirus	Poliomyelitis
Rhinoviruses	Common cold
Coxsackievirus A16	Foot-and-mouth disease
***Retroviridae* (RNA, enveloped)**	
HIV type 1	AIDS
Human T-cell leukemia virus type 1	Human T-cell leukemia
***Orthomyxoviridae* (RNA, enveloped)**	
Influenza viruses A, B, and C	Influenza, pharyngitis
***Hepadnaviridae* (DNA, enveloped)**	
Hepatitis B virus	Hepatitis
***Poxviridae* (DNA, enveloped)**	
Variola virus	Smallpox
Vaccinia virus	Smallpox vaccine
***Rhabdoviridae* (RNA, enveloped)**	
Rabies virus	Rabies, paralysis
Vesicular stomatitis virus	Similar to foot-and-mouth disease; flu-like
***Coronaviridae* (RNA, enveloped)**	
Human coronavirus	Severe acute respiratory syndrome, colds
Mouse hepatitis virus	Wasting syndrome
***Herpesviridae* (DNA, enveloped)**	
Herpesvirus (herpes simplex virus types 1 and 2)	Conjunctivitis, gingivostomatitis, genital herpes, meningitis
Varicella-zoster virus	Chickenpox/shingles

(nonenveloped DNA viruses). Viruses that infect fungi (e.g., the nonenveloped RNA viruses barnavirus and chryovirus) and bacteria (bacteriophages) (Fig. 1.12) have also been described.

Bacteriophages (commonly known as phages) are mostly DNA viruses (e.g., the T3, T7, and lambda [λ] phages are *E. coli* viruses), although some RNA viruses have been described (e.g., nonenveloped MS2 and enveloped φ6 *E. coli* phages). Bacteriophages have been studied for many years as genetic-engineering tools, but they have other practical applications, including uses in typing of bacteria and as indicators of fecal contamination in water and limited medical applications (such as antibacterials). *Lactobacillus* phages are a significant contamination concern in the dairy industry. Phages are considered to be resistant to biocides, like other animal and plant viruses, and are therefore used to investigate biocidal activities (e.g., MS2 phage) and modes of action. They can be routinely cultured and purified in most bacteriology laboratories.

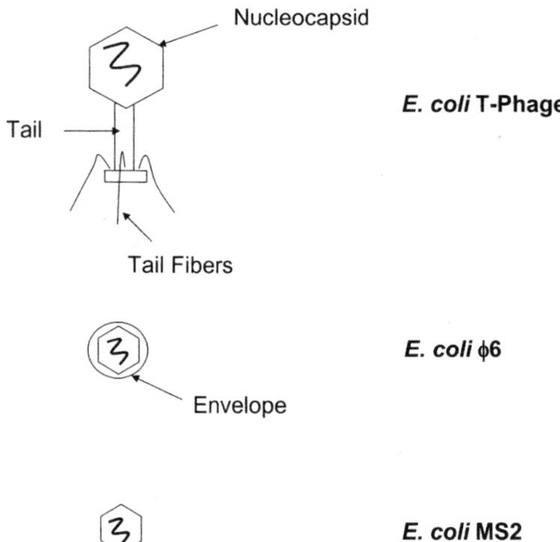

FIGURE 1.12 *E. coli* bacteriophages. The T-phages are complex DNA viruses; MS2 and ϕ6 are RNA viruses, with ϕ6 enveloped.

Two other groups of infectious agents are also considered "viruses" but have unique morphologies. The first are viroids, which are devoid of protein and appear to consist of naked RNA molecules. The second are proposed to be devoid of a nucleic acid and are termed "prions"; these are discussed in further detail in section 1.3.6. Viroids are known to infect only higher plants and have been identified as the causes of a number of crop diseases. Examples are potato spindle tuber viroid, coconut cadang-cadang viroid, and tomato apical stunt viroid. They consist only of small, circular RNA sequences that range in size from 246 to 375 nucleotides. It is interesting that their sequences do not encode proteins and that they are dependent on the host for replication in the cell nucleus. Although at first it would seem that these agents would not survive well in the environment, their structures are somewhat protected by forming double-stranded portions (by base pairing) within their circular, single-stranded structures. Although no human viroids have been identified, hepatitis D (delta) virus is similar to a viroid and is known as a satellite virus. A satellite virus is an agent that consists of a nucleic acid and that depends on the coinfection of a host with another virus, which is required for its replication. Hepatitis delta virus appears to be a defective transmissible pathogen that is dependent on hepatitis B virus. It consists of a circular RNA molecule (~1,680 bp), but unlike a true viroid, it does encode a capsid protein. The virus consists of a nucleocapsid of 60 proteins surrounding the RNA molecule and an external envelope of lipid and hepatitis B surface antigens.

1.3.6 Prions

Prions are unique infectious agents that are composed exclusively of protein and do not appear to have an associated nucleic acid. The protein in question is a normal cellular protein (cellular prion protein [PrP^c]) that is expressed in many body tissues and in all vertebrates, including humans and animals. The proteins are produced in cells as long chains of amino acids (known as the primary structure), which then fold to make structural and functional (e.g., enzyme) forms (e.g., secondary and tertiary structures). The exact function of the PrP protein is unknown, but it is known to be a eukaryotic cell membrane-associated glycoprotein. Like other cellular proteins, PrP is manufactured by the cell and can be subsequently broken down by normal cellular processes (Fig. 1.13).

However, PrP appears to be able to change its conformational secondary structure into

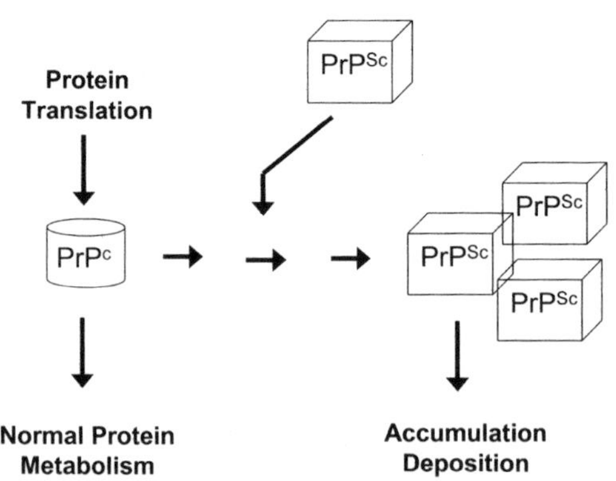

FIGURE 1.13 Theory of prions as infectious proteins. PrP^c is the normal form of the protein, and PrP^{Sc} the abnormal form.

insoluble, "infectious" forms (PrP^{Sc}). The conformational change to PrP^{Sc} renders the protein highly resistant to normal cellular degradative processes, leading to accumulation and cell damage or death, with particular consequences to neural tissues. More specifically, an insoluble portion of the protein (PrP^{27-30}, a 27- to 30-kDa protein) accumulates to form amyloid deposits in the brain. Therefore, the protein primary structure does not change, but the protein secondary structure is radically altered to give an overall greater proportion of β-sheets over α-helices in the folded protein structure (Fig. 1.14). What triggers this reaction is currently unknown; PrP^{Sc} itself has been shown to be involved in the transition, but it may also require other, yet unidentified factors.

Prions are the causative agents in a group of diseases known as transmissible spongiform encephalopathies. Animal (scrapie in sheep and bovine spongiform encephalopathy in cattle) and human (classical Creutzfeldt-Jakob disease [CJD] and variant CJD) diseases have been shown to be infectious prion diseases. Some forms have also been found to be inherited, e.g., familial CJD is responsible for ~10% of CJD cases and Gerstmann-Sträussler-Scheinker syndrome, due to modifications in the PrP-encoding gene. Human diseases are considered very rare; for example, CJD is the most common human transmissible spongiform encephalopathy, with an approximate rate of 1 to 1.5 cases per 1,000,000 population. Animal diseases are considered more widespread; for example, scrapie is estimated to affect 4 to 8% of sheep. Prions have been shown to be transferred in contaminated tissues (including infected foods, neural tissues, and blood) and on the surfaces of contaminated instruments (surgical devices). Zoonotic transmission to humans has been reported, with bovine spongiform encephalopathy now widely accepted as the source of variant CJD in humans. Finally, some researchers have speculated that other diseases that are associated with the deposition of protein (for example, the neurodegenerative diseases Parkinson's and Alzheimer's diseases) could also be linked to infectious agents; these reports, however, remain to be substantiated.

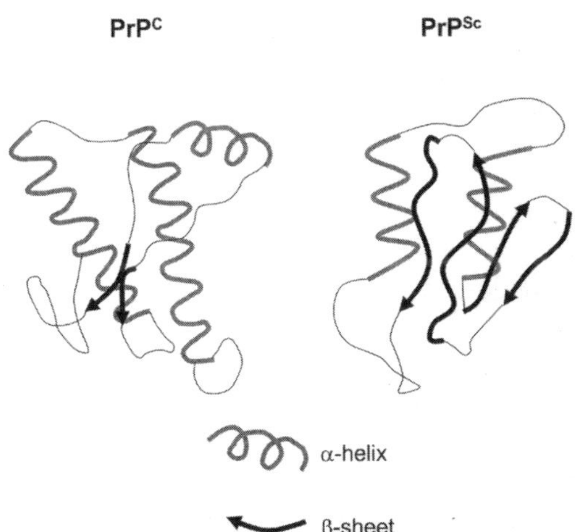

FIGURE 1.14 Representation of the proposed structural changes in PrP.

1.3.7 Toxins

Toxins are microbial substances that are able to induce damage to host cells, an immunogenic or allergic response, and/or fever. Fever is an abnormal rise in body temperature often associated with acute microbial infections. As toxins are released from the microorganism, either during normal cell metabolism or on cell death, they can have dramatic effects on a susceptible host away from the actual site of infection or microbial growth; in some cases, the toxins can remain present despite the removal or inactivation of the microorganism. Although many toxins may be inactivated by various biocidal processes used to control microorganisms, in some cases toxins are considered heat and/or chemical resistant and require special consideration.

Many toxins are potent poisons and are important factors in the pathogenic nature of bacteria, fungi, and algae (Table 1.15).

Many toxins are macromolecules, in particular, proteins, polysaccharides, and LPSs, but can also include chemical toxins, as in the cases of many fungal and algal toxins. They can be classified in many ways, including by their sites of activity (e.g., neurotoxins, affecting neural tis-

TABLE 1.15 Examples of bacterial, fungal, and algal toxins

Toxin class and producing microorganism	Toxin	Effect or disease
Bacterial exotoxins		
Campylobacter jejuni	Enterotoxin, cytotoxin	Food-borne illness; cell toxicity
Clostridium botulinum	Neurotoxins	Paralysis (relaxed muscles); botulism
Clostridium tetani	Neurotoxin	Paralysis (tensed muscles); tetanus
Escherichia coli (some entero-pathogenic strains)	Enterotoxins	Food poisoning, including diarrhea
Bacillus anthracis	Three-protein-component toxin (protective antigen, lethal factor, and edema factor)	Anthrax
Vibrio cholerae	Enterotoxin	Cholera
Corynebacterium diphtheriae	Two-protein-component toxin	Diphtheria
Bacterial endotoxins		
Escherichia coli, Shigella, Salmonella	Endotoxin	Fever, diarrhea, inflammation
Fungal toxins		
Aspergillus flavus	Aflatoxins	Hepatic disease and known carcinogens; often associated with contaminated foods and feeds
Penicillium rubrum	Rubratoxins	Liver and kidney toxicity; often associated with contaminated foods and feeds
Stachybotrys spp.	Mycotoxins (e.g., trichothecenes)	Respiratory effects, headaches, flu-like illness, allergic reactions; associated with water-damaged buildings
Algal toxins		
Gonyaulax	Saxitoxins	Food-borne illness (associated with shellfish)
Microcystis	Hepatoxins	Liver damage; associated with contaminated water

sue, and enterotoxins, affecting the small intestine), their structures, and their mechanisms of action.

Bacterial toxins are categorized as exotoxins when they are actively produced and released from the bacterial cell during growth and as endotoxins when they are a normal part of the cell wall structure but are toxic when released following damage to the cell wall or on cell death.

The most widely studied bacterial exotoxins are proteins (ranging in size from 50 to 1,000 kDa) that are released from actively growing gram-positive and gram-negative bacteria. As proteins, they are generally heat sensitive, although some have been shown to survive heat treatment processes. Many exotoxins are potent poisons at relatively low concentrations and are important virulence factors in bacterial diseases, such as anthrax, tetanus, cholera, and food poisoning. Their toxic effects can include cell damage (AB toxins), cell lysis (cytotoxic toxins), and an inflammatory response (superantigen toxins). Examples of exotoxins and their effects on host cells are given in Table 1.16.

By definition, endotoxins can be any cell-bound toxin that is released upon cell damage or cell death, although the term is generally used to refer to the LPS component of the cell walls of gram-negative bacteria, including *E. coli*, *Salmonella*, *Shigella*, and *Pseudomonas* (see section 1.3.4.1). LPS contains a lipid portion (known as lipid A) that forms part of the external surface of the outer membrane, which is

TABLE 1.16 Common examples of bacterial exotoxins

Type	Example	Microorganism	Effects
AB toxins (component toxins that cause cell damage)	Diphtheria toxin	*Corynebacterium diphtheriae*	Inhibition of protein synthesis
	Tetanus and botulism toxins	*Clostridium tetani, Clostridium botulinum*	"Neurotoxins"; block neurotransmitters
	Cholera toxin	*Vibrio cholerae*	"Enterotoxin"; secretion of fluids from small intestine
Cytotoxic toxins (cause cell lysis)	α, β, and γ toxins	*Corynebacterium perfringens*	Cell lysis, including damage to cell membrane
	α toxin	*Staphylococcus aureus*	Cell lysis
Superantigen toxins (cause an immunological response and inflammation)	Toxic shock syndrome toxin	*Staphylococcus aureus*	Septic shock
	Erythrogenic toxin	*Streptococcus pyogenes*	Scarlet fever rash

linked to an external polysaccharide (containing a core and an O-polymer of sugars) (Fig. 1.15). The exact fatty acid and sugar structures of LPS vary among gram-negative species. In general, the polysaccharide can contain various types of sugars and the lipid A portion consists of fatty acids attached to a disaccharide of *N*-acetylglucosamine phosphate.

Endotoxins can have a variety of biological activities when introduced directly into the blood and are therefore an important consideration in various pharmaceutical, medical-device, and water purification applications. LPS is pyrogenic (fever causing) and induces an inflammatory response, which can lead to septic shock, diarrhea, and, under some circumstances, death. The polysaccharide component is considered responsible for fever and inflammation, while the lipid A component is linked to the toxicity effect on host cells. Overall, the toxic effects of LPS are considered to be less than those of exotoxins. Endotoxins are notably heat resistant.

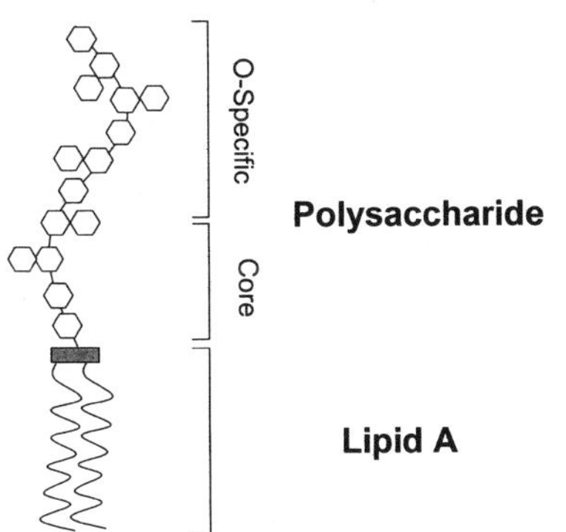

FIGURE 1.15 The general structure of lipopolysaccharide. The lipid A component is integrated into the outer membrane of the gram-negative cell wall, with the polysaccharide portion extending to the outside of the cell.

Mycotoxins are produced by fungi, in particular, molds like *Aspergillus*, *Fusarium*, *Stachybotrys*, *Penicillium*, and *Chaetomium*. They are usually produced during the late exponential and/or stationary phase of growth and, like other secondary metabolites (e.g., antibiotics), provide competitive advantages to the fungus in its environment. They can be associated with the vegetative mold, its spores, or surrounding mold growth. Most of these toxins are chemical in nature, and they include aflatoxins, ochratoxins, trichothecenes, and gliotoxins; an example of a fungal aflatoxin is shown in Fig. 1.16.

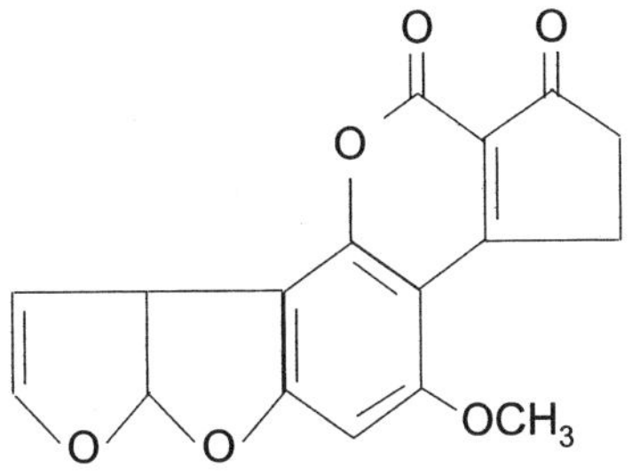

FIGURE 1.16 Typical fungal aflatoxin structure.

Mycotoxins also have multiple effects on target cells, including membrane damage, cell death, and free-radical damage. Aflatoxins have been particularly associated with food and feed (grain) contamination and have been shown to be carcinogenic. Some fungal cell wall components (like β-1,3-glucan) are also considered toxins and can cause allergic reactions, including coughing and other respiratory effects.

Many algae also produce toxins, which are often associated with contaminated water. These include hepatoxins (in particular, from blue-green algae), neurotoxins, cytotoxins, and endotoxins (similar to gram-negative bacteria, the LPS from the outer membrane of the algal cell wall).

1.4 GENERAL CONSIDERATIONS

1.4.1 Microbial Resistance

Different types of microorganisms vary in their responses to antiseptics, disinfectants, and sterilants. This is hardly surprising, in view of their different cellular structures, compositions, and physiologies (see section 1.3). Traditionally, microbial susceptibilities to biocides have been classified based on these differences (Fig. 1.17). Bacterial spores are generally considered the organisms most resistant to antiseptics, disinfectants, and sterilants, although prions have shown marked resistance to many physical and chemical processes (see section 8.9). It is important to note that this classification is considered only a general guide to antimicrobial activity and can vary depending on the biocide, formulation, or process under consideration. For example, while the profile shown in Fig. 1.17 may be considered applicable to heat-based processes, some fungal spores can demonstrate greater resistance to non-ionizing-radiation methods, and some protozoan oocysts are relatively sensitive to heat but resistant to chemical sporicides. Some extremophiles can also show atypical patterns of resistance to various biocides (see section 8.3.10). The resistance of microorganisms to biocides is considered in more detail in chapter 8.

In addition, it is clear that the resistance of a microorganism also depends on direct contact with the biocide and is affected by many other associated variables, including the following:

- The actual microbial strain and culture conditions for growth
- The growth phase of the microbial culture (population and exponential- versus stationary-phase growth)
- The type of associated surface and/or medium (water, plastic, metals, paper, etc.)
- The presence of organic and/or inorganic soils
- Presence within its normal environmental conditions, e.g., within a biofilm (see section 8.3.8)

A range of microorganisms can be chosen to establish the broad-spectrum activity of a product or process, depending on the required or desired application. For example, a sterilizing agent is expected to be effective against viruses, fungi, protozoa, mycobacteria, and other bacteria, including bacterial spores. Bacteria (including spores), fungi, mycobacteria, and to a lesser extent viruses are most commonly used as test microorganisms. Considering the multitude of microorganisms and applications, it is common to use surrogates as test organisms to establish the broad-spectrum efficacy of a product or its antimicrobial activity against a class of microorganisms (Table 1.17). Despite acceptance of these surrogates, in some cases the specific test organisms are used, or are required to be used, to verify the claimed antimicrobial activity.

1.4.2 Evaluation of Efficacy

The antimicrobial activity of a biocide or a biocidal process can be investigated using a variety of methods that can range from simple laboratory tests to evaluation under actual use conditions. These tests not only are important in the investigation of biocides and the development of products and processes but are also the basis for the regulatory clearance, labeling, and use of antiseptics, disinfectants, and sterilization processes. The various tests and requirements

	Microorganism	Examples
More Resistant	Prions	Scrapie, Creutzfeldt-Jakob disease, chronic wasting disease
↑	Bacterial spores	*Bacillus, Geobacillus, Clostridium*
	Protozoal oocysts	*Cryptosporidium*
	Helminth eggs	*Ascaris, Enterobius*
	Mycobacteria	*Mycobacterium tuberculosis, M. terrae, M. chelonae*
	Small, nonenveloped viruses	Poliovirus, parvoviruses, papillomaviruses
	Protozoal cysts	*Giardia, Acanthamoeba*
	Fungal spores	*Aspergillus, Penicillium*
	Gram-negative bacteria	*Pseudomonas, Providencia, Escherichia*
	Vegetative fungi and algae	*Aspergillus, Trichophyton, Candida, Chlamydomonas*
	Vegetative helminths and protozoa	*Ascaris, Cryptosporidium, Giardia*
	Large, nonenveloped viruses	Adenoviruses, rotaviruses
	Gram-positive bacteria	*Staphylococcus, Streptococcus, Enterococcus*
Less Resistant	Enveloped viruses	Human immunodeficiency virus, hepatitis B virus, herpes simplex virus

FIGURE 1.17 General microbial resistance to biocides and biocidal processes. This classification can vary depending on the biocide or biocidal process under consideration.

can vary considerably, and there are currently no standardized requirements that apply to all situations. Most countries specify particular test methods to verify antimicrobial activity, but these also vary for the particular application (e.g., medical, dental, agricultural, water disinfection, or industrial), type of biocide or process, and use of the formulation or process (e.g., preservation, antisepsis, disinfection, or sterilization).

TABLE 1.17 Examples of surrogate microorganisms used to test and verify antimicrobial activities of biocides, products, and processes

Efficacy claim	Surrogate	Example(s) of use
Sporicidal	*Bacillus atrophaeus, Bacillus cereus, Clostridium sporogenes*	General disinfectant and sterilant testing; sterility assurance testing for sterilization processes
Fungicidal	*Trichophyton mentagrophytes, Aspergillus niger, Candida albicans*	General disinfectant testing
Bactericidal	*Staphylococcus aureus, Pseudomonas aeruginosa, Salmonella enterica* serovar Choleraesuis, *Enterococcus hirae, Escherichia coli, Serratia marcescens*	General antiseptic and disinfectant testing
Virucidal	Poliovirus, adenovirus, herpesvirus, bacteriophages (e.g., *Lactococcus* phage F7/2)	General antiseptic and disinfectant testing
Mycobactericidal	*Mycobacterium bovis, Mycobacterium terrae, Mycobacterium smegmatis*	General disinfectant testing
Oocysticidal	*Cryptosporidium parvum*	General disinfectant testing

1.4.2.1 SUSPENSION TESTING

Suspension tests are widely used under laboratory conditions in the development, verification, and registration of biocidal products. The simplest test is the determination of the MIC—the lowest concentration of a biocide that inhibits the growth of a test organism—which is widely used in the evaluation of antibiotic activity against bacteria. A series of biocide dilutions (usually in growth media specific for the test organism) are inoculated with a known concentration of the test organism and then incubated to determine the MIC. This method is useful for evaluating the efficacies of biocides against a wide range of vegetative organisms, such as bacteria and fungi, and in the development of product preservation. MICs are limited, as many biocides react with organic and inorganic constituents of the growth media and are therefore not available for activity against the test organism; examples of this include oxidizing agents, halogens, and aldehydes. As biocide MICs are generally at relatively low levels, they have limited use in demonstrating the various formulation effects that can enhance the efficacy of an antiseptic or disinfectant. Similar to MIC determination, the minimum microbicidal concentration (e.g., the minimum bactericidal concentration) can be determined by exposing the test organism to biocide or biocidal-product dilutions for a fixed time and then determining at what concentration no growth is observed. These tests are not widely used to evaluate biocidal activity.

Time-kill, or *D*-value, determinations are used to study the effects of a biocidal product over time. In their simplest form, the test organism at a known concentration is added to the product, and samples are removed over time to determine the concentration of test organisms remaining (Fig. 1.18). An important consideration in these tests (as for any microbicidal test) is the need to stop the activity of the biocide at a required exposure time, which is referred to as neutralization. With chemical biocides, neutralization can be by physical removal (the most obvious method being filtration), dilution, or chemical sequestration or inactivation. Filtration is achieved by passing the sample through a 0.1- to 0.4-μm-pore-size filter, trapping the organisms (usually bacteria and fungi), and allowing the biocide to pass through into the filtrate. Chemical neutralizers include sodium thiosulfate (for some oxidizing agents

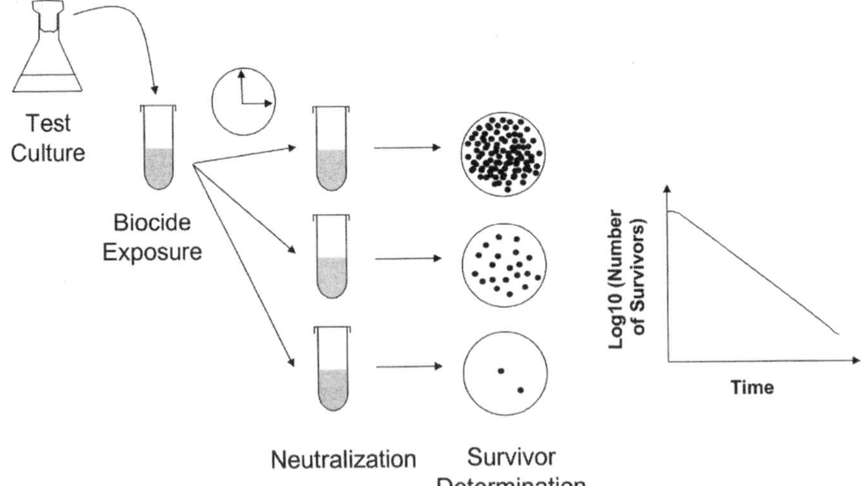

FIGURE 1.18 Typical time kill, or *D*-value, determination. A known concentration of the test culture is exposed to the biocide, samples are withdrawn at various times and neutralized, and the population of survivors is determined by incubation on growth medium. The actual exposure can be conducted at various temperatures, in the presence or absence of test soils, or under other test conditions.

and halogens), Tween and lecithin (for quaternary ammonium compounds [QACs] and chlorhexidine), and sodium sulfite or glycine (for glutaraldehyde). It is important that, other than the neutralization of the biocide, no inhibitory substances (including the neutralizer itself) be present or formed that could inhibit the growth of the test organism on incubation; for example, chlorhexidine has affinity for certain filter materials, which can subsequently inhibit the growth of the test organism on incubation of the filter on growth media. It is therefore important that positive, negative, and neutralization growth controls be included to ensure the correct interpretation of results.

Following exposure and neutralization of the biocide, the survivor population can be determined qualitatively or quantitatively. Quantitative methods determine the number of survivors by direct enumeration, e.g., by plating onto growth agar for bacteria and fungi (as shown in Fig. 1.18). The data from this analysis can be plotted as a time-log reduction relationship (Fig. 1.19).

From this plot, the decimal reduction time, or *D* value, can be calculated; it is defined as the time (e.g., in minutes or seconds) at a given temperature required to kill 1 log unit (or 90%) of a given microbial population under stated test conditions (Fig. 1.19). It is usual for the average *D* value to be determined as the negative reciprocal of the slope (*m*) of the plotted relationship (−1/slope):

$$m = \Delta \log N / \Delta T$$

$$D \text{ value} = -1/m$$

where $\Delta \log N$ is the change in $\log_{10}$ microbial population, ΔT is the change in time, and m is the slope of the survivor curve.

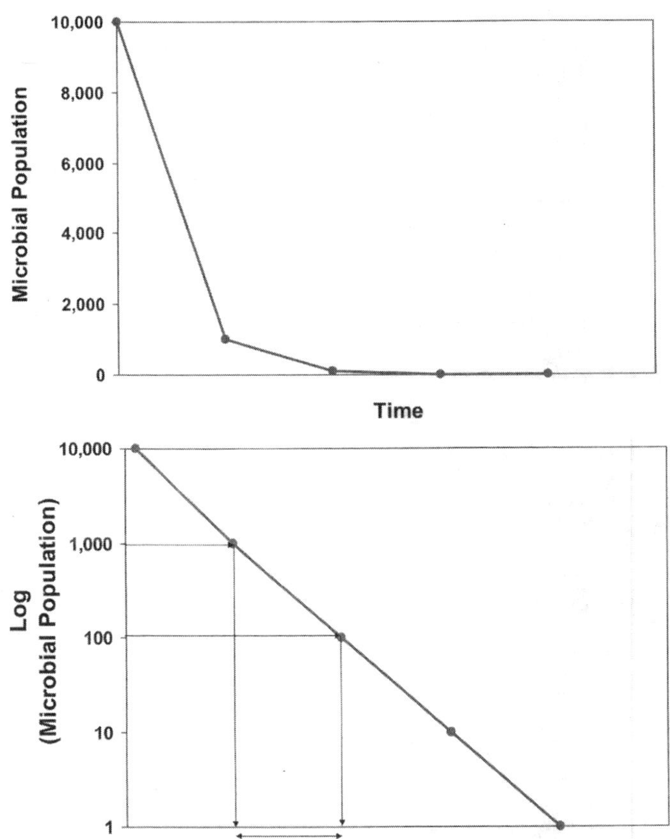

FIGURE 1.19 Determination of the *D* value on microbial exposure to a biocide.

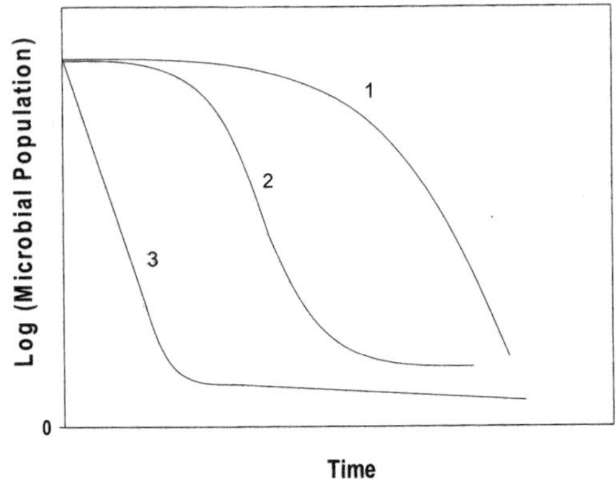

FIGURE 1.20 Typical survivor curves on biocide exposure. Curve 1 is concave downward, curve 2 is sigmoidal, and curve 3 is concave upward.

Graphical presentation of the microbial response to a biocide over time can also be useful for analysis of the biocide–microbial-population interaction. Although the data presented in Fig. 1.19 demonstrate a linear relationship, typical biocide survivor curves are often found to be nonlinear (examples are shown in Fig. 1.20). Practically, these data can have many interpretations. For example, curve 1 suggests an initial lag phase in biocidal activity that could be due to the presence of interfering soils or microbial clumping, which limits biocide access to the test microorganism. Curve 3 may be indicative of insufficient biocide concentration or the presence of a microbial subpopulation (or mixed population) with greater resistance to the biocide.

Qualitative methods simply determine the presence or absence of growth in a sample, although the data from the analysis can be used to estimate the actual population present by serial dilution if it is accepted that the microbial population is randomly distributed (i.e., not clumped) (Fig. 1.21).

By serial dilution of the initial sample (in this case, using 10-fold dilutions) in growth media and monitoring of growth, the highest dilution demonstrating growth must have contained ≤0 viable cells and can be used to estimate the most probable number in the initial sample (Fig. 1.22). This analysis is also referred to as a "fraction-negative" determination. In certain situations, these methods can be used to estimate D values (a representation of a test is shown in Fig. 1.22).

In this case, the fraction of observed growth or no growth can be used to estimate the number of survivors in the sample at a specific exposure time. Different mathematical equations are used, for example, the Halvorson-Ziegler equation (to estimate the surviving population):

$$N_t = 2.303 \log_{10} (n/r)$$

where N_t is the population at time t, n is the number tested, and r is the number sterile.

Therefore, if we take the example from Fig. 1.22, we can generate the following table:

Time	n	r	n/r	N_t
1	4	1	4	1.4
2	4	2	2	0.7
3	4	3	1.3	0.3

From this analysis, the D value can be estimated by plotting (as described above) or using

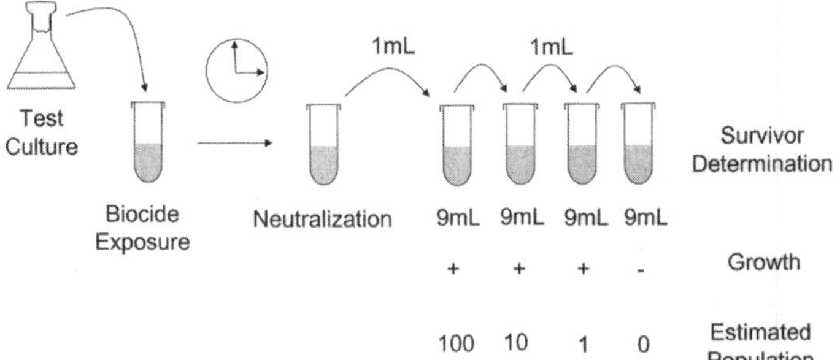

FIGURE 1.21 Qualitative and semiquantitative population determinations.

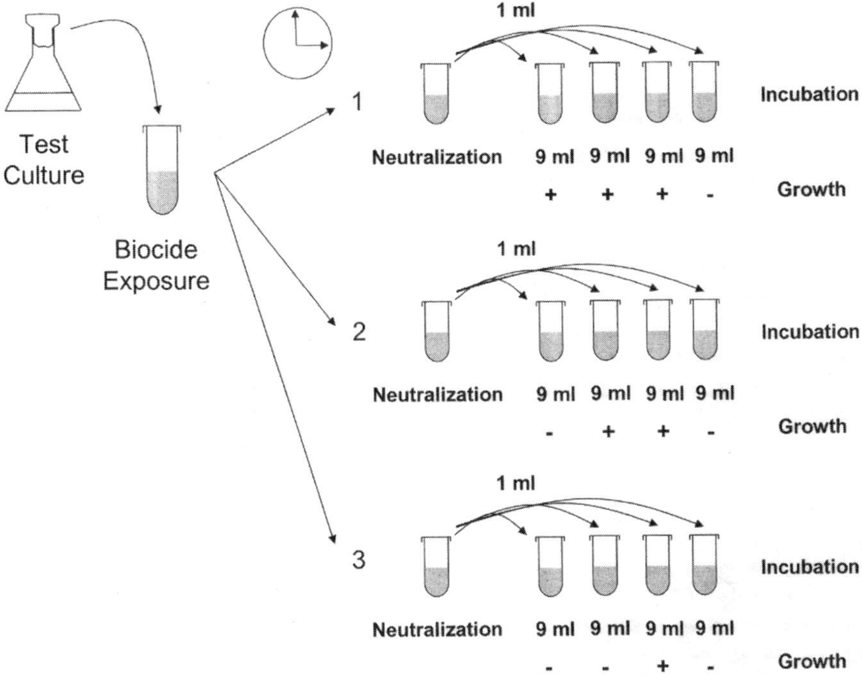

FIGURE 1.22 *D*-value estimation using most probable number estimations.

mathematical equations, like the Stumbo-Murphy-Cochran equation:

$$D \text{ value at } t = t/(\log_{10} N_0 - \log_{10} N_t)$$

where t is the exposure time, N_0 is the initial population, and N_t is the population at time t.

Clearly fraction-negative methods are relatively restrictive, but they are often used in combination with direct-enumeration methods to estimate the number of survivors in the quantal (10^2 to 10^{-2} CFU/ml) range of the survivor curve (see section 1.4.3).

The effects of various types of physical and chemical variables can be tested by using suspension methods. Physical effects include the product temperature and pH, while chemical effects include the biocide concentration or dilution, formulation type, and interfering substances, such as organic (e.g., serum and blood) and inorganic (e.g., heavy metals and hard water) soils. These effects are often important considerations in the practical use of the biocidal product.

Examples of some standardized suspension tests are given in Table 1.18.

1.4.2.2 SURFACE TESTING

Surface tests are used to verify the antimicrobial activity of a product or process on a test surface. This is an important consideration in the use of many surface antiseptics, disinfectants, and sterilants. Tests can be considered to belong to three types: carrier tests, simulated-use testing, and in-use testing.

In carrier methods, the test microorganism is inoculated onto a defined carrier material, in the presence or absence of interfering soils, and is then exposed to the biocidal process or product. The carrier material can simply consist of a coupon (a piece) of any test surface (including paper, stainless steel, glass, or plastic) or a defined test carrier; for example, stainless steel and porcelain penicylinders are widely used in the United States to test the surface-disinfectant efficacies of products. For antiseptic testing, sections of ex vivo skin have been used as test

TABLE 1.18 Examples of standardized suspension tests

Reference[a]	Title	Summary
AOAC Official Method 955.11	*Testing Disinfectants against Salmonella typhi* (includes phenol coefficient method)	Tests the bactericidal activity in comparison to known concentrations of phenol (also used to standardize test cultures) using *Salmonella typhi*, *Staphylococcus aureus*, and *Pseudomonas aeruginosa*
ASTM E1052-96 (2002)	*Standard Test Method for Efficacy of Antimicrobial Agents Against Viruses in Suspension*	Guidelines on testing of the virucidal activity of a product in suspension
ASTM E1891-97 (2002)	*Standard Guide for Determination of a Survival Curve for Antimicrobial Agents Against Selected Microorganisms and Calculation of a D-Value and Concentration Coefficient*	Guidelines on the determination of survival curves and calculation of *D* values
USP XXIII	*Antimicrobial Preservatives—Effectiveness Protocol*	Guidelines to confirm the preservative effectiveness in a formulated product by inoculation of *Staphylococcus aureus*, *Escherichia coli*, *Pseudomonas aeruginosa*, *Candida albicans*, and *Aspergillus niger*; determines that a product does not promote but prevents microbial growth over time
EN 1040:1997	*Chemical Disinfectants and Antiseptics. Basic Bactericidal Activity. Test Method and Requirements (Phase 1)*	Testing for the basic bactericidal efficacy of a disinfectant or antiseptic using *Pseudomonas aeruginosa* and *Staphylococcus aureus*; required to observe $\geq 10^5$-log-unit reduction in 60 s
EN 1650:1997	*Chemical Disinfectants and Antiseptics. Quantitative Suspension Test for Evaluation of Fungicidal Activity of Chemical Disinfectants and Antiseptics Used in Food, Industrial, Domestic and Institutional Areas. Test Method and Requirements, (Phase 2, Step 1)*	Testing for fungicidal activity of a disinfectant or antiseptic using *Candida albicans* and *Aspergillus niger* in the presence of hard water (if dilution is required) and organic soil (albumin, skim milk, and other components); required to observe $\geq 10^4$-log-unit reduction in 15 min
EN 13610:2002	*Chemical Disinfectants. Quantitative Suspension Test for the Evaluation of Virucidal Activity against Bacteriophages of Chemical Disinfectants Used in Food and Industrial Areas. Test Method and Requirements (Phase 2, Step 1)*	Testing for virucidal activity using *Lactococcus lactis* F7/2 bacteriophage; required to show $\geq 10^4$-log-unit reduction in 15 min

[a]AOAC, Association of Official Analytical Chemists; ASTM, American Society for Testing and Materials; USP, U.S. Pharmacopeia; EN, European Norm, from the CEN (European Committee for Standardization).

surfaces. Following exposure, the test coupons are retrieved (with neutralization if required) and tested for the survival of the test microorganism. This can also be performed qualitatively (by immersion into growth medium and incubation, followed by observation of growth or no growth) or quantitatively (by elution of the test culture and direct enumeration or fraction-negative determination, as described in section 1.4.2.1). Examples of various types of standardized carrier tests are given in Table 1.19. Some of the most widely used carrier tests are defined biological and chemical indicators used for various sterilization process tests, which are described in more detail in section 1.4.2.3.

Simulated-use tests are also laboratory based; an artificial inoculum is applied to a surface to simulate the actual use of the product or process in a typical application. Examples are the use of an artificial inoculum on the skin or on various surfaces, such as medical devices. In these methods, it is important to validate the test methods, including the inoculation method and neutralization and recovery methods, to ensure that

TABLE 1.19 Examples of standardized carrier tests

Reference[a]	Title	Summary
AOAC Official Methods 991.47, 991.48, 991.49	*Hard Surface Carrier Test*	Bactericidal activities of disinfectant/sterilants against *Pseudomonas aeruginosa*, *Staphylococcus aureus*, and *Salmonella enterica* serovar Choleraesuis quantitatively inoculated onto glass penicylinders; carriers tested for growth/no growth following exposure
AOAC Official Method	*Tuberculocidal Activity of Disinfectants*	Porcelain penicylinders contaminated with *Mycobacterium bovis* and exposed to the product; carriers tested for growth/no growth following exposure
AOAC Official Method 966.04	*Sporicidal Test Method*	*Clostridium sporogenes* and *Bacillus subtilis* cultures (including spores) dried onto porcelain penicylinders and suture loop carriers; exposed to the test disinfectant/sterilant for the required time and incubated to detect the presence/absence of growth; includes an HCl resistance test to confirm the acid resistance of the spores
ASTM E1053	*Standard Test Method for Efficacy of Virucidal Agents Intended for Inanimate Environmental Surfaces*	Guidelines on testing of the virucidal activity of a product on an inanimate surface
ASTM E2111	*Standard Quantitative Carrier Test Method To Evaluate the Bactericidal, Fungicidal, Mycobactericidal and Sporicidal Potencies of Liquid Chemical Germicides*	Carrier (glass vials) test for the potencies of liquid disinfectants against bacteria and fungi
EN 13697	*Chemical Disinfectants and Antiseptics. Quantitative Non-Porous Surface Test for the Evaluation of Bactericidal and/or Fungicidal Activity of Chemical Disinfectants Used in Food, Industrial, Domestic and Institutional Areas. Test Method and Requirements*	Various bacteria (e.g., *Pseudomonas aeruginosa* and *Enterococcus hirae*) and fungi (*Candida albicans* and *Aspergillus niger*) inoculated onto stainless steel discs in the presence/absence of interfering soil and exposed to the test disinfectant/antiseptic; must demonstrate a $\geq 10^4$ reduction of bacteria in 5 min and $\geq 10^3$ reduction of fungi in 15 min

[a]AOAC, Association of Official Analytical Chemists; ASTM, American Society for Testing and Materials; EN, European Norm, from the CEN (European Committee for Standardization).

they are reproducible and reliable. As well as direct application of the test culture to a surface, in some situations, the microbial culture can be inoculated onto a carrier or inserted into the test equipment at a worst-case location (e.g., in the internal channel of a lumened device), exposed to the product or process, and recovered for evaluation. Recovery methods can include elution, swabbing, air filtering, and use of contact plates. Examples of various simulated-use test guidelines and standards are given in Table 1.20.

Finally, in-use testing is designed to test the product or process under the actual conditions of use. These tests can be designed to test biocidal efficiency on a given surface, including routine microbial sampling of a surface using a recovery method (e.g., a swabbing or elution method). The efficiency can be determined before and after the application of a product or process with the estimation of the associated bioburden, which is defined as the population of viable microorganisms on or in a product, surface, or area. In some applications, in-use

TABLE 1.20 Examples of simulated-use and/or in-use tests and/or guidelines[a]

Reference[b]	Title	Summary
ASTM E1837-96	*Standard Test Method To Determine Efficacy of Disinfection Processes for Reusable Medical Devices*	Simulated-use testing for the effectiveness of a disinfection process for reprocessing reusable medical devices using bacteria, viruses, and/or fungi
ISO 11737-1	*Sterilization of Medical Devices—Microbiological Methods—Part 1: Estimation of Population of Microorganisms on Products*	In-use testing guidelines for estimation of the population of viable microorganisms (or the bioburden) on a medical device
ISO 14698-1	*Cleanrooms and Associated Controlled Environments—Biocontamination Control, Part 1: General Principles and Methods*	In-use testing guidelines for the assessment and control of biocontamination within a cleanroom environment
WHO	*Guidelines for Drinking-Water Quality*	Guidelines for the microbial and chemical safety of drinking water, including water-testing methods for monitoring water disinfection efficacy
ASTM E1174-94	*Standard Test Method for Evaluation of Healthcare Personnel Handwash Formulations*	Simulation to test the activity of an antiseptic on the hands using an artificial inoculum of *Serratia marcescens*
ASTM E1173-01	*Standard Test Method of an Evaluation of Preoperative, Precatheterization, or Preinjection Skin Preparations*	In-use test for the activity of an antiseptic to reduce the resident microbial flora of the skin

[a]Simulated testing uses an artificial inoculum, and in-use testing uses the normal bioburden present on a surface or device.
[b]ISO, International Standards Organization; ASTM, American Society for Testing and Materials; WHO, World Health Organization.

testing is recommended to actively monitor the success or failure of a product or process over time. Examples include the routine sampling of a reusable medical device, swabbing of a food contact surface, and verification of the operation of disinfection and/or sterilization equipment (examples of test methods are given in Table 1.20).

1.4.2.3 BIOLOGICAL, CHEMICAL, AND OTHER INDICATORS

Indicators are routinely used to check the effectiveness of various cleaning, disinfection, and sterilization processes. They include biological, chemical, and other (e.g., mechanical) indicators.

Biological indicators (Fig. 1.23) consist of a standardized population of microorganisms inoculated onto a carrier material. They are particularly widely used in the monitoring and

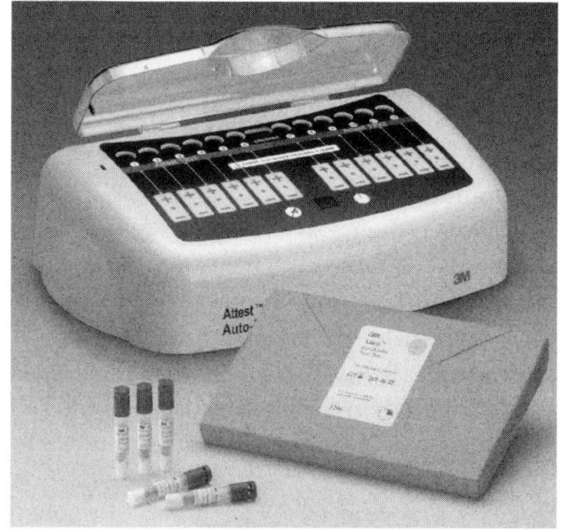

FIGURE 1.23 Example of a self-contained biological indicator. The 3M Attest 1292 Rapid Readout Biological Indicator is used to monitor steam sterilization cycles. Reproduced with permission of 3M Health Care.

validation of sterilization processes. Bacterial endospores are commonly used as the test microorganisms, as they are generally nonpathogenic and stable and demonstrate high resistance to various sterilization processes (Table 1.21). Defined bacterial strains, obtained from standard culture collections (e.g., the American Type Culture Collection), are used. The intrinsic resistance of the inoculated spore population can vary depending on the culturing methods used and other variables. Therefore, to standardize the use of biological indicators, manufacturers test each batch of indicators to determine the population and the relative resistance to a given sterilization process (e.g., *D*-value determination at 121°C with saturated steam and at 55°C, 800 mg of ethylene oxide/liter, and 70% relative humidity for ethylene oxide). Depending on the application, other microorganisms may be used, but to a much lesser extent.

The carrier can consist of any material, with typical examples being paper, stainless steel, glass, and plastics. In its true definition, a biological indicator consists of the inoculated coupon placed into a "primary pack," which can be a protective envelope or pouch, or within an assembled vial or ampoule. In their simplest form, biological indicators are present within a protective envelope, and following exposure to a given sterilization process, the inoculated coupon is aseptically removed from its pack and incubated in a specified growth medium to determine the presence or absence of spore viability. Due to the release of dipicolinic acid (see section 8.3.11) upon germination and outgrowth of the spores, pH indicator dyes can be used in the growth media to indicate the presence of viability before visible growth (turbidity) is observed. To minimize aseptic handling, self-contained biological indicators that include the inoculated carrier within a vial containing a sealed ampoule of growth medium have also been developed (Fig. 1.23). Following exposure, the medium ampoule is broken to allow incubation without handling of the coupon. Further "rapid-review" biological indicators are available that detect the presence of certain endospore enzymes (e.g., α-D-glucosidase) whose destruction by heat correlates with the loss of viability of the spore; the presence of enzyme activity can be detected fluorimetrically and can give a rapid indication of spore viability (usually within 1 to 4 h). In addition, these indicators are further incubated to demonstrate the presence or absence of growth, as for traditional biological indicators. Various standards that define the requirements for and use of biological indicators are given in Table 1.22.

TABLE 1.21 Bacterial-endospore species used to monitor and validate sterilization processes

Sterilization process	Biological indicator
Moist heat	*Geobacillus stearothermophilus*
Dry heat	*Bacillus atrophaeus*
Irradiation	*Bacillus pumilus*
Ethylene oxide	*Bacillus atrophaeus*
Low-temperature steam formaldehyde	*G. stearothermophilus*
Hydrogen peroxide vapor	*G. stearothermophilus*

Chemical indicators change color (or provide another visible change) on exposure to a given disinfectant or sterilization process (Fig. 1.24). They can range from simple process indicators that indicate exposure to a given process parameter (e.g., exposure to heat, but not necessarily at the right temperature and for the right amount of time) to more specific integrator indicators, which change color only on exposure to multiple variables (e.g., temperature and time for steam sterilization and concentration or time, temperature, and humidity for ethylene oxide sterilization). They can be classified in various ways, and an example is given in Table 1.23.

Chemical indicators are widely used, as they give an instant result and in some cases (as with some integrators) can be correlated to a biological indicator result. Applications include specific direct parameters that are required for disinfection or sterilization (e.g., verification of the presence of a minimal concentration of a biocidal formulation prior to use or that a range of conditions have been met in a sterilizer), but also other, indirect variables that are important to the efficacy of the process (e.g., Bowie-Dick

TABLE 1.22 Examples of biological-indicator standards

Reference[a]	Title	Summary
ISO 11138-1	*Sterilization of Health Care Products—Biological Indicators—Part 1: General Requirements*	General requirements for production, labeling, test methods, and performance characteristics of biological indicator systems to be used in the validation and routine monitoring of sterilization processes
ISO 11138-2	*Sterilization of Health Care Products—Biological —Part 2: Biological Indicators for Ethylene Oxide Sterilization Processes*	Specific requirements for biological indicators used for ethylene oxide sterilization, including test organism and performance criteria
ISO 11138-3	*Sterilization of Health Care Products—Biological Indicators—Part 3: Biological Indicators for Moist Heat Sterilization Processes*	Specific requirements for biological indicators used for moist-heat (steam) sterilization, including test organisms and performance criteria
ISO 14161	*Sterilization of Health Care Products—Biological Indicators—Guidance for the Selection, Use and Interpretation of Results*	Guidance for the selection, use, and interpretation of results of biological indicators used in the development, validation, and routine monitoring of sterilization processes
EN 866-1	*Biological Systems for Testing Sterilizers and Sterilization Processes. Part 1—General Requirements*	General requirements for production, labeling, test methods, and performance characteristics of biological indicator systems to be used in the validation and routine monitoring of sterilization processes
USP XXIII	*Biological Indicators—Resistance Performance Tests*	Testing of the resistances and population of biological indicators
EP 5.1.2	*Biological Indicators of Sterilization*	Requirements for biological indicators, including population and resistance

[a]ISO, International Standards Organization; EN, European Norm, from the CEN (European Committee for Standardization); USP, United States Pharmacopeia; EP, European Pharmacopoeia.

tests are used to confirm the adequate removal of air in prevacuum-type steam sterilizers [see section 5.2]). Examples of various standards that define the requirements for and use of chemical indicators are given in Table 1.24.

Other, miscellaneous indicators include mechanical indicators, such as gauges or sensors that measure temperature, concentration, pressure, time, etc., that are used to monitor various physical parameters during a given process and cleaning indicators that use artificial test soils inoculated onto a surface to test (generally by visual inspection) physical removal during a cleaning process or cycle. Mechanical indica-

TABLE 1.23 A typical classification of chemical indicators

Class	Type	Description
1	Process indicators	Indicate exposure to minimal process conditions; used to differentiate exposed from unexposed items (e.g., autoclave tape)
2	Indicators for use in specific tests	Indicate that a specific process is obtained, which is linked to the sterilization process (e.g., a Bowie-Dick test indicates the adequate removal of air from a prevacuum steam sterilizer)
3	Single-parameter indicators	Indicate a change on exposure to one parameter (e.g., concentration of a biocide or temperature).
4	Multiparameter indicators	Indicate a change on exposure to at least two parameters
5	Integrating indicators	Indicate a change on exposure to all the critical parameters of a given process (e.g., ethylene oxide sterilization with temperature, biocide concentration, relative humidity, and time)

FIGURE 1.24 Example of a chemical-indicator color change.

tors play an important role in the parametric release of a product or process as an alternative to the use of chemical and biological indicators for routine monitoring of sterilization processes (see section 1.4.2.4).

1.4.2.4 PARAMETRIC CONTROL

The concept of parametric control (or release) as a method to verify the effectiveness of a biocidal process is based on the understanding of all the key physical parameters that can affect its success or failure. Although theoretically this could be applied to any disinfection or sterilization process, it is generally restricted to well-characterized sterilization methods, including steam, dry heat, ethylene oxide, and ionizing radiation. An example is steam sterilization. The efficacy of steam is affected by the temperature and time, but also by the presence of air (see section 5.2). These parameters are reasonably well understood and can be physically measured (by using mechanical indicators [see section 1.4.2.3]) to ensure that the correct conditions have been met during a given steam sterilization cycle. In addition to monitoring these conditions, a series of in-process tests and controls are also conducted to provide further assurance that the sterilization process has been efficient. However, the concern with parametric release as an alternative to biological monitoring is in the control of other variables that can affect the effectiveness of the process. In the case of steam, these include the quality of the steam (see section 5.2), variations in the load being sterilized, and in the case of reusable devices, if the cleaning process has been sufficient prior to sterilization (see section 1.4.8). In most cases, disinfection and sterilization processes are routinely tested and monitored using a combination of biological and chemical indicators in parallel with mechanical indicators for parametric control.

TABLE 1.24 Examples of chemical-indicator standards

Reference[a]	Title	Summary
ISO 15882	*Chemical Indicators—Guidance on the Selection, Use, and Interpretation of Results*	Guidance for the selection, use, and interpretation of results of chemical indicators used in process definition, validation, and routine monitoring and control of sterilization processes
ISO 11140-1	*Sterilization of Health Care Products—Chemical Indicators—Part 1: General Requirements*	General requirements for production, labeling, test methods, and performance characteristics of chemical indicators to be used in the validation and routine monitoring of sterilization processes
ISO 11140-3	*Sterilization of Health Care Products—Chemical Indicators—Part 3: Class 2 Indicators for Steam Penetration Test Sheets*	Specific requirements for class 2 steam penetration test indicators
EN 867-1	*Non-Biological Systems for Use in Sterilizers—Part 1: General Requirements*	General requirements for indicators that are used to monitor the presence or attainment of one or more sterilization process variables
ANSI/AAMI ST60	*Sterilization of Health Care Products—Chemical Indicators—Part 1: General Requirements*	Requirements for chemical indicators intended for use with sterilization processes employing steam, ethylene oxide, irradiation, or dry heat

[a]ISO, International Standards Organization; EN, European Norm, from the CEN (European Committee for Standardization); ANSI/AAMI, American National Standards Institute/Association for the Advancement of Medical Instrumentation.

1.4.2.5 MICROSCOPY AND OTHER TECHNIQUES

Other specific methods are used to evaluate the efficacies of biocidal processes and products. These are generally used due to restrictions on the cultivation of various microorganisms under laboratory conditions. Microscopy or other detection (biochemical and genetic) methods for the presence of microbial contaminants have been used; however, these methods can identify the presence of an organism but may not necessarily detect its actual viability. A specific example of the use of microscopy is in the determination of the viability of protozoan (oo)cysts or helminth eggs. In the case of protozoa, the viability of cysts can be determined in vitro by suspension in a specific medium under controlled conditions (including temperature) to cause the cysts to excyst and release their vegetative forms (see section 1.3.3.4); this can be monitored microscopically and is considered a reasonable indication of cyst viability. Cell culture methods (using mammalian cells) have also been developed to determine cyst viability and are also widely used to culture viruses and some bacteria. In many of these cases, in vitro methods are not sufficiently developed to determine microbial viability, and the use of in vivo (animal) models is required. An example of this is the case of prions (see section 1.3.6), which are proposed to be infectious proteins; although the biochemical detection of the protein can be used as an initial indicator of inactivation and cell culture assays are currently under development, in vivo infectivity models are highly recommended to confirm activity against these unusual agents.

1.4.3 Disinfection versus Sterilization

In the consideration of biocides and biocidal processes, there is an important distinction between disinfection and sterilization. Disinfection is the reduction by an antimicrobial of the number of viable microorganisms to a level previously specified as appropriate for intended further handling or use; however, "safe to handle" does not necessarily mean that all microorganisms are killed or removed, and different levels of disinfection can be defined, including pasteurization, sanitization, and high-, intermediate-, or low-level disinfection (see chapters 2 and 3). In contrast, sterilization is defined as a validated process used to render a surface or product free from viable organisms, or "sterile." These include physical (e.g., heat and radiation [see chapter 5]) and chemical (e.g., ethylene oxide gas [see chapter 6]) processes. Disinfection efficacy can be demonstrated by using various surface and suspension tests (see section 1.4.2), many of which are specified to meet local requirements for product registration (e.g., in the United States with Food and Drug Administration- or Environmental Protection Agency-registered disinfectants). Sterilization processes require investigations that are more detailed. They include an analysis of the sterilizing agent itself and the definition of the use of the agent in a standardized sterilization process for specific applications.

Characterization of any sterilizing agent should include the following:

- Definition of the sterilization agent (e.g., generation, stability, physical chemistry, and safety)
- Detailed antimicrobial studies (see below)
- Identification of the variables that can affect the antimicrobial activity of the agent, including temperature, humidity, time, distribution, penetration, and (for some applications) the presence of soil

The sterilization process should be shown to be effective against a broad range of microorganisms, including bacteria, mycobacteria, viruses, fungi, protozoa, and bacterial spores. From this analysis, specific resistant microorganisms (usually bacterial spores [see section 1.4.2.3]) are chosen to establish the mathematical relationship on exposure to the sterilizing agent. This can be determined by using the various suspension and surface tests (direct enumeration and fraction negative) specified in section 1.4.2 and by plotting the number of

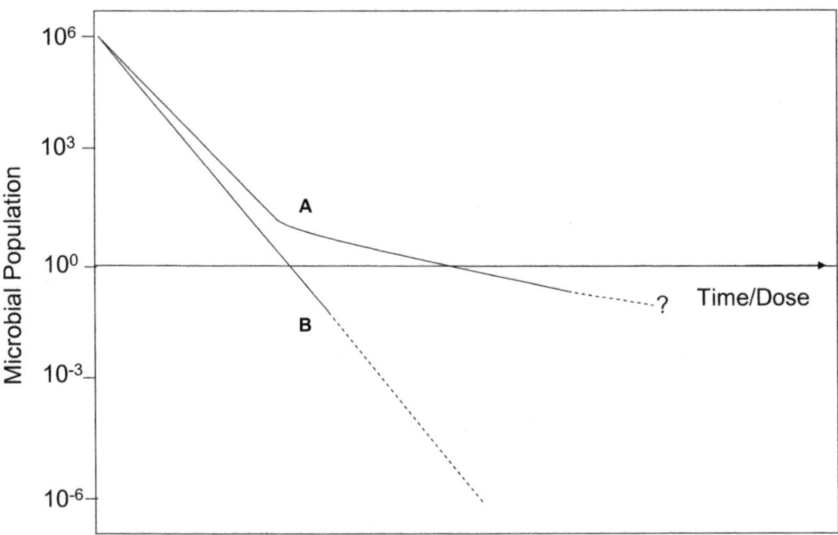

FIGURE 1.25 Rate of microbial inactivation on exposure to sterilization processes. In this case, the test microorganism (generally bacterial spores) at a starting population of 10^6 is exposed to the sterilizing agent under two conditions (A and B). The number of microorganisms can be determined over contact time or dose using a combination of direct-enumeration and fraction-negative methods (solid lines). In process A, "tailing" is observed, which may not allow the extrapolation of the kill curve to a defined probability of survival (known as an SAL). In process B, the kill curve is linear, allowing extrapolation (dotted line) to an SAL of 10^{-6}.

microbial survivors on exposure to the sterilizing agent over time (Fig. 1.25).

This analysis allows the determination of the probability of a microorganism surviving the sterilization process, when the microbial reduction has been shown to be predictable (linear). Because it is difficult to confirm that sterility has been achieved with a given process, the concept of the sterility assurance level (SAL) is used. The SAL can be defined as the probability of survival of a viable microorganism after a sterilization process (generally expressed as 10^{-n}). For example, it is common in health care applications to use an SAL of 10^{-6}, implying a chance of less than one in a million that an item may be contaminated when a starting population of 10^6 test organisms is present on the test surface.

When the sterilizing-agent conditions are understood experimentally, they can then be applied in actual sterilization processes, which include specific loads for treatment (like packaged liquids and devices) in equipment used to provide and control the required conditions (e.g., steam sterilizers or radiation exposure chambers [see chapters 5 and 6]). These processes are also required to be tested to ensure that the minimum sterilizing conditions are met within the load. There are two basic methods recommended: overkill and bioburden-based methods. Overkill methods are probably the most widely used, in particular with sterilization of reusable medical devices. In these methods, a test microorganism (generally a resistant spore at a given population either directly in or on a product, or using a biological indicator) is placed at worst-case locations within the load, and the minimum time or dose to give a complete kill is determined; this time or dose is then at least doubled to give a conservative sterilization cycle. A typical overkill method is shown in Fig. 1.25B, giving an SAL of 10^{-6}. Bioburden-based methods are based on knowledge of the population size and resistance of microorganisms present on or in a product; similarly, the reduction of the bioburden over time or dose is determined and extrapolated to give the minimum conditions for the required SAL. In some cases, these methods can be combined in the validation of a specific sterilization process for a specific application.

1.4.4 Choosing a Process or Product

At least three factors should be considered in the choice of a biocidal process or product for a given application: antimicrobial efficacy, safety, and compatibility. For antimicrobial efficacy, the requirements and choice of biocide for a preservation application (generally bacteriostatic and fungistatic activity) vary from that of a sterilization process which should render a product sterile and free from microbial contamination. The spectrum of antimicrobial activities for various physical and chemical biocides are considered further in chapters 2 to 6. The choice of biocidal treatment will often depend on the risk associated with the level and type of contamination on the surface or in a given product. An example is the Spaulding classification for reusable medical devices, which defines them as critical, semicritical, or noncritical based on the risk of infection with the presence of contamination. Critical devices demonstrate the greatest risk because they are introduced directly into the human body, with contact with the bloodstream or other normally sterile areas of the body; due to the risks associated with contamination, it is recommended that critical devices be sterilized. Semicritical devices present a lower risk, as they may contact intact mucous membranes or nonintact skin during use, and therefore a minimum requirement for high-level disinfection is recommended. High-level disinfectants are considered effective against all microbial pathogens, with the exception of large numbers of bacterial spores. Finally, noncritical devices present the lowest risk of transmission of infection, i.e., they contact intact skin only, and at a minimum should be reprocessed with intermediate- or low-level disinfectants. A similar risk assessment can be used in the choice of any antiseptic, disinfectant, or sterilization process for a given application.

Safety aspects include hazards in the use of the product, residues that remain on or in a treated product following application, environmental concerns, and reactivity on mixing with other agents. For this reason, biocides and biocidal products are usually provided with safety data sheets (e.g., material safety data sheets) that contain information regarding ingredients, hazards, first aid measures, personnel protection, stability and reactivity, toxicology, and ecological (e.g., bioaccumulation) concerns. For automated processes, these details should also be provided in equipment manuals and are often specified in various guidelines and standards. These safety aspects should be reviewed and considered prior to the use of a biocidal product or process. In many countries, the specific use of certain biocides may be restricted due to health and environmental concerns.

Finally, compatibility with the surface or product is important to ensure that unexpected damage does not occur. Compatibility may be defined as the suitability of a biocidal product or process to be used on a surface or in a solution without causing unacceptable interactions, damage, or other undesirable effects. It is for this reason that a restricted number of biocides are used on foods or on the skin (as antiseptics) (see chapter 4). A wider range of biocides are used on hard surfaces, but they also vary in compatibility (e.g., some heat-based processes cannot be used for temperature-sensitive surfaces or products). Other considerations will depend on the specific application and include reproducibility, ease of use, cycle or application time, cost, guidelines and standards (which are further considered in section 1.4.5), and specific regulatory requirements.

1.4.5 Guidelines and Standards

Various guidelines and standards are available that assist in the choice, use, testing, and validation of biocidal processes and products (examples of these are given in Table 1.25). They include international and country-specific requirements, many of which are mandatory for the use of the product or process in certain countries.

1.4.6 Formulation Effects

Unlike many therapeutic antimicrobials (such as antibiotics), most biocides are provided in formulation with other ingredients as products. Formulation may be defined as the combina-

TABLE 1.25 Examples of standards and guidelines for antisepsis, disinfection and sterilization

Reference[a]	Title	Summary
Standards		
ISO 14937	*Sterilization of Healthcare Products—General Requirements for Characterization of a Sterilizing Agent and the Development, Validation and Routine Control of a Sterilization Process*	Basic requirements for any sterilization process, including characterization of the sterilizing agent and validation of specific sterilization processes
ISO 11137-1	*Sterilization of Healthcare Products—Requirements for the Development, Validation and Routine Control of a Sterilization Process for Medical Devices—Radiation—Part 1: Requirements*	Requirements and tests for radiation sterilization processes, including radionucleotides, X rays, and electron beams
EN 285	*Sterilization: Steam Sterilizers. Large sterilizers*	Requirements and tests for large steam sterilizers primarily used in health care facilities
ISO 13408-1	*Aseptic Processing of Healthcare Products. Part 1: General Requirements*	Requirements and guidance for processes, programs, and procedures for the validation and control of aseptically processed health care products in cleanrooms and barrier isolator systems
Guidelines		
FDA 21 CFR880.6885	*Guidance on the Content and Format of Premarket Notification (510(k)) Submissions for Liquid Chemical Sterilants/High Level Disinfectants, and User Information and Training*	Guidance on the requirements for the registration of a liquid chemical sterilant/high-level disinfectant with the FDA
HC-HPFBI (2001)	*Process Validation: Moist Heat Sterilization for Pharmaceuticals*	Guidelines for the steam sterilization of pharmaceutical dosage forms
TGO-TGA		Guidelines for the registration or listing of disinfectants and sterilants in Australia
EPA, DIS-TSS 01	*Disinfectants for Use on Hard Surfaces*	Efficacy data requirements for the registration of disinfectants for use on hard surfaces with the EPA (01 and associated guidelines)
EC Council Directive 98/8/EC	*Biocidal Products Directive*	Requirements for the use of biocidal products in the European Union, including disinfectant and preservative safety and efficacy
APIC	*Guideline for Hand Washing and Hand Antisepsis in Health-Care Settings*	Guidelines on the types and uses of various antiseptics in health care applications
WHO, 1999	*Infection Control Guidelines for Transmissible Spongiform Encephalopathies*	Guidelines for infection control practices against prion diseases, including decontamination

[a]ISO, International Standards Organization; EN, European Norm, from the CEN (European Committee for Standardization); APIC, Association for Professionals in Infection Control and Epidemiology (United States); EPA, U.S. Environmental Protection Agency; FDA, U.S. Food and Drug Administration, HC-HPFBI: Health Products and Food Branch Inspectorate of Health Canada; EC, European Commission; TGO-TGA, Therapeutic Goods Order-Therapeutic Goods Administration, Australia; WHO, World Health Organization.

tion of ingredients, including active (biocides) and inert ingredients, into a product for its intended use (e.g., cosmetics, antiseptics, and disinfectants). Inert (or excipient) ingredients include water, nonaqueous solvents, emulsifiers, chelating agents, and corrosion inhibitors. The functions of these various ingredients are summarized in Table 1.26.

The formulation of a biocide can be a complex task to ensure the optimization of antimicrobial efficacy, compatibility, required characteristics, and aesthetics of the final product. The first consideration is the choice of the biocide itself, which must have an optimal range of concentration, pH, temperature, solubility, stability, and spectrum of activity. It is also clear that the desired performance attributes of the product also need to be considered during its formulation (e.g., the effect of water quality if the product is diluted prior to use, compatibility with surfaces, and improved antimicrobial activity by synergy with other biocides or excipients). These considerations allow the choice of various formulation ingredients (Table 1.26). The basic components of many formulations are water and other solvents (such as alcohols); although many biocides and other excipients are soluble (ionic or hydrophilic) in water, many are insoluble (hydrophobic). Biocides are therefore often mixed with emulsifiers, including soaps and detergents, to increase their solubility or dispersion in a for-

TABLE 1.26 Various constituents of formulated biocidal products

Ingredient	Purpose	Examples
Biocide	Antimicrobial or preservative activity	QACs, phenolics, biguanides
Solvent	A solvent is a substance (usually liquid) that is capable of dissolving other substances, with water being the most common. Solvents are used for dissolution and dilution of the biocide and other ingredients.	Deionized water, isopropanol, propylene glycol, urea
Emulsifiers, surfactants	Emulsifers are ingredients (including surfactants) that allow the formation of stable mixtures (emulsions) of water- and oil-soluble ingredients. Surfactants ("surface-acting agents") can be used as emulsifiers. but also to reduce surface tension, improve wettability of a surface, disperse contaminants, and inhibit foam formation.	Sodium lauryl sulfate, potassium laurate, lecithin, nonionic and other surfactants (see section 3.16)
Thickeners	A substance used to increase the viscosity of a formulation	Polyethylene glycol; polysaccharides, like pectin, gums, and alginates
Chelating agents or sequestrants	Binding metals (like calcium and magnesium) and inhibiting their precipitation; water softening and prevention of mineral deposition	Ethylenediamine, EDTA, EGTA
Alkali or acid	pH stabilization. Alkalis are used as "builders" to optimize the activities of surfactants, including emulsification of soils. Acids are also used to prevent mineral deposition and for water softening.	Alkalis (NaOH, KOH, silicates); acids (acetic acid, citric acid, phosphoric acid)
Buffer	Maintaining pH over time and increasing alkalinity	Disodium phosphate
Corrosion inhibitors	Reducing the corrosion rates and protecting the surfaces of metals	Nitrates, phosphates, molybdates, ethanolamine
Others	Aesthetic qualities	Colors and fragrances

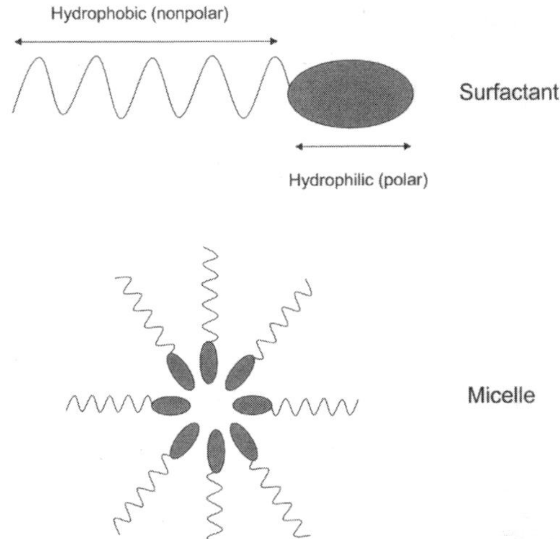

FIGURE 1.26 Basic structures of surfactants and soaps and micelles (a water-in-oil micelle is shown).

mulation. Emulsifiers form micelles, which are aggregated units of surface-active molecules (Fig. 1.26). Soaps are water-soluble salts or fatty acids, which are made by reactions of fats and/or oils with an alkali (e.g., sodium hydroxide). Detergents are mixtures of surfactants, which are defined as surface-active agents. Surfactant molecules act in low concentrations to change the properties of a liquid at its surface or interface with a surface. This increases the wettability of the liquid by breaking its surface tension, the force that holds the surface molecules together, and allowing it to spread over a surface better. Surfactants are further defined as nonionic (no charge), anionic (negatively charged), cationic (positively charged), and amphotheric (positively and negatively charged), and many possess antimicrobial activity (see section 3.16). Surfactants form micelles (Fig. 1.26), which are useful for the solubilization, dispersion, or emulsification of incompatible materials, as well as aiding in cleaning processes by the removal and dispersion of hydrophobic soils from a surface.

Other formulation ingredients, including thickeners, buffers, chelating agents, and fragrances, allow further optimization of the stability, efficacy, and compatibility of the product. Due to the variety of ingredients that can be present in a given formulation, the preservative and/or antimicrobial activity can vary considerably. For this reason, users should pay close attention to the instructions (or labeling) provided with the product for its intended use, including the shelf life, application, dilution (if required), contact time for antimicrobial efficacy, spectrum of activity, safety, and compatibility.

1.4.7 Process Effects

Just as the antimicrobial activity of a biocidal product can vary depending on various formulation effects, it is also affected by various process effects, including variables like temperature, humidity, pressure, time, and biocide concentration. This is particularly true in the development and optimization of processes. Important process variables in various disinfection and sterilization techniques are given in Table 1.27; they are discussed in further detail in chapters 2, 5, and 6.

The activity of a biocide is usually greater as the contact time, temperature, or concentration increases. The effect of contact time is often demonstrated by studying the loss of microbial viability over time, for example, *D*-value determinations (see section 1.4.2.1). Some biocidal applications are required to be rapid in action due to their practical use, as in the case of hand washing or surface disinfection. In contrast, preservative applications are only required to control microbial growth within a product over a longer exposure time or within a given shelf life. Temperature itself can be a reliable method of disinfection and sterilization, depending on the contact time and temperature for a given application (see section 2.2). In most cases, the activities of chemical biocides are also increased as the temperature increases; however, in the case of higher temperatures, increased degradation can also be observed, depending on the biocide type and the temperature conditions. Various materials or applications may also be restricted to low-temperature exposure condi-

TABLE 1.27 Examples of process variables in various disinfection/sterilization techniques

Biocidal process	Variables
Steam (moist heat)	Temperature, time, pressure, quality of steam (including saturation), biocide penetration
Ethylene oxide	Formulation, temperature, humidity, biocide concentration, vacuum, time, biocide penetration
Liquid peracetic acid	Formulation, temperature, biocide concentration, time, biocide penetration (e.g., directed flow)
Hydrogen peroxide vapor	Temperature, biocide concentration, time, humidity, biocide penetration (vacuum or directed flow)
Radiation	Radiation dose, penetration, exposure time

tions, for example, in the case of thermosensitive materials or due to safety concerns.

Antimicrobial activity is also greater as the concentration of biocide is increased but also varies depending on the biocide and its application. A notable example is alcohols, where less bacteriocidal activity is observed at concentrations greater than 90% alcohol in water, and the optimal range is actually within 60 to 80%; efficacy is dramatically less at lower concentrations. Further, despite the alcohol concentration, little to no efficacy has been reported against bacterial spores. The optimization of a biocide concentration is an important consideration in various disinfection and sterilization processes. Higher biocide concentrations can lead to unwanted effects, including material incompatibility and safety risks, in particular with gas-based applications. In the case of liquid applications, as discussed in section 1.4.6, the efficacy of a biocide can be dramatically enhanced or reduced by various formulation effects that should also be appreciated. These effects include pH (for biocide efficacy and stability), the quality of water, and the presence of excipients, like surfactants.

The control of relative humidity is an important consideration for many gas-based chemical biocidal processes, including the use of ethylene oxide and formaldehyde. Other effects include the state of the biocide (in liquid or gaseous form) and its delivery (to ensure that all site are contacted). Many physical and chemical sterilization processes are conducted under vacuum (e.g., ethylene oxide and plasma-hydrogen peroxide vapor), in vacuum or pressure cycles (e.g., steam), or under specific directed-flow conditions (with liquids and gases) to optimize the penetration of the biocide to all contact sites within a given load.

1.4.8 The Importance of Cleaning

Cleaning is the removal of contamination from an item to the extent necessary for its further processing and its intended subsequent use. In many applications, it is important to ensure the removal of residues following the use of a reusable surface, for example, to prevent cross-contamination between pharmaceutical manufacturing batches, to reduce the level of bioburden on the surface, and particularly, to ensure that a subsequent biocidal process can be effective. Various surfaces require routine cleaning, including manufacturing vessels, equipment, or areas; food-handling surfaces; and reusable medical, veterinary, and dental devices. The presence of various organic (including lipids, proteins, and carbohydrates) and/or inorganic (including various heavy metals like calcium and iron) soils on these surfaces can often dramatically interfere with the activity of a biocide.

Cleaning is generally achieved by a combination of physical and chemical processes. Physical effects include simple immersion, manual cleaning (brushing and wiping), and automated

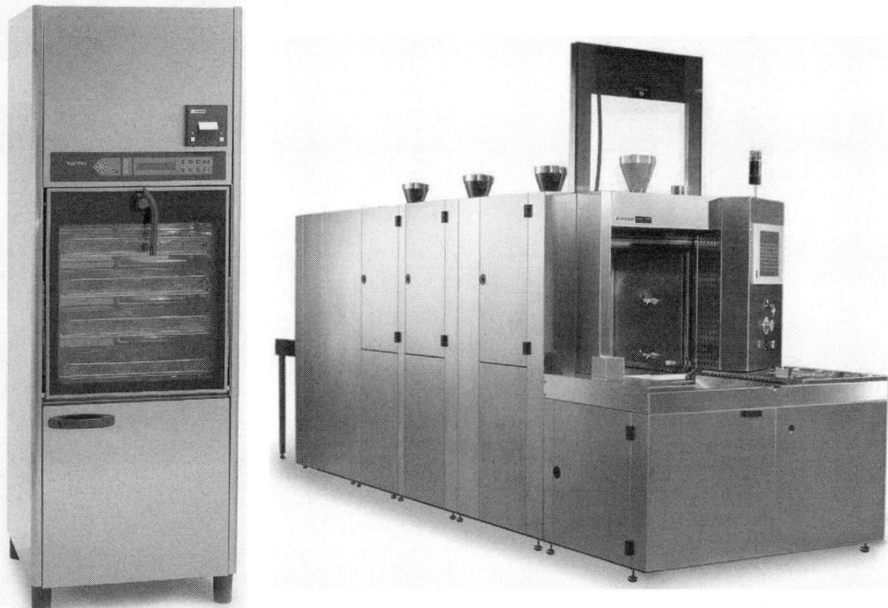

FIGURE 1.27 Examples of single (left)- and multiple (right)-chamber washer and washer-disinfector machines. Washer-disinfectors can come in a variety of shapes and sizes, depending on their required uses.

cleaning. Automated cleaning includes the use of washers (or washer-disinfectors [Fig, 1.27]) and clean-in-place systems. Clean-in-place systems are integral to manufacturing equipment (such as reaction vessels), which can be automatically cleaned without disassembly. Automated washing machines allow the placement of items into the washing chamber for exposure to a cleaning process. They can be used for washing only or as washer-disinfectors, which are used to clean and disinfect (using heat and/or chemicals) devices and other articles. They can consist of single- or multiple-chamber washers and provide physical cleaning by agitation, directed flow, spraying, and ultrasonics (where the items are immersed and exposed to sound waves that aid in the physical removal of soil).

Chemical cleaning is achieved using various types of cleaning chemistries (Fig. 1.28). Similar to formulation of biocides (see section 1.4.6), cleaning formulations can contain a variety of components that aid in the chemical removal of soils from a surface (Table 1.28). Cleaning chemistries can be classified into various types, including enzymatics and nonenzymatics. Enzymatic formulations contain active enzymes that degrade various organic-soil components over time, including lipases (lipids and oils), proteases (proteins), and amylases (starch and other carbohydrates). Nonenzymatic formulations can be further subclassified into neutral, acidic, and alkaline cleaning formulations. Acid cleaners are particularly used for the removal of scale and mineral deposits, while alkaline cleaners are particularly effective at removing and degrading protein-based soils. Neutral cleaners, depending on their formulations, usually have the widest compatibility with various types of surfaces. In some applications, simpler cleaning chemistries are employed, including alcohol wipes and high-quality water (such as water for injection [see section 5.2]).

The choice of physical and chemical cleaning processes depends on the types and levels of

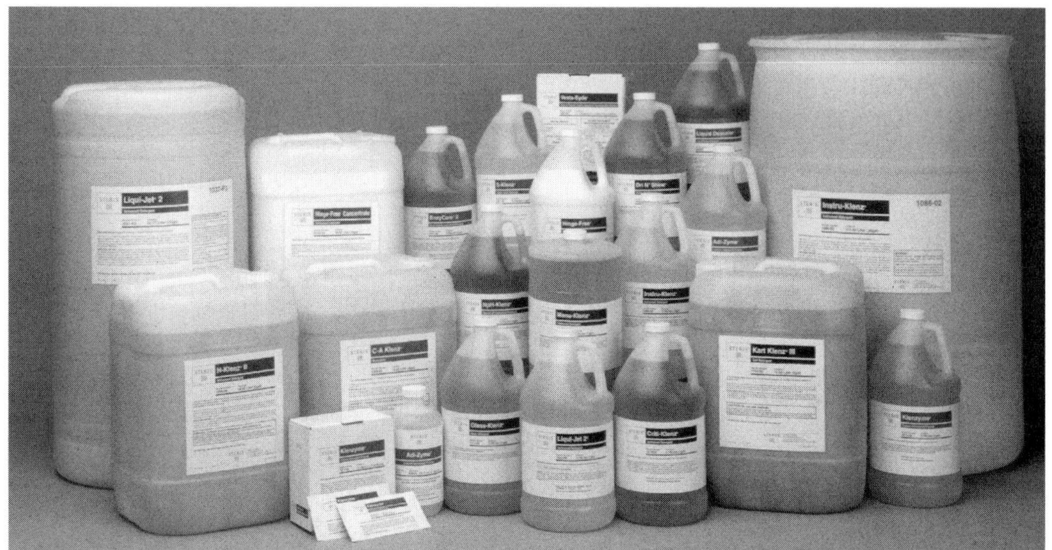

FIGURE 1.28 Various types of cleaning chemical formulations.

soils that are present on a surface. The overall efficacy and efficiency of these processes can be optimized for a given application by consideration of the cleaning contact time, chemical concentration, temperature, and efficiencies of physical effects.

1.4.9 Water Quality

Water is an important component of many antiseptic, disinfectant, and sterilization applications. Typical uses of water include:

- Biocidal-product formulation (as a solvent)

TABLE 1.28 Various components of cleaning formulations

Ingredient	Purpose
Solvent, including water	A solvent is a substance (usually liquid) that is capable of dissolving other substances, water being the most common. Solvents are also used for solubilization of various soil components.
Emulsifiers, surfactants	Emulsifiers are ingredients (including surfactants) that allow the formation of stable mixtures (emulsions) of water- and oil-soluble ingredients. Surfactants ("surface-acting agents") can be used as emulsifiers, but also to reduce surface tension, improve the wettability of a surface, disperse contaminants, and inhibit foam formation.
Chelating agents or sequestrants	Binding metals (like calcium and magnesium) and inhibiting their precipitation; water softening and prevention of mineral deposition
Enzymes	Digestion of soil components, including proteases (protein digestion), lipases (lipid/oil digestion), and amylases (carbohydrate, e.g., starch, digestion)
Alkali	pH stabilization; alkalis are used as "builders" to optimize the activities of surfactants, including emulsification of soils and degradation of proteins.
Acid	pH stabilization; acids are also used to prevent and remove mineral deposits and for water softening.
Dispersants	Suspending solids
Corrosion inhibitors	Reducing the corrosion rates and protecting the surfacs of metals
Others	Aesthetic qualities, like perfumes and colors, and biocides as preservatives

- Biocidal-product dilution on use (e.g., antiseptics and disinfectants)
- Cleaning alone or in combination with cleaning formulations prior to disinfection or sterilization
- Pharmaceutical-product preparation (e.g., dilution for injection)
- Rinsing to remove residuals following cleaning or disinfection
- As a disinfectant (moist heat) or sterilization agent (steam)
- Humidification as part of sterilization processes (e.g., with ethylene oxide or formaldehyde)
- Steam sterilization

In addition to these applications, water itself is a source of microbial contamination (e.g., enteric protozoa, such as *Cryptosporidium* and *Giardia*; bacterial pathogens, such as *E. coli*, *Legionella*, and *Vibrio*; and toxins, such as endotoxins), requiring the use of various biocidal products and processes to render it safe for its intended use. The most important of these are the use of halogens (like chlorine and bromine [see section 3.11]), oxidizing agents (like chlorine dioxide and ozone [see section 3.13]), moist heat (boiling and steam distillation [see sections 2.2 and 5.2]), irradiation (such as UV treatment [see section 2.4]), and filtration (see section 2.5).

Water can include various dissolved and suspended contaminants, many of which have negative effects on antiseptic, disinfectant, and sterilization applications (Table 1.29).

Overall, the qualities of water used for particular applications vary, including the following:

- Potable water (water that is considered safe for human consumption, which in many countries is tap water)
- Pretreated water (e.g., "softened" to remove hardness due to calcium or magnesium ions)
- Disinfected (e.g., by UV radiation [see section 2.4])
- Filtered to remove gross particulates or pretreated to remove contaminants (e.g., with activated carbon or sodium bisulfite to remove chlorine)
- Sterile filtered (to physically remove microorganisms [see section 2.5])
- Purified (e.g., by reverse osmosis, deionization, and distillation [see sections 2.5 and 5.2])

TABLE 1.29 Examples of common water contaminants and their effects

Contaminant	Examples	Concerns
Inorganic salts	Hardness (dissolved compounds of calcium and magnesium)	Inhibits activities of cleaners and biocidal products; can also cause the buildup of scaling over time or "spotting" on a surface
	Heavy metals (metallic elements with high atomic weights, e.g., iron, chromium, copper, and lead)	Can inhibit the activities of cleaners and biocidal products; cause damage to some surfaces (e.g., corrosion); in some cases, toxic and bioaccumulative
Organic matter	Trihalomethanes	Toxic chlorine disinfection byproducts
	Proteins, lipids, polysaccharides	Can leave harmful residues, including protein toxins and endotoxins (lipopolysaccharide [see section 1.3.7]); can also reduce the effectiveness of biocides
Biocides	Chlorine, bromine	Can cause corrosion and rusting on surfaces (in particular, when carried in steam)
Microorganisms	*Pseudomonas*, *Salmonella*, and oocysts of *Cryptosporidium*	Biofilm formation and biofouling; deposition onto surfaces or products and cross-contamination
Dissolved gases	CO_2, Cl_2, and O_2	Can cause corrosion and rusting (in particular, when carried in steam); noncondensable gases, like CO_2 and O_2, can inhibit the penetration of steam in sterilization processes.

In some applications, the quality of water required will be specified, including microbiological and chemical limits that should be considered to ensure the safety and effectiveness of biocidal products and processes.

FURTHER READING

American National Standards Institute. 2006. *Sterilization of Health Care Products—Vocabulary.* ISO/TS 11139:2006. American National Standards Institute, Washington, D.C.

American National Standards Institute. 2000. *Sterilization of Health Care Products—General Requirements for Characterization of a Sterilizing Agent and the Development, Validation and Routine Control of a Sterilization Process for Medical Devices.* ISO 14937:2000. American National Standards Institute, Washington, D.C.

Ascenzi, J. M. 1996. *Handbook of Disinfectants and Antiseptics.* Marcel Dekker, New York, N.Y.

Block, S. S. 2001. *Disinfection, Sterilization, and Preservation*, 5th ed. Lippincott Williams & Wilkins, Philadelphia, Pa.

Collier, L., and J. Oxford. 2000. *Human Virology*, 2nd ed. Oxford University Press, New York, N.Y.

Flick, E. W. 1999. *Advanced Cleaning Product Formulations*, vol. 5. Noyes Publications, Norwich, N.Y.

Fraise, A. P., P. A. Lambert, and J.-Y. Maillard. 2004. *Russell, Hugo and Ayliffe's Principles and Practice of Disinfection, Preservation and Sterilization,* 4th ed. Blackwell Publishing, Malden, Mass.

Greenwood, D., R. Slack, and J. Peutherer. 2002. *Medical Microbiology, a Guide to Microbial Infections: Pathogenesis, Immunity, Laboratory Diagnosis and Control.* Churchill Livingstone, New York, N.Y.

Holt, J. G., N. R. Krieg, P. H. A. Sneath, J. T. Staley, and S. T. Williams (ed.). 1994. *Bergey's Manual of Determinative Bacteriology*, 9th ed. Williams & Wilkins, Baltimore, Md.

Hurst, C. J., R. L. Crawford, J. L. Garland, D. A. Lipson, A. L. Mills, and L. D. Stetzenbach (ed.). 2007. *Manual of Environmental Microbiology*, 3rd ed. ASM Press, Washington, D.C.

International Society for Pharmaceutical Engineering. 2001. *Baseline Guide*, vol. 4. *Water and Steam Systems.* International Society for Pharmaceutical Engineering, Tampa, Fla.

Kanegsberg, B., and E. Kanegsberg. 2001. *Handbook for Critical Cleaning: Aqueous, Solvent, Advanced Processes, Surface Preparation, and Contamination Control.* CRC Press, Boca Raton, Fla.

Kohn, W. G., A. S. Collins, J. L. Cleveland, J. A. Harte, K. J. Eklund, and D. M. Malvitz. 2003. Guidelines for infection control in dental health-care settings. *Morb. Mortal. Wkly. Rep.* **52**(RR-17): 1–61.

LeBlanc, D. A. 2000. *Validated Cleaning Technologies for Pharmaceutical Manufacturing.* Interpharm Press, Denver, Colo.

Madigan, M. T., J. M. Martinko, and J. Parker. 2003. *Brock Biology of Microorganisms*, 10th ed. Pearson Education, Upper Saddle River, N.J.

Montville, T. J., and K. R. Matthews. 2005. *Food Microbiology: an Introduction.* ASM Press, Washington, D.C.

Murray, P. R., E. J. Baron, M. A. Pfaller, F. C. Tenover, and R. H. Yolken (ed.). 2003. *Manual of Clinical Microbiology*, 8th ed. ASM Press, Washington, D.C.

Prusiner, S. B. 2004. *Prion Biology and Diseases*, 2nd ed. Cold Spring Harbor Laboratory Press, Woodbury, N.Y.

Russell, A. D., W. B. Hugo, and G. A. J. Ayliffe. 1992. *Principles and Practice of Disinfection, Preservation and Sterilization*, 2nd ed. Blackwell Science, Cambridge, Mass.

Sehulster, L., and R. Y. W. Chinn. 2003. Guidelines for environmental infection control in health-care facilities. *Morb. Mortal. Wkly. Rep.* **52**(RR-10):1–42.

van Doorne, H. 2004. *A Basic Primer on Pharmaceutical Microbiology.* PDA, Bethesda, Md.

Von Rheinbaben, F., and M. H. Wolff. 2002. *Handbuch der viruswirksamen Desinfektionen.* Springer-Verlag, New York, N.Y.

PHYSICAL DISINFECTION

2

2.1 INTRODUCTION

Disinfection is the antimicrobial reduction of the number of viable microorganisms on or in a product or surface to a level previously specified as appropriate for its intended further handling or use. This chapter considers the most widely used methods of physical disinfection, including heat (moist- and dry-heat methods), cold, radiation, and filtration. Filtration methods are not considered truly "biocidal," as the basic principle of action is the physical removal of microbial contamination from liquids and gases (including air) rather than its inactivation; despite this, some consideration is given to filtration as a method of physical disinfection or sterilization. Physical biocidal methods include high and low temperatures; heat-based processes are among the most efficient and convenient techniques of disinfection, including specific and widely utilized processes, like pasteurization for the treatment of solid and liquid foods. Nonionizing-radiation methods, including low-energy UV light, are also considered disinfectants; ionizing radiation technologies are further considered in chapter 5, since they are primarily used as sterilization methods.

2.2 HEAT

Types. Physical methods using heat are among the most widely used and reliable techniques for disinfection and sterilization. Heat is a form of energy that can be transferred from one system to another due to a difference in their temperatures. Heat can be transferred by conduction (energy transfer from a surface), by convection (transfer by liquid or gas), or by radiation (energy transfer in the form of electromagnetic waves or particles). Here, we are primarily concerned with heat convection and conduction, with further consideration of radiation (for disinfection) in section 2.4.

Heat-based methods can be separated into two basic types:

1. Wet (moist) heat
   - **a.** Heating of liquids, including pasteurization and boiling (disinfection)
   - **b.** Steam under atmospheric pressure (disinfection)
   - **c.** Steam under subatmospheric pressure, or "low-temperature" steam (disinfection)
   - **d.** Steam (or water) under pressure (sterilization)

2. Dry heat
   a. Incineration (sterilization)
   b. Hot air (disinfection and sterilization)

Wet and dry sterilization techniques are discussed in chapter 5; disinfection is considered further here. Wet heat is the most effective method, as it uses water in a liquid or gaseous (steam) form, which has a higher capacity to carry and transfer heat to a surface than dry air. Dry heat is rarely used as a true disinfection process but has been useful for some applications at <140°C; higher temperatures are defined as sterilization processes (see section 5.3). Moist-heat disinfection methods include immersion in hot water, the direct use of steam, and heating of a liquid or suspension (e.g., pasteurization).

Heat is essentially lethal to all microorganisms, but each will have its own intrinsic tolerance. For example, many common bacterial pathogens (including *Staphylococcus* and *Streptococcus*) are inactivated at moist-heat temperatures of 55 to 60°C, while some spore-producing bacteria are unaffected even at 100°C. The mechanisms behind these resistance profiles are discussed in more detail in section 8.1. Furthermore, lethality will be affected by the initial microbial population, temperature distribution, contact time, and materials surrounding the microorganisms (including organic [e.g., protein] and inorganic [e.g., salts] soils).

At the minimum temperature at which a microorganism is sensitive to thermal inactivation by heat, the rate of microbial lethality is generally considered to be logarithmic and can be plotted as a time-log reduction relationship (Fig. 2.1).

From such a plot, the decimal reduction time, or D value, can be calculated, defined as

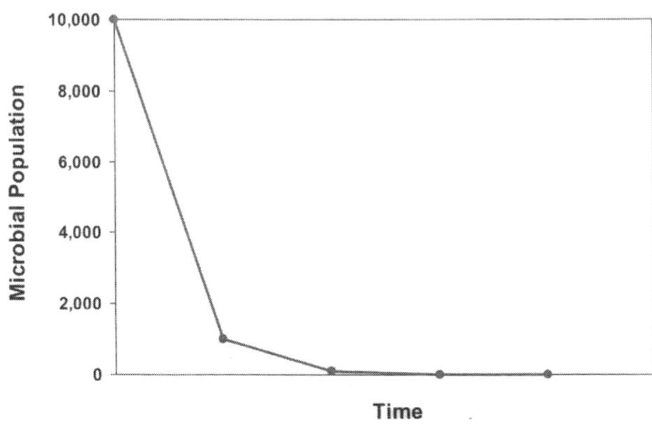

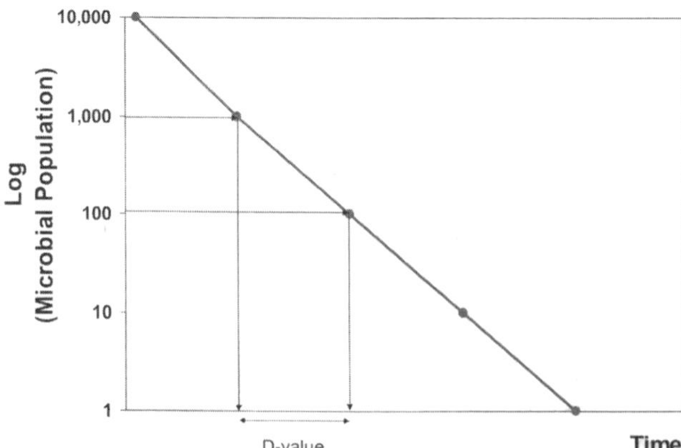

FIGURE 2.1 Typical microbial sensitivities to moist-heat disinfection.

the time (in minutes or seconds) at a given temperature required to kill 1 log unit (or 90%) of a given microbial population under stated test conditions. From the graph, the average D value can also be determined as the negative reciprocal of the slope of the plotted relationship (–1/slope). With the knowledge of the initial population of the target organism, the thermal-death time can be determined as the time required to achieve a population of zero (no remaining viable organisms) at the test temperature for a given application. It is expected that as the temperature increases, so does the lethal effect on the test microorganism, thereby reducing the D value and the thermal-death time. Therefore, a further relationship that can be determined is the effects of various temperatures on the D value (Fig. 2.2). This relationship is also considered logarithmic, and from it can be calculated the Z value, which is defined as the temperature change required to give a change in the D value by a factor of 10. Therefore, the D value is expressed as a time and the Z value as a temperature.

The D and Z values are the bases for determining the heat sensitivities of microorganisms. For heat-based disinfection processes, it is typical to choose a test organism with the highest resistance to heat and to determine the D and Z values for it. For example, *Mycobacterium tuberculosis* or *Coxiella burnetii* may be used in determining the values for pasteurization processes, *Enterococcus* or *Legionella* species for device disinfection, and *Geobacillus stearothermophilus* spores for sterilization processes. From these values, the disinfection time can be determined, depending on the desired (or tolerated) temperature and the required level of microbial log reduction. As the chosen test organism demonstrates greater resistance than other

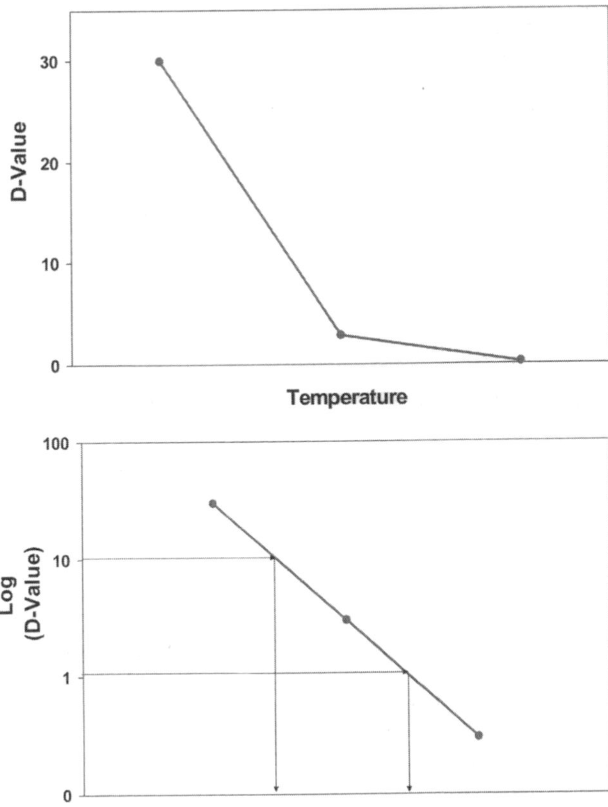

FIGURE 2.2 Effect of temperature on microbial lethality and Z-value determination.

organisms that would typically be present, it is expected that the disinfection process will be efficient for the intended application.

As water is heated to 100°C at atmospheric pressure, steam is formed. Steam is also used as a direct disinfecting agent or as a source of heat for other methods. The temperature at which steam is formed is dependent on the pressure. For example, when the pressure is reduced (by creating a vacuum or under "subatmospheric" conditions), the temperature at which steam is formed is lowered; equally, as the pressure is increased, the temperature of steam rises. These processes require special chambers to achieve the necessary pressure levels, with steam under pressure as the basis of steam sterilization, which is discussed in more detail in section 5.2.

Applications. Moist-heat-based disinfection can be routinely obtained by heating to temperatures greater than 60 to 65°C, at which most bacteria, viruses, fungi, and other pathogens or unwanted microbial contaminants are inactivated (see Fig. 2.4), with the exception of some bacterial spores. Simple applications include the boiling of drinking water or immersion of surgical instruments or other materials into heated water for the required disinfection time. The boiling of instruments in water for ≥5 min is a useful process for rapid disinfection, in particular in emergency situations. Hot water is the method of choice for routine disinfection of heat-resistant materials. Applications include automated washer-disinfector machines (for reusable surgical devices, bedpans, and other materials) (section 1.4.8) and laundry disinfection. In general, the disinfection time will depend on the temperature. Recommended examples of overkill moist-heat disinfection times for medical or veterinary surgical devices include the following:

100 min at 70°C
10 min at 80°C
1 min at 90°C
0.1 min at 100°C

Pasteurization is considered a mild disinfection process and is generally applied to foods or other liquids to reduce the risk of the presence of pathogens and to improve the shelf life of the product by reducing the presence of food spoilage organisms. It is widely used for the treatment of milk and milk products, beer, juices, and vaccines and as an alternative to boiling for device disinfection in water (Fig. 2.3).

Typical pasteurization processes are developed at a temperature and for a time that will not destroy the product but will provide a level of disinfection acceptable for the subsequent use of the product (e.g., human consumption). Examples are traditional processes at 63 to 66°C for ≥30 min and "flash" pasteurization processes at 71 to 72°C for ≥15 to 16 s. Pasteurization can be performed as a batch or continuous-duty process. Following heat treatment, the product shelf life can be further extended by storing the product at a low temperature (<10°C), which inhibits the growth of spoilage organisms. An alternative to pasteurization for food products is ultra-high-temperature processing. The product is treated at a temperature of ≥100°C (e.g., 140°C for 4 s) and then aseptically placed into presterilized storage containers. Ultra-high-temperature processes are generally performed as continuous-duty processes by the direct injection of steam under pressure (convection) or indirectly via heated surfaces (conduction).

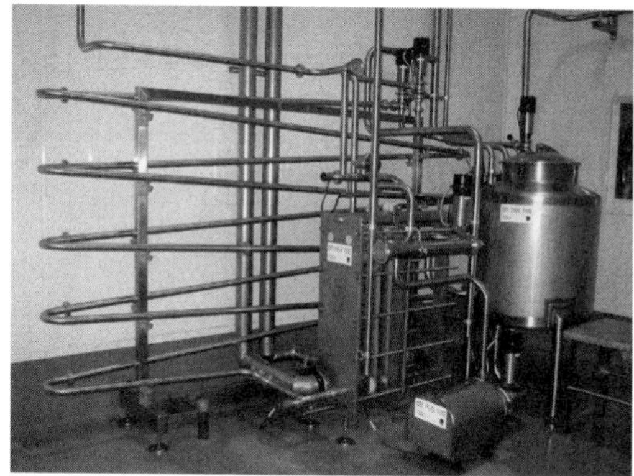

FIGURE 2.3 A pasteurizer for heat treatment of liquids. Courtesy of System Products Ltd.

Steam may be used directly for rapid disinfection of general surfaces (e.g., steam cleaning). Low-temperature steam (or steam under vacuum) can be used for the disinfection of fabrics and temperature-sensitive instruments, generally at 70 to 95°C. It is also used as a rapid humidification process prior to exposure to chemical sterilants and fumigants, including ethylene oxide, formaldehyde, chlorine dioxide, and ozone (see chapters 3 and 6). A specific method known as tyndallization is used for disinfection of liquids, in particular temperature-sensitive liquids that contain proteins or carbohydrates. This process involves repeated cycles of heating (by conduction or direct injection of steam) and cooling over 3 days to allow initial disinfection of vegetative organisms, germination of any spore-forming bacteria or fungi, and subsequent redisinfection.

Dry heat is rarely used as a true disinfection process but can be useful for the treatment of resistant materials, including glassware and metal materials, at temperatures of <140°C. While dry heat has some direct antimicrobial effect, it also causes drying of (or the removal of moisture from) microorganisms, which is biostatic and even biocidal to many bacteria and viruses. Drying is a useful method of preserving the sterility or disinfected state of surfaces and reducing the risk of subsequent microbial growth.

Finally, heat plays an essential role in the overall efficacy of cleaning and biocidal disinfection processes. Most cleaning processes are more effective at temperatures of >30 but <60°C, at which point proteins can coagulate and become difficult to remove from contaminated surfaces. An example is the use of enzyme-based cleaners, which are typically more active in the 40 to 60°C range (see section 1.4.8). The role of humidification has already been described as being required for the antimicrobial activities of many chemical biocides. It is also used in combination with other biocides to enhance their activities; in general, as the temperature increases, the antimicrobial effect will also increase, although in some cases, higher temperature may also cause greater biocide degradation. Examples of various standards and guidelines for heat disinfection are given in Table 2.1.

Spectrum of Activity. In general, as temperature increases, so does activity against microorganisms, with variable intrinsic and acquired mechanisms of resistance to heat (Fig. 2.4).

TABLE 2.1 Examples of various standards and guidelines for heat disinfection

Reference[a]	Title	Summary
FDA/CFSAN	*Grade "A" Pasteurized Milk Ordinance*	Regulations for the safety and sanitation of milk
FDA/CDRH	*Class II Special Controls Guidance Document: Medical Washers and Medical Washer-Disinfectors*	Guidance on the content and format for registration of washer-disinfectors, including disinfection testing
ISO 15883-1	*Washer-Disinfectors, Part 1: General Requirements, Definitions and Tests*	Requirements for washer-disinfectors, including heat disinfection testing and requirements
AS 4187	*Cleaning, Disinfecting and Sterilizing Reusable Medical and Surgical Instruments and Equipment, and Maintenance of Associated Environments in Health Care Facilities*	Guidelines for disinfection and sterilization practices in health care facilities
CFIS (2001)	*Recommendations for the Production and Distribution of Juice in Canada*	Recommendations for the heat treatment and pasteurization of juices

[a]FDA/CFSAN, Center for Food Safety and Applied Nutrition, U.S. Food and Drug Administration; FDA/CDRH, Center for Devices and Radiological Health, U.S. Food and Drug Administration; ISO, International Standards Organization; AS, Australian standard; CFIS, Canadian Food Inspection Agency.

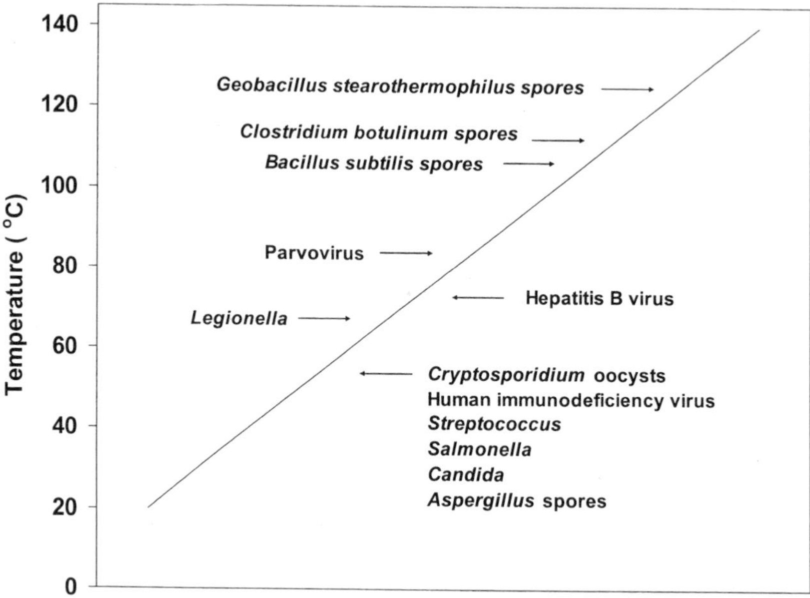

FIGURE 2.4 Moist-heat resistance of microorganisms.

Most pathogenic and spoilage microorganisms are readily inactivated at temperatures greater than 65°C. Some vegetative bacteria and viruses demonstrate unusual tolerance to heat; these microorganisms are known as thermophiles and may be defined as microorganisms that can live at or survive temperatures above 45 to 50°C (see sections 8.3.9 and 8.3.10). Some examples are *Legionella*, *Enterococcus*, *Coxiella*, and *Mycobacterium* species, as well as viruses like parvoviruses and noroviruses. In general, the thermophiles are readily inactivated at 70 to 90°C, although the overall tolerance to heat will be affected by the suspension media and growth conditions, as well as specific developmental responses in bacteria and fungi to heat treatment (e.g., the heat shock response [see section 8.3.3]). A dramatic developmental response is the production of spores, which consist of a central dormant cell surrounded by multiple protective layers that present a significant barrier to the effects of chemical and physical agents (the development, structure, and resistance of spores are discussed in greater detail in section 8.3.11). Fungi and many bacteria produce spores, but bacterial spores, including those of *Bacillus*, *Geobacillus*, and *Clostridium*, are considered the most resistant to heat, requiring temperatures in excess of 100°C for processes to be effective. A further group of thermophiles (known as extreme thermophiles, or "hyperthermophiles"), which are capable of growing and surviving at temperatures of >80 to 90°C, have also been described (see section 8.3.10). These include archaeal species, like *Thermocrinis ruber*, *Thermotoga maritima*, and *Thermus aquaticus*, which have been isolated from hot springs and deep-sea vents. Some species have been described as growing at temperatures up to 160°C, and they owe their resistance to unique protective mechanisms, including protein design, DNA repair and protection functions, and unique cell wall/cell membrane structures. These organisms are not considered to be feasible pathogens or contaminants and are not considered a concern for routine disinfection and sterilization processes.

Although many bacterial and fungal toxins are readily inactivated by heat, bacterial endotoxins are resistant to moist and dry heat, with high dry-sterilization temperatures required for effective destruction. Prions have also shown dramatic resistance to heat-based processes, although these results may be due to protective effects (like fixed protein and lipids) preventing heat penetration. In particular, prions are highly resistant to dry heat, but their infectivity has been shown to be dramatically reduced by boiling in water. Hydration appears to play an important role in the activities of heat-based processes against prions.

Advantages. Heat disinfection methods (in particular moist heat) are easy to use, flexible for various applications, readily available, and cost-effective. They are the methods most widely accepted as being reliable and broad spectrum and are well described. With *D* and *Z* value determinations, heat-based methods can be predictive and allow simple verification of efficiency by temperature monitoring. Pasteurization methods reduce the risk of contamination of foodstuffs by pathogens and extend the shelf lives of products. Moist heat is an effective method for the humidification and heating of materials for subsequent sterilization by heat and/or chemicals, while dry heat is effective for drying surfaces after disinfection and sterilization. Finally, heat is a synergistic agent for many chemical biocidal processes.

Disadvantages. Care should be taken in the use of heating methods or handling of treated materials and surfaces due to the risk of burning. Surfaces and liquids should be allowed to cool down before use. In the case of surgical devices that have been boiled, they should be used immediately following cool down and should not be stored prior to use. Heating can cause damage to liquids (especially if they contain biological materials, like proteins, that need to be preserved) and surfaces, such as many temperature-sensitive polymers. Damage can also occur to temperature-resistant materials by stress cracking, warping, and corrosion. Pasteurization can change the taste of foodstuffs, but this can generally be controlled by process optimization. Dry-heat disinfection can be used only for inanimate surfaces, like metals and glass.

It is necessary to ensure that all surfaces are exposed to the minimum disinfection temperature for the required disinfection time. Similarly, the temperature distribution in a liquid needs to be uniform, as cold spots can occur, and they may not be adequately disinfected. The quality of the water may affect the efficacy and safety of moist-heating processes (see section 1.4.9). Heat disinfection can cause the release of endotoxins, which are resistant to disinfection temperatures, from some gram-negative bacteria; endotoxins can cause pyrogenic reactions (i.e., fever) if introduced directly into the bloodstream (see section 1.3.7). The efficacy of heat can be reduced in the presence of organic and inorganic soils, in particular, dried salts, due to lack of heat penetration to the target microbial population.

Mode of Action. Heat clearly has multiple effects on the viability of microorganisms. High temperatures can initially cause the denaturation of structural and functional proteins, unwinding of nucleic acids, and destabilization of surface structures, including cell walls, cell membranes, and viral envelopes. These effects alone cause the release of cytoplasmic materials and can accumulate and lead to cell death or loss of viral infectivity. As the temperature increases further, proteins and other biomolecules will precipitate, leading to further loss of structure and/or function and cell lysis. Higher temperatures are required to penetrate the multiple protective layers of bacterial spores and have an effect on the more sensitive inner core. Heat treatment leads to the release of dipicolinic acid and calcium from spores; dipicolinic acid and calcium are considered to play roles in protecting proteins in the inner core from heat damage and are examples of the multiple resistance mechanisms that protect spores from the effects of heat (they are discussed further in section 8.3.11).

2.3 COLD TEMPERATURES

Cold temperatures—cooling to temperatures of <10°C and freezing at <0°C—have biostatic and some biocidal effects. At a minimum, cold conditions can prevent or reduce the growth of microorganisms due to the need for specific temperatures for the activities of cellular enzymes. They are generally considered effective preservative methods and are widely used (e.g., refrigeration and freezing for the storage of microbial cultures). However, some bacteria, including *Listeria*, and fungi can multiply at refrigeration temperatures (4 to 10°C); these microorganisms are known as psychrophiles. In most cases, microorganisms will remain viable under these conditions and will grow when the necessary temperatures and growth conditions are restored.

Freezing as a microbial-preservation method includes storage at −10 to −80°C, usually in the presence of a stabilizer, like glycerol and dimethyl sulfoxide, or freeze-drying, a process of removing water from a frozen product directly into a gas by a process known as sublimation. Immersion in liquid nitrogen (at −196°C) is also used as a rapid freezing process. Freeze-thaw cycles can cause inactivation of proteins and cell wall/membrane structure damage or lysis (due to ice crystal formation), leading to death of the microbes.

2.4 RADIATION

Radiation is energy in motion and refers to a natural process in which unstable atoms of an element emit (or "radiate") excess energy in the form of particles or electromagnetic waves. For the purpose of this discussion, radiation sources will be considered to be isotopes (naturally occurring or manufactured unstable atoms) or other sources of electromagnetic radiation. Electromagnetic radiation is energy transmitted in the form of waves or rays, including X rays and UV and infrared (IR) radiation, which are considered to be within the electromagnetic spectrum.

Isotopes. In its simplest form, an atom is a unit of matter that is indivisible by chemical means. It is made up of a nucleus, consisting of positively charged protons and neutral neutrons, surrounded by negatively charged electrons contained within defined orbits, or energy levels, around the central nucleus (Fig. 2.5).

There are at least 112 known elements (as listed in the periodic table of elements), including the building blocks of biological materials, like carbon, hydrogen, and oxygen, which have an overall neutral charge, as in each atom the number of protons equals the number of electrons. When there is an overall positive or negative charge, the atom is known as an isotope (e.g., ^{35}S, ^{32}P, and ^{60}Co). Isotopes are unstable and spontaneously decay, causing the release of radiation (Fig. 2.5) from an atom in the form of streaming particles (α or β radiation) or electromagnetic waves (for example, γ radiation). These energy particles or waves have lethal effects on microorganisms, but their energies and penetration vary. α particles consist of two protons and two neutrons (essentially the helium nucleus, ^{4}He) and have a +2 charge. α radiation, although reactive, is not considered further here as a disinfection method, since it is not highly penetrating; for example, α radiation does not pass through paper or skin. β particles, when accelerated, and γ radiation are widely used for industrial processes, including sterilization, deinfestation, food preservation, and

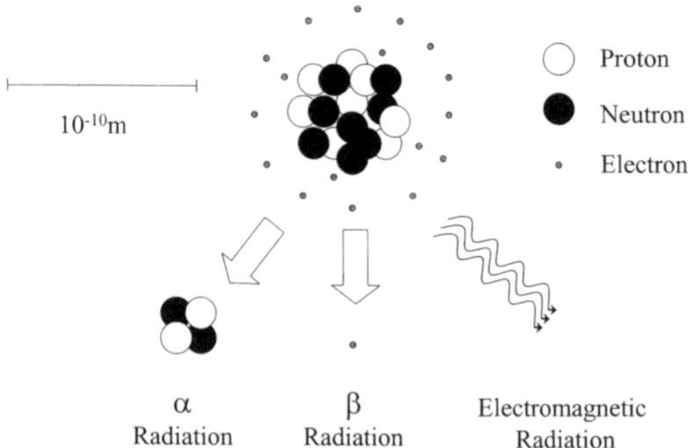

FIGURE 2.5 Atomic structure and the source of radiation.

decontamination of medical devices and materials (e.g., bandages), cosmetics, and foodstuffs. β particles are electrons (with a −1 charge), which demonstrate greater penetration than α particles but can still be blocked by soft metals, like aluminum. β-radiation-emitting isotopes (e.g., ^{32}P) are not generally used as direct sources for disinfection, but β particles can be more readily produced from an electron gun (e.g., a heated filament) and are then accelerated by passage through an electrical field to enhance their penetration capabilities. Radioisotopes, including ^{60}Co and ^{137}Cs, which release γ radiation at specific energies, are direct sources of γ radiation. γ radiation is a high-energy form of electromagnetic radiation and is used for disinfection, sterilization, and deinfestation. Both β- (accelerated) and γ-radiation methods are considered in more detail in section 5.4 as sterilization processes, while other sources of electromagnetic radiation are considered here.

Electromagnetic Radiation. Electromagnetic radiation is by definition light waves or, more specifically, fluctuations of electric and magnetic fields in space. The basic unit, or particle, of electromagnetic radiation is the photon, which (unlike particle radiation) has no mass or electric charge and travels at the speed of light in a wavelike pattern. There are many types of photons, ranging from radio waves to γ waves, which differ and are classified by their respective energies and wavelengths (Fig. 2.6). A wavelength can be defined as the length in meters of a single wave of photon energy, or the distance between the two adjacent wave peaks. As the wavelength (given as λ) becomes shorter, the frequency (the number of waves that pass a given point in a given time, recorded in hertz) increases. For example, radio waves have very long wavelengths, low frequencies, and low energy, in contrast to γ rays, which have very short wavelengths, high frequency, and high energy (Table 2.2).

As disinfection agents, higher-energy radiation is clearly more effective and penetrating. For disinfection purposes, the electromagnetic spectrum can be divided into ionizing and non-

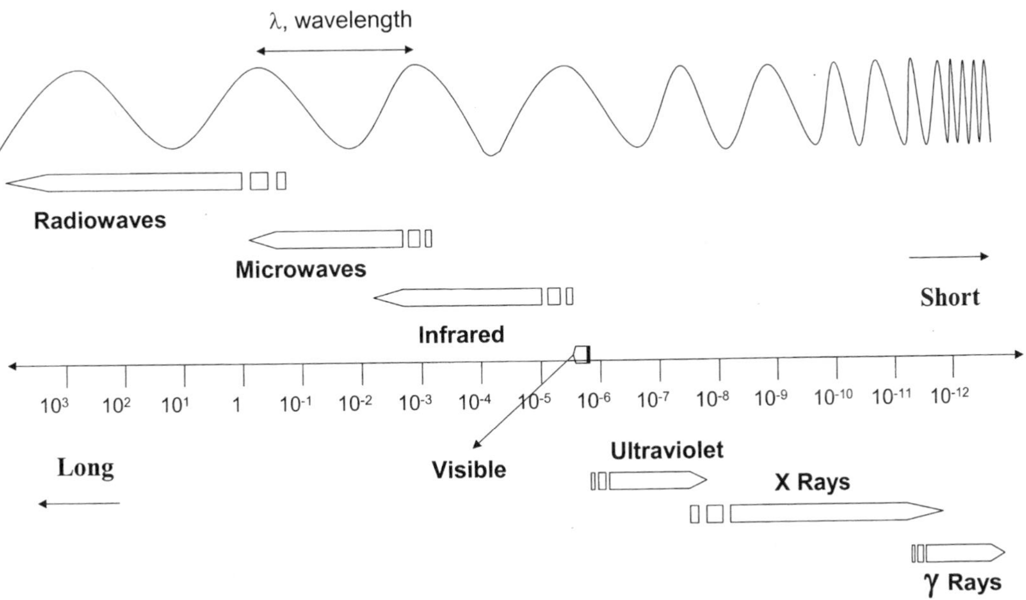

FIGURE 2.6 The electromagnetic spectrum. The range of wavelengths is shown on the axis in meters, with the longest wavelengths (radio waves) on the left and shortest (γ rays) on the right.

TABLE 2.2 Wavelengths and energies of types of electromagnetic radiation

Radiation	Wavelength (λ) (m)	Energy (J)
Nonionizing		
Radio waves	$>1 \times 10^{-1}$	$<2 \times 10^{-24}$
Microwaves	1×10^{-1}–1×10^{-3}	2×10^{-24}–2×10^{-22}
IR	1×10^{-3}–7×10^{-7}	2×10^{-22}–3×10^{-19}
Visible light	7×10^{-7}–4×10^{-7} (violet........blue)	3×10^{-19}–5×10^{-19}
UV	4×10^{-7}–1×10^{-8}	5×10^{-19}–2×10^{-17}
Ionizing		
X rays	1×10^{-8}–1×10^{-11}	2×10^{-17}–2×10^{-14}
γ rays	$<1 \times 10^{-11}$	$>2 \times 10^{-14}$

ionizing radiation. Ionizing radiation has enough energy to cause the release of electrons from the target atom, which therefore becomes charged. Both γ and X rays are ionizing radiation; they differ in that γ radiation causes electron release from the atom nucleus, while X rays cause release of the orbiting electrons. Nonionizing radiation causes the excitation of electrons and, in some cases, electron transitions from one orbit to another, which can lead to an increase in temperature, depending on the exposure time and energy. Types of nonionizing radiation used for disinfection include UV and IR radiation and microwaves. Visible light itself can be antimicrobial with excessive exposure, but it is not generally used as a disinfection method (with the exception of pulsed-light technology, discussed in section 5.6.2).

Types. Ionizing radiation (γ and X rays) is used for disinfection and deinfestation but is further considered in this book as a means of physical sterilization (see section 5.4). Nonionizing-radiation methods used for disinfection include UV and IR radiation and microwaves. Nonionizing radiation is emitted from atoms when electrons in an excited stage transition from a higher to a lower energy state to give off photons in their respective wavelength/energy ranges (Table 2.2).

UV. The main sources of UV radiation are simple UV lights, including mercury vapor lamps, fluorescent lights, pulsed UV lamps, and "black-light" lamps. A typical mercury vapor lamp is shown in Fig. 2.7. Lamps can vary in diameter and length, for example, 15 to 25 mm and 100 to 1,200 mm, respectively. A typical lamp consists of a sealed tube of a UV-transmitting material (e.g., quartz) with an electrode on each end and contains a small amount of mercury and an inert gas (typically argon) under pressure. UV light is produced by applying electricity (voltage) to the lamp to cause an electric arc and the subsequent excitation of the electrons in the available mercury vapor. When these excited electrons return to their ground state, they release photons within the UV wavelength range (~350 to 100 nm). The inert (argon) gas has only secondary functions, including extending lamp life and reducing thermal loss (note that heat is another form of energy and reduces the light output).

A variety of UV lamps are available, including the following:

- Low-pressure mercury lamps (Fig. 2.7) contain a small amount of mercury vapor maintained at very low internal lamp pressure (typically <0.001 kPa). Some designs include small amounts of other metals (such as gallium and indium), which can increase the UV output. These are probably the most widely used UV sources and

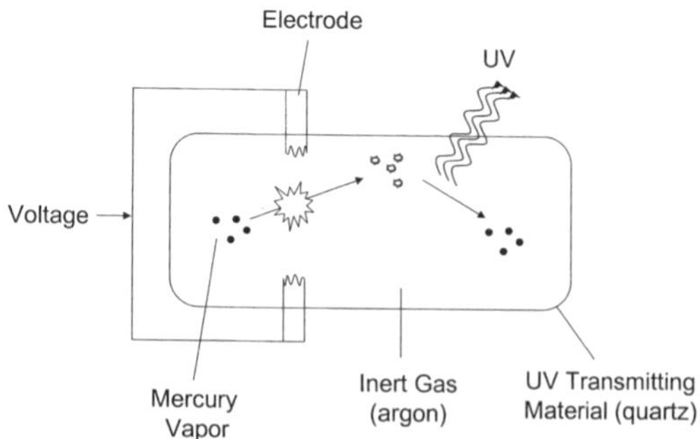

FIGURE 2.7 A representation of a typical UV (low-pressure UV mercury) lamp and the generation of UV radiation.

TABLE 2.3 Types of UV radiation

UV type	Common name	Wavelength range (nm)	Comments
UV-A	Long wave	315–400	Fluorescent light, black light
UV-B	Medium wave	280–315	Responsible for sunburn
UV-C	Short wave	200–280	Germicidal range

have a standard output of UV at 254 nm (primarily) and 185 nm. The energy output is considered low, but they are efficient and have a long effective life. Typical operating temperatures are 40 to 100°C.

- Medium-pressure mercury lamps are fundamentally the same design as low-pressure lamps but contain a larger amount of mercury maintained at or near atmospheric pressure and emit a wider range of wavelengths (200 to 400 nm). These lamps characteristically have a higher UV output but a shorter usable life.
- "Flash" lamps are usually operated above atmospheric pressure and also emit a wide range of wavelengths (170 to 400 nm). They include pulsed-light and eximer lamps. Pulsed-light lamps typically contain xenon gas and require a high voltage supply pulse (up to 30 times a second) to provide a high output of UV light. Similar eximer lamps use rare gas-halogen mixtures, including KrCl (which emits at 222 nm) and XeBr (which emits at 281 nm). Flash lamps have a shorter life, require greater power, and are less often used than low- and medium-pressure lamps.

Not all UV wavelengths are effective against microorganisms (Table 2.3). The most effective range is the UV-C, or "short" UV wavelengths, in the 200- to 280-nm range. The most effective wavelength has been found to be 265 nm.

IR. IR radiation spans the ~0.7- to 1,000-μm wavelength range and can be further subdivided into near, middle, and far IR (Table 2.4). The near (or short to medium)-IR range is the most widely used for heating and disinfection purposes. Even within this range, IR does not tend to cause electron transitions and is absorbed only by atoms with small energy differences in their orbiting electrons. Therefore, IR is used for surface treatments only and provides a source of heat directly on those surfaces, which can range from 50 to 1,000°C, depending on the wattage of the source lamp. Therefore, IR can be considered a method of dry-heat disinfection/sterilization (see section 5.3). IR (or "heat") lamps consist of single or multiple heated filaments, which use low energy and heat quickly to release radiation in the desired wavelength in the IR range. The lamp itself can be made of red or clear glass, but the IR light emitted is not visible to the human eye (as it is below the red wavelength range of the visible spectrum). In more complicated lamp sources, the released light can be reflected (for example, by aluminum and ceramics) to focus the light from the source, and due to the high heat output, the lamps may be cooled by air or water.

Microwaves. Microwaves are electromagnetic radiation within the wavelength range of ~1 mm to 1 m. Although microwaves may have direct, if negligible, antimicrobial activity, the primary action is due to the rapid transfer of heat, and microwaves can therefore also be considered a heat disinfection method (see section 2.2). Microwaves can be conveniently produced in widely available ovens at a typical frequency

TABLE 2.4 IR wavelength range

IR type	Wavelength range (μm)
Near	0.7–2.5
Middle	2.5–50
Far[a]	50–1,000

[a]Far IR is often further subdivided into far and far-far ranges.

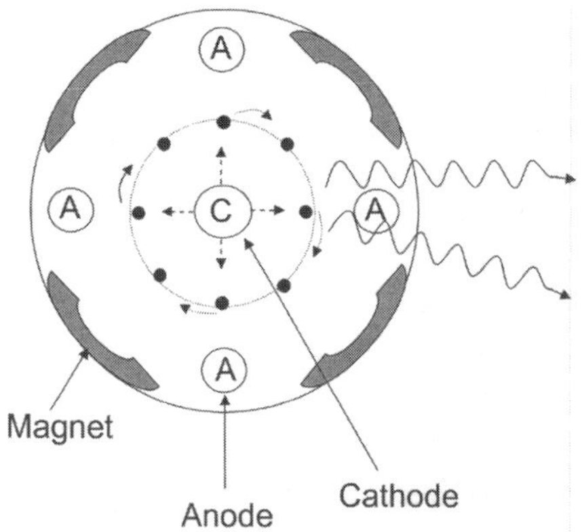

FIGURE 2.8 Simple structure of a magnetron used for the production of microwaves. Voltage applied to a central cathode causes the release of electrons (shown in black), which are forced to circulate by attraction to the anode and the effect of the surrounding magnetic field. Microwaves are released as the circulating electrons lose their energy.

of ~2,500 MHz. In these ovens, a standard electricity supply (or voltage) is transformed into a higher voltage (~3,000 V) and supplied to a magnetron tube, which generates microwaves that are released into the oven interior. The magnetron tube is a simple device consisting of a central cathode surrounded by anodes and contained within an electrical field (Fig. 2.8). When voltage is applied to the cathode, it heats up to release electrons, which, being negatively charged, attempt to travel to surrounding anodes but are prevented by an applied magnetic source. The electrons therefore travel in a circular path around the central cathode and release electromagnetic energy within the microwave wavelength range. Dry items can be placed in the oven for treatment, but the antimicrobial process is more effective in the presence of water. Within the oven, it is optimal for items to be circulated, usually on a rotating table, to ensure even heat distribution.

Applications

UV. UV light is used for a variety of germicidal applications, including liquid, air, and surface disinfection. Typical continuous or batch liquid applications involve the close passage of the liquid past a UV-emitting source for a controlled exposure time, determined by the flow and output of the UV source. These simple systems are normally encased in a protective metal enclosure to prevent direct human exposure (Fig. 2.9).

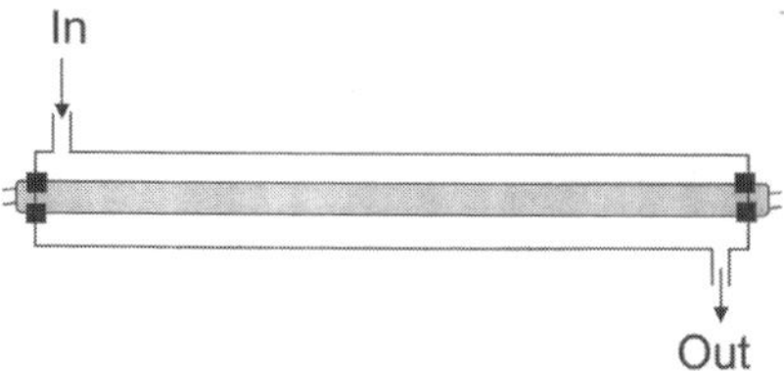

FIGURE 2.9 A simple continuous-duty UV disinfection system for liquids. The UV light is encased centrally in a chamber through which the liquid flows.

Liquids that can be routinely disinfected with UV light include water (drinking water and wastewater), emulsions, and liquid foods. UV treatment of water is particularly used in the treatment of drinking water in Europe at typical dosages ranging between 16 and 40 mJ/cm^2. The type of UV lamp used depends on the quality of the water and the flow rate required: higher-capacity lamps are required for higher flow rates and water of low quality. Multiple low-pressure lamps may also be used, depending on the application. In addition to antimicrobial effects, UV radiation can also be used for deodorization, dechlorination, deozonation, and organic-pollutant control. UV is also used for area decontamination, including isolators, laminar-flow cabinets, drying cabinets, chambers, rooms (including surgical suites and food-processing areas), and air conditioning/air handling systems. These systems are easy to apply and cost-effective. They can be as simple as installing UV lamps at various positions within a room or ductwork. It is particularly important that all areas be exposed to the UV light in large-area applications to ensure that the right UV dose is applied to all surfaces. This can be effectively monitored using a series of UV intensity sensors, which can monitor the exposure dose applied to a given surface or liquid or ensure that the UV intensity is sufficient at the source.

Other applications include the direct treatment of food and packaging materials and use in combination with other decontamination methods. Examples are air-handling control in combination with air filtration and hydrogen peroxide vapor (see section 3.13) and as an activator for surfaces coated with titanium dioxide (TiO_2) or zinc oxide (ZnO). When TiO_2 is activated with UV light, it produces active oxygen species, including hydroxyl radicals and superoxide ions, which are effective against microorganisms (in particular, bacteria and viruses) and also in the reduction of organic pollutants, like ethylene vapors (see section 3.17.2). Flash lamps have also been successfully employed for limited sterilization applications, including aseptic filling lines (blow-fill-seal aseptic applications) and simple medical devices. The use of pulsed light is further considered as a sterilization method in section 5.6.2.

IR. IR radiation is used for a variety of applications, including detection, monitoring, therapeutic applications, and data transmission. For decontamination, IR lamps can be used in large areas for heating and disinfection or in ovens for disinfection and sterilization applications. The heat absorbed by surfaces can then be transferred by convection or conduction. The efficacy of a given process depends on the temperature imparted to a surface and can range from disinfection at a temperature of <100°C and sterilization at temperatures typically in the 120 to 200°C range, although high-wattage lamps can provide much higher temperatures required by industrial applications. Typical applications have included the treatment of glass, ceramics, and other temperature-sensitive materials. Sterilization processes for glass syringes have been described in which the product was passed through an IR oven on conveyor belts for the required exposure time, although such processes are not widely used. Disinfection processes are used for a variety of surfaces, including inanimate objects and food. IR ovens are used as an alternative to the dry-heat oven described in sections 2.2 and 5.3. Due to the transfer of heat, IR irradiation can be an efficient method of drying or heating surfaces and/or areas.

Microwaves. Microwave radiation is routinely used as a household method for rapid and controlled heating of foods and liquids. The rapid application of heat is itself antimicrobial to the levels discussed in section 2.2. Microwave ovens may be used as a flash disinfection method for wet devices and laboratory utensils, although these applications have not been widely used or investigated. Systems are available for the treatment (disinfection) of medical waste as an alternative to incineration. In these processes, the waste is initially shredded, sprayed with water or steam to moisten it, and heated to ~95°C using microwaves. Other applications that have been described include low-level disinfection of contact lenses in water, antifungal treatment of paper, and as an alternative energy source for other antimicrobial processes (e.g., electrode-free UV lights can use microwaves for activation, with applications in water, air, and surface decontamination).

Spectrum of Activity

UV. UV radiation (at the optimal germicidal wavelengths within the UV-C range) is an effective broad-spectrum antimicrobial, with the level of activity dependent on the exposure time and the output of the UV source (Table 2.3). In both room and liquid applications, UV is an effective bactericide against pathogenic gram-positive and gram-negative bacteria at typical doses of >5 mJ/cm^2 (a measure of UV intensity as the energy per unit surface area). Higher-than-minimal doses are recommended, as many bacteria can reverse the damage caused by UV radiation to nucleic acids under bacteriostatic exposure conditions and subsequently reactivate to become viable; this intrinsic mode of resistance is discussed further in section 8.3.12.

Important bactericidal applications for UV radiation include the control of *Legionella*, which can be transmitted in water and in aerosols, and of *M. tuberculosis*, which can be transmitted by aerosols. Some bacteria, for example, *Deinococcus radiodurans*, have notable resistance to radiation, presumably due to multiple protective mechanisms, including efficient repair processes (see section 8.3.9); similar resistance mechanisms can decrease the sensitivity of other bacteria, including *Escherichia coli*, to UV radiation. Efficacy has also been reported against *Cryptosporidium* oocysts and *Giardia* cysts at 5 to 10 mJ/cm^2, which has led to the greater acceptance of UV radiation as a method of potable-water disinfection. Fungi and viruses, in particular nonenveloped viruses, demonstrate greater resistance, with higher dosage levels (>20 mJ/cm^2) required for effectiveness. Bacterial spores are also quite resistant to UV-C, but sporicidal effects are observed at longer exposure times and at greater energy outputs, as with fungi. *Bacillus pumilus* spores are often used to monitor the effectiveness of UV radiation treatments. There may be differences in the intrinsic resistances of microorganisms in water and when dried on surfaces; this may be related to the protection of target organisms in organic and/or inorganic soils, which can prevent the penetration of UV waves. These protective effects can be reduced by using medium-pressure and flash lamps, which have greater germicidal activity and demonstrate greater efficacy for higher flow rates in liquid applications.

IR. IR radiation is a source of heat for dry-heat disinfection and sterilization and therefore shows a typical profile for antimicrobial efficacy, depending on the temperature and time (as discussed in section 2.2). Under these conditions, dry heat is an effective bactericide, fungicide, and virucide, with higher temperatures and longer contact times required for sporicidal activity in sterilization processes.

Microwaves. As the mode of action of microwaves is thought to be primarily through the action of heat transfer, the spectrum of activity is dependent on the temperature achieved over time (as discussed in section 2.2). Therefore, efficacy has been described against bacteria, fungi, and viruses, with little or no activity against bacterial spores that demonstrate extreme heat resistance (e.g., *G. stearothermophilus* spores). Sporicidal activity can be achieved, as monitored by *Bacillus subtilis* subsp. *niger* spore activity (which is more sensitive to heat than *G. stearothermophilus*) in microwave-based waste disposal systems. Efficacy is significantly more efficient in the presence of water than on dry surfaces.

Advantages

UV. UV radiation is a broad-spectrum antimicrobial. Its use for the treatment of water, air, and surfaces is preferred over chemical methods due to the lack of chemical residuals or by-products, in particular as an alternative to chlorine (for water disinfection) and formaldehyde (for area fumigation). UV is easy to handle, and applications are usually compact and can be monitored to ensure that an effective dose is applied over time and the life of the UV lamp source. Safety switches that reduce the risk of exposure to UV radiation can be employed. In addition to antimicrobial activity, UV radiation can also be used for the removal of chlorine, ozone, and organic pollutants, especially with medium-pressure and flash lamps.

IR. IR lamps are convenient, cheap, and economical sources of heat. As heat sources, their antimicrobial effects have been well described. The efficacies of processes can be easily monitored by temperature profiling. In general, it is easy to control applications and to minimize risks of exposure.

Microwaves. Microwaves are cheap and easy to produce in conveniently available ovens. As a method of heat transfer, microwaves are rapid, with significantly less heat-up time than conventional dry ovens. They can also be used to enhance drying, and due to their specific reactions with water and other biological molecules, microwaves may cause less damage to metals, plastics, and other materials due to nonabsorption or reflection. Microwaves are a useful source of energy for other processes (including UV light production) and may be used synergistically with other chemical antimicrobials.

Disadvantages

UV. UV radiation can cause damage to the skin and eyes on direct exposure over time, depending on the wavelength, dosage time, and output. In general, these effects are delayed and not permanent, but UV radiation can cause skin burns and irreversible damage to eye tissue. Some damage to surfaces can be observed (including color bleaching and effects on plastics), which is primarily thought to be due to the localized production of ozone or reactive radicals, especially at maximum germicidal wavelengths. These effects appear to be more pronounced with long exposure times and lower-energy lamps. Efficacy is dramatically reduced in the presence of organic or inorganic soils, due to lack of contact with the target microorganisms. This is particularly important in the treatment of water, because of the presence of iron, hardness, and total dissolved solids, or in the presence of high contamination levels, where dead microorganisms can shield viable organisms from receiving an effective dose. Overall, UV radiation has low penetration and is also absorbed by glass, plastics, and metals, which limit applications to direct exposure to a surface or liquid. Effective dose outputs can also be reduced at high temperatures (in particular, low-pressure lamp applications, due to loss of heat energy instead of release of radiation energy) and, in air and surface applications, high relative humidity. UV radiation does not leave any residual activity, which increases the risk of downstream contamination following UV disinfection of water or air, as in the case of air-handling duct work. Resistance mechanisms (in bacteria and fungi) can allow the reactivation of microorganisms following UV treatment by repairing damage and permitting multiplication.

IR. IR radiation has limited penetration; only exposed surfaces are adequately treated, although heat can be subsequently transferred by convection or conduction. Care should be taken to ensure that all surfaces are exposed and not shielded from the light. Uneven heat distribution can cause damage to surfaces, so that only temperature-sensitive materials can be adequately disinfected. Furthermore, cold spots in a given load may not permit the required disinfection times and temperatures. High-temperature sources should be adequately controlled to limit any potential exposure, which can cause severe burns.

Microwaves. Microwaves can produce uneven temperature distribution, depending on the density and type of load or the material treated. Hot spots can be damaging to the treated material, while cold spots will not be adequately disinfected. The presence of moisture or other absorbing materials is essential to ensure sufficient heat distribution; therefore, dry materials may not be adequately disinfected. The rapid transfer of heat can also be difficult to control, and heat conduction to temperature-sensitive plastics and other materials can lead to damage. With the exception of some waste disposal processes, microwave applications have not been widely tested or validated. Care should be taken to minimize any exposure to microwave energy, due to the risk of internal-organ damage from localized heating.

Mode of Action

UV. The main targets for UV radiation, as with other sources of electromagnetic radiation, are nucleic acids, like DNA and RNA, especially at 280 nm. UV is specifically known to causes photochemical reactions, particularly with pyrimidine bases, to form covalent linkages between adjacent bases (cytosine and thymine dimers) in the DNA helical structure, as well as other structural damage due to absorption of energy and excitation of atomic structures (see section 7.3 for a discussion of the structure of DNA). This prevents the normal functions of DNA—transcription and replication—which prevents cell multiplication and viral infection. Higher doses of photons also cause protein damage (in particular, at 260 nm), leading to loss of structure and function and cell lysis.

IR. The mode of action of IR radiation is predominantly, if not totally, due to the transfer of heat to a surface or microorganism. The effects of heat (see section 2.2) culminate in cell death and loss of infectivity.

Microwaves. Little is known about the direct antimicrobial effects of microwaves, as application to surfaces causes heat transfer, which is thought to be primarily responsible for biocidal activity. Microwaves are an efficient method of heating. At typically used frequency ranges, microwaves are rapidly absorbed by water and other molecules, including fats and sugars, to cause heating and disruption of structure and function. In contrast, many materials, like plastics, glass, and ceramics, do not absorb the energy, and some metals cause deflection. For further discussion, refer to section 2.2.

2.5 FILTRATION

Types and Applications. Filtration is one of the oldest and most widely used physical methods for the removal of contaminants from liquids and gases (Fig. 2.10). Filtration methods are not true biocidal processes, as they are based on the physical removal of microorganisms rather than their inactivation; however, in some cases, biocides or biocidal processes have been integrated into filters, and they can be used for air quality control, disinfection, or sterilization applications. Filtration is therefore only briefly described here.

The liquid or gas can be passed through a variety of types of filter (or membrane), which retard the passage of contaminants based on the sizes of their molecules (Fig. 2.11).

A wide variety of filters are available, consisting of flat sheets (often pleated), hollow fibers,

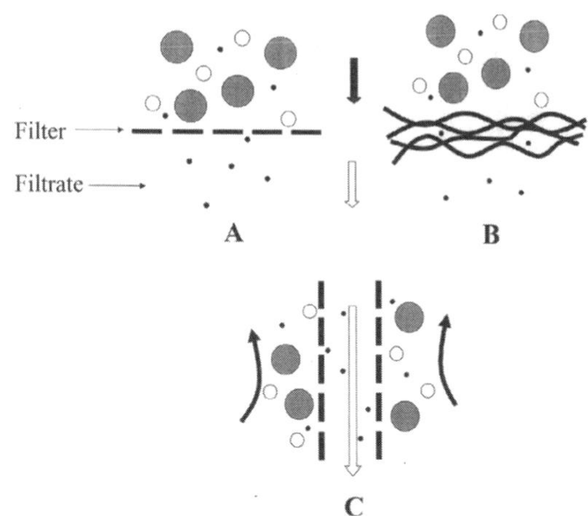

FIGURE 2.10 The theory of filtration. Various types of filtration processes are shown, with larger particles being retained by the filter and smaller particles allowed through the filter. Dead-end (A and B) and cross-flow (C) filters are shown. (A) Simple screen filter; (B) depth screen filter; (C) cross-flow filter.

or coated tubes in a range of media types. These include inorganic (e.g., glass, ceramics, and metals) and organic materials. Organic materials further encompass natural polymers (e.g., polysaccharides and polypeptides) and synthetic polymers, including plastics. Filter types can also be classified as screen or depth filters (Fig. 2.10). Simple screen filters prevent the passage of particles due to a given dead-end pore size, while depth filters prevent passage through a matrix. Because these filters can quickly become blocked, filter life can be extended by periodically (e.g., "back flowing," or reversing the flow across the filter) or constantly ("cross-flow" filtration) removing contaminants from the filter surface (Fig. 2.10).

Due to their flexibility and ease of use, filters are widely used for the decontamination of liquids, including water, and gases, including air (Table 2.5 and Fig. 2.12).

Liquid filtration is widely used for the pretreatment, disinfection, or sterilization of water. Pretreatment applications include reduction of the microbial load and generation of water for steam production. Critical applications include the production of water for injection and for

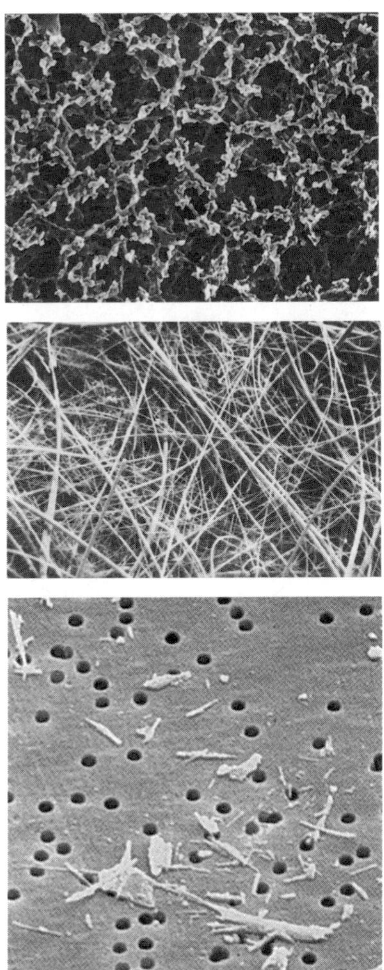

FIGURE 2.11 The microscopic structures of the surfaces of three filter materials. Reproduced with permission of Whatman International Ltd.

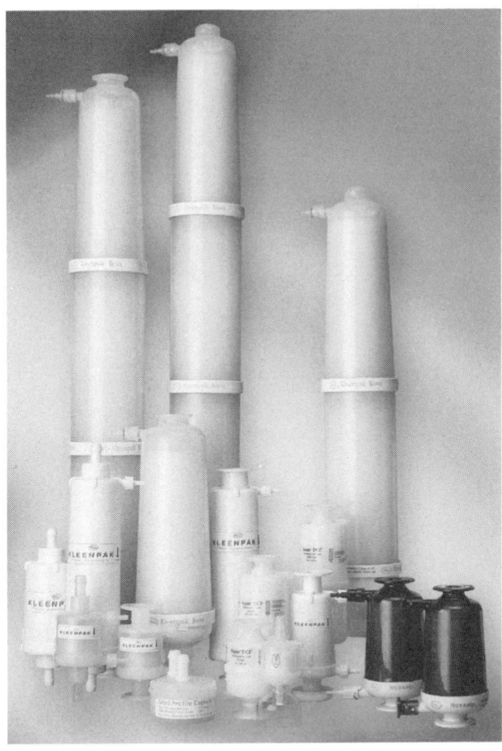

FIGURE 2.12 Examples of a variety of liquid filter types. Reproduced with permission from the Pall Corporation.

dialysis and sterile water for rinsing of manufacturing vessels or medical devices (e.g., following chemical disinfection). Similarly, many temperature-sensitive materials can be filtered to reduce the risk of contamination; examples are the sterile production of antibiotics, vaccines, and other pharmaceuticals or the concentration of (or removal of the water from) a product. Filters are also widely used to test liquids and air for the presence of contaminants for the purpose of quality control. Filtration is equally widely used for gas, especially air, decontamination. Air contamination control is

TABLE 2.5 Typical uses of filtration for liquid and gas applications

Liquid applications	Gas applications
Sanitization or disinfection of water or other liquid	Clean rooms, isolators, and work cabinets
Sterile-water production	Ventilators, operating theaters
Sterilization of temperature-sensitive products, e.g., antibiotics, tissue culture media, and vaccines	Odor control
Determination of contamination	Air sampling
Sample concentration	Medicinal-gas delivery

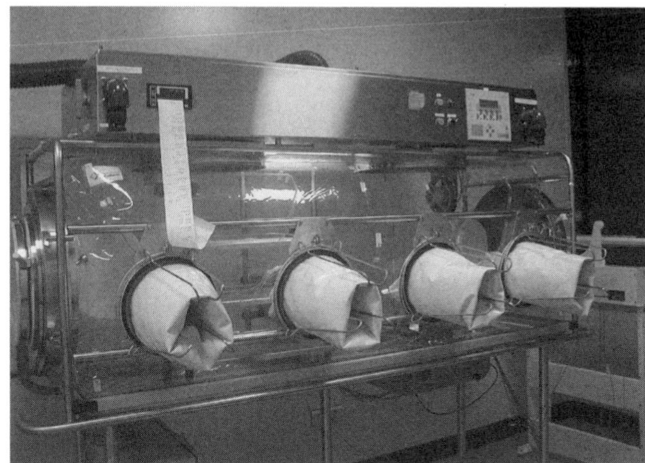

FIGURE 2.13 An example of a rigid-walled isolator system, with glove access ports on the front and transfer hatches on either side.

simply the reduction of the presence of pathogens or other contaminants in noncritical or critical areas. Many microorganisms can be spread in aerosols (e.g., *M. tuberculosis*) and/or in a dry state (e.g., bacterial or fungal spores). The control of these contaminants is particularly important to prevent cross-infection, product contamination, and spoilage. Typical examples are the use of clean rooms or separative enclosures (e.g., isolators) by pharmaceutical, hospital dispensing, semiconductor, and other facilities for contamination control. Clean rooms are defined as rooms in which the concentration of airborne particles is controlled and maintained. Separative enclosures provide the same control within a defined, enclosed area and include different types of isolators, such as barrier systems, which separate a process or activity from the operator and/or external environment (Fig. 2.13).

Other applications of air filtration are the use of filter vacuuming for the reduction of surface contamination, for medicinal gas (e.g., oxygen) delivery, and for the venting of air from or into various processes (e.g., washer-disinfectors and sterilizers).

Filters are also used to reduce the potential for cross-contamination in critical hospital environments (operating rooms and ventilators) or research laboratories (containment rooms and laminar-flow cabinets) for the protection of both a patient or sample and those working in the environment. Similar to liquid filters, this can be achieved by both physical retention by and/or electrostatic interactions of the filter. The most widely used air filters are high-efficiency particulate air (HEPA) filters, which are fiberglass depth filters of various efficiencies. These are generally rated as microfilters (see below) to remove contaminants of ≥0.3 μm and have also been reported to remove smaller virus particles (0.1 μm) due to adsorption.

In addition to the use of filters, the design of the air-handling system in a given room or enclosed area (e.g., a cabinet or isolator) is important for microbial control. The first consideration is air pressure (Fig. 2.14).

When an area is placed under negative pressure, contamination may be kept within the area (as air is drawn into the area), which is an important consideration when handling high concentrations of pathogenic organisms. The opposite is true for areas under positive air pressure, which keeps contamination out of the area and is important in the design of clean rooms or operating rooms.

The next consideration is the control of air flow in the area in a uniform way, which can be used to maintain the room at a given microbial level. This is the concept behind the laminar-flow principle, which controls the flow of air at a standard velocity and direction

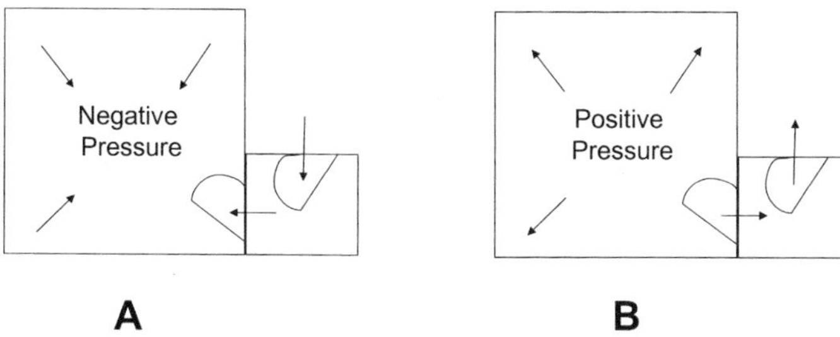

FIGURE 2.14 Air pressure in environmentally controlled enclosed areas. (A) Rooms under negative pressure draw air into the room, maintaining microorganisms within the room. Negative pressure is typically used in rooms or cabinets where pathogenic organisms are manipulated. (B) Rooms under positive pressure force air out of the room to reduce the risk of contaminants entering the room. Uses of positive pressure include clean rooms and sterility control isolators.

within an enclosed area while minimizing air turbulence.

Enclosed areas under positive pressure, including clean rooms and isolators, can be maintained at various levels, depending on the risks associated with potential contamination in the area. This can be achieved by the area design, the air velocity, and the efficiency of the filters. The quality of air in a given environment can be classified based on the maximum number of particles (e.g., of ≥0.5 μm) in a given volume of air. Various classification systems for clean rooms have been described; they are compared in Table 2.6.

Biological control or safety cabinets use the same principles to reduce the levels of contaminants in a smaller enclosed environment. They include simple designs that pass HEPA-filtered air over a given work area, either away from or toward a user, depending on the use of the cabinet. More complicated designs are used for critical applications. For example, various classes of biological safety cabinets can be designated based on their design and intended use (Fig. 2.15).

Biological safety cabinets of classes I, II, and III are all run under negative pressure and are designed to protect the user of the cabinet from

TABLE 2.6 Classification of clean rooms based on number of ≥0.5-μm particles detected within a given volume of air

Maximum no. of particles detected per m^3 (per ft^3)[a]	Classification		
	FDA FS 209[b]	ISO 14644[c]	EU GGMP[d]
35 (1)	1	3	
352 (10)	10	4	
3,520 (100)	100	5	A, B[e]
35,200 (1,000)	1,000	6	
352,000 (10,000)	10,000	7	C
3,520,000 (100,000)	100,000	8	D

[a]One cubic meter is approximately equal to 35 ft^3.

[b]Federal Standard 209, *Cleanroom and Workstation Requirements, Controlled Environments*, U.S. Food and Drug Administration, 1992. (Withdrawn in 2001 but still widely cited.)

[c]ISO 14644, *Cleanrooms and Associated Environments*, ISO, 2001.

[d]European Union Guide to Good Manufacturing Practices, European Union, 1997.

[e]Classes A and B differ in permissible particle counts when the room is "in use" or "at rest."

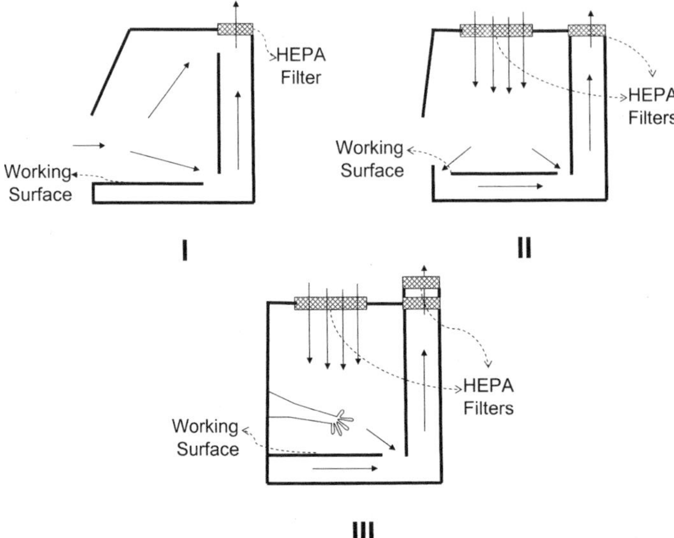

FIGURE 2.15 Biological safety class I, II, and III cabinets. Class I cabinets provide the lowest level of biological control, with all air that leaves the cabinet passing through a HEPA filter. Class III cabinets provide the highest level of control; they are totally enclosed, with access via a glove port, as shown.

the microorganism under investigation. In class I cabinets, the air is drawn into the cabinet and exhausted away from the user and through a microbiological-grade filter. For class II cabinets, the user and the specimen under investigation are protected, as the incoming air is also filtered and a laminar flow of air is passed over the working area; the air is then directed out of the cabinet through a further filter. Finally, class III cabinets are totally enclosed and airtight. They are used for the handling of high-risk pathogens. The agent is handled through gloves or a half-suit, and the air leaving the cabinet is passed through two filters. These designs may also include special handling pass-through ports or be directly connected to an autoclave to allow the safe handling of materials inside and outside of the cabinet.

Examples of standards and guidelines on the use of filtration for disinfection and sterilization are given in Table 2.7.

Spectrum of Activity. Filters can be used to remove a variety of contaminants, including microorganisms, biological molecules (e.g., proteins and endotoxins), and chemicals, such as metals and salts. Filtration methods can be defined based on the size range of contaminants they can remove (Fig. 2.16).

Coarse filters are generally used as prefilters to remove gross contaminants, including high-molecular-weight substances. Typical filter materials used include sand, activated carbon (charcoal activated with oxygen), cotton, polypropylene, and cellulose. In addition to gross physical removal, other contaminants can be reduced in the filtrate by chemical interactions; for example, activated-carbon filters can also remove low-molecular-weight microorganisms and halogens (including chlorine) due to affinity adsorption to the filter surface.

Microfiltration can remove particles as small as 0.05 μm, depending on the filter type, and therefore it is widely used to remove a broad range of pathogenic organisms, including parasitic cysts, bacteria, fungi, and many viruses. Typical filters used for bacterium-free water filtration include 0.2- and 0.1-μm filters. Surface and depth filters can be used; they are manufactured from a variety of materials, including

TABLE 2.7 Examples of standards and guidelines for disinfection and sterilization filtration applications

Reference[a]	Title	Summary
ISO 13408-2	*Aseptic Processing of Health Care Products. Part 2: Filtration*	Requirements for sterilizing filtration as part of aseptic processing of health care products, including requirements for setup, validation, and routine operation of a sterilizing filtration process
ISO 13408-6	*Aseptic Processing of Health Care Products. Part 6: Isolator Systems*	Requirements for isolator systems used for aseptic processing, including guidance on qualification, biodecontamination, validation, operation, and control
ISO 14644-1	*Cleanrooms and Associated Controlled Environments. Part 1: Classification of Air Cleanliness*	Guidelines for the classification of air quality used in clean rooms and other environments
ISO 14698-1	*Cleanrooms and Associated Controlled Environments, Biocontamination Control. Part 1: General Principles and Methods*	Principles and basic methodology for assessing and controlling biological contamination when clean-room technology is applied for that purpose
EN 12901	*Products Used for Treatment of Water Intended for Human Consumption. Inorganic Supporting and Filtering Materials. Definitions*	Definitions for the use of filtration in the treatment of drinking water
PDA Technical Report 26	*Sterilizing Filtration of Liquids*	Guidelines for the use of filtration in sterilization of liquids, including validation and integrity testing
ASTM F2101-01	*Standard Test Method for Evaluating the Bacterial Filtration Efficiency (BFE) of Medical Face Mask Materials, Using a Biological Aerosol of Staphylococcus aureus*	Test method used to measure the bacterial-filtration efficiencies of medical face mask materials

[a]ISO, International Standards Organization; EN, European Standard (Norm); PDA, Parenteral Drug Association; ASTM, American Society for Testing and Materials.

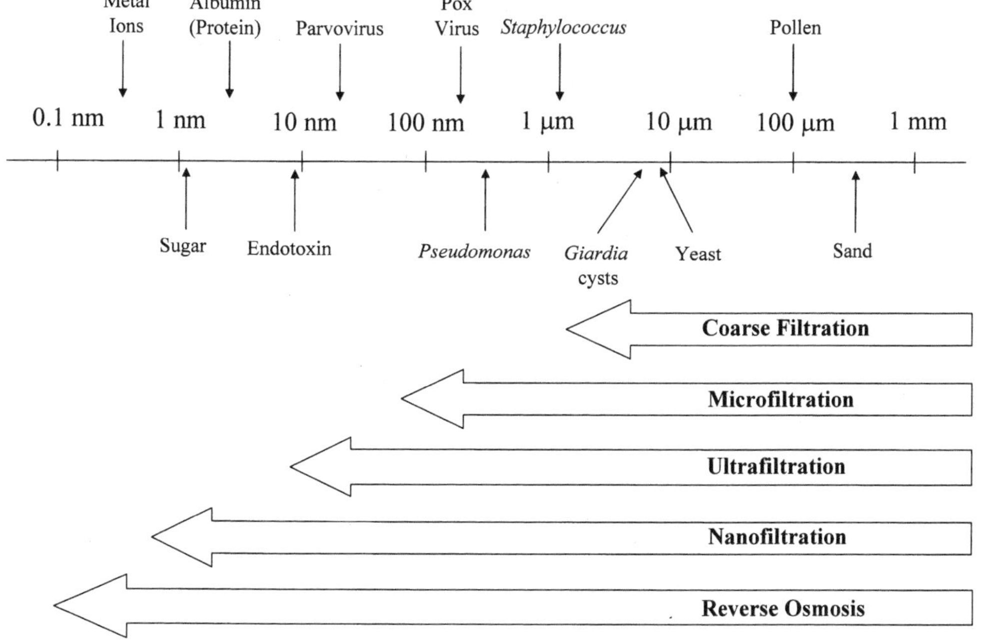

FIGURE 2.16 Range of filtration methods and reference size exclusion capabilities. Note that the size ranges are shown on a log scale.

polymers (polycarbonate, polypropylene, polyethylene, and polytetrafluoroethylene (PTFE), as well as ceramics and metals (e.g., silver). To increase the effectiveness of surface filters, the surface area for liquid-gas contact can be increased by preparing the filter material in folds or pleats. Similarly, depth filters can be optimized by having a gradient of pore sizes (from larger to smaller) through the filter to prevent premature clogging of the smaller pores and thereby increasing the life of the filter. Microfilters are generally rated as "absolute" or "nominal," depending on their retentive capabilities. Absolute filters should not allow the passage of any particle greater that the rated pore size, while nominal filters could allow some passage over time; for example, a nominal depth filter could allow organisms to pass by working through the torturous path of the filter matrix over time.

Contaminants of less than 0.1 to 0.05 μm can be removed by ultrafiltration, nanofiltration, and reverse osmosis (RO). These are all cross-flow filtration methods (Fig. 2.10). The filters are composed of semipermeable membranes in a variety of configurations; the liquid is passed over the filter surface under pressure to allow filtration, and unfiltered molecules are subsequently swept away to prevent fouling of the filter surface. The filter pore size dictates the filtration method. Ultrafiltration methods remove most organic molecules but do not remove salts or other inorganic contaminants. Nanofiltration, in addition, also removes endotoxins and other pyrogens, as well as some salts (e.g., it reduces water hardness). Finally, RO is considered the ultimate filtration method, removing nearly all organic molecules and high-efficiency inorganic salts. RO is actually a combination of filtration and electrochemical interaction; the filter membranes have extremely small pore sizes but are also highly adsorptive. Typical membranes used for RO include cellulose acetate and polyamide polymers. RO methods are used as alternatives to physical or chemical purification. Physical methods include water distillation (or the condensation of steam), and chemical methods include deionization (which uses a bed of synthetic resins that can adsorb cations or anions).

Advantages. Filtration can be a simple and cost-effective method for reducing contamination loads in heat-sensitive materials (e.g., pharmaceutical preparations) and to reduce or maintain the contamination levels in enclosed environments, like clean rooms and laminar-flow cabinets. Filtration methods can also be used for efficient sterilization, and many may also include the removal of other chemical contaminants (e.g., RO removes chemical and microbiological contamination as a method of water purification). Some filters may contain impregnated biocides that combine physical removal with biocidal activity (see section 3.17.2).

Disadvantages. It should be noted that in general, filtration methods can only remove, but not necessarily inactivate, microorganisms. Some filter technologies are available that incorporate the presence of biocides to reduce the microbes or that can be routinely sterilized, using chemicals or heat. Although coarse and microfiltration methods are cost-effective, as the filter pore size is decreased, the cost of filtration increases. Nominal filters may allow the passage of contaminants over time; in addition, absolute filters have also been reported to allow the "grow through" of microorganisms over extended use. To reduce this possibility, it is recommended that the filters be routinely changed and/or periodically treated with heat or chemicals. Finally, the efficiency of filtration can be affected by chemicals present in the gas or liquid due to damage to the filter. Filters should be routinely checked for integrity; widely used methods include microbiological sampling or retention tests (e.g., retention of 10^7 CFU of *Brevundimonas diminuta*/cm^2), the bubble point test, and smoke tests.

Mode of Action. Filters allow the physical removal of contaminants from gases, fluids, and solids based on their rated pore sizes. Some filtration materials and processes may also allow the removal of chemical and/or smaller-than-expected microbial contaminants by adsorption and other chemical interactions.

FURTHER READING

Block, S. S. (ed.). 1991. *Disinfection, Sterilization, and Preservation*, 4th ed. Lea & Febiger, Philadelphia, Pa.

Block, S. S. (ed.). 2001. *Disinfection, Sterilization, and Preservation*, 5th ed. Lippincott Williams & Wilkins, Philadelphia, Pa.

Carlberg, D. M. 2005. *Cleanroom Microbiology for the Non-Microbiologist*, 2nd ed. CRC Press, Boca Raton, Fla.

Gardner, J. F., and M. M. Peel. 1998. *Sterilization, Disinfection and Infection Control*, 3rd ed. Churchill Livingstone, Edinburgh, United Kingdom.

Jornitz, M. W., and T. H. Meltzer. 2004. *Filtration Handbook: Liquids.* PDA, Bethesda, Md.

Lewis, M. J., and N. J. Heppell. 2000. *Continuous Thermal Processing of Foods: Pasteurization and UHT Sterilization*. Springer, Cambridge, Mass.

Ljungqvist, B., and B. Reinmüller. 1996. *Clean Room Design: Minimizing Contamination through Proper Design*. PDA, Bethesda, Md.

Russell, A. D., W. B. Hugo, and G. A. J. Ayliffe. 1992. *Principles and Practice of Disinfection, Preservation and Sterilization*, 2nd ed. Blackwell Science, Cambridge, Mass.

CHEMICAL DISINFECTION

3

3.1 INTRODUCTION

Chemical biocides are used for various applications due to their ability to inhibit or inactivate microorganisms. In this chapter, biocides are classified according to their general chemical types, including alcohols, aldehydes, antimicrobial metals, and halogens. For each chemical group, the major types of biocides used are described, with consideration of their applications, spectra of activity, advantages, disadvantages, and what is known about their modes of action. The modes of action of biocides are considered further in chapter 7, and the specific uses of some chemical biocides in sterilization processes are discussed in chapter 6. Examples of various guidelines and standards that describe the use and testing of chemical disinfectants are given in Table 3.1.

3.2 ACIDS AND ACID DERIVATIVES

Types. Acids are defined as substances that dissociate in water to provide hydrogen ions (H^+), which are measured on the pH scale as <7. Acids form salts when they are mixed with an alkali, or base (see section 3.3). A variety of acids and acid salts are used as preservatives and, to a lesser extent, disinfectants. They include short-chain-length acids (acetic and propionic acids), long-chained acids (sorbic and citric acids), and other acid derivatives, including phenolic derivatives (benzoic acid and salicylic acid) and esters. An ester is an organic compound that is formed in the reaction of an acid and an alcohol; the most widely used esters are the *p*-hydroxybenzoic esters. They include methyl, ethyl, propyl, butyl, and benzyl derivatives.

Strong acids, such as hydrochloric acid (HCl) and sulfuric acid (H_2SO_4), readily dissociate in solution to give hydrogen ions, for example:

$$HCl \rightarrow H^+ + Cl^-$$

Although strong acids possess antimicrobial activity, they are limited in use due to concerns about safety and material compatibility. Similarly, strong bases, or alkalis, such as sodium hydroxide (NaOH), readily dissociate in water to provide hydroxyl ions (OH^-) and are measured on the pH scale as >7; the exception is the use of 1 to 2 N NaOH as a method for prion decontamination (see section 3.3). In contrast, the weaker acids do not readily dissociate in water and depend on the pH of the solution, e.g., with benzoic acid (Fig. 3.1).

Benzoic acid is usually applied in the salt (sodium benzoate) form. In solution, as the pH

TABLE 3.1 Examples of various guidelines and standards on the use and application of chemical disinfectants

Reference[a]	Title	Summary
AAMI TIR7 (1999)	*Chemical Sterilants and High Level Disinfectants: a Guide to Selection and Use*	Guidelines on the types and uses of disinfectants in health care settings
APIC (1996)	*Guideline for Selection and Use of Disinfectants*	Guidelines on the types and uses of disinfectants in health care settings
CDC HICPAC (2003)	*Guideline for Environmental Infection Control in Health-Care Facilities*	Environmental infection control guideline on strategies for the prevention of environmentally mediated infections, particularly among health care workers and immunocompromised patients
FDA (2000)	*Content and Format of Premarket Notification [510(k)] Submissions for Liquid Chemical Sterilants/High Level Disinfectants*	Guidance on the content and format for registration of liquid chemical sterilants/high-level disinfectants intended for the sterilization and/or high-level disinfection of reusable heat-sensitive critical and semicritical medical devices
EPA (1982) DIS/TSS-1	*Efficacy Data Requirements: Disinfectants for Use on Hard Surfaces*	Testing and labeling requirements for disinfectants
HC Sanitation Code for Canada's Food Service Industry	*Hand Washing, Cleaning, Disinfection and Sterilization in Health Care*	General guidelines on the types and uses of disinfectants in health care facilities
MDA	*MAC Manual*	Guidance on the principles, protocols and procedures for decontamination, including disinfection and sterilization
TGO 54 Standard for Disinfectants and Sterilants	*Guidelines for the Evaluation of Sterilants and Disinfectants*	Guidelines on the information to be supplied for the registration or listing of disinfectants and sterilants in Australia
AS 4187	*Cleaning, Disinfecting and Sterilizing Reusable Medical and Surgical Instruments and Equipment, and Maintenance of Associated Environments in Health Care Facilities*	Guideline on disinfection and sterilization practices in health care facilities
ASTM E1837-96	*Standard Test Method to Determine Efficacy of Disinfection Processes for Reusable Medical Devices (Simulated Use Test)*	Method for testing the effectiveness of a disinfection process for reprocessing reusable medical devices when challenged with vegetative cells, including mycobacteria
EN 14885	*Chemical Disinfectants and Antiseptics—Application of European Standards for Chemical Disinfectants and Antiseptics*	Guideline on the testing of chemical disinfectants and antiseptics
DPC Guideline 9	*Fundamentals of Cleaning and Sanitizing Farm Milk Handling Equipment*	Guideline on the cleaning and disinfection/sanitization of milk-handling equipment

[a]AAMI, Association for the Advancement of Medical Instrumentation; APIC, Association for Professionals in Infection Control and Epidemiology; CDC HICPAC, Centers for Disease Control and Prevention, Healthcare Infection Control Practices Advisory Committee; FDA, Food and Drug Administration; EPA, Environmental Protection Agency; HC, Health Canada; MDA MAC, Medical Devices Agency, Microbiology Advisory Committee, United Kingdom Department of Health; TGO, Therapeutic Goods Order, Australia; AS, Australian Standard; ASTM, American Society for Testing and Materials; EN, European Standard (Norm); DPC, Dairy Practices Council.

increases, the acid demonstrates greater dissociation, while at lower pH values, a greater concentration of the undissociated form is observed; in parallel, the antimicrobial efficacy of the acid increases at lower test pH values. The widely used antimicrobial acids include acetic acid, propionic acid, benzoic acid, citric acid, and sorbic acid. While acetic acid is used directly, propionic

$H_3C—COOH$

Acetic Acid

Benzoic Acid (ring–COOH)

$H_3C—H_2C—COOH$

Propionic Acid

$H_3C—HC{=}HC—HC{=}HC—COOH$

Sorbic Acid

OH (ring) COOX*

X*
Methyl CH_3
Ethyl C_2H_5
Butyl C_4H_9 etc.

p-hydroxybenzoic acid esters

acid, due to its corrosive nature, is generally used as a sodium or calcium salt form. Salicylic acid is considered in more detail as a phenolic compound below (see section 3.14). The *p*-hydroxybenzoic esters consist of various chain lengths to give methyl, ethyl, and other derivatives, which are commonly known as the parabens. They are colorless, odorless, stable, low cost, and relatively safe—factors that contribute to their widespread use as preservatives.

Applications. The primary uses of acids and acid derivatives are as preservatives for foods, pharmaceuticals, cosmetics, soaps, and other products. The parabens are among the most widely used preservatives in cosmetics at typical concentrations of ≤0.4% and often in various combinations. They are commonly added to cosmetics, eye drops, lotions, powders, pastes, drugs, and foodstuffs. Many types of acids are also used as preservatives. Acetic acid is commonly used as a food preservative, for example, at 1 to 8% in the pickling of vegetables and at lower concentrations in products such as salad dressings; vinegar, which contains ~4% acetic acid, is widely used in the food industry. Propionic acid is more often used in baked goods and other foods at concentrations ranging from 0.1 to 0.5%. Benzoic acid is widely used as a preservative in the pharmaceutical, food, and other industries and also as an antiseptic in combination with other biocides; it

$$C_6H_5COOH \leftrightarrow H^+ + C_6H_5COO^-$$

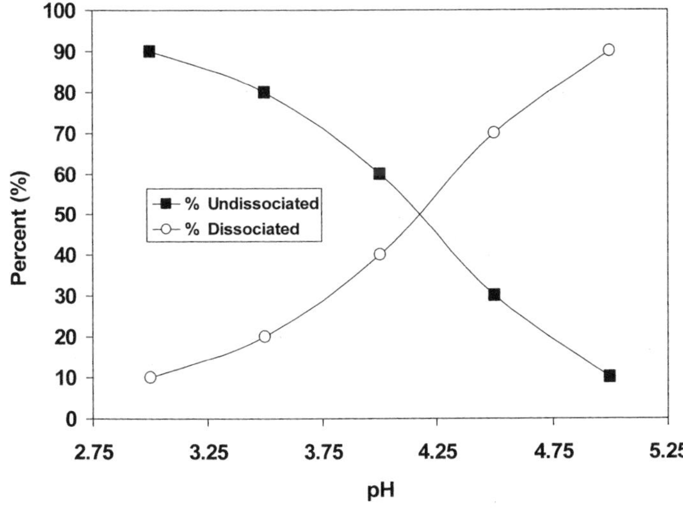

FIGURE 3.1 Dissociation of benzoic acid. As the pH increases, the dissociation of the acid also increases.

shows greater efficacy in low-pH (2.5 to 4.0) foods, such as fruit juices.

Maleic, sorbic, citric, and hydrochloric acids are among the other acids used for synergistic antiseptics, disinfectants, and/or preservative activities. A combination of citric acid and hydrochloric acid is recommended as a hard-surface disinfectant against some enveloped viruses (e.g., the foot-and-mouth disease virus). Formulations of citric acid with concentrations ranging from 2.5 to 8% are used as broad-spectrum disinfectants, with claimed efficacy against viruses, fungi, bacteria, and mycobacteria; citric acid is also used as a preservative in beverages (e.g., fruit juices and wines) and as an effective cleaning agent. The acid works in synergy with certain biocides, presumably because of its ability to increase the permeability of gram-negative cell walls (probably due to chelation and disruption of the cell wall structure [see section 8.6]). The stronger acids, such as HCl and H_2SO_4, have had little use as disinfectants or liquid sterilants, but some limited veterinary applications have included the inactivation of the spores of *Bacillus anthracis* on surfaces, such as animal hides.

Other acid biocides used as preservatives are dehydroacetic acid, undecenoic acid, and vanillic acid esters. Acidic cleaners, based on formulations containing phosphoric, acetic, citric, lactic, and other acids, are used for removing mineral deposits, including those due to water hardness (calcium carbonate).

Spectrum of Activity. The acids and acid derivatives demonstrate a range of antimicrobial activities, which also depend on their solubility in water or oil/lipid. These effects are important for their use in various emulsions and other formulations. The parabens are bacteriostatic against gram-positive bacteria and fungistatic against yeasts and molds, including *Candida, Saccharomyces, Trichophyton, Penicillium,* and *Aspergillus*, at ~100 to 200 μg/ml. Higher concentrations are required for gram-negative bacteria, particularly *Pseudomonas* spp., whose tolerances vary (up to ~1,000 μg/ml), although greater efficacy is observed against *Pseudomonas* with the methyl and ethyl esters. The parabens can also be sporistatic by inhibiting the germination of bacterial spores. In general, the shorter-chained parabens (methyl and ethyl derivatives) are less effective than the longer-chained parabens; however, the solubilities of the biocides in water decrease as their lengths increase. They remain effective within a wide pH range (between pH 4 and 8), which makes them attractive as preservatives; the antimicrobial efficacy decreases at pHs higher than 8 due to increased ionization of the biocide.

The acids also show variable activities. For example, acetic acid is more effective against bacteria and yeasts than against molds, in contrast to propionic acid, which is fungistatic with little or no activity against yeasts and bacteria. Some yeasts, molds, and bacteria can even use acids, such as lactic and citric acids, as carbon sources for growth. Benzoic acid is particularly active against yeasts at very low concentrations (0.01 to 0.02%), while sorbic acid inhibits the growth of yeast, molds, and bacteria to a lesser extent. Overall, the antimicrobial activity tends to be microbistatic, with greater activity observed with greater chain length, but similar to the parabens, as the chain length increases the solubility in water decreases. The decrease in pH alone is inhibitory to most bacteria and fungi at pH <4.5, with the exception of acidophilic microorganisms. Viruses are particularly sensitive to extremes of pH, as evidenced by the use of citric and hydrochloric acids against enveloped viruses; the spectra of activity of acids and parabens against viruses have not been well investigated, although some citric acid formulations have been shown to be effective (e.g., against rhinoviruses).

Advantages. The acids and esters are quite flexible as preservatives, depending on the required application. The parabens vary in water solubility, while the acids are mostly highly soluble in water. Various ester-acid mixtures can be broad-spectrum preservatives for many products. In addition, most of these biocides are nontoxic, nonirritating, and not known to be carcinogenic. For example, most of the acids, including acetic acid, propionic acid, benzoic acid, and sorbic acid, are naturally broken down in the body or the environment and therefore are widely designated as safe for use directly on foodstuffs intended for consumption. Some longer-chained acids, e.g., sorbic acid, can irritate the mucous membranes at 0.2% or higher concentrations. They are also widely available and inexpensive. The parabens are colorless, odorless, and stable. Overall, the acids and parabens are useful microbistatic agents.

Disadvantages. At the concentrations most often used, these biocides are considered only bacteriostatic or fungistatic; the exceptions are at higher concentrations in some antiseptic and disinfection applications (for example, citric acid at 2 to 8%). Some bacteria and fungi can use the acids or parabens as carbon sources and can therefore degrade the biocide or preservative over time and develop overgrowth within products; this can be prevented with the use of more than one active agent or, in some cases, by adding a higher concentration of the active agent. The parabens have lower water solubility than the acids and are also inactivated by nonionic surfactants. At higher concentrations, some of these biocides can be irritating and can cause allergic reactions. Acetic acid at higher concentrations has a strong pungent odor, which can be undesirable.

Modes of Action. When the modes of action of acids are considered, the reduction in pH alone can have a dramatic effect on microbial surfaces. With strong acids in particular, H^+ ions are attracted to microbial surfaces; the effect on bacterial and fungal cell structures initially is to disrupt the proton motive force (see section 8.3.4), thereby restricting the uptake of essential cell nutrients, oxidative phosphorylation, ATP synthesis, and other essential cell wall and membrane functions. It is also clear that changing the environmental pH disrupts the structures of essential surface and intracellular macromolecules (in viruses, protozoa, and other microorganisms); the effects are on the secondary and tertiary structures of proteins, lipids, carbohydrates, and nucleic acids, leading to loss of structure and functions. However, the mode of action is clearly not that simple with the weaker acids. As shown in Fig. 3.1, the increased accumulation of the undissociated acid with decreased pH also correlates with the antimicrobial activity; therefore, as the concentration of the undissociated form increases, so does the antimicrobial activity. This may be due to the pH effect alone or, more likely, in combination with direct effects on the structure and function of the microbial cell surface by the undissociated acid. The main effects in these cases have been studied in bacteria and have been shown to prevent the uptake of essential nutrients due to disruption of the proton motive force, which provides the energy for active uptake (see section 8.3.4). The parabens have demonstrated a similar mode of action, with further inhibition of electron transport and other proton motive force-related functions. Specific inhibition of various surface and internal enzymes has been reported for various acids and ester derivatives; sorbic acid has been reported to covalently bind to sulfhydryl groups (-SH) in proteins, which causes inactivation. Further, disruption of cell permeability (particularly for the longer-chained acids) and inhibition of respiration and of nucleic acid and protein synthesis have also been reported. These may be due to direct interaction with lipid membranes, cell walls, and proteins, leading to disruption of these structures and functions.

3.3 ALKALIS (BASES)

$NaOH$	KOH
Sodium Hydroxide	Potassium Hydroxide
Na_2SiO_3	$NaHCO_3$
Sodium Metasilicate	Sodium Bicarbonate

Types. Alkalis (or "bases") are defined as substances capable of forming hydroxide (OH^-) ions when dissolved in water and are measured at pH >7. They are therefore the opposite of acids (see section 3.2). Some limited disinfection methods use high concentrations of strong alkalis, such as NaOH (commonly known as caustic soda or soda lye) and KOH (also known as lye), while lower concentrations of these and weaker alkalis, such as sodium bicarbonate (baking soda) and sodium metasilicate, are used in various cleaning applications. Other biocides, such as the acridines, are considered weak bases (see section 3.7).

Applications. High concentrations (0.5 to 2.0 N) of NaOH and KOH are used for the routine cleaning and disinfection of various manufacturing surfaces, including purification and separation equipment, like chromatography columns and fractionation vessels used, e.g., in the fractionation of blood. These are considered aggressive processes to clean surfaces and inactivate/remove various microorganisms, particularly viruses and prion contamination. Prions have the greatest known resistance to disinfection and sterilization methods (see sections 1.3.6 and 8.9); it is recommended that surfaces be decontaminated with 1 to 2 N NaOH, typically for 1 h, to ensure priocidal activity. Applications include the decontamination of manufacturing equipment (especially those types that contact human- or animal-derived materials) and reusable medical equipment. Some investigators have recommended boiling in 1 N NaOH as the most effective process against prions, including high-temperature or high-pressure systems for the destruction of contaminated whole animals. Alkaline cleaning formulations include a variety of bases at much lower concentrations, such as NaOH, KOH, sodium bicarbonate, and sodium metasilicate, which are effective cleaners due to their ability to emulsify and saponify lipids and fats. In addition, they are effective for protein removal from surfaces and can break down proteins into peptides; some of these formulations have also been shown to be effective against prions and some enveloped viruses, presumably due to synergism between the lower concentration of alkali present and other formulation effects (including surfactants, chelating agents, and phosphates). Sodium metasilicate is widely used as a source of alkalinity in mild alkaline cleaners, as it protects various surfaces from damage by corrosion, often associated with other alkalis. Sodium bicarbonate is also used as a deodorizer. Alkalis are used in the manufacture of soaps and detergent; soaps, for example, are made by reacting alkali (particularly NaOH) with the fatty acids from various fats and oils. Alkaline conditions have been shown to increase the activities of some biocides, including phenols, glutaraldehyde, and the sporicidal activity of hypochlorites; bacterial spores are more sensitive to heat inactivation under alkaline conditions, presumably due to destabilization of the spore coat structure (see section 8.3.11).

Spectrum of Activity. Extremes of alkalinity are inhibitory to microorganisms, with the exception of certain extremophiles (alkaliphiles [see section 8.3.10]). In general, pH values of ≥9 are restrictive for the growth of most vegetative microorganisms, including bacteria and fungi. Low concentrations are generally inhibitory, while higher concentrations are bactericidal and fungicidal. The antimicrobial activities of NaOH and KOH against viruses have been particularly well studied, due to their use in studies of viral clearance. Typical virucidal concentrations are 1 to 2% NaOH and at least 4% sodium carbonate; enveloped viruses (due to envelope disruption) are more sensitive than nonenveloped viruses. High concentrations of NaOH (1 to 2 N) are recommended for the inactivation of prions.

Advantages. Alkalis are widely available and inexpensive but are rarely directly used as biocides. They can be used at lower concentrations as preservatives, and at higher concentrations, they show some microbicidal activity. They are widely used as formulation ingredients and demonstrate synergistic antimicrobial activity with various biocides. They are the basic ingredients in cleaning formulations, providing excellent cleaning efficacy, particularly against stubborn protein-based (solubilization and peptidization) and lipid-based (emulsification and solubilization) soils.

Disadvantages. Alkalis are damaging to various surfaces, depending on the concentration of alkali used and the formulation pH. Concentrated solutions should be handled carefully; for example, NaOH and KOH are extremely damaging to the skin and mucous membranes and can cause severe burns; they are also corrosive to hard surfaces, including metals (stainless steel, copper, brass, and aluminum) and various plastics. Reactions with some metals can, under certain circumstances, lead to the release of flammable (hydrogen) gases, and when they are mixed with certain other organic or inorganic chemicals, they can cause violent reactions. These effects can be minimized by using lower concentrations and combinations with other formulation effects.

Modes of Action. Alkaline conditions inhibit the growth of microorganisms by restricting various metabolic processes; the structures and functions of some macromolecules, including enzymes, are particularly affected. At higher concentrations, alkalis cause the solubilization of bacterial cell walls and membranes and viral envelopes. Studies with enveloped paramyxoviruses have shown disruption of the viral envelope at pH 9 to 11. The reactions of alkalis with the various types of lipids (including phospholipids) in these membranes can be compared to their reactions with fatty acids in lipids and oils to cause salt (soap) formation. Membrane disruption leads to cell wall destabilization (in the case of gram-negative bacteria) and loss of membrane structure and function, including disruption of the proton motive force (see section 8.3.4) and leakage of cytoplasmic materials. Alkali also causes breakage of peptide bonds and the breakdown of proteins, which is presumed to be the major mechanism of action against prions (see section 8.9).

3.4 ALDEHYDES

Types. Three aldehydes are widely used as disinfectants and/or sterilants: glutaraldehyde, orthophthaldehyde (OPA), and formaldehyde.

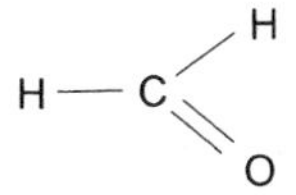

H—C(H)=O

Formaldehyde

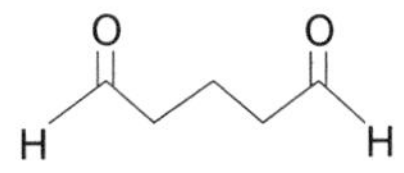

Glutaraldehyde

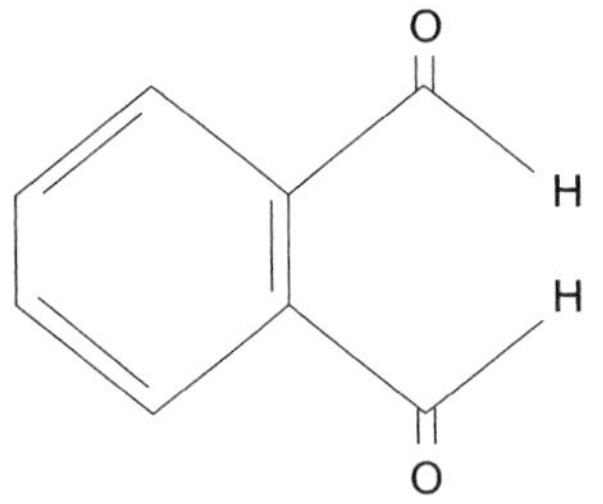

Ortho-phthaldehyde

Applications

Glutaraldehyde and OPA. Glutaraldehyde (1,5-pentanedial) and OPA formulations are widely used as low-temperature liquid disinfectants for temperature-sensitive medical devices (e.g., flexible endoscopes) and, in the case of glutaraldehyde, as a general surface disinfectant. Examples of glutaraldehyde and OPA solutions are shown in Fig. 3.2.

In addition to its antimicrobial applications, glutaraldehyde is used for many industrial applications and as a fixative for electron microscopy. OPA is used as a detection agent for protein, which turns grey or black on contact when OPA is used alone, or to provide fluorescence when used in conjunction with a sulfhydryl compound. Glutaraldehyde is a simple molecule with two aldehyde groups that are the keys to its mode of action. Formulations are usually provided at 1.5 to 3.5% (generally at 2%) under acidic conditions and are subsequently activated (or made alkaline to ~pH 8) prior to use. Glutaraldehyde is a reactive, cross-linking biocide that can be dramatically affected in

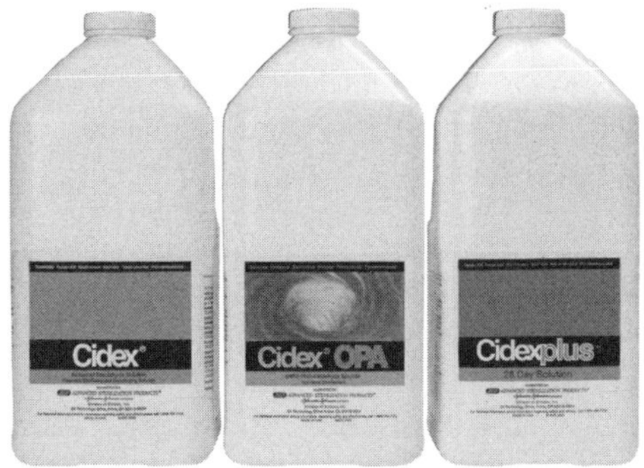

FIGURE 3.2 High-level disinfectants for medical-device disinfection based on 2.4% alkaline glutaraldehyde and 0.55% OPA. Reproduced with permission from Advanced Sterilization Products, a Johnson & Johnson company.

efficacy and stability based on formulation effects, particularly product pH. As the pH increases from 4 to 9, an increase in antimicrobial activity is observed, but with a concomitant reduction in shelf life; however, glutaraldehyde solutions also have much shorter useful lives at alkaline pHs, due primarily to increased condensation, as the biocide cross-links (or polymerizes) with itself. Stabilized acidic formulations, which do not require activation and have increased sporicidal activity, are also available. Glutaraldehyde solutions are colorless, although many contain a dye to give an amber color, and have a characteristic strong "rotten-apple" odor. A commercial ready-to-use OPA formulation is available at 0.55% and pH 7.5 for disinfection of temperature-sensitive devices at 20°C, with improved efficacy observed at 35°C. Similarly, a concentrated solution of OPA is also used specifically for dilution in automated washer-disinfectors to provide a final concentration of at least 0.055% OPA for disinfection at 50 to 55°C. In contrast to glutaraldehyde, OPA is stable over a wide pH range (pH 3 to 9) and does not autopolymerize under alkaline conditions. Further, due to a lower vapor pressure, OPA is odorless and less irritating to users. Its antimicrobial activity has been tested over 0.05 to 1% (wt/wt), but solutions at 1% (pH 6 to 8) are required for sporicidal activity, with over 10 h of exposure.

Formaldehyde. Formaldehyde (methanal [CH_2O]) is used in aqueous or gaseous form for a variety of applications. Formaldehyde itself is a monoaldehyde that exists as a freely water-soluble colorless gas with a pungent odor. Formaldehyde aqueous solutions (formalin) contain ca. 34 to 40% (wt/wt) CH_2O in water with methanol (8 to 15%) to delay polymerization. Formaldehyde is also available in polymeric form, as paraformaldehyde, a white, crystalline powder. Four to 8% formaldehyde solutions in water or alcohol (70% ethanol) are used as hard-surface disinfectants, primarily in laboratory applications. Formaldehyde solutions in alcohol were used in the past for device disinfection but are now generally contraindicated due to toxicity and corrosion concerns. Formalin is widely used to fix histological preparations and as a preservative (e.g., in embalming solutions). Formaldehyde is also widely used in many manufactured products, such as resins and adhesives, and in vaccine (poliovirus) production.

Formaldehyde gas is produced by heating paraformaldehyde, heating formalin solutions, or mixing formalin with potassium permanganate crystals. Formaldehyde is used in gaseous form as an area (laboratories, rooms, incubators, etc.) fumigant and in combination with "low-temperature" steam as a device sterilization process. A typical recommended fumigation process uses 6 g of formalin in 40 ml of water for every cubic meter; it is vaporized by being heated, held in the room for 7 h, and then subsequently aerated for up to 2 days, depending on the application. The antimicrobial effects of the gas are dependent on the presence of humidity (>70%), but condensation should be avoided, as formaldehyde rapidly dissolves and becomes significantly less effective, which restricts efficacy in the area.

Novel processes have also utilized formaldehyde-releasing agents for antisepsis, preservation, and other applications (Fig. 3.3). They include a large number of cyclic and acyclic compounds, including noxythiolin (oxymethylenethiourea), taurolin (a condensate of two molecules of the aminosulfonic acid

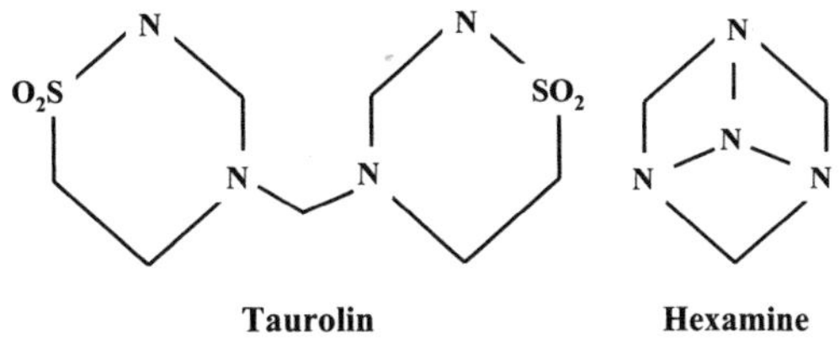

FIGURE 3.3 Examples of formaldehyde-releasing agents.

taurine with three molecules of formaldehyde), and hexamine (hexamethylenetetramine, or methenamine). Hexamine, for example, is a widely used chemical in adhesives and for other industrial purposes. Its primary antimicrobial use is as a preservative or as a urinary tract antiseptic. Other hexamine derivatives are also used as preservatives and antiseptics. All of these agents are claimed to be microbicidal due to the release of formaldehyde. However, many of them actually demonstrate greater antimicrobial effects than formaldehyde alone, which may be due to direct or indirect (synergistic) effects. Low- and high-temperature formaldehyde processes have also been developed for medical, dental, and industrial sterilization applications (see sections 6.3 and 6.4).

Spectrum of Activity

Glutaraldehyde and OPA. Glutaraldehyde has a broad spectrum of antimicrobial activity; it is fungicidal, virucidal, and bactericidal in <10 min at 2%, with longer contact times required for sporicidal activity. Acidic formulations demonstrate greater activity at higher temperatures (35°C). Initial reports of protozoal activity in vitro could not be verified in vivo. Other reports of microbial resistance to 2% glutaraldehyde include strains of *Mycobacterium chelonae, Mycobacterium avium-M. intracellulare*, and some fungi. OPA has a similar efficacy profile, with the notable exception of little or no sporicidal activity; improved mycobactericidal efficacy has been observed, including some efficacy against glutaraldehyde-resistant mycobacteria, which may be linked to its less cross-reactive nature and (due to its lipophilic nature) greater penetration into bacterial cell walls. OPA has also been shown to be rapidly bactericidal, virucidal, and fungicidal.

Formaldehyde. Formaldehyde is virucidal, bactericidal, mycobactericidal, fungicidal, and also sporicidal with longer contact times. Typical concentrations used range from 5 to 50 mg/liter. There has been some debate about the extent of sporicidal activity and whether the effect is primarily sporistatic; however, this uncertainty could be due to variations in experimental test methods, particularly relative humidity levels. It is known that the activity of formaldehyde is significantly less effective in the presence of contaminating soil or microorganism clumping. This has been shown in preparations of viral vaccines (poliovirus), where particle clumping protected infectious viruses from inactivation by formaldehyde; such preparations subsequently caused disease in immunized subjects. Similarly, considering the mode of action, formaldehyde has been shown to be ineffective against prions. In a notable clinical case of medical-device (neurological-electrode) transmission of Creutzfeldt-Jakob disease, the material was fixed onto the device surface and remained infectious over time, transmitting the disease to patients and experimental animals. Some bacterial species have demonstrated increased tolerance of formaldehyde, due to alterations in the outer cell surface structure (*Pseudomonas*) and plasmid-mediated expression of formaldehyde dehydrogenase (*Escherichia*), which degrades the biocide. Formaldehyde gas has been shown to be ineffective against some protozoal cysts and helminth eggs, although these studies require further investigation.

Advantages

Glutaraldehyde and OPA. Glutaraldehyde formulations provide rapid low-temperature (generally room temperature, ~20 to 25°C) disinfection of heat-sensitive medical devices and other surfaces. Particularly notable is its noncorrosive nature and lack of deleterious effects on sensitive materials, including plastics, lenses, and rubbers. Many formulations are available and are low cost. OPA-based products are more expensive but provide good compatibility with materials. OPA has greater mycobacterial activity, including against glutaraldehyde-resistant strains. No activation is required prior to use, and formulations are considered more stable, increasing the number of times the product can be reused. OPA is a weaker fixative than glutaraldehyde and, due to its lower vapor pressure, is less noxious than glutaraldehyde solutions.

Formaldehyde. Fumigation with formaldehyde gas is cost-effective and easy, with no specific apparatus required. It has traditionally been used for control of microorganisms in enclosed areas. Formaldehyde, via conversion to formic acid, breaks down in the environment into carbon dioxide and water, with a typical half-life of a few hours. Liquid and vapor applications demonstrate broad-spectrum activity, including against spores. The biocide is compatible with a range of metals and plastics.

Disadvantages

Glutaraldehyde and OPA. Glutaraldehyde fumes are notably irritating and toxic to skin, mucous membranes, and, in particular, the respiratory tract. Respiratory tract irritation is observed at concentrations as low as 0.3 ppm. Therefore, good ventilation, preferably a vented fume cabinet, is strongly recommended when glutaraldehyde is used. There is conflicting evidence on mutagenicity associated with the biocide. A further consideration is the absorption of glutaraldehyde into plastics and rubbers, which can cause localized toxicity (e.g., colitis with the use of flexible endoscopes). This can be avoided by adequate rinsing in water for about 2 min, or longer where multiple glutaraldehyde exposures have occurred. Surfaces should be meticulously cleaned prior to treatment, due to the potential of glutaraldehyde to fix material onto a surface. OPA has been less studied but is considered less cross-linking and less toxic than glutaraldehyde; however, due to the mode of action, similar precautions in its use should be taken. The discovery of waterborne mycobacteria with increased levels of resistance to the biocide is of some concern. OPA has little or no activity against bacterial spores and protozoan cysts. The biocide stains surfaces (particularly protein-containing surfaces, including clothing, hard surfaces, and skin) grey or black, which can be undesirable; it can also be considered a benefit in the detection of residual soil, although this can limit the efficacy of the biocide.

As for many biocides, the activities of aldehydes are dramatically reduced in the presence of contaminating or residual soil (particularly the presence of amines), presumably due to reactions with the soil and protection of the microorganism from biocidal activity. Many countries (or areas therein) have restricted the disposal of aldehyde wastes in sewer systems or waterways due to toxicity concerns.

Formaldehyde. The biggest disadvantage of formaldehyde is the safety concerns: formaldehyde is considered a strong irritant, toxic, mutagenic, and also carcinogenic. The data about its carcinogenic properties are conflicting, and current data are associated with the gaseous form. Permanent damage to olfactory (smelling) tissues and other mucous membranes can occur at toxic levels. Allergic reactions to lower concentrations are not uncommon. Formaldehyde can cause eye and mucous membrane irritation at 0.05 ppm, with a proposed safety limit of 0.75 ppm over a typical workday; control and monitoring of these levels can be difficult. Further, chemicals used to generate the biocide or deposited on surfaces following fumigation can be equally hazardous to the user. For example, formalin is an irritant, toxic, and caustic, and formalin-permanganate reactions are violently exothermic (heat producing). Close attention should be paid to ensure that humidity levels are maintained as required for efficacy and, where surfaces can absorb formaldehyde, that sufficient time is allowed for an area to aerate prior to reentry. Corrosion of some materials may occur. Some countries restrict the venting of formaldehyde into the environment without prior neutralization (e.g., by ammonia or ammonium hydroxide). Removal of gross soil prior to fumigation will ensure better efficacy.

Mode of Action

Glutaraldehyde and OPA. The major mode of action of glutaraldehyde is by cross-linking with proteins and inhibition of the synthesis of DNA, RNA, and other macromolecules. Glutaraldehyde is predominantly a surface-reactive biocide. The specific mode of action is due to alkylation reactions with amino groups (primary amines) and sulfhydryls, which form bridges or cross-links. Some amino acids (as the primary building blocks in proteins) have free, exposed amino groups (e.g., lysine and arginine), which are the direct targets of coupling reactions with aldehydes like glutaraldehyde. It is believed that cross-linking of these groups on cell surface proteins leads to rapid inhibition of essential cell functions.

Glutaraldehyde is more active at alkaline than at acidic pH. As the external pH is altered from acid to alkaline, amino groups at the cell surface are converted to the free amine forms and readily react with glutaraldehyde, leading to a more rapid bactericidal effect. The resulting cross-linking prevents the cell from undertaking most, if not all, of its essential functions, particularly cell wall- and membrane-related functions. Novel acidic glutaraldehyde formulations (as alternatives to alkaline glutaraldehyde products) have been produced that benefit from the greater inherent stability of the aldehyde at lower pH. The improved sporicidal activities claimed for these products may be due to agents that potentiate the dialdehyde. Glutaraldehyde is also mycobactericidal. Unfortunately, no critical studies have as yet been undertaken to evaluate the nature of this action. A number of recent reports have described the identification of *Mycobacterium chelonae* strains with dramatically increased resistance to glutaraldehyde; although the specific resistance factors remain to be identified, differences in the structures of the cell walls in these isolates, particularly in the cell wall-associated carbohydrates and lipids, have been described.

Although most studies have been of bacteria, similar modes of action are expected for fungi (interaction with chitin), viruses, and spores. Spore-forming bacteria become more resistant to glutaraldehyde as spore development proceeds. Mature spores bind the biocide to their surfaces, but uptake has been debated and may be pH dependent, with alkaline formulations thought to have greater penetration. It has been suggested that changes in pH may also affect the cell surface itself, freeing more amino groups for cross-linking at alkaline pH. The presence of glutaraldehyde can cause spore swelling and inhibits subsequent spore germination. Viruses are sensitive to relatively low concentrations; however, it has been noted that free nucleic acid (for example, poliovirus RNA) is more resistant, suggesting a predominantly capsid (surface) interaction. Inhibition of protozoa has also been shown, although the mode of action is unknown.

OPA has a mode of action similar to that of glutaraldehyde but is considered a less aggressive cross-linking agent. OPA covalently binds with proteins via Schiff's base formation with side terminal amino groups and side chain amino groups from lysine and arginine residues, while glutaraldehyde can react with other amino groups in biomolecules. Further, the benzene ring structure of OPA limits its ability to interact with adjacent reactive groups due to stearic hindrance. OPA demonstrates rapid mycobactericidal activity, presumably due to greater penetration of the lipophilic cell wall structure. OPA has been shown to be more penetrating than glutaraldehyde and to be effective on proteins within bacterial and fungal cell walls and membranes. This may be due to differences in the structure of OPA under the hydrophilic conditions observed at the external surface of the cell; it adopts a "locked" structure with unexposed aldehyde groups and allows penetration of the biocide into the cell. Once within a hydrophobic environment, typical of the cell wall or membrane, it is proposed to assume a more open, exposed form with reactive aldehyde groups (see section 7.4.3).

Formaldehyde. Formaldehyde is an extremely reactive chemical that interacts with protein, DNA, and RNA in vitro. It is considered sporicidal by virtue of its ability to penetrate into the interiors of bacterial spores. The interaction with protein results from combination with the primary amide, as well as with the amino groups. Formaldehyde is considered mutagenic, presumably by reaction with carboxyl, sulfhydryl, and hydroxyl groups. Formaldehyde also reacts extensively with nucleic acids, which form cross-links that inhibit DNA and RNA activities. Lower concentrations of formaldehyde are sporistatic and inhibit germination. A similar mode of action is expected for other microorganisms. Overall, it is difficult to pinpoint accurately the mechanisms responsible for formaldehyde-induced microbial inactivation. Clearly, its interactive and cross-linking properties play a considerable role in this activity. Further, hydration is a key, as the antimicrobial activity of formaldehyde is dependent on the presence of water or humidity (>60%).

3.5 ALCOHOLS

Types. Alcohols are compounds with a hydroxyl group (-OH) attached to a saturated carbon atom. A variety of alcohols are used for many chemical and industrial purposes. As antiseptics and disinfectants, the most widely used alcohols are isopropanol (isopropyl alcohol, propan-2-ol, or "rubbing alcohol"), ethanol ("alcohol"), and *n*-propanol (propan-1-ol). Many products list "methylated spirits," or IMS, as the biocide, which is simply a mixture of 95% ethanol and 5% methanol. The alcohols used as antiseptics and disinfectants are short-chained alcohols, which are both water and lipid soluble. Alcohols are actually less effective in the absence of water, with typical in-use concentrations ranging from 50 to 90%, the optimum being 60 to 70%. Some alcohols are also used as preservatives at low concentrations, particularly phenoxyethanol. Phenoxyethanol is a glycol ether and is provided as an oily, viscous liquid.

$$CH_3.CH_2.OH$$

Ethanol

$$(CH_3)_2CHOH$$

Isopropanol (Propan-2-ol)

Applications. Alcohols are used for cleaning, drying, disinfection, and antisepsis. They are good choices for cleaning (particularly for lipids or lipid-soluble soils), as they dry rapidly following treatment of a surface; however, protein- and carbohydrate-based soils can coagulate on treatment. They are often used in combination as cleaners and disinfectants (Fig. 3.4).

They are probably the oldest known antiseptic, used for intact or broken (wounded) skin. They are commonly used for routine skin disinfection in hospitals and other facilities, by direct application or using alcohol-impregnated wipes (Fig. 3.4).

In formulation, increased surface activity can be achieved by retarding the evaporation rate,

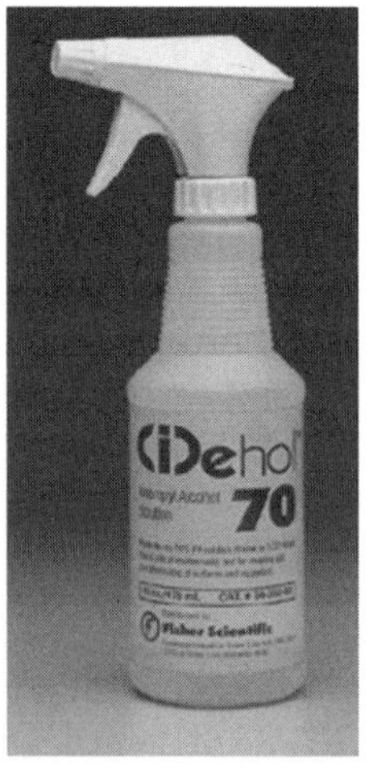

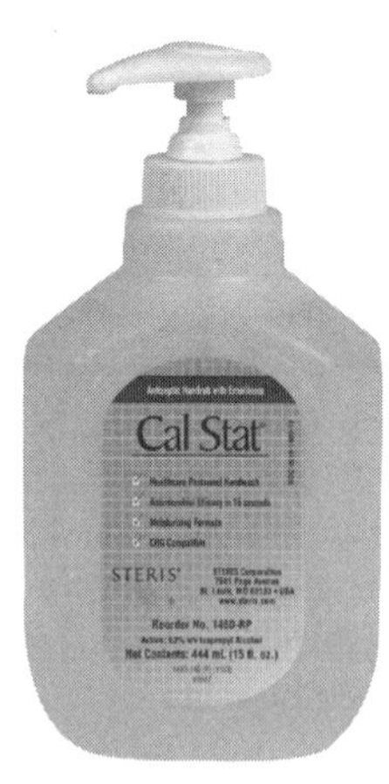

FIGURE 3.4 Examples of an alcohol-based disinfectant (left) and an alcohol-based antiseptic (right).

thereby increasing the contact time. Alcohols are also used as preservatives and solvents in formulation, as well as in synergy with other biocides (e.g., chlorhexidine, hydroxides, and hydrogen peroxide). Phenoxyethanol is particularly used as a preservative in a variety of products, including cosmetics, ophthalmological solutions, and pharmaceuticals (e.g., vaccines) at between 0.1 and 2% and usually in combination with the parabens (see section 3.2).

Spectrum of Activity. Alcohols have rapid bactericidal and mycobactericidal activities (e.g., 70% ethanol within 30 s). Efficacies against fungi and viruses are variable and slower (>2 min with 70% ethanol), with greater activity against enveloped viruses. Alcohols, in their own right, demonstrate little or no activity against bacterial spores but are sporistatic. Sporicidal activity can be demonstrated in synergy with other biocides (e.g., surfactants and hydrogen peroxide). There is minimal information on activity against protozoa. The propanols demonstrate greater activity than ethanol. Phenoxyethanol is primarily a bacteriostatic and fungistatic biocide with a limited spectrum of activity; its activity is particularly marked against gram-negative bacteria, including *Pseudomonas*.

Advantages. Alcohols are fast-acting, broad-spectrum antimicrobials with no residues or environmental concerns following application. Cleaning and disinfection can be combined, leaving a dry surface. They are relatively stable, with little odor, inexpensive, nontoxic, and have good compatibility with surfaces (including skin and inanimate surfaces). They are excellent solvents and are used as preservatives at low concentrations. Phenoxyethanol is stable over a wide pH range (pH 3 to 8.5) and at elevated temperatures and is not considered toxic at the preservative concentrations typically used; at these concentrations, phenoxyethanol is nonirritating to the eyes, skin, and mucous membranes and is not considered a sensitizer.

Disadvantages. Alcohols demonstrate little or no sporicidal activity. At high concentrations, flammability risks should be controlled. Repeated use on the skin and certain inanimate surfaces can cause drying and cracking over time, and they are irritating (stinging) to broken skin. Phenoxyethanol is primarily microbistatic and thus is used mainly as a preservative. Despite a good toxicity record, irritation and allergic reactions have been reported, often related to higher concentrations than those used for preservation.

Modes of Action. Little is known about the specific mode of action of alcohols on microorganisms, but multiple toxic effects on structure and metabolism are suspected, primarily due to protein denaturation and coagulation. The reactive hydroxyl (-OH) group readily forms hydrogen bonds with proteins, which lead to loss of structure and function, causing protein and other macromolecules to precipitate. Specific inhibition of enzymes in vitro and in whole cells has been described. The hydrogen bonds in the tertiary structure of proteins are particularly sensitive: the alcohol disrupts the amino acid-amino bond to form an amino acid-alcohol hydrogen bond. It is believed that in more concentrated (>80% alcohol) solutions the alcohol rapidly coagulates the protein on the outside of the cell wall and prevents further penetration into the cell, thereby limiting its antimicrobial activity; at 60 to 80% alcohol, greater penetration of the bacterial or fungal cell wall is expected, with further effects on cell membrane and cytoplasmic proteins and enzymes. Alcohols also disrupt the structures of any surface lipid-based cell membranes, cell walls, and viral envelopes to cause loss of integrity and function. Alcohols overall lead to cell lysis but have been shown to directly interfere with metabolite production (and therefore cell division). Although not effective against bacterial spores, alcohols do inhibit spore germination and are therefore sporistatic. Phenoxyethanol appears to primarily target cell membranes. Low concentrations specifically interrupt the membrane proton motive force and cause leakage of cytoplasmic constituents, although these effects have been shown to be reversible in *Escherichia coli*; higher concentrations cause more gross effects on the membrane structure and penetrate into the cytoplasm, with observed inhibition of enzymes and other functions, including DNA replication.

3.6 ANILIDES

Types. The anilides are derivatives of salicylanides and carbanilides. The most successful derivatives are halogenated, including the carbanilide-based triclocarban (3,4,4′-trichlorocarbanilide) and salicylanilide-based tribromsalan (3,4′,5-tribromosalicylanide).

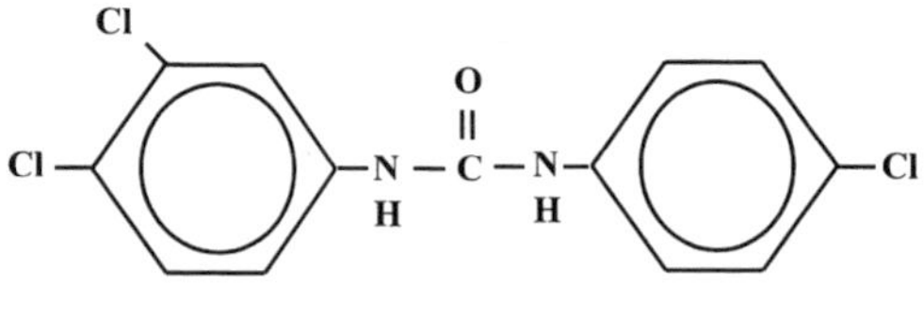

Triclocarban

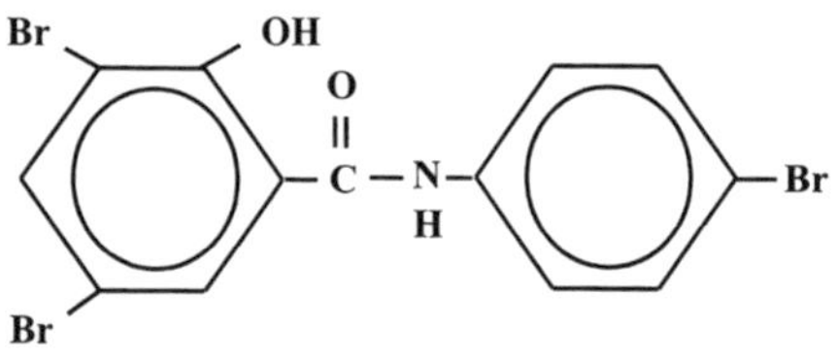

Tribromsalan

Applications. The salicylanilides, particularly tribromsalan, are used as preservatives in paper, plastics, and paints. They are also used to a lesser extent in antiseptic soaps and cosmetics. Triclocarban has been used as a cosmetic preservative and is still used in consumer antimicrobial soaps and deodorants. Overall, their use has been limited due to a restrictive spectrum of activity in contrast to other antiseptic biocides. They have also had limited use as agricultural preservatives or pesticides.

Spectrum of Activity. Anilides, particularly the halogenated derivatives, are especially effective bacteriostatic and fungistatic agents. Their specific microbicidal activities vary depending on the biocide and its formulation, but in general, they have limited fungicidal activity and some bactericidal activity. Triclocarban is particularly active against gram-positive bacteria, many of which are important pathogenic or odor-causing bacteria on the skin. Bacteriostatic activities are observed at ~1 μg/ml, but higher concentrations are required for fungistatic activity. Triclocarban has little efficacy against gram-negative bacteria and fungi; the exceptions are some of the fungal skin pathogens (*Trichophyton, Epidermophyton,* and *Microsporum*), which are inhibited at concentrations below 10 μg/ml. It also lacks appreciable substantivity (persistence) on the skin. The substantivity of an antiseptic may be defined as its property of adsorbing to the skin during washing and subsequently remaining available for antimicrobial activity. Tribromsalan demonstrates persistency on the skin, inhibiting the growth of bacteria and fungi, but has seen limited use in antiseptics because it causes irritation. Little or no activity has been reported against viruses or other microorganisms.

Advantages. Some anilides, particularly triclocarban, have reasonable safety profiles; others are restricted in use due to toxicity concerns. Triclocarban and tribromsalan are useful preservatives at relatively low concentrations against a variety of bacterial and fungal species. They are also particularly effective against gram-positive bacteria. Tribromsalan is persistent on the skin and can provide residual bacteriostatic and fungistatic activity following antiseptic washing.

Disadvantages. Triclocarban is not persistent on the skin, which is a desired attribute in many other biocides used in antiseptics. In contrast, tribromsalan is persistent but is sensitizing and irritating. Anilides have a limited spectrum of activity, which has restricted their use as preservatives and antiseptics; they are generally considered only reasonable bacteriostatic and fungistatic biocides.

Mode of Action. The anilides are thought to act by adsorbing to and destroying the semipermeable character of the cytoplasmic membrane, leading to cell death. The disruption of bacterial surface activities has been particularly investigated. Anilides have been shown to cause disruption of the proton motive force across the bacterial surface and interruption of key membrane functions, including active transport and energy metabolism. These effects may be due to interference with proteins or the phospholipid bilayer of the membrane to disrupt its structure and function. Greater antimicrobial activity is observed with increased halogenation of the anilides; the reactions of these groups with various macromolecules appear to contribute to their mode of action.

3.7 ANTIMICROBIAL DYES

Types. A variety of antimicrobial dyes have been used as traditional antiseptics and in some cases for water disinfection. They include the acridines and a variety of other dyes. The acridines were first introduced as systemic and topical antimicrobials in the early 1900s, but their use decreased following the introduction of antibiotics. The basic acridine structure is shown below, along with derivatives with various antimicrobial or toxic properties. They are essentially heteroaromatic dyes, which have been investigated by a variety of modifications, including the addition of amino groups (known as aminoacridines), halogenation, and nitrification. Various early investigations into specific acridine modifications led to the identification of many therapeutic antiprotozoal drugs, including quinoline and quinacrine (see section 7.2.4). Further, naturally occurring acridines have been identified, e.g., the acridine alkaloids extracted from plants. The acridines most widely used as antiseptics are the aminoacridines, which include proflavine, euflavine (or "acriflavine"), and aminacrine (Fig. 3.5). Acriflavine exists in two forms, an acid form (euflavine, shown in Fig. 3.5) and a neutral form; the latter is more widely used due to less irritancy.

Other dyes are the triphenylmethane dyes (particularly crystal violet and malachite green), the quinones (1,4-naphthaquinone and chloranil), and methylene blue (a phenothiazinium dye).

Applications. Acridine derivatives have been and are being used in therapeutic and topical applications. Proflavine and euflavine were among the first to be used as wound antiseptics, particularly proflavine, which is less irritating to the skin. They may be applied in powders or ointments or in soaked gauze. Proflavine, in particular, has been used in wound dressings. Older studies showed that proflavine (and other acridine derivatives) were photosensitive dyes that demonstrated increased activity against bacterial and fungal skin infections when the infections were first treated with the dye and then with various wavelengths of light. It has been suggested that these applications be reinvestigated as logical treatments for antibiotic-resistant bacterial wound infections. Various acridines are also added to water for the surface

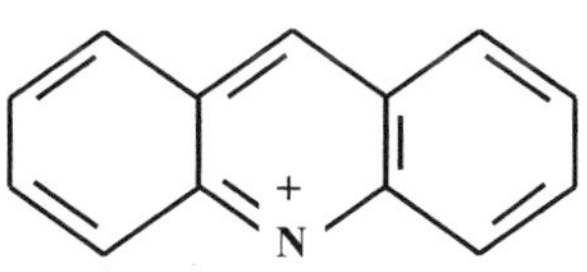

N+

Acridine

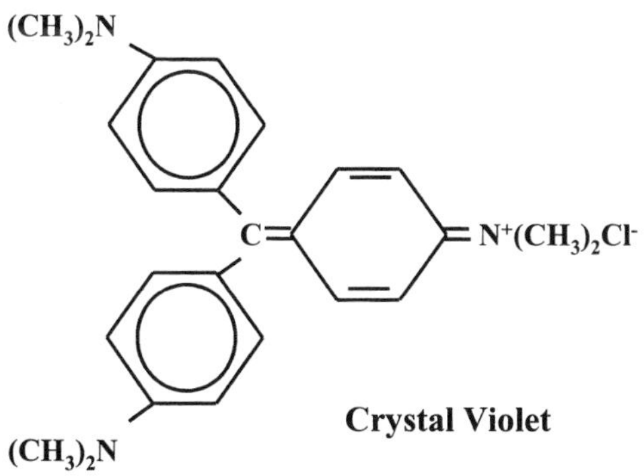

$(CH_3)_2N$

C

$N^+(CH_3)_2Cl^-$

$(CH_3)_2N$

Crystal Violet

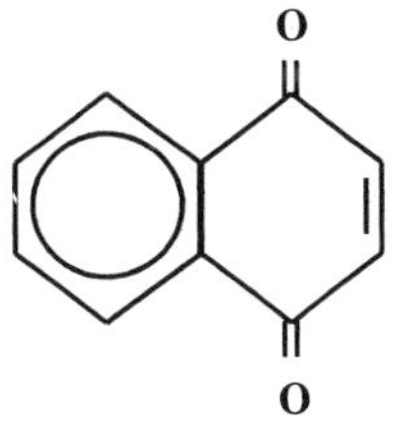

O

O

1,4-Naphthaquinone

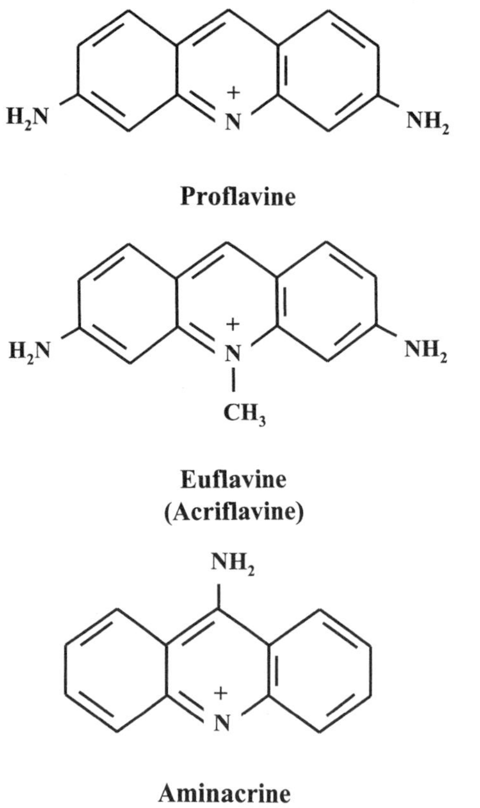

Proflavine

Euflavine (Acriflavine)

Aminacrine

FIGURE 3.5 Aminoacridines commonly used as antiseptics.

treatment of fish or fish egg infections, including surface fungal, bacterial, and protozoal infections. An example is the use of acriflavine at 5 to 10 ppm in water for the treatment of open wounds and surface protozoal infections in fish. Aminacrine is still used for the prevention and treatment of mucous membrane infections, including as vaginal suppositories in the treatment of *Trichomonas* infections or as a topical antiseptic. Recent research has focused on the development of new acridine derivatives, due to their use as anticancer agents. Many of the acridines developed may also show variable activities against bacterial, fungal, and protozoan pathogens and may have future applications as therapeutic antiseptics.

Other dyes, such as malachite green and crystal violet, have similar antiseptic applications; these dyes have also been used as topical local antiseptics, particularly in wound applications in animals, but they are not widely used on humans. Triphenylmethane dye preparations have been used for the topical treatment of persistent tinea skin infections, such as ringworm and athlete's foot. Typical applications include localized treatment with a dye tincture or addition of a few drops of a dye preparation to a water sample, which is then used for skin or mucous membrane washing. In addition to specific treatment of infections, a variety of these dyes are also used as general preservatives in aquaculture applications (including fish tanks) to prevent the overgrowth of bacteria, algae, and other microorganisms. Others, such as the quinones, are used as agricultural bactericides and fungicides, including the naphthaquinones and chloranil.

Many of these dyes are also widely used for cytological and microbiological staining; examples are the use of crystal violet to differentiate bacterial types by Gram staining and fluorescent acridine dyes used for the staining of chromosomes and other nucleic acid structures.

Spectrum of Activity. The spectra of activity of the various acridines vary depending on their chemical structures and preparation. The dyes that form cations in solutions demonstrate the greatest antimicrobial activities. Cationic acridines are particularly broad spectrum and retain activity in the presence of organic soils. In general, they are effective against gram-positive and gram-negative bacteria to various degrees and over time. The triphenylmethane dyes are more effective against gram-positive than gram-negative bacteria; it has been proposed that this is due to the increased peptidoglycan layer in gram-positive bacteria (see section 8.5). Increased resistance in some bacteria has been shown to be due to reduced uptake and efflux mechanisms (see section 8.3.4). Most are fungistatic and also fungicidal against yeasts and molds. The acridine dyes have been used for the specific treatment of fungal infections, including those caused by *Trichophyton* and *Microsporum* and tinea, for example, in the topical treatment of athlete's foot.

Their effects against viruses have not been well studied, but some reports have shown activity against enveloped viruses. Acridines and other dyes have varying activities against protozoans, including *Amoeba*, *Leishmania*, and other surface-related parasites. They are often used as preservatives at low concentrations to prevent fungal and algal growth in water tanks. Little or no sporicidal activity has been described, although the dyes are sporistatic.

Advantages. Many of the antimicrobial dyes are effective against a wide range of microorganisms at relatively low concentrations, even in the presence of serum or other organic soils, making them useful as antiseptics. Many are odorless and readily soluble in water. Their ranges of toxicity vary; for example, proflavine is less toxic or irritating to the skin than acriflavine. They are generally stable in preparations and formulations, with characteristically long shelf lives. In aquaculture, they can be used for the treatment of fish pathogens or surface diseases, as well as in preventing the growth of microorganisms, without significant harm to fish or other aquatic life. Nonstaining acridine dyes have also been developed (e.g., aminacrine).

Disadvantages. One of the biggest disadvantages of dyes is aesthetic: the dye colors the skin and mucous membranes, which is often undesirable. This is not a concern with newer acridines, including aminacrine and salacrine. Like other biocides, their antimicrobial activities vary; for example, acriflavine is less effective against fungi and lacks sufficient biocidal activity under acidic (pH <7) conditions. Many of the dyes are toxic at higher concentrations, particularly as the concentration of the dye is increased from preservative to microbicidal levels. Malachite green is toxic to fish but not to fish eggs. There have been concerns over the use of some acridines due to evidence of mutagenicity in bacteria and in cell culture experiments. Aminacrine is actually used as an experimental mutagen. The potential for mutagenicity may not be surprising considering their mode of action (intercalation of nucleic acid), but they are also photosensitive, which can lead to irritation (dermatitis) of the skin and other toxic effects. Photosensitization is a process by which a photosensitive molecule (in this case the acridine) adsorbs light radiation to cause a photochemical alteration. In some applications, further investigation into the carcinogenic nature of some dyes is required. Another cited disadvantage of some acridines is the ability of some bacteria, such as *Staphylococcus*, to acquire increased tolerance to the biocide due to energy-dependent efflux mechanisms; however, it is interesting that this has been reported for some acridines (including proflavine) but not for others, such as the aminacrine derivatives.

Mode of Action. The modes of action of the acridines have been well studied, particularly that of the aminoacridines. The primary site of acridine activity is double-stranded nucleic acids. The polycyclic, flat structure of the acridine molecule appears to be well suited to intercalate between adjacent nucleotide base pairs of DNA and other double-stranded nucleic acid structures. This alone disrupts the structure of DNA, but further interactions with the phosphate backbone and the nucleotides also cause the disruption of DNA unraveling, which is required for replication and transcription. The position of the amino group in the aminoacridines appears to be important in these interactions and in the overall activity of the molecule. It is for this reason that the acridines have been investigated as potential anticancer drugs; however, during these investigations, different modes of action have also been described. Interactions with specific DNA-related (including topoisomerases) and other (cytoplasmic kinases) enzymes have also been described. Multiple effects have been observed in bacterial studies, including inhibition of separation during cell division and strong binding to the bacterial cell envelope. It is clear that other surface effects may contribute to the mode of action. This may be important in the modes of action of other dyes that have been less studied. Many antimicrobial dyes are also believed to result in catalytic production of reactive radicals during intracellular reactions. Intercalation into the bacterial peptidoglycan or interaction with other microbial surfaces appears to play an important role. For example, the triphenylmethane dyes (including crystal violet) are more active against gram-positive bacteria, which may be linked to the greater proportion of peptidoglycan in their cell wall structure (see section 8.5). These dyes are difficult to remove from the cell wall surface following application (as demonstrated by the Gram stain). This leads to disruption of structure and function. Further penetration into the cell membrane and cytoplasm is also expected, with effects similar to those of general toxic substances. Although not described, these effects clearly affect the survival of fungi, some viruses, and other microorganisms.

3.8 BIGUANIDES

Types. Biguanides are compounds that contain the $C_2H_5N_7$ ligand. Chlorhexidine (a bisbiguanide) is insoluble in water and is therefore supplied in salt forms, consisting of the chlorhexidine base reacted with an acid. The chlorhexidine molecule itself consists of a central lipophilic hexamethylene chain with a basic chlorophenyl guanide group on either end reacted with an acid. Chlorhexidine gluconate, known as CHG, is widely used, but other salts include chlorhexidine diacetate and dihydrobromide. Alexidine differs chemically from chlorhexidine in possessing ethylhexyl end groups. Other, similar chemicals, including octenidine, have been described but are less used. A newer class is the polymeric biguanides, which are heterodisperse mixtures of polyhexamethylbiguanides (PHMBs); as an example, the general structure of PHMB chlorides is shown below. Vantocil is a heterodisperse mixture of PHMBs with a molecular weight of approximately 3,000.

Applications. Chlorhexidine is probably the most widely used biguanide, with a range of applications, including use as the biocide in antimicrobial soaps (antiseptics, including the widely used Hibiclens and Hibiscrub formulations), biocidal wound dressings, mouth washes, hair care products, and surface disinfectants and as a preservative (e.g., in contact lens storage solution). Chlorhexidine (at 0.5 to 4%) is primarily used as an antiseptic for high-risk applications, including in hospital surgical scrubs and hand washes for health care personnel (Fig. 3.6).

The wide use of chlorhexidine is due to its minimal skin irritation (which can be formula-

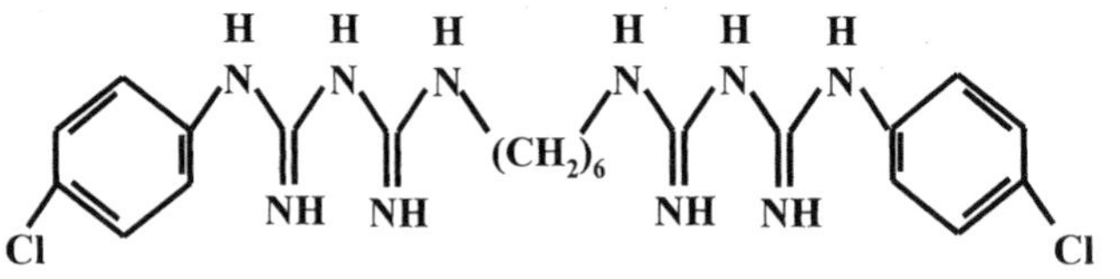

Chlorhexidine

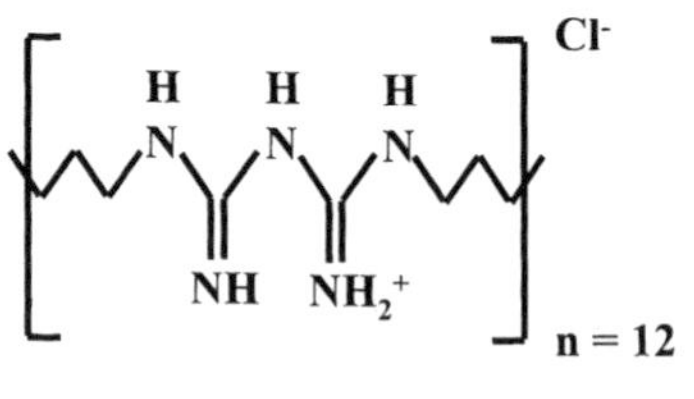

PHMB

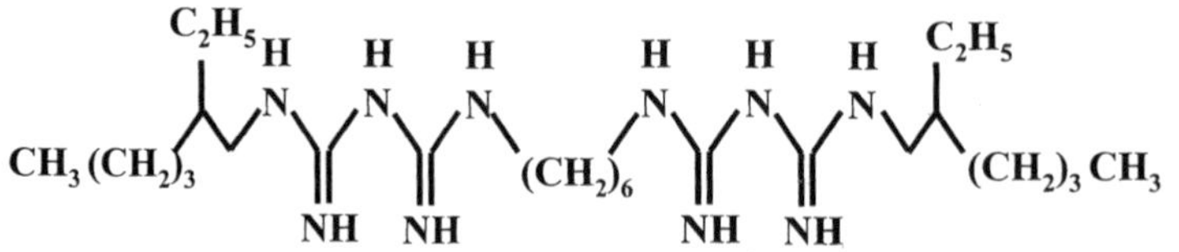

Alexidine

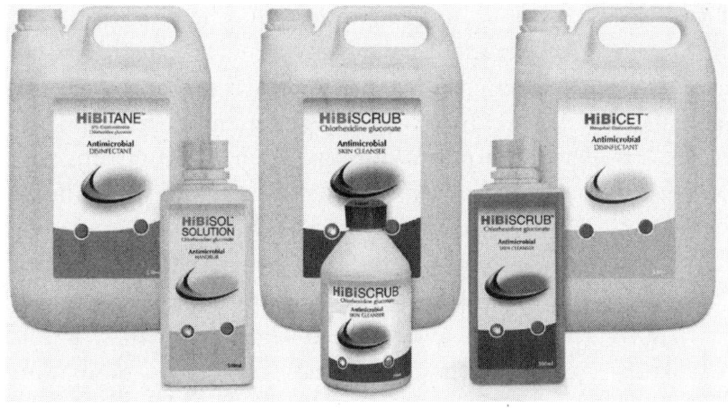

FIGURE 3.6 Examples of chlorhexidine-based antiseptics and disinfectants. Courtesy of Regent Medical Ltd.

tion dependent) and its substantivity on the skin and mucous membranes. Irritation is markedly higher with alexidine and octenidine. The broad-spectrum activities of biguanides can be enhanced in combination with other biocides, particularly alcohols and quaternary ammonium compounds (QACs) (also known as "quats"; see section 3.16), and can be dramatically affected by pH (they are more active at pH 5 to 7). PHMBs have had wide application for surface disinfection and water sanitization, particularly as an alternative to chlorine and bromine in swimming pools and water spas. Some biguanides have also been used therapeutically; for example, dimethylbiguanide (metformin) has been used since medieval times for the control of non-insulin-dependent diabetes and as a malarial prophylactic (e.g., proguanil).

Spectrum of Activity. Biguanides are broad-spectrum bactericidal biocides, showing rapid action against gram-positive and gram-negative bacteria. The PHMBs are also active against gram-positive and gram-negative bacteria, although *Pseudomonas aeruginosa* and *Pseudomonas vulgaris* are less sensitive. In general, biguanides are more active against gram-positive bacteria, even in the presence of interfering soils, such as blood or serum. They are less active against fungi, including yeasts and molds, although their activities can be enhanced by synergy with other active agents or by formulation effects. Although chlorhexidine and alexidine have similar spectra of activity, alexidine is more rapid in its action. Overall, the formulation of these active agents is important in optimizing their antimicrobial activities. They are not sporicidal, but they do inhibit the outgrowth (but not the germination) of spores, and some sporicidal activity can be achieved in combination with other biocides or at higher temperatures (>70°C). They have limited activity against viruses, with some activity against the lipid-enveloped viruses (including significant nosocomial pathogens, such as human immunodeficiency virus and influenza virus) due to disruption of the viral envelope, and little activity against nonenveloped viruses. As with other biocides, mycobacteria are more resistant than other bacteria, presumably due to lack of penetration through their unique cell wall structures, but their growth can be inhibited at low concentrations, similar to bacteria. Biguanides also cause damage to active protozoal life stages (including trophozoites and amoebae) but have little or no effect on the viability of cysts or eggs, and they have been reported to be algistatic.

Advantages. Biguanides, in particular chlorhexidine, have been widely used for antisepsis due to little irritation of skin, wounds, and mucous membranes. Skin absorption has also been reported as being minimal. They have similar advantages, as alternatives to chlorine and bromine, in swimming pool maintenance. They are particularly effective in the control of hand transmission of pathogens in hospitals, including that of antibiotic-resistant bacteria, such as methicillin-resistant *Staphylococcus aureus*, and in the treatment of wounds. As chlorhexidine and alexidine can be present at bacteriostatic concentrations on the skin following washing, they can control the subsequent regrowth or contamination of the skin; this may be particularly important in the prevention of bacterial overgrowth on the skin when it is under occlusion (for example, when gloves are used) during surgical procedures.

Disadvantages. Some bacterial strains have developed increased tolerance of biguanides, which has been linked to plasmid-mediated cross-resistance to antibiotics. Although these changes may not be significant enough to allow growth at the bacteriostatic concentrations of biguanides, they have been speculated to promote antibiotic resistance (see section 8.7.3). Although limited, some cases of sensitivity (including anaphylactic shock) to biguanides have been reported, and contact with the eyes should be avoided. Chlorhexidine and other biguanides can be inactivated by nonionic surfactants, which can be present in some soaps and hand creams, natural soaps, and inorganic water contaminants (such as phosphates and chlorine). For PHMBs with limited broad-spectrum activity, the growth of algae, water-based molds, or bacterial biofilms can selectively develop over time in treated water.

Modes of Action. The mechanism of antimicrobial activity of chlorhexidine against bacteria and yeast has been well studied. Biguanides primarily act on cell membranes, causing loss of structure and function. Their biguanide chemical structure allows rapid absorption through bacterial and fungal cell walls and damage to the inner cell membranes (at higher concentrations), causing cytoplasm leakage and precipitation of proteins and nucleic acids. Direct insertion and interaction with the lipids in the cell membrane is the proposed primary mechanism. The proposed sequence of events during biguanide interaction with the gram-negative cell envelope is as follows. (i) There is rapid attraction toward the negatively charged bacterial cell surface, with strong and specific adsorption to phosphate-containing compounds. (ii) The integrity of the outer membrane is impaired, and further penetration toward the inner membrane occurs. (iii) Direct insertion into the membrane or binding to the phospholipids occurs, with an increase in inner-membrane permeability (K^+ loss), accompanied by bacteriostasis. In the cases of alexidine and the polymeric biguanides, the attraction to and interaction with the membrane lipids lead to the formation of lipid domains, with dramatic effects on membrane permeability due to loss of structure. (iv) Complete loss of membrane function follows, with precipitation of intracellular constituents and a bactericidal effect.

Mycobacteria are unique in their cell wall structure (see sections 1.3.4.1 and 8.4) and demonstrate varied resistances to chlorhexidine. *M. avium-M. intracellulare* is considerably resistant, while other species are inhibited at lower concentrations. This may be due to differences in the various cell wall structures that limit penetration of the biocide into the primary cell membrane target. The trophozoites, or "vegetative" forms of protozoa, such as *Acanthamoeba castellanii*, are sensitive to chlorhexidine due to membrane damage; however, the dormant cysts are much less sensitive, presumably due to limited penetration of the biocide. Similarly, chlorhexidine is effective against vegetative forms of bacteria but not bacterial spores. Even at high concentrations of the biguanide, no effects on the viability of *Bacillus* spores were observed at ambient temperatures, although at elevated temperatures a marked sporicidal effect was achieved. Presumably, sufficient changes occur in the spore structure to permit an increased uptake of the biguanide and interaction with internal constituents. Chlorhexidine does not inhibit germination but does inhibit the outgrowth of bacterial spores.

The antiviral activity of chlorhexidine is variable. Studies with different types of bacteriophages have shown that chlorhexidine has no effect on MS2 or K coliphages. High concentrations also failed to inactivate *P. aeruginosa* phage F116 and had no effect on phage DNA within the capsid or on phage proteins; the phage transduction process was more sensitive to chlorhexidine and other biocides than the phage itself. Chlorhexidine is not always considered a particularly effective antiviral agent, and its activity is restricted to the lipid-enveloped viruses. This appears to be due to disruption of the lipid viral envelopes, which can render the virus noninfectious. Chlorhexidine does not inactivate nonenveloped viruses, such as rotaviruses, hepatitis A virus, or polioviruses. Its activity appears to be restricted to the nucleic acid core or the outer coat, although it is likely that the latter is a more important target site.

3.9 DIAMIDINES

Types. The diamidines are a small group of antimicrobial agents with similar structures. The most widely used as antiseptics are propamidine and the halogenated dibromopropamidine. They are both provided in the isethionate salt form in drop, ointment, or cream formulations.

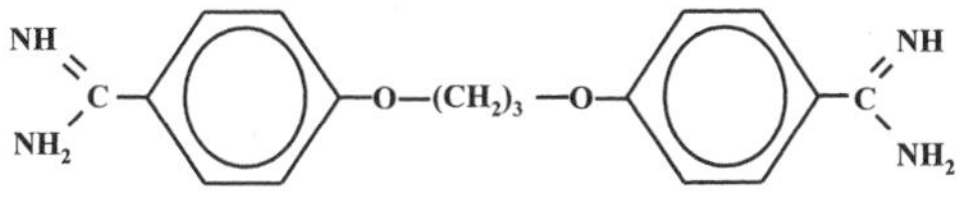

Propamidine

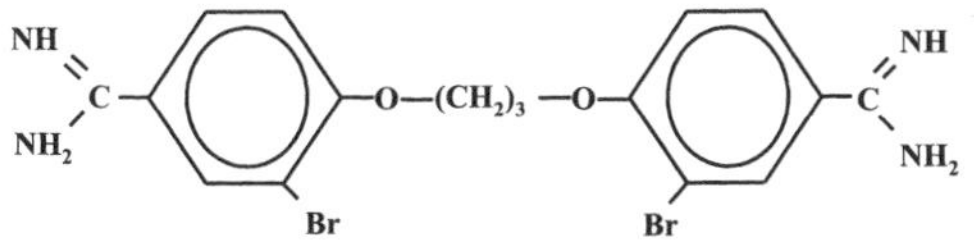

Dibromopropamidine

Applications. The diamidines are primarily used therapeutically in the treatment of skin, wound, or eye infections. Examples are creams and ointments containing up to 0.15% propamidine or dibromopropamidine, which are used for prevention or topical treatment of wounds. Other uses are in eye drops or ointments in the treatment of conjunctivitis (bacterial, fungal, and viral) and keratitis due to the amoeba *Acanthamoeba*, which is frequently implicated in contact lens contamination. Therapeutically, the diamidines are used for systemic infections with trypanosomes, *Leishmania* and *Pneumocystis*. Diamidine derivatives are the focus of research for further antiparasitic chemotherapy.

Spectrum of Activity. Propamidine and dibromopropamidine have similar spectra of activity. They are effective against bacteria, fungi, and parasites. Antibacterial activity is particularly marked against gram-positive bacteria, with a typical MIC range of 0.2 to 25 μg/ml; higher concentrations are required to inhibit the growth of gram-negative bacteria (25 to 500 μg/ml) and fungi (100 to 1,000 μg/ml). Many *Pseudomonas* species have demonstrated high resistance to diamidines. Activities against *Leishmania*, *Trypanosoma*, and *Pneumocystis* have also been investigated. The diamidines are effective against amoebae, including *Acanthamoeba*, but are poorly cysticidal (except when combined with 30% dimethyl sulfoxide as a carrier in formulation).

Advantages. The diamidines are not considered toxic in antiseptic applications and are safe for direct use in the eye (depending on the concentration used). They demonstrate broad-spectrum activity against bacteria and fungi and maintain activity in the presence of organic soils.

Disadvantages. Bacteria, fungi, and parasites resistant to diamidines have been described, including *Pseudomonas* species, which are common water contaminants. The activities of diamidines are dramatically affected under acidic (low-pH) conditions. In some cases, diamidines have caused skin irritation; side effects of renal and hepatic toxicity have also been reported, but primarily in chemotherapeutic applications.

Mode of Action. The mechanisms of action of the diamidines are considered similar to those of cationic surfactants (see section 3.16), due to their bipolar structure with interference in cell membrane structure and function. Their exact mechanism of action is unknown, but diamidines have been shown to inhibit membrane uptake, modify cell permeability, and induce leakage of amino acids. Their charge and hydrophobicity allow interaction with microbial cell surfaces and affinity with the negatively charged phospholipids of the cell membrane and other intracellular components (e.g., nucleic acids). Specific disruption and damage to the cell surfaces of *P. aeruginosa* and *Enterobacter cloacae* and the plasma membranes of amoebae have been described. It is clear that the diamidines (also similar to cationic surfactants) can further penetrate into the cytoplasm to cause denaturation and coagulation of proteins and enzymes; specific inhibition of various enzymes, including membrane-associated (e.g., ATPase) and intracellular (e.g., topoisomerases and decarboxylases) proteins, has been reported. The mode of action of diamidines has also been shown to include interaction with DNA, RNA, and nucleoside-containing compounds, leading to their precipitation. Interactions with DNA appear to be preferably at adenine-thymine tracts (referred to as "minor" grooves in the structure of DNA). In addition to primary effects on microbial membranes, the diamidines clearly inhibit DNA and RNA functions and those of proteins and enzymes.

3.10 ESSENTIAL OILS AND PLANT EXTRACTS

Types. The essential oils are a complex mixture of chemicals that are extracted from plants by concentration or distillation. They are widely distributed and are isolated from various plant parts, including flowers, leaves (or needles), wood, and roots (Table 3.2).

As secondary metabolites from plants, they have been ascribed various functions, including as natural biocides for the protection of plant cells from pathogens. Chemical analysis of these oils has shown that they consist of a range of terpenes, terpenoids, and oxides. Terpenes are hydrocarbons with the molecular formula $(C_5H_8)_n$ and are classified based on the number of repeating isoprene (five-carbon) units that they contain, such as monoterpenes (two isoprene units, e.g., pinene and camphor) and sesquiterpenes (three units, e.g., nerolidal). The terpenoids are oxygen-containing analogues, such as alcohols (geraniol and citronellol), phenols (thymol), aldehyde (neural and citronellal), and ketones (camphor). The oxides include various acids and sulfur compounds (e.g., eucalyptol). Tea tree oil, for example, contains over 100 compounds, including monoterpenes, sesquiterpenes, and various alcohols; the major biocide has been found to be the alcohol

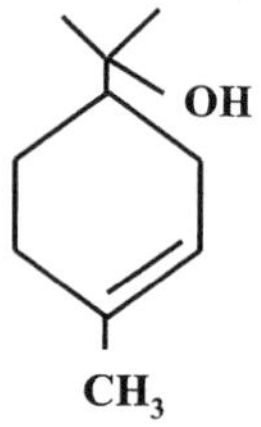

OH
CH_3
Terpineol

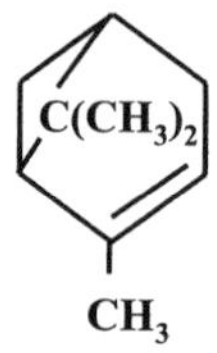

$C(CH_3)_2$
CH_3
Pinene

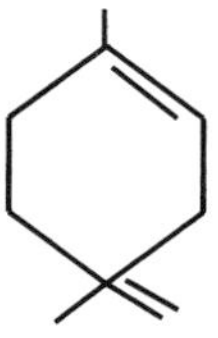

Limonene

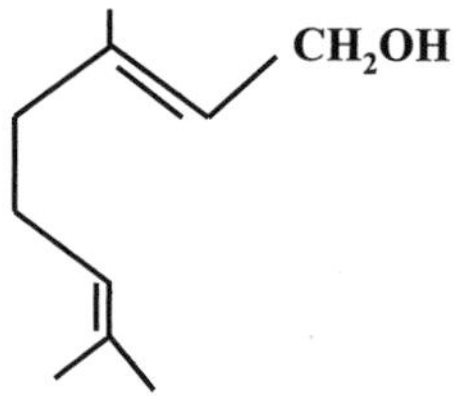

CH_2OH
Geraniol

TABLE 3.2 Various types and sources of essential oils

Oil	Source	Major biocides
Tea tree	*Melaleuca alternifolia*	Terpinen-4-ol (>30%), cineole (3%)
Pine	*Pinus* species	Pinene, terpineol
Lemon	*Citrus limon*	Limonene (90%)
Thyme	*Thymus vulgaris*	Thymol (20–30%)
Geranium	*Cymbopogan* species	Geraniol (85–90%)
Eucalyptus	*Eucalyptus globulus*	Cineol (>70%), various terpenes

terpinen-4-ol (generally present at ≥30%). Pine oil is isolated by steam distillation from wood chips and/or pine needles from various species of *Pinus*, and the major biocides identified are pinene and terpineol.

Applications. Essential oils have characteristic strong yet pleasant odors and have been used in various cleaners and deodorizers (Fig. 3.7). They are widely used as fragrances and traditionally as food preservatives (e.g., herbs and spices). Some have been used in antiseptics, including hand washes and mouthwashes and for acne treatment; they include tea tree oil, which has been particularly well studied and is used for various antiseptic applications. Pine oil has been widely used in cleaning and disinfection formulations. Its "fresh" smell is often associated with cleanliness; however, in its own right, it has little antimicrobial activity and is usually formulated with other biocides (particularly phenolics, including chlorophenols) for disinfectant applications. Similarly, lemon oil (containing ~90% limonene) and other citrus oils are used in cleaning and disinfection formulations. In addition to their biocidal properties, a variety of other chemotherapeutic and medicinal applications have been proposed for essential oils and their components.

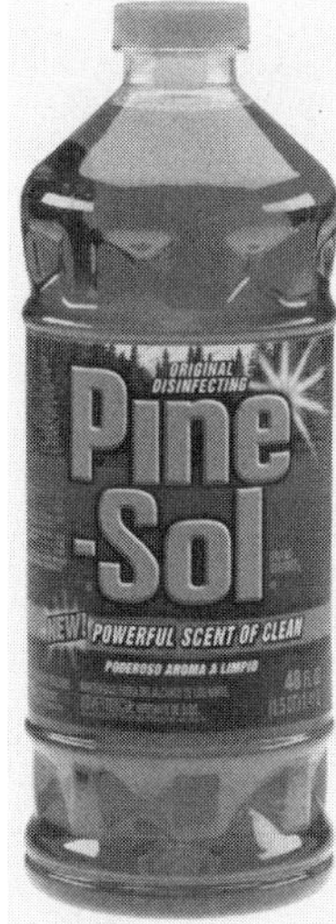

FIGURE 3.7 An example of an essential-oil-containing disinfectant.

Spectrum of Activity. Given the range of essential oils, their spectra of activity can vary considerably, from potent bactericidal or fungicidal activity to only narrow bacteriostatic or fungistatic activity and, in some cases, no appreciable biocidal activity. In general, essential oils demonstrate greater activity against gram-positive bacteria than gram-negative bacteria, with *Pseudomonas* and *Listeria* strains showing the greatest resistance; exceptions include the activity of pine oil against *Pseudomonas* (although less for some gram-positive bacteria) and the broad bactericidal activity of tea tree oil. The biocidal activity of tea tree oil has been particularly well studied; bactericidal activity has been described within the 0.25 to 0.5% range, with *Pseudomonas* being the most resistant. Tea tree oil is also effective against various fungi, particularly yeasts and dermatophytes (including *Candida* and *Trichophyton*, which can be commonly isolated from the skin or mucous membranes), with fungistatic activity at 0.03 to 0.5% and fungicidal activity at 0.06 to 1%. The main compounds with biocidal activity in tea tree oil appear to be terpin-4-ol, linalool, and α-terpineol. Some oils have been shown to inhibit the production of fungal alpha-toxins (e.g., geranium oils). The virucidal potentials of various oils have not been investigated in any detail, although some reports of tea tree oil have suggested activity against some enveloped viruses (such as herpes simplex viruses, associated with cold sores and other mucous membrane infections), but not the more resistant nonenveloped viruses. Some essential oils have been found to be mycobacteriostatic and sporistatic.

Advantages. Most essential oils demonstrate bacteriostatic and fungistatic activities at relatively low concentrations. Some oils also have broad bactericidal and fungicidal activities, with little associated irritancy at the concentrations typically used. They have pleasant odors and are considered biodegradable. Many have good compatibility with various treated surfaces, including skin and hard surfaces. Tea tree oil and other oils used on the skin have been shown to have some persistency, remaining active on the skin over time.

Disadvantages. The antimicrobial activities of essential oils are dependent on correct formulation, and product efficacies can range considerably. At high concentrations, they can be flammable and combustible. In some cases, skin irritancy has been described, and allergic reactions are common; there have been some concerns over skin and mucous membrane toxicity, with excessive use leading to poisoning. In some disinfectant applications, incompatibility with various elastomers (such as silicon rubber and polyvinyl chloride) has been described.

Modes of Action. The mechanisms of action of essential oils can be complex, depending on the hydrophobicity or hydrophilicity of the oil and the various biocidal components that can be present, including the potential synergism. Overall, they appear to cause effects similar to those described for phenolics (see section 3.14), particularly the predominantly hydrophobic oils (including terpenes). The major site of action is the cell membrane (including the outer membrane in gram-negative bacteria). Electron microscopy has shown the cell membrane structure to be disrupted, with parallel interference with various membrane functions, including disruption of the proton motive force (see sections 7.4.5 and 8.3.4) and leakage of cytoplasmic materials. Thymol and tea tree oil have been specifically shown to disrupt the outer and inner membranes of *E. coli*, leading to cytoplasmic leakage and eventual cell lysis; similar effects have been observed in gram-positive bacteria. As general cell poisons, other effects have been observed, including protein coagulation, cell wall disintegration, and inhibition of RNA, DNA, protein, and carbohydrate synthesis in bacteria and fungi. Specific studies with the fungus *Cladosporium herbarum* with eugenol and carvacrol have shown similar morphological changes, with lower concentrations affecting the activities of various cell wall-associated enzymes, reduced growth rates, and inhibition of stationary-phase phenomena, such as sporulation and secondary-metabolite production.

3.11 HALOGENS AND HALOGEN-RELEASING AGENTS

Types. Halogens are a group of elements that are physically distinct but show similarities in their chemical reactivities. They include fluorine (F_2), chlorine (Cl_2), bromine (Br_2), and iodine (I_2). Chemically, they have high electronegativity and are highly reactive as oxidizing agents, in the order $F_2 > Cl_2 > Br_2 > I_2$. Physically, at room temperature and atmospheric pressure, iodine is a solid, bromine is a liquid, and fluorine and chlorine are both gases. Chlorine, iodine, and bromine are widely used as disinfectants and antiseptics.

I - I
Iodine

Br - Br
Bromine

Cl - Cl
Chlorine

Iodine (I; atomic weight, 126.9) is a bluish-black shiny solid that is readily soluble in organic solvents (such as alcohol or chloroform) but only slightly soluble in water. It can also sublime into a purple-blue gas with an irritating odor. It is found naturally in seawater and subterranean brines and can be synthesized by reaction of potassium iodide with copper sulfate. The chemistry of iodine in water is complicated by the formation of various iodine-containing species (Fig. 3.8), but only two contribute to the overall antimicrobial activity: "free," or "molecular," iodine (I_2) and hypoiodous acid (HOI).

Simple iodine solutions are prepared by dissolving iodine, potassium iodide, or sodium

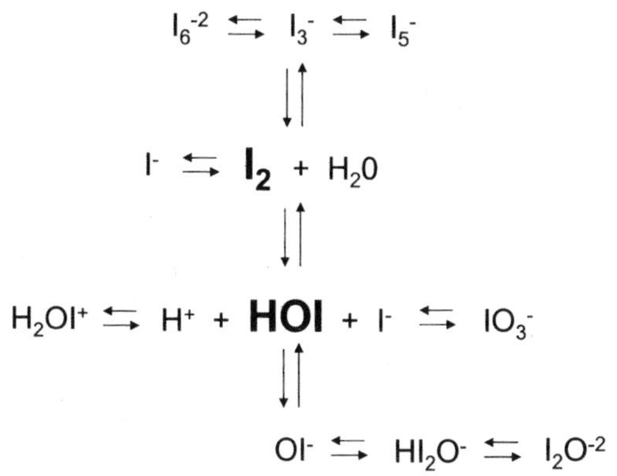

$$I_6^{-2} \rightleftharpoons I_3^- \rightleftharpoons I_5^-$$
$$\updownarrow$$
$$I^- \rightleftharpoons \mathbf{I_2} + H_2O$$
$$\updownarrow$$
$$H_2OI^+ \rightleftharpoons H^+ + \mathbf{HOI} + I^- \rightleftharpoons IO_3^-$$
$$\updownarrow$$
$$OI^- \rightleftharpoons HI_2O^- \rightleftharpoons I_2O^{-2}$$

FIGURE 3.8 Simplified chemistry of iodine in water, demonstrating those species important for biocidal activity.

iodide in water or alcohol. Examples are tincture of iodine (2% iodine and 2.4% potassium iodide in ethanol) and Lugol's solution (5% iodine and 10% potassium iodide in water). Alternatively, elemental iodine can be complexed or bound with high-molecular-weight neutral polymers, including alcohol, amide, and sugar polymers. These complexes are known as iodophors and have the benefit of increasing the solubility and stability of iodine by allowing the active iodine species to be slowly released over time. The most widely used iodophor is poly(*N*-vinyl-2-pyrrolidone), which is complexed with iodine in the triiodide form (povidone-iodine [PVPI]) (Fig. 3.9). PVPI solutions or formulations can be prepared in an aqueous (water) or organic (e.g., alcohol) base; for example, a 10%

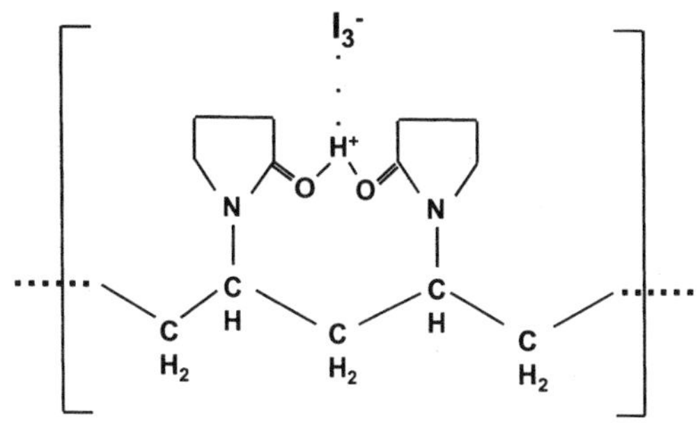

PVPI

FIGURE 3.9 The structure of PVPI. The polymer consists of repeating units of the base structure shown, with particle sizes of 90 to 140 μm.

PVPI solution in water gives an active iodine (I_2) concentration of 0.03 to 0.04% (Fig. 3.10). A further example of an iodophor is poloxamer-iodine.

Chlorine (Cl; atomic weight, 35.45) is a yellow-green gas with a strong, irritating odor. It is found in reduced forms in nature as sodium (NaCl, or common salt), calcium, and potassium salts. For antiseptic and disinfection purposes, "chlorine" refers to the presence of active, or "oxidized," chlorine compounds, which are formed in water (Fig. 3.11). They include Cl_2 (elemental chlorine), OCl^- (hypochlorite ion), and HOCl (hypochlorous acid).

The antimicrobial activity of "chlorine" in water (or "free available chlorine") is a combination of Cl_2, HOCl, and OCl^- but is predominantly due to HOCl. Chloride ions (Cl^-) are

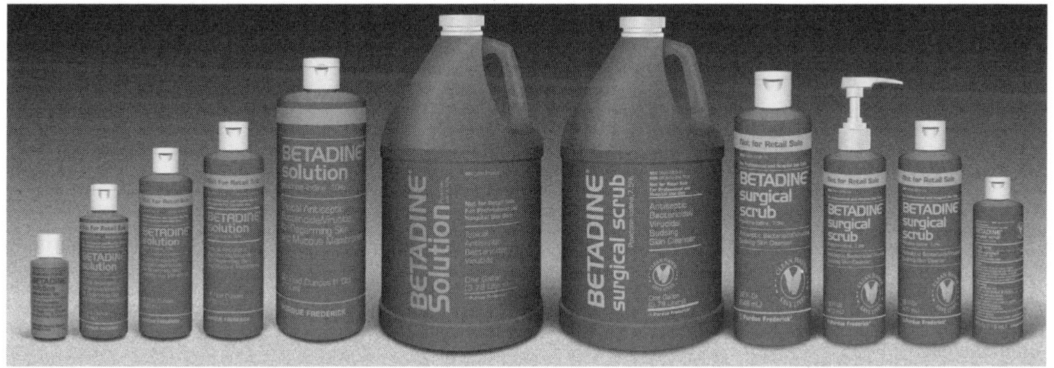

FIGURE 3.10 Various types of PVPI antiseptic products. Reproduced with permission from Purdue Products L.P.

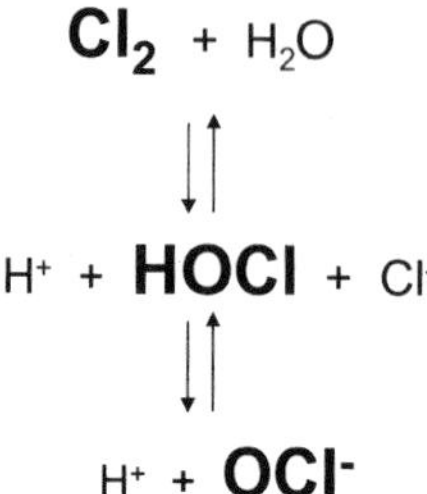

FIGURE 3.11 Simplified chemistry of chlorine in water, demonstrating those species important for biocidal activity.

inactive. Inorganic chloramines or other nitrochloro compounds may also be formed by the reaction of chlorine with ammonia and other nitrogen-containing compounds. They include monochloramine (NH_2Cl) and dichloramine ($NHCl_2$), which can act as chlorine-releasing agents but are considered weak disinfectants. The antimicrobial activity of available chlorine varies depending on the concentration, temperature, and pH. As for other biocides, the efficacy increases with temperature and concentration. In addition, the dissociation of HOCl increases at higher pH, with greater production of OCl^- and less antimicrobial efficacy; the optimal pH for activity is 4 to 7, under which conditions HOCl is the dominant species. Further, the presence of reducing agents, such as iron and copper ions, catalyzes dissociation and reduces the available chlorine. Similar decreases in activity can be observed in the presence of protein, other organic material, and UV light.

The most important sources of chlorine are chlorine gas, hypochlorites, and chloramines. Chlorine gas is provided as a compressed, amber-colored liquid, which rapidly forms a gas on release at atmospheric pressure and room temperature. It is extremely irritating and corrosive, with a detectable odor at a concentration as low as 3.5 ppm, and it is fatal at 1,000 ppm. It can be directly added to water to form HOCl and is rarely used as a fumigant gas due to safety risks. Hypochlorites are the most widely used sources of chlorine and include powders and liquid preparations. Powders or tablets contain sodium and potassium hypochlorites mixed with trisodium phosphate. Calcium hypochlorite [$Ca(OCl)_2$] is a dry white solid used in powdered or tablet form that can be added directly to a surface or in water. Liquid forms include sodium or potassium hypochlorite solutions, which typically contain 1 to 15% available chlorine. Sodium hypochlorite (NaOCl) solutions have a clear to light-yellow color (depending on the concentration) with a distinctive chlorine odor. They include household bleach solutions, which are generally at ~5% and contain product stabilizers.

A variety of chloramines (as liquids and powders) also possess antimicrobial activity, although to a lesser extent than hypochlorite. They include inorganic chloramines, such as monochloramine and dichloramine (discussed above), and organic chloramines, including chloramine T (sodium *p*-toluene sulfonchloramide), sodium dichloroisocyanurate, and halazone (*p*-sulfondichloramidobenzoic acid) (Fig. 3.12). Organic chloramines are formed by the reaction of HOCl with amine or imine compounds. In general, they are less irritating and more stable but release lower concentrations of active chlorine in solution. Other chlorine-releasing compounds are interhalogens, such as bromine chloride (in which bromine is actually the key antimicrobial when added to water) and the *N*-halamines. The *N*-halamines are nitrogen-containing compounds with anchored chlorine or bromine atoms, which can be released on contact with microorganisms. They can be used integrated into antimicrobial surfaces (as polymers) or as water-soluble monomers, which can subsequently be reactivated by applying a chlorine- or bromine-containing liquid formulation. Chlorine-releasing examples are 1-chloro-2,2,5,5-tetramethyl-1,3-imidazolidin-4-one (water soluble and monomeric) and poly-1,3-dichloro-5-methyl-5-(4′-vinylphenyl) hydantoin (water insoluble and polymeric). Chlorine has also been successfully used in synergism with other halogens, such as low concentrations of iodine and bromine (e.g., *N*-bromo-*N*-chlorodimethylhydantoin). Newer methods of chlorine production include

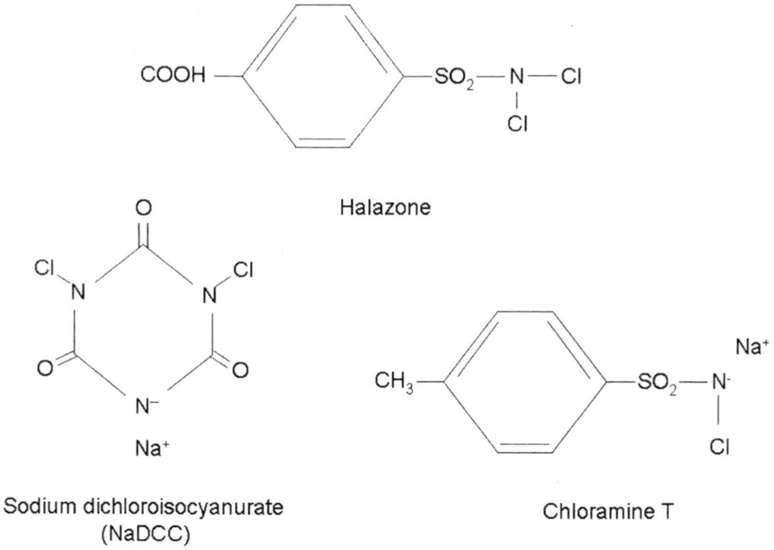

Halazone

Sodium dichloroisocyanurate (NaDCC)

Chloramine T

FIGURE 3.12 Examples of organic chloramines.

the use of electrolysis of sodium chloride (or other chloride salts) to form chlorine compounds and other oxidizing agents, which have rapid antimicrobial activities. Another important chlorinated compound is chlorine dioxide, which is considered in section 3.13 below.

Bromine (Br; atomic weight, 79.9) is a volatile reddish-brown liquid that can give off a red vapor with an unpleasant and irritating odor. Care should be taken in the handling of liquid bromine, as it poses a serious health risk. Bromine occurs naturally and is extracted in the form of bromide from seawater as a sodium salt (NaBr). When bromine is dissolved in water, hypobromous acid (HOBr) and the hypobromite ion (OBr^-) are formed; both are responsible for the antimicrobial activity observed. Further reaction of bromine with ammonia or nitrogen compounds produces bromamines, which also contribute to the microbicidal activity. The bromide ion (Br^-) itself is inactive but can be reactivated to active bromine species (Br_2, HOBr, and OBr^-) by reaction with a strong oxidizer, such as chlorine species and potassium peroxymonosulfate. Typical bromine sources for water or liquid disinfection include liquid bromine, sodium bromide (NaBr, together with an activating agent), bromine chloride (BrCl), and bromine-releasing agents (Fig. 3.13), such as BCDMH (1-bromo-3-chloro-5,5-dimethylhydantoin; $BrClC_5H_6O_2N_2$), DBDMH (1,3-dibromo-5,5-dimethylhydantoin; $C_5H_6Br_2N_2O_2$), STABREX (a stabilized liquid of oxidized bromide), and bronopol (2-bromo-2-nitro-1,3-propanediol; $C_3H_6BrNO_4$). Typical bromine-releasing agents, including BCDMH, are supplied as tablets, which when dissolved in water release HOBr and HOCl, in which the available chlorine can further activate bromide species (Br^-) to give other active HOBr and OBr^- species. Similarly, sodium bromide is usually provided in a two-step method, first with the addition and dissolution of NaBr in water to produce Br^-, which is subsequently activated by a strong oxidizer. More recent applications have included the impregnation of bromine into resins or polymers, e.g., polyethylenimine, poly(4-vinyl-*N*-alkylpyridinium bromide), and bromine-based *N*-halamines (Fig. 3.13). An example is poly-1, 3-dibromo-5-methyl-5-(4′-vinylphenyl)hydantoin (PSHB), which is a water-insoluble polymeric *N*-halamine (Fig. 3.13). Bromine-based com-

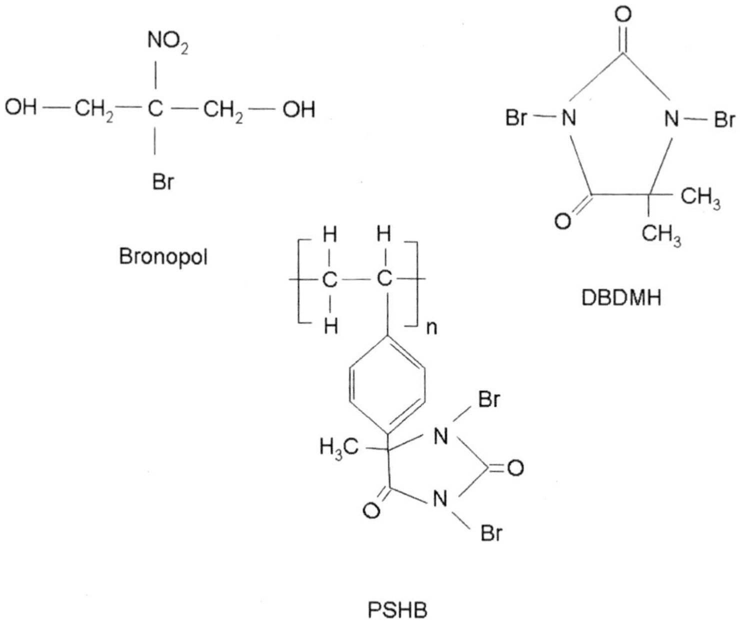

Bronopol

DBDMH

PSHB

FIGURE 3.13 Typical bromine-releasing agents. PSHB is an example of a water-insoluble polymeric *N*-halamine.

pounds are also used as corrosion inhibitors in biocide formulations, e.g., benzoltriazole. Methyl bromide (CH_3Br) is used for restrictive applications as a stable gas, on its own or in combination with chloropicrin. At typical concentrations, it is colorless, tasteless, odorless, and nonflammable. It is supplied as a compressed liquid, which rapidly vaporizes on release at room temperature. Due to safety and environmental concerns, methyl bromide is not widely used and requires special handling for fumigation applications, e.g., as an insecticide in soil.

Fluorine (F; atomic weight, 18.99) is one of the most reactive chemicals known. It is a pale-yellow gas with a pungent odor, detectable at very low concentrations (in the part-per-billion range). It is widely used for industrial purposes, including the production of uranium and fluorochemicals, including antibiotics (fluoroquinolones), plastics, and refrigerants. Its presence in water as fluoride (at <1 mg/liter) is claimed to reduce the incidence of dental cavities by direct reaction with tooth enamel hydroxyapatite and some minor bacteriostatic effect. A variety of fluoride compounds are used for water treatment, laundry detergents, toothpastes, mouthwashes, and varnishes. They include silicofluorides (e.g., sodium fluorosilicates), stannous fluoride, and amine fluorides. Oral antiseptic treatments may play a role in controlling periodontal (below the gum line) infections. Sodium and potassium fluoride have been used as preservatives, but concerns with toxicity have limited their used. These compounds are not considered further.

Applications

Iodine. Iodine has been particularly widely used as an antiseptic. Its uses include the reduction of the microbial population on intact skin in preoperative preparation or surgical scrubs and for therapeutic applications on wounds and burns. Traditional solutions in water or alcohol are still used for wound or other topical localized applications. They include tincture of iodine and Lugol's solutions. However, these solutions can be irritating, particularly in repeated applications. Iodophors have allowed greater flexibility in the use of iodine in antiseptic and disinfectant liquids, dry powders, and lotions. A variety of formulations are available, including solutions with surfactants and buffers, which are used as surgical scrubs, preoperative preparations, shampoos (antidandruff), and wound cleansers (for further discussion, see section 4.5). Iodophor formulations are also used as general surface sanitizers and disinfectants, especially in agricultural and veterinary applications and for equipment, walls, and floors. They are less used for medical-device disinfection, and generally only for noncritical applications. "Iodination" is defined as the use of iodine for water disinfection, including drinking water, wastewater, and swimming pool treatment. Low-level iodination (at 1 ppm) is recommended in urgent cases, which include the addition of iodine-releasing tablets or direct addition of a few drops of an iodine solution to drinking water. Some synergistic applications are the addition of inactive iodide (I^-), which is activated by reaction with another oxidizing agent, such as hypochloride (HOCl). Air fumigation with iodine vapor has been described, but applications have been limited due to the risks of severe irritation and respiratory damage.

Chlorine. Available chlorine has been particularly widely used for water disinfection. In fact, drinking water chlorination has been responsible for the control of formerly widespread diseases, such as cholera (caused by *Vibrio cholerae*) and typhoid (caused by *Salmonella enterica* serovar Typhi). Typical concentrations for drinking water range from 0.5 to 1 mg of available chlorine/liter, usually provided by addition of elemental chlorine or calcium hypochlorite. Chloramines, such as sodium dichloroisocyanurate, have been recommended as alternatives to hypochlorites due to delayed release of chlorine and greater activity in the presence of contaminating soils. Hypochlorites are also used as bleaching agents for laundry or other applications. Other water applications are recreational water (swimming pools and hot tubs) and wastewater, both typically at higher concentrations of 1 to 3 mg of available chlorine/liter. In addition to microbial control, chlorine and chloramines are useful for neutralizing sulfide odors due to oxidation of compounds such as hydrogen sulfide and dimethyltrisulfide and for masking other odors. Chlorine is also widely used for the sanitization of water supply systems and pipe work. Hypochlorites, particularly liquid sodium hypochlorite or "bleach" solutions, are commonly used for hard-surface disinfection in households, hospitals, and food-handling establishments and other industrial settings (Fig. 3.14). They include direct applications (sprays and wipes) and indirect fogging methods. Direct application to food has also been shown to be effective in reducing the risk of pathogen contamination, including *Salmonella* and *Listeria*. Chlorine has also been used in the past for wound or mucous membrane antiseptics, including calcium hypochlorite powders, chloramine T, and Dakin's solution (based on sodium hypochlorite). The *N*-halamines and other chlorine-releasing agents have been incorporated into surface polymers (such as clothing, bench tops, and filters) to provide intrinsic antimicrobial activity; the *N*-halamines have the advantage of being regenerated by application of a hypochlorite solution.

In some applications, it is necessary to remove residual chlorine following disinfec-

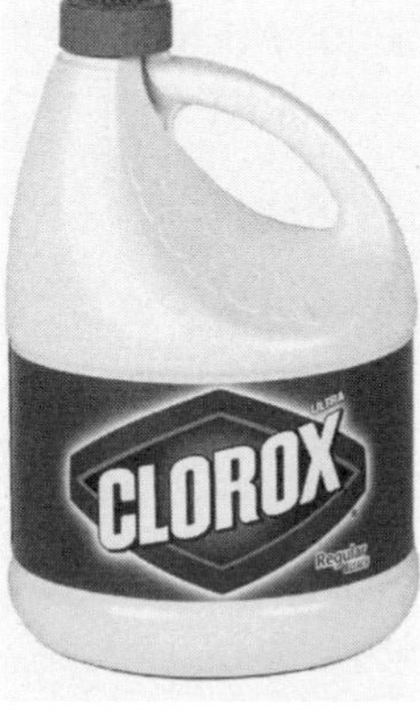

FIGURE 3.14 Sodium hypochlorite (bleach)-based disinfectant. A concentrate (which is diluted in water prior to use) is shown. Courtesy of The Clorox Sales Company.

tion; an example is the use of water to produce steam, where the presence of chlorine gas causes corrosion of stainless steel and other metals. This can be achieved by reaction with neutralizers, including activated carbon, sodium metabisulfite, sodium bisulfite, and sulfur dioxide.

Bromine. Applications for bromine and bromine-releasing agents are primarily restricted to recreational- and industrial-water disinfection, including swimming pools, baths, and cooling systems and towers. Other applications are wastewater treatment and odor control, and to a lesser extent drinking water. Typical applications are at 2 to 4 mg/liter over wide temperature (5 to 45°C) and pH (pH 6.5 to 9.5) ranges. Bromine has also been used as a broad-spectrum disinfectant, including fogging applications, or for control of fungal diseases of plants. Methyl bromide has limited applications as a fumigant, particularly as an insecticide, nematocide, herbicide, and fungicide for crops, plants, and soil. The gas can be used on its own or in combination with 2 mg of chloropicrin/liter. Typical applications use methyl bromide at 16 to 24 g/m^3 at room temperature (15 to 25°C) for 12 to 24 h. Primary applications are generally restricted to agriculture, including foodstuffs, clothing, soil fumigation, and plants. Similar to chlorine-based *N*-halamines, bromine *N*-halamines have been integrated into various surfaces to provide an antimicrobial barrier.

Spectrum of Activity. The halogens have similar broad-spectrum antimicrobial profiles, depending on the concentration and control of the application.

Iodine. Molecular iodine (I_2) and, to a lesser extent, hypoiodous acid are broad-spectrum biocides, with potent bactericidal, fungicidal, tuberculocidal, and virucidal activities. Activity has also been reported against actinomycetes and rickettsias. Reports vary, depending on the formulation and test conditions (pH, temperature, etc.). Aqueous iodine solutions are more active under acidic pH, due to the optimal presence of molecular iodine species, with the prevalence of other ions at alkaline pH. Iodophors can be formulated over a wider pH range, due to the slow release of iodine. Although the antimicrobial activity is maintained, iodophors are considered less active against certain fungi and spores than tinctures. Iodine can be sporicidal, particularly in hard-surface disinfectants, but generally not at the concentrations used for antiseptic applications. For example, vegetative bacteria are rapidly killed at 0.01 to 1 mg of available iodine/liter in 1 min but require 10 mg/liter for bacterial spore activity with up to 5 h of contact time. Nonenveloped viruses, as with other halogens, demonstrate the greatest resistance to iodine but are generally sensitive at concentrations as low as 15 μg/liter. The microbicidal effects can be improved by various formulation effects, particularly for application on hard surfaces. Activity has been reported against the encysted form of *Giardia*, with a much smaller effect against the oocysts of *Cryptosporidium*. Iodine has poor algicidal activity but is an effective insecticide and nematocide.

Chlorine. Available chlorine is well established as a broad-spectrum biocide. Vegetative bacteria are readily sensitive to very low concentrations of chlorine (0.1 to 0.3 mg/liter within 30 s), but mycobacteria, fungi, protozoan cysts, algae, viruses, and bacterial spores are significantly more resistant. Chlorine has also been used for the removal and disinfection of biofilms common in water systems in order to control pathogens such as pseudomonads and *Legionella*. Chlorine is effective against enveloped and nonenveloped viruses, even in the presence of soil contamination. Other forms of life, including fish, frogs, and plants, are also affected at higher concentrations. Special consideration should be given to the control of protozoan cysts, particularly *Cryptosporidium* oocysts, and parasitic worm eggs, which demonstrate greater tolerance of chlorine but are sensitive to higher concentrations in drinking water. Chlorine is slowly effective in the control of algal growth. *N*-Chloro compounds, including chloramines, are considered less effective than hypochlorites, with greater activity under acidic conditions and in the presence of organic soils. Sodium hypochlorite solutions (at 2.5%, or 25,000 mg of available chlorine/liter) have been shown to be effective against prions.

Bromine. Bromine demonstrates broad-spectrum activity, including bactericidal, mycobactericidal, fungicidal, slimicidal, cysticidal, and virucidal activities. Viruses and bacteria are sensitive at relatively low concentrations (0.3 mg/liter); in the case of viruses, higher concentrations (10 to 20 mg/liter) are required to achieve total inactivation and degradation of the viral structure and nucleic acid. Bromine has algicidal activity similar to that of chlorine, and protozoan (*Entamoeba*) cysts were inactivated at 1.5 mg/liter. Bromine has also been used for biofilm control (removal and disinfection) in water systems.

Advantages

Iodine. As topical biocides, iodine solutions are widely available and easy to prepare. They demonstrate broad-spectrum antimicrobial activity at relatively low concentrations on the skin and may have some short-lived persistent activity, remaining on the skin after application to provide residual antimicrobial activity. Iodophors present the greatest advantages, as they are generally nonstaining and water soluble, have little or no odor, increase the stability of iodine in solution, and minimize the concentration of iodine required for antimicrobial activity. Minimal concentrations of iodine reduce any toxicity, discoloration, or irritation. As disinfectants, iodophors and iodine solutions can tolerate the presence of contaminating soils, as seen with other halogens, such as chlorine. As water disinfectants, they have little or no odor or taste and are not irritating to the eyes at typical concentrations; iodine is generally used for water treatment only in emergencies.

Chlorine. Chlorine is well accepted as an antimicrobial with reliable broad-spectrum activity. For water and surface disinfection, it is colorless, cost-effective, and easy to handle. It retains some activity in the presence of some organic materials and at high water hardness levels, depending on the chlorine and soil concentrations. Chlorine-releasing agents are relatively stable and allow demand release over time for preservation efficacy. At typical concentrations, chlorine is not toxic and can be routinely monitored. In addition to microbicidal activity, chlorine also oxidizes some unwanted and harmful organic and inorganic compounds that may be present, particularly for sulfide odor control. At lower concentrations, chlorine is an efficient wound cleanser. Due to its bleaching activity, chlorine solutions are used for removing stains on surfaces and clothing.

Bromine. Bromine compounds are well-established, broad-spectrum antimicrobials. In comparison to chlorine, bromine is considered less volatile and less toxic to aquatic life, but with a similar level of irritation. Bronopol, in particular, has a lower toxicity profile. It is also less corrosive, odorless, relatively safe to use, and easy to handle. Residual bromide ions (Br^-) formed following the reaction of active bromine species with microorganisms can be reactivated by use of a strong oxidizer. Bromine is more effective at higher pH than chlorine and demonstrates good algicidal activity at lower concentrations than other halogens. Methyl bromide is a particularly efficacious and low-cost fumigant.

Disadvantages

Iodine. Iodine causes brown stains on surfaces, including skin, clothing, and porous materials, such as plastics. Iodine solutions are poisonous at high concentrations (>5%) and can be irritating to broken skin and mucous membranes, particularly in combination with alcohol. Surface compatibility can be a concern with some metals (corrosion) and plastic surfaces. It should be noted that many of these disadvantages are significantly reduced with the use of iodophors, such as PVPI. Although it is not substantiated, there has been some speculation regarding health complications, e.g., thyroid function; this is considered unlikely with the concentrations typically used.

Chlorine. Chlorine is an aggressive chemical that can promote corrosion of metal surfaces, particularly at higher concentrations. This is especially important when water is heated, which can cause the release of chlorine gas, which is particularly corrosive. At higher concentrations, chlorine is irritating and can lead to hypersensitivity. This is primarily due to the production of inorganic chloramines on reaction with ammonia and nitrogen-containing compounds, which are also responsible for strong chlorine odors from treated water. Further, chlorine can be toxic to fish and other aquatic species. Concentrated solutions should be handled with care, as they can be toxic to humans. Reaction of chlorine with some organic molecules can lead to the production of disinfection by-products, such as trihalomethanes (THMs), including chloroform and bromodichloromethane. THMs are potential carcinogens and are monitored for acceptable levels in drinking water. Typical chlorine odors are detected at ~0.3 mg/liter, with further odorous by-products that can be formed by reactions with phenols (chlorophenols), and amino acids or peptides (aldehydes, including methional and acetaldehyde). Contaminating protein, inorganic ions (including iron), and reducing agents neutralize chlorine but can be compensated for by increasing the biocide dosage. Chlorine antiseptics are not widely used due to concerns over delayed healing and wound irritation.

Bromine. The formation of bromate, THMs, and haloacetic acids as by-products of water disinfection are a concern, since they have been labeled potential human carcinogens. Although it is less toxic than chlorine, high concentrations of bromine are considered a hazard to aquatic life. Bromine, similar to other halogens, is degraded by UV light and the presence of reducing agents, which can decrease the overall efficacy of disinfection. In general, bromine is more expensive than chlorine for water disinfection. Bromine is considered less corrosive than chlorine but can still result in significant surface damage over time and at higher concentrations. Methyl bromide has been banned in certain countries due to occupational risks related to respiratory damage and long-term accumulation in body tissues, leading to severe damage. It is also known to be a delayed neurotoxin. Its ability to damage the ozone layer is another concern.

Mode of Action

Iodine. Active iodine species, as reactive oxidizing agents, have multiple effects on the cell surface (cell wall and membrane) and in the cytoplasm. As with other halogens, the exact modes of action are unknown. Iodine has a dramatic effect on microbial surfaces but also rapidly penetrates into microorganisms. Reactive iodine species have been shown to attack amino acids (particularly lysine, histidine, cysteine, and arginine) to cause protein disruption and loss of structure and function. Iodine reacts with and substitutes for various functional groups on these amino acids. Further, iodine reacts with nucleic acids, lipids, and fatty acids (including those in the cell membrane structures). These effects culminate in loss of cell function and death. Less is known about iodine's antiviral action, but nonlipid viruses and parvoviruses are less sensitive than lipid-enveloped viruses. It is likely that iodine attacks the surface proteins of enveloped viruses, but it may also destabilize membrane fatty acids by reacting with unsaturated carbon bonds. Similar effects are observed against nonenveloped viruses. The effects of iodine and iodophors against protozoan parasites and prions have not been well investigated.

Chlorine. The mode of action of chlorine has been investigated, and it clearly has multiple modes of action by oxidation of proteins, lipids, and carbohydrates. This is expected, as chlorine and chlorine-releasing agents are highly active oxidizing agents. Potentiation of oxidation may occur at low pH (pH 4 to 7), where the activity of chlorine is maximal, although increased penetration of outer cell layers may be achieved in the neutral state. Hypochlorous acid has long been considered the active moiety responsible for bacterial inactivation, with the OCl^- ion having a minute effect compared to HOCl. This correlates with the observation that chlorine activity is greatest when the percentage of HOCl is highest. This concept also applies to chlorine-releasing agents. The primary mode of action is believed to be against structural and functional proteins, both on the microorganism surface and internally. Sulfhydral groups of essential enzymes appear to be particularly targeted, as well as nitrogen interactions on amino acids. Even low concentrations have a dramatic effect on the activities of metabolic enzymes in vitro. Direct protein degradation into smaller peptides and precipitation have been shown and are believed to be the main modes of action against prions. Other observed effects are cell wall and membrane disruption by attacking structural proteins, lipids, and carbohydrates. Hypochlorous acid has also been found to disrupt oxidative phosphorylation and other membrane-associated enzyme activities. Further effects have been reported on nucleic acids, including the formation of chlorinated derivatives of nucleotide bases. Studies of specific effects on the growth of *E. coli* have shown inhibition of bacterial growth by hypochlorous acid. At relatively low concentrations (~50 μM, or ~3 ppm active chlorine), growth inhibition was observed within 5 min, with nearly complete inhibition of DNA synthesis but only partial inhibition of protein synthesis and no obvious membrane disruption, suggesting that intercellular DNA synthesis was a particularly sensitive target at inhibitory concentrations of chlorine. Specific effects on viral nucleic acids are expected and have been reported. Direct degradation of poliovirus RNA into fragments has been observed, in addition to severe morphological changes and disintegration of the viral capsid.

Direct effects on macromolecules are probably responsible for the observed sporicidal activity of chlorine. Direct studies of chlorine's effect on spores have shown that they lose refractivity, followed by separation of the spore coats from the cortex and inner-cortex lysis. Further studies have also reported increased permeability of the normally resistant spore coat, which leads to biocide penetration and spore death.

Bromine. Similar to other halogens, bromine oxidizes organic molecules, including proteins, nucleic acids, and lipids. It is generally accepted that the culmination of the resulting structural and functional damage is cell death and loss of viral-particle infectivity. Direct reaction with viral coats and nucleic acids has been described. Methyl bromide has been shown to react with the sulfhydryl groups of proteins and enzymes, which leads to the inhibition of cellular biochemical processes.

3.12 METALS

Types. Metals are a group of elements that may be chemically defined as having a shiny or lustrous surface and are generally good conductors of electricity and heat. Metals form positive ions (cations) in water, which is the basis of their antimicrobial and toxic effects. It should be noted that many metals (including sodium, potassium, calcium, and iron) are essential for life, but at high concentrations, they are toxic by disruption of cellular functions and structure. The metals that are specifically used as antiseptics and disinfectants are often called "heavy" metals. This is a vague term that does not have a precise chemical definition, but generally, it is used to describe metallic elements with a specific density greater than 4 or 5, with the corresponding "light" metals (such as calcium and sodium) having lower densities. The heavy metals include known toxic elements, such as mercury, cadmium, arsenic, and lead, as well as the less toxic and more widely used silver and copper-containing compounds. Many metals have been traditionally used as biocides, but bioaccumulation and toxicity concerns have limited their recent applications. For example,

Ag^{2+}	Cu^{2+}
Silver	Copper

mercury is unique as a liquid metal and has been used in various forms (including elemental mercury, organic compounds, and inorganic compounds) as an antiseptic, disinfectant, and preservative. Examples are merbromin, nitromersol, and mercurochrome. Other examples are arsenic and tin compounds; tin compounds, including tributyltin oxide and tributyltin acetate, are considered less toxic than mercury for preservative applications. Due to their decreased use, these metals are not further considered in detail.

The most widely used biocidal metals are copper and silver compounds. Copper (Cu; atomic weight, 63.55) in minute quantities is an essential element for plants, animals, and other forms of life. It is commercially available in a variety of forms, with a typical copper (yellow-brown) color. Elemental copper is rarely used, with copper sulfate ($CuSO_4$) and other copper-containing compounds (including cupric chloride, copper-8-quinolinolate, copper naphthenate, and cuprous oxide) more frequently used. Copper sulfate pentahydrate is a blue crystalline solid that is readily soluble in water. The copper ion (Cu^{2+}) is the actual biocide, but it may be used in synergy with other active agents.

Silver (Ag; atomic weight, 107.87) is not an essential element. Widely used biocidal silver compounds are silver nitrate ($AgNO_3$) and silver sulfadiazine (AgSD), in which the silver ion (Ag^{2+}) is the active species. Silver nitrate is a white crystalline powder that readily dissolves in water. Silver sulfadiazine (Fig. 3.15) is generally provided as a cream or liquid solution. It is essentially a combination of two antibacterial agents, silver and sulfadazine. Silver (as metallic silver, silver nitrate, or silver oxide) has also been integrated into polymers, filters, and other surfaces to allow its slow release over time. Synergistic preparations have included chlorhexidine, cerium nitrate, and combination with copper ions.

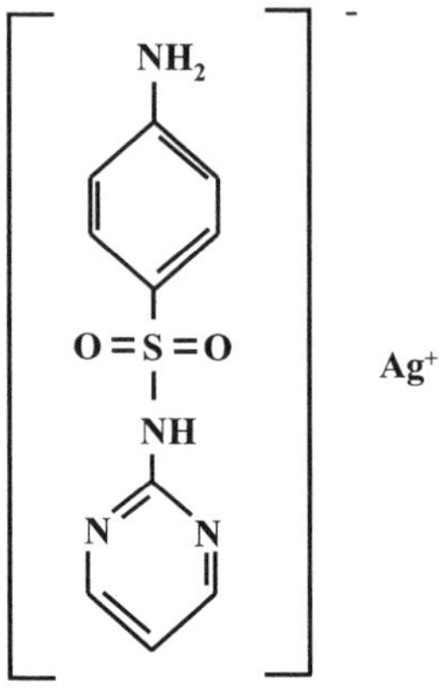

Silver sulfadiazine

FIGURE 3.15 Silver sulfadiazine.

Applications

Copper. Copper has been widely used as a fungicide for agricultural applications, including direct application to plants. An example is the Bordeaux mixture (first used in France on grape vines), a mixture of copper sulfate and calcium hydroxide, which is used as a crop spray. Other applications are water treatment and preservation. Copper is an effective water disinfectant at low concentrations, including drinking and recreational water. A typical application for swimming pools is at <3 μg of copper sulfate/ml, particularly for control of algae. Electrolytic generators may also be used, such as for *Legionella* control in hospital and industrial hot- and cold-water supply pipes, as an alternative to chlorine treatment. They consist of an electrode cell with copper-containing anodes to which a current is supplied to cause the release of copper ions into the water flow. Typically, these generators are provided with copper and silver anodes to produce effective ion concentrations at approximately 0.4 and 0.04 mg/liter, respectively. The ion levels can be controlled by varying the current applied to the cell. An example of a copper-silver ionization system is shown in Fig. 3.16.

Copper compounds are also used as preservatives in paints, cement, fabrics, and wood; higher concentrations in some paints may be used to provide an antimicrobial barrier on surfaces, especially for fungal control. Some older antiseptics have been used for topical treatment

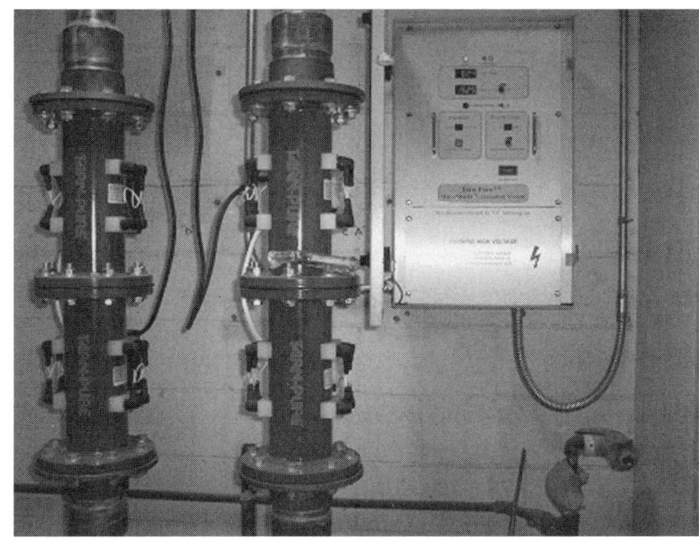

FIGURE 3.16 A typical copper-silver ionization system. The electrode cell consists of copper and silver electrodes and a central titanium electrode. Reproduced by kind permission of Tarn-Pure.

of humans and animals. Metallic copper- or copper alloy-containing surfaces can release a low concentration of copper over time, which has been used to prevent the attachment and growth of microorganisms.

Silver. Topical (antiseptic) silver applications include 1% silver sulfadiazine cream or solutions for direct application to chemical or heat burns and 1% silver nitrate solutions for instillation into the eye and for cleaning wounds or mucous membranes and preventing infections. These applications have been used for the prevention of wound infections by *S. aureus* and *Pseudomonas* and mixed bacterial infections of the eye in newborns. Silver has also been used for disinfection of drinking water (particularly in Europe) and recreational water (including swimming pools) and as a food preservative at a typical concentration range of 0.02 to 10 μg/ml. Examples are the silver-copper ionization systems (which use copper and silver electrodes as sources of ions when an electrical current is applied) for *Legionella* control in water, as described for copper above. Surfaces impregnated with metallic silver or silver compounds (including polymers, like polyethylene and nylon) have been used for wound dressings and on the surfaces of indwelling medical devices, such as catheters, which are prone to bacterial colonization and infection. The slow release of silver (at 1 to 2 μg/ml) from these surfaces can reduce the attachment and proliferation of bacteria (like *S. aureus*) on these surfaces. Typically, surfaces are impregnated with metallic silver or silver salts, such as silver chloride and silver calcium phosphate, or silver-containing zeolites (zeolites are microporous crystals of aluminosilicate that retain and slowly release cations).

Other heavy-metal-based compounds (including mercury- and tin-based compounds) are used as effective preservatives for clothing, paints, pharmaceuticals, and cosmetics at relatively low concentrations.

Spectrum of Activity

Copper. Copper is particularly bactericidal at very low concentrations and is effective against fungi (yeasts and molds), being both fungistatic and fungicidal. Copper is also an effective algicide and molluscicide; the control of molluscs (slugs and snails) in the part-per-million range is important for the indirect control of carriers of parasites (e.g., in the control of schistosomiasis in humans and liver flukes in animals). Copper is an effective virucide against enveloped and nonenveloped viruses. Copper is not considered sporicidal but is sporistatic at typical concentrations.

Silver. Silver is an effective bacteriostatic and bactericidal agent at relatively low concentrations, particularly against gram-positive bacteria. Less activity is observed against yeasts and molds. Silver is algistatic and algicidal, although little viricidal activity (except some activity against enveloped viruses) has been reported at typical concentrations.

Advantages

Copper. Copper is a powerful, stable biocide at relatively low concentrations. It is cost-effective, easy to use, and colorless and odorless at typical concentrations. Copper-silver ionization methods are not considered corrosive as alternatives to chlorine water treatment. They are easy to install and cost-effective to maintain.

Silver. Silver is particularly active against bacteria and is not irritating to skin or mucous membranes at effective concentrations. Side effects are rarely reported, particularly with silver sulfadiazine. Silver has affinity for many surfaces and can provide a residual, sustained antibacterial and fungistatic barrier. As described for ionization methods with copper, silver is less aggressive on surfaces as an alternative to chlorine treatment of water.

Disadvantages

Copper. Copper is considered toxic at high concentrations, including skin irritancy. It is stable in the environment and can be bioaccumulated by aquatic life. Some bacteria, fungi, and protozoa, including *E. coli*, *Legionella*, *Candida*, and *Paramecium,* can develop resistance to copper ions. This can develop due to conversion to nontoxic forms, sequestration, or uptake reduction (e.g., efflux); these are considered in more detail in section 8.3. At high concentrations in water supplies, copper can react with other chemicals to form unwanted deposits on surfaces, including medical devices. Levels of contaminants, including phosphates, protein, and chlorides, can reduce the activity of copper ions by neutralization or sequestration. Copper is less effective at pH >8.

Silver. Overuse of silver (at high concentrations) can cause burns to the skin and mucous membranes and may impede the healing of wounds. Silver nitrate causes black discoloration of the skin and other materials, as well as electrolyte loss in patients with extended use, which should be monitored. At high concentrations, silver can cause a blue-grey discoloration of the skin (argyria) and severe toxicity, although these have been rarely reported. The long-term effects of silver are unknown. In addition to limited activity against fungi, which can also cause wound infections or biofouling, the development of resistance has been described in bacteria, including active efflux (in *E. coli*) and complex formation (in *Pseudomonas stutzeri*); this is discussed in more detail in section 8.3. Levels of phosphates, calcium (e.g., water hardness), protein, and chlorides can reduce the activity of silver in water treatment.

Mode of Action

Copper. The mode of action of copper is similar to those of other heavy metals. Positively charged ions have a rapid affinity for negatively charged microbial surfaces. Proteins are a particular target, where ions can disrupt tertiary and secondary structures required for functional (enzymatic) and structural activities. Thiol (sulfhydryl; -SH) groups are particularly sensitive. Further reactions (copper-mediated catalysis) can lead to the production of hydroxyl radicals, which also damage proteins, lipids, and nucleic acids. Cell surface attack can lead to altered permeability and disruption of cell wall and membrane functions. Lower concentrations of copper are growth inhibitory (and also reversible), but higher concentrations lead to protein denaturation and precipitation, the cumulative effects of which are cell death and loss of infectivity. Copper has been shown to bind to the phosphate group backbone of

DNA, causing unraveling of the helix and subsequent degradation.

Silver. Silver ions are rapidly attracted to the surfaces of microorganisms, which can lead to disruption of cell wall and membrane functions by affecting the structures and functions of proteins. Silver binds to sulfhydryl, amino, and carboxyl groups on amino acids, which leads to protein denaturation. Sulfhydryl (thiol; -SH) groups appear to be particular targets, as demonstrated with amino acids, such as cysteine (CySH), while other compounds containing thiol groups, such as sodium thioglycolate, neutralize the activity of silver ions against bacteria. In contrast, amino acids containing disulfide (S-S) bonds, non-sulfur-containing amino acids, and sulfur-containing compounds, such as cystathione, cysteic acid, L-methionine, taurine, sodium bisulfite, and sodium thiosulfate, are all unable to neutralize silver activity. These and other findings imply that the interaction of silver with thiol groups in enzymes and proteins plays an essential role in bacterial inactivation, although there may be other cellular components involved. They include other amino acid groups and effects on hydrogen bonding. Specific interference with protein structure is believed to be responsible for increased permeability of the cell membrane, as observed with release of potassium from target cells. Virucidal and fungicidal properties might also be explained by binding to sulfhydryl groups. Silver has been shown to specifically inhibit cell wall metabolism, respiration (cytochromes *b* and *d*), and electron transport (e.g., disruption of the proton motive force). It also has been shown to bind to DNA (specifically the nucleotide bases) and to inhibit replication and transcription. These effects are overall responsible for the various morphological changes in microorganisms that have been observed. These include deposition of silver in vacuoles and as granules in the cell wall of the fungus *Cryptococcus neoformans*, damage to bacterial cell walls and cell division, increase in size, and other structural abnormalities. The mode of action of silver sulfadiazine may be a synergistic effect of silver and sulfadiazine. Differences in the mode of action in comparison to that of silver nitrate have been observed, particularly on the surfaces of bacteria, indicative of cell wall and membrane damage. Unlike the action of silver ions alone, silver sulfadiazine produces surface and membrane blebs in susceptible bacteria, suggesting greater damage to the cell wall and membrane. Silver sulfadiazine also binds to cell components, including DNA. The polymeric structure of the biocide, which is proposed to consist of six silver atoms linked to the six sulfadiazine molecules of nitrogen, binds to sufficient base pairs in the DNA helix to inhibit transcription and replication. A similar effect may contribute to the mode of action against microorganisms, including viruses.

3.13 PEROXYGENS AND OTHER FORMS OF OXYGEN

Types. Oxidation may be defined as the process of electron removal, while oxidizing agents (or oxidants) are substances that accept these electrons. In addition to many chemical uses, oxidizing agents have potent antimicrobial activities. Many oxidizing agents are used, including halogens (chlorine, bromine, and iodine [see section 3.11]), peroxygens, and other forms of oxygen.

Peroxygens are an important group of oxidizing agents that includes hydrogen peroxide, peracetic acid (PAA), and chlorine dioxide.

Hydrogen peroxide is a strong oxidizing agent and is probably one of the most widely used biocides for medical, industrial, and household applications. It is commercially available as a colorless liquid at various dilutions (generally 3 to 90%) in water. Pure hydrogen peroxide is relatively stable, but most dilutions contain a stabilizer (e.g., acetanilide or phenol) to prevent decomposition. Peroxide is considered environmentally friendly, as it decomposes into water and oxygen on exposure to increased temperature and various catalysts, including organic molecules, enzymes (e.g., catalase or peroxidases), and most metals (e.g., iron, copper, and manganese). Some organic peroxides

Hydrogen Peroxide

Peracetic Acid

Chlorine Dioxide

Ozone

are also used as biocides, with the most prevalent being benzoyl peroxide (Fig. 3.17).

Many other oxygen- and/or hydrogen peroxide-releasing compounds are used for various industrial and biocidal applications; examples are given in Table 3.3.

PAA is commercially available as a colorless liquid, with a strong, pungent (vinegar-like) odor at 5 to 37%. It is significantly less stable than hydrogen peroxide solutions and is therefore provided in equilibrium with water, hydrogen peroxide, and acetic acid. For example, 35% PAA is provided with 7% hydrogen peroxide, 40% acetic acid, and 17% water; in some cases, a stabilizer (sodium pyrophosphate or hydroxyquinolone) may be added. For most medical disinfection and sanitization purposes, PAA is used in formulation with hydrogen peroxide and other components to improve its stability and compatibility with a wider range of material surfaces. Formulations may contain either one or two components (the PAA-hydrogen peroxide component separated from the base formulation), with the latter requiring mixing prior to use. PAA may also be produced in situ by reaction of sodium perborate or sodium percarbonate with an acetyl donor, such as acetylsalicylic acid (aspirin) or tetraacetyl ethylene diamine (Fig. 3.18). Such formulations have longer shelf lives, as they are supplied dry and are activated by dilution in water prior to use.

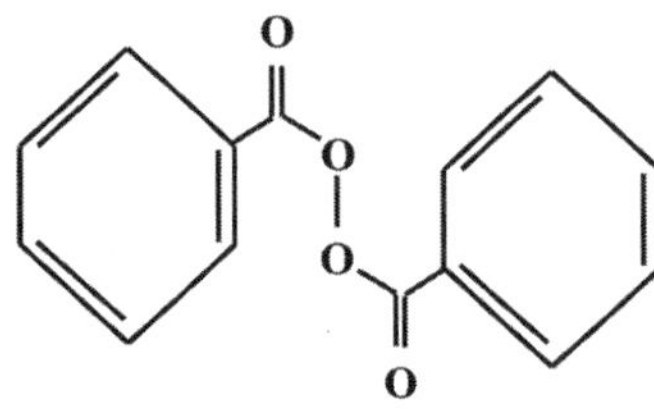

Benzoyl Peroxide

FIGURE 3.17 Structure of benzoyl peroxide.

Some other peroxygen compounds have also been used, including performic and perpropionic acids, with efficacies and compatibility profiles similar, if not inferior, to those of PAA.

Chlorine dioxide is a water-soluble gas that exists as a reactive free radical. Due to its unstable and explosive nature (at high concentrations), it is manufactured at the site of use. A variety of methods are used for its generation, particularly from sodium chlorite ($NaClO_2$) or sodium chlorate ($NaClO_3$) by acidification with HCl, H_2SO_4, or organic acids; reaction with chlorine or sodium hypochlorite; and electrolysis. Typical examples are shown in Fig. 3.19.

These methods may be conducted with chlorine in a gaseous state (e.g., by passing chlorine gas through columns of sodium chlorite) or as a liquid (e.g., by mixing a solution of sodium chlorite with acids, in some cases including sodium hypochlorite) and subsequently supplied to air or water. In addition to direct generation in water or liquid, typically for surface disinfection, applications are provided in two-part systems, which can include

TABLE 3.3 Other oxygen- and hydrogen peroxide-releasing compounds

Compound	Formula	Characteristics	Applications
Potassium monopersulfate (potassium peroxymonosulfate)	$KHSO_5$	White powder, readily soluble in water; releases oxygen on contact with moisture	Sanitization and organic-waste removal ("shocking") in pools and spas; disinfection formulations; bleaching applications
Ammonium, potassium, and sodium persulfates	$(NH_4)_2S_2O_8$, $K_2S_2O_8$, $Na_2S_2O_8$	Colorless crystals or white powders; liberate oxygen on contact with moisture; react with hydrogen peroxide to boost oxidative process	Skin and hair bleaching; deodorizers
Sodium percarbonate	$2Na_2CO_3{\cdot}3H_2O_2$	Dry, white powder that contains ~30% (wt/wt) hydrogen peroxide; releases hydrogen peroxide when dissolved in water	Cleaning and disinfection formulations; food and laundry bleaching
Sodium perborate	$NaBO_3{\cdot}H_2O$ (monohydrate)	White crystalline granules; releases hydrogen peroxide when dissolved in water	Cleaning, disinfection, and antiseptic formulations; dental and industrial bleaching; deodorizer
Calcium peroxide	CaO_2	White/yellow solid; slowly decomposes to release oxygen on contact with moisture	Remediation (including soil and water); disinfection and cleaning formulations (in particular, agricultural applications); bleaching

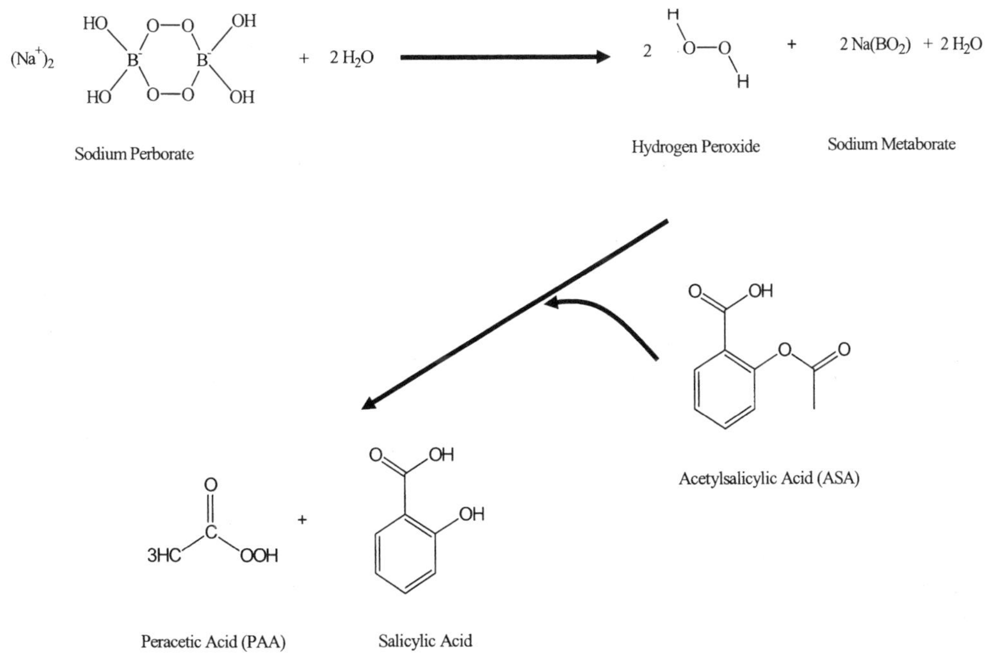

FIGURE 3.18 Example of the generation of PAA from sodium perborate and acetylsalicylic acid.

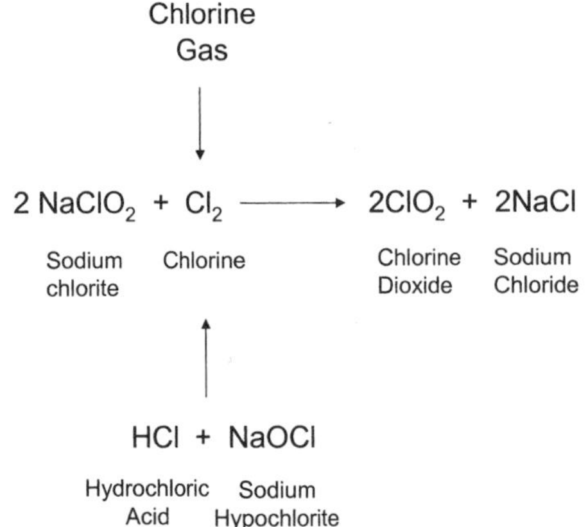

FIGURE 3.19 Examples of the production of chlorine dioxide from chlorine.

formulation excipients, such as preservatives, buffers, and corrosive inhibitors to improve efficacy, stability, and surface compatibility. Dry or stabilized mixtures that are activated on mixture with water are also available. In the gaseous state, chlorine dioxide is reactive and short-lived, breaking down into chlorine gas and oxygen. It can be much more stable in water, depending on the presence of light, the concentration, the temperature, the presence of neutralizing agents, and formulation effects.

Chlorine dioxide boils at 11°C and is therefore a gas at room temperature, with a slight yellow-green color (similar to that of chlorine gas) and a pungent, irritating chlorine odor. In solution, a similar color is observed, but it can vary in color (e.g., light red, amber, or blue) depending on the concentration in water and formulation effects. It is soluble in water and can be stored at up to 10 g/liter at 4°C (depending on the partial pressure in air and the temperature), although typical disinfection concentrations are $<$500 mg/liter in liquid and $<$2 mg/liter in gas.

A consideration of the chemistry of oxygen is also useful, as many active oxygen species are responsible for the antimicrobial activities of mixed-oxidant (or "activated") gases and liquids. Elemental oxygen is found abundantly as a diatomic molecule ("dioxygen," or O_2). As an allotropic element (i.e., existing in two or more forms), it is also naturally found as atomic oxygen (O) and as ozone (O_3), both of which are highly reactive and unstable oxidizing agents. Ozone is a naturally occurring water-soluble gas. For example, the upper atmospheric ozone layer protects the earth from damaging UV radiation from the sun. At low concentrations ($<$0.01 mg/liter), it is colorless and odorless, but at higher concentrations, it has a slight blue color ($>$5 mg/liter) and a distinctive, fresh, acrid odor ($>$0.1 mg/liter). Ozone is relatively stable in clean air over a few hours but rapidly degrades on contact with surfaces or in water. Other reactive forms of oxygen are formed by electron acceptance of oxygen to give various other reactive, short-lived species, including superoxide (O_2^-) and peroxide (O_2^{2-}) ions. Further, by protonation, other species are generated, including the hydroxyl ($^{\bullet}OH$) and hydroperoxyl (HO_2) radicals. All of these species are highly reactive and can damage microorganisms, culminating in cell death.

Applications

Ozone. Due to its reactive, unstable nature, ozone is produced at the point of use. Ozone generators effectively pass air (which is ~20% oxygen) or, in cases where high concentrations are required, pure oxygen through a high-energy source. The resulting physicochemical reaction leads to the formation of ozone, which can then be used directly for area or surface decontamination or, when bubbled or injected into water, for liquid disinfection. Widely used high-energy sources include a simple UV light, electrochemical cells, or, more commonly, a corona discharge. A corona is formed by an electrical discharge (or spark) around a gas, which causes ionization and ozone production. It should be noted that a corona is therefore a plasma in its formative stage (see section 5.6.1). Ozone production is most effective in a temperature-controlled environment, since the stability of ozone decreases as the temperature increases. A variety of generators are available for applications as diverse as odor control, taste and color remediation, preservation and saniti-

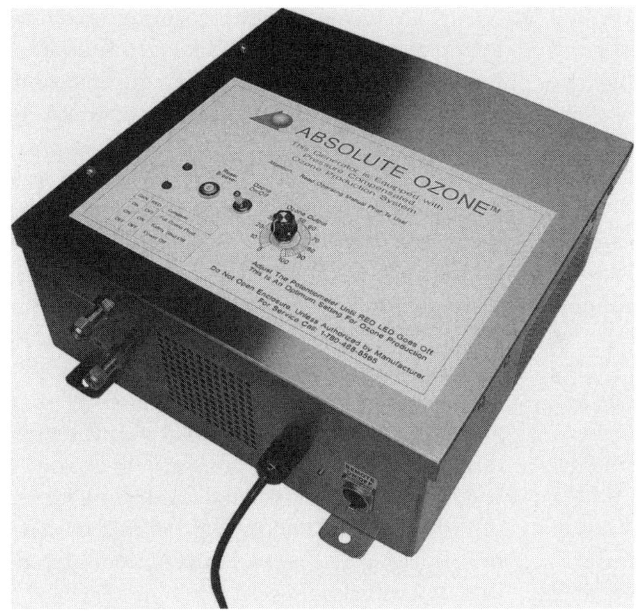

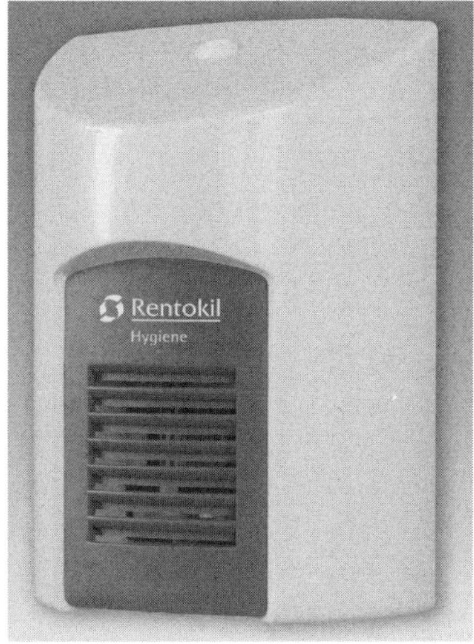

FIGURE 3.20 Examples of ozone generators. Courtesy of Absolute Systems (left) and Rentokil (right).

zation of foods, area fumigation, and sterilization (Fig. 3.20).

Ozone disinfection of water and wastewater is widely used worldwide, with applications increasing in the United States. The typical concentrations used range from 0.2 to 0.4 mg/liter at pH 6 to 7, with up to 5 mg/liter required for wastewater treatment due to the increased organic load, which readily reacts with ozone. Currently, due to restrictions on maintaining high concentrations in a given area (0.5 to 3 mg/liter), ozone is used primarily for odor control fumigation. A typical decontamination cycle includes area humidification (to 70 to 80%), ozone decontamination (while maintaining humidity levels), and aeration (to below 0.1 ppm). The recommended safe level of ozone is 0.1 ppm over a typical 8-h workday, with a minimum short-term exposure level of 0.3 ppm for 15 min. Cycle times vary depending on the area size, desired level of decontamination, and area contents. The difficulty of maintaining effective ozone concentrations limited its use in the past, but recent advances in generator technology have seen an increased use of ozone for both water- and air-based systems. A number of medical-device sterilization systems have also recently been developed (see section 6.6.4).

Although they are generally not referred to as "ozone generation," it is clear that ozone plays an important part in the overall efficacy observed in many mixed-oxidant generation systems. Mixed-oxidant ("oxygenated") species are similarly formed by passing liquids or gases through any high-energy source, including electrochemical cells, ionizing radiation, or corona and plasma generation systems. These species not only have direct antimicrobial activity, but also react with other air and water components (including chlorine) to form other active species; however, many of the generated species may also have undesirable attributes (such as material incompatibility).

Hydrogen peroxide. Hydrogen peroxide is used as a preservative, antiseptic, disinfectant, fumigant, and sterilant. Direct application as a liquid or a gas, and also in synergistic combinations with other biocides, can be considered.

Liquid peroxide is generally stored in vented plastic (polyethylene) containers to allow the release of oxygen over time. It is typically used as an antiseptic at 3 to 3.5% in water or in creams and gels; interestingly, it has been proposed for cancer therapy, but few clinical data are available to support this application.

Inorganic and organic peroxides have been used for various industrial biocidal applications, with benzoyl peroxide being one of the most widely used for treatment of acne vulgaris. Acne is a common skin condition in young adults and is often associated with *Propionibacterium acnes* and other bacteria on the skin. Benzoyl peroxide is also used as an antifungal antiseptic with typical concentrations in the 1 to 10% range in many different formulations of creams, lotions, gels, and cleansing solutions.

Five to 6% peroxide is used as a bleaching agent (e.g., for hair and paper). Higher liquid concentrations are used for a variety of industrial and medical purposes. Typical concentrations include 35 and 50%, with higher concentrations generally not used for biocidal applications due to increased safety considerations. General industrial applications include pollution control and chemical manufacture. Due to its rapid degradation into innocuous by-products, hydrogen peroxide is widely used in the food industry for general- or critical-surface disinfection and sterilization. As a rapidly active biocide and sporicidal agent, it is also used as a general surface and water disinfectant. Formulations at 7.5% alone and in combination with PAA are used for low-temperature medical-device disinfection. High-speed sterilization processes use liquid peroxide at 35 to 50% and up to 70 to 80°C. Preservative and immersion disinfection applications include contact lens solutions and control of bacteria and algae in water. The generally low rate of microbicidal action of hydrogen peroxide-based liquids can be accelerated by various formulation effects, including the addition of certain detergents and the inclusion of anticorrosive agents to improve material compatibility.

The antimicrobial activity of hydrogen peroxide gas is much greater at lower concentrations than that of the liquid form, and it is used for odor control, fumigation, and sterilization processes (Table 3.4). Typical concentrations range from 0.1 to 10 mg/liter (0.00001 to 0.001%), depending on the exposure temperature, which ranges from 4 to 80°C. For example, a >6-log-unit reduction in bacterial spores is observed within 10 s with peroxide at 4.5 mg/liter and 45°C at atmospheric pressure. Peroxide gas can be simply produced by heating or pulling a vacuum on a peroxide solution. For fumigation applications, peroxide gas is flash-vaporized by applying liquid directly to a heated (>100°C) surface, which forms a mixture of peroxide and water gases. Gas generator and control systems are used for the fumigation of critical environments (e.g., aseptic production isolators and clean rooms), rooms, buildings, and vehicles (Fig. 3.21).

These systems connect directly to an enclosed area and introduce peroxide gas by controlling the flow of air through the system in a closed loop (Fig. 3.22).

A typical fumigation cycle consists of four phases: dehumidification, conditioning, decontamination, and aeration. During the initial phase, the relative humidity in the area is generally reduced to below 50%, followed by the introduction of peroxide gas to a level to initiate decontamination. As the concentration of peroxide and water increases, it will reach a point (the dew point, condensation point, or saturation), depending on the temperature in the area, where condensation will occur. It is optimal to maintain the concentration of peroxide

TABLE 3.4 Comparison of sporicidal efficacies of liquid and gaseous hydrogen peroxide at 20 to 25°C against bacterial spores

Bacterial spore	*D* value[a]	
	Liquid peroxide (250,000 mg/liter; 25%)	Peroxide vapor (1.5 mg/liter; 0.00015%)
Geobacillus stearothermophilus	1.5	1–2
Bacillus atrophaeus	2.0–7.3	0.5–1
Clostridium sporogenes	0.8	0.5–1

[a]Time to kill 1 log unit of test organism in minutes.

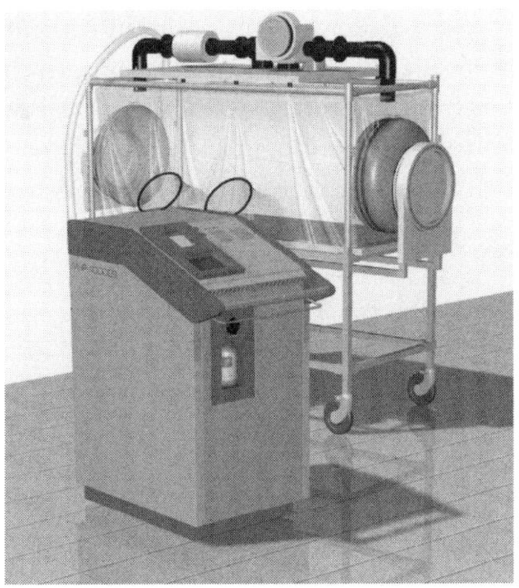

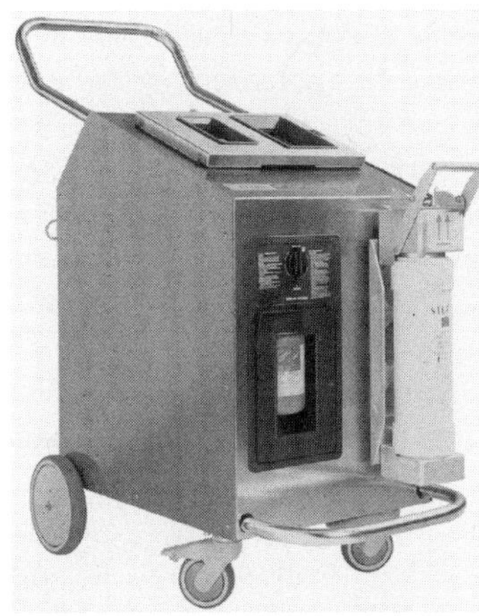

FIGURE 3.21 Examples of vaporized hydrogen peroxide (VHP) generators. The example on the left shows a large generator connected to a flexible-walled isolator for decontamination. On the right is a smaller generator system. Generators can be mobile (as shown) or integrated into a facility. VHP is a registered trademark of STERIS Corporation.

and water below the condensation point, which is achieved by consistently removing and replenishing the gas mixture in the area during the conditioning and decontamination phases. This is particularly important, as peroxide breaks down on contact with surfaces, causing the buildup of water vapor and reduced efficacy. In some applications, the concentration of peroxide and water is deliberately increased over the condensation point to allow the deposition of high concentrations of liquid peroxide (>70%) on the surface, which is also antimicro-

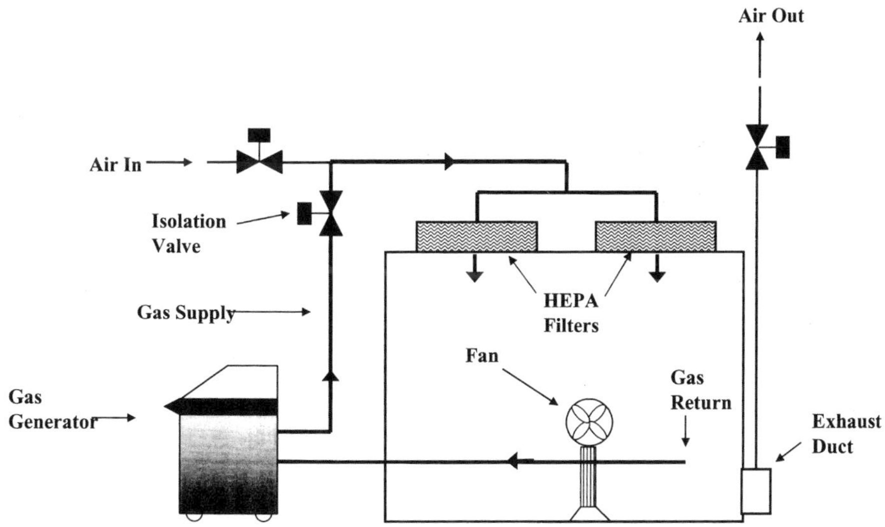

FIGURE 3.22 Typical room fumigation setup with a hydrogen peroxide gas generator. During fumigation, the air-handling system for the room is turned off and the gas is fed into the room. In the case shown, fumigation included the room, as well as the air-handling ductwork. Alternatively, the generator can be placed directly into the room.

bial but requires tight control to be effective and safe. Following decontamination, the area is aerated to remove the peroxide gas to a safe level (generally to 1 to 2 ppm).

Hydrogen peroxide gas diffuses passively when introduced into a given area, and therefore, constant movement of the gas is required to ensure that all surfaces are contacted. This can be aided at atmospheric pressure by using fans or air-handling systems or by introducing a slight positive or negative pressure in the area being fumigated. For sterilization methods, it is more effective to introduce the gas under vacuum, which ensures greater penetration of the biocide into a given load. Hydrogen peroxide gas sterilization systems are used for industrial and medical applications. These include simple peroxide gas cycles and combination systems with other agents, particularly plasma (these systems are described in more detail in section 6.5).

Many novel formulations and processes using liquid hydrogen peroxide in combination with other biocides or processes have been described. These are considered synergistic, as the efficacy of a given concentration of hydrogen peroxide may be greater in the presence of these active agents. Synergism with hydrogen peroxide has been shown in both the liquid and gaseous phases. These applications can be in simple combination with heat, as well as in combination with other chemical and physical agents (Table 3.5).

PAA. Liquid PAA is used industrially for chemical manufacture (e.g., for epoxidation), as a catalyst, and in paper bleaching. It is also widely used both directly and in formulation for cleaning, sanitization, disinfection, and sterilization. As mentioned above, all solutions and formulations are provided with PAA in synergy with hydrogen peroxide, water, and acetic acid. PAA can also be produced in situ by dilution of dry formulations in water (Fig. 3.18). Formulation effects, including anticorrosives, surfactants, and chelating agents, are important for the stability, efficacy, and material compatibility of PAA, which vary considerably based on these effects. Stability can be improved at lower pH and higher concentrations of hydrogen peroxide and by storage at lower temperatures. The overall efficacies of these formulations increase at higher concentrations of PAA and at higher

TABLE 3.5 Hydrogen peroxide-based synergistic formulations and processes

Synergistic agent	Application	Description
Copper, iron, manganese	Reaction with liquid or gas	Results in the production of free radicals (including ·OH)
Heat	Heating up to 80°C	As the temperature increases, the activity of peroxide increases, but in parallel to some increase in the degradation rate of peroxide. As a gas, the higher the temperature, the greater the concentration of peroxide (and thus, antimicrobial activity) that can be maintained in air without condensation.
UV	Reaction in liquid or gas	Results in the production of free radicals (including ·OH)
Ultrasonics[a]	Applied in liquid	Unknown; proposed to increase the production of free radicals and to increase the penetration of peroxide into target cells; may also cause cells to disassociate to allow direct contact with the biocide
Peracetic acid	Combined in formulation or as a gas	Unknown, but both active agents are powerful oxidizing agents; may promote the production of free radicals
Ozone	Combined in liquid or as a gas	Unknown, but both active agents are powerful oxidizing agents; may promote the production of free radicals
Plasma	Combined as a gas and also proposed in liquid	Plasma causes the breakdown of peroxide, giving a higher concentration of free radicals, in combination with the effects of plasma itself.

[a]Ultrasonics is the generation of high-frequency sound waves in liquid.

temperatures; however, the degradation rate of PAA also increases at higher temperatures.

Typical concentrations of PAA used for disinfection are <0.35% (or 3,500 mg/liter). Due to its natural breakdown into water and a low concentration of acetic acid, it is extensively used in the food industry, directly on food and for sanitization of food contact surfaces; many applications do not require rinsing, which is an advantage. For medical applications, PAA formulations have become popular alternatives to glutaraldehyde for low-temperature disinfection of reusable medical devices, including flexible endoscopes. Formulations include 7 to 1% hydrogen peroxide and 0.25 to 0.1% PAA, as well as in situ generation formulations based on acetylsalicylic acid. A liquid-PAA-based sterilization process is discussed in section 6.6.1. Other medical applications include solid and liquid waste treatment, hemodialyzer machine reprocessing, and tissue (e.g., bone) decontamination. PAA is also used directly on surfaces for general environmental disinfection, due to its rapid antimicrobial (including sporicidal) activity; this is particularly important for critical environments, such as clean rooms and aseptic isolators. Other applications have included the treatment of ointments and lotions (at 0.05 to 0.1%), sewage treatment, biofilm removal (due to its powerful oxidizing-agent activity, which improves cleaning, particularly for lipid material), and water or water surface disinfection and remediation (e.g., for *Legionella* control). In addition to hydrogen peroxide, synergistic formulations at low concentrations of PAA with alcohols have also been reported to provide sporicidal activity for skin antisepsis.

Gaseous PAA has been used less than liquid applications. This is primarily due to the corrosive nature of PAA, which can be better controlled in liquid formulations, and its pungent odor. Similar to hydrogen peroxide, the efficacy of gaseous PAA is greater at lower concentrations than in liquid; overall, efficacy should be considered as a combination of those of PAA and peroxide vapors. Applications have included enclosed-area fumigation, food sanitization, and medical-device sterilization. The use of PAA-plasma sterilization is considered in section 6.6.3.

Chlorine dioxide. Chlorine dioxide is used in liquid form and, to a lesser extent, as a gas. Industrial uses include paper bleaching and potable-water, wastewater (e.g., slime reduction), and water contact surface disinfection. As an alternative to chlorine, chlorine dioxide does not leave a residual taste or odor in water applications; typical concentrations used range from 0.1 to 5 mg/liter. Due to the degradation of phenols, cyanides, aldehyde, and other undesirable compounds, it has also been used to improve water taste and potable quality. It is particularly utilized in the food industry (both directly and in formulation) for food contact surface and food surface sanitization and disinfection. A similar variety of formulations have been used in some countries for low-temperature medical-device disinfection (Fig. 3.23). Typical concentrations used for critical applications (including sporicidal activity) are 200 to 500 mg/liter for 5 to 30 min, but they vary depending on the formulation and its use.

Chlorine dioxide gas is more effective at lower concentrations (with the typical concentrations used varying from 0.5 to 30 mg/liter). As a gas, it is used for odor control, area fumigation, remediation, and sterilization. A brief description of the use of chlorine dioxide under vacuum for biomedical and industrial sterilization processes is given in section 6.6.5. Atmospheric applications include the fumigation of manufacturing and laboratory equipment, isolators, and rooms (including clean rooms) and for large-area remediation. For example, chlorine dioxide gas (at >65% relative humidity) has been successfully used for the remediation of contaminated buildings (at ~2 mg/liter, or 750 ppm, and >65% humidity for 12 h). Mobile and fixed generator systems that allow automation of these applications are commercially available (Fig. 3.24).

A typical fumigation process includes humidification of the area (generally, 70 to 80% humidity is preferred), exposure to chlorine

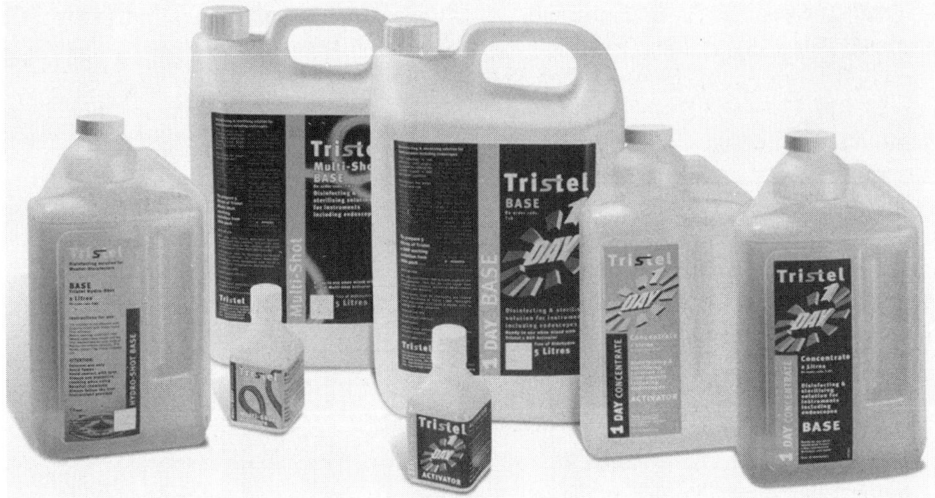

FIGURE 3.23 A range of chlorine dioxide-based liquid formulations for medical-device disinfection. Courtesy of The Tristel Co.

dioxide, and subsequent aeration to below the safe level of 0.1 ppm (Fig. 3.25). Aeration can be safely achieved by neutralization of the gas through sodium bisulfite.

Chlorine dioxide has also been used at low concentrations as an antiseptic, including for skin disinfection (e.g., mastitis control) and in mouthwashes and toothpastes. An example is the activation of 0.1% sodium chlorite with 0.3% mandelic acid for immediate use as a preoperative preparation.

Spectrum of Activity

Ozone. At the concentrations typically used (0.2 to 0.5 mg/liter), ozone is an effective bactericide and virucide, with greater resistance observed with mycobacteria and bacterial spores. For gas-based processes, sporicidal activity requires high levels of relative humidity (75 to 95%) to be effective. Yeasts and molds have been reported to have a wide range of resistance profiles but are generally less resistant than bacterial spores. Similar spectra of activity have been reported for other mixed-oxidant systems. A range of studies with ozone have focused on protozoal and cysticidal activities, due to a number of notable outbreaks of *Giardia* and *Cryptosporidium* in contaminated water. Ozone was reported as being the most effective water disinfectant, in comparison to chlorine dioxide, chlorine, and monochloramine, with *Cryptosporidium* oocysts demonstrating the highest resistance. Ozone has also been used for treatment of wastewater, which is often heavily contaminated, including control of algae. Higher concentrations are generally required due to interaction with and neutralization by the high organic load. For fumigation or surface sterilization applications, antimicrobial activity is dependent on the presence and maintenance of 70 to 80% relative humidity, below which little or no activity is observed. Ozone, under these conditions, has some activity in neutralizing protein toxins, including mycotoxins, and preliminary reports have suggested some activity against prions.

Hydrogen peroxide. Hydrogen peroxide demonstrates broad-spectrum efficacy against viruses, bacteria, mycobacteria, fungi, and bacterial spores. Greater efficacy is seen at much lower concentrations of hydrogen peroxide gas than of the liquid (Table 3.4). Higher concentrations of liquid peroxide (10 to 55%) and longer contact times are required for sporicidal activity, in contrast to the gaseous phase. Peroxide is more effective against gram-positive than gram-negative bacteria; however, the presence

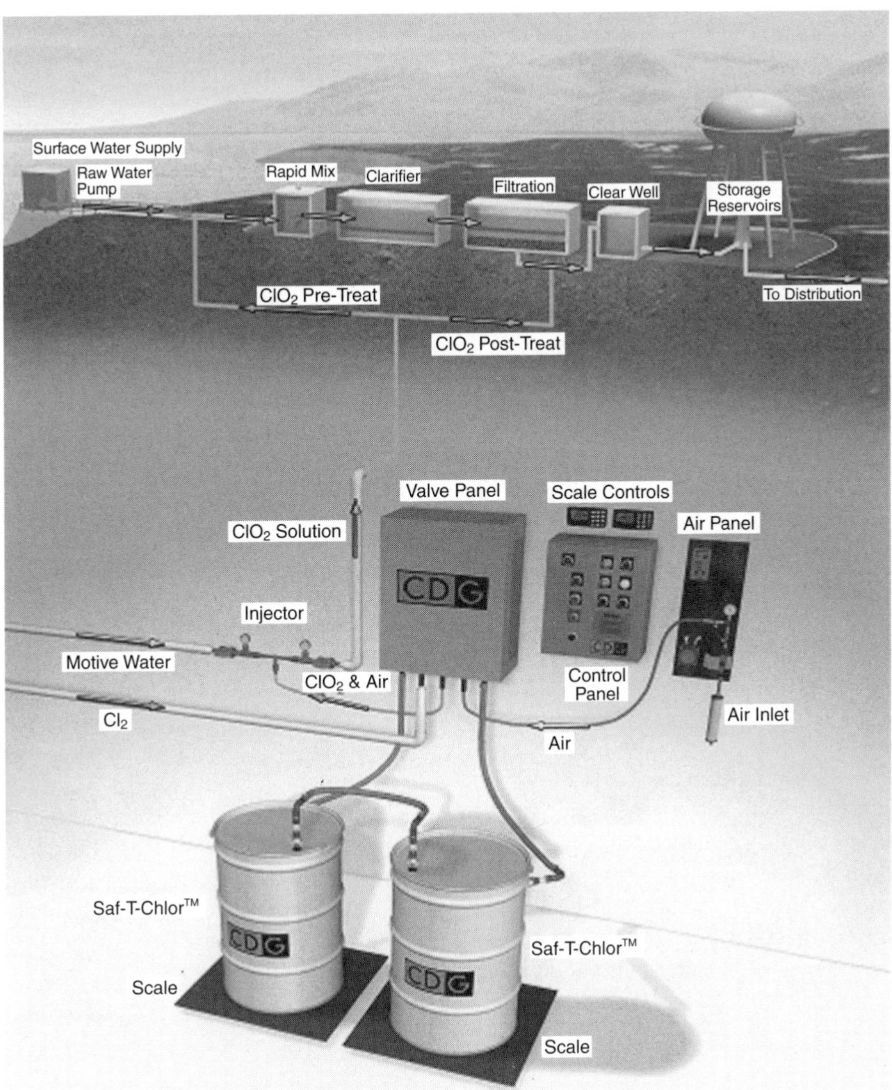

FIGURE 3.24 A chlorine dioxide gas generator for liquid applications. Courtesy of CDG.

of catalase or other peroxidases (particularly in gram-positive bacteria, such as *Staphylococcus*) allows increased tolerance of peroxide, due to enzymatic degradation. In general, concentrations of peroxide above 3% are bactericidal, and concentrations below 3% demonstrate good bacteriostatic, fungistatic, and algistatic activities. Efficacy against *Cryptosporidium* and *Giardia* has also been described at 6 to 7% liquid, and in the gaseous form at 1 to 6 mg/liter; 3% peroxide, which is used for contact lens disinfection, has been shown to be effective against *Acanthamoeba* over 4 h. Hydrogen peroxide gas has also been shown to be effective against parasite eggs (including those of *Caenorhabditis*, *Enterobius*, and *Sphacia*). Although liquid peroxide has been shown to have little or no effect on prions, gaseous peroxide has been effective. This may be linked to the ability of gaseous peroxide to break down proteins; similar efficacy has been reported against protein toxins and bacterial endotoxins. In addition to biological applica-

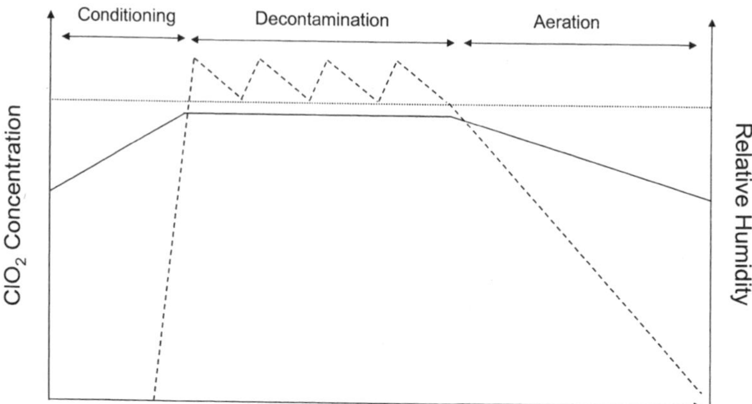

FIGURE 3.25 A typical chlorine dioxide fumigation cycle. The biocide concentration is shown as a dashed line, and the humidity is shown as a solid line. The dotted line indicates the minimum concentration of chlorine dioxide required for activity, which depends on the application. As chlorine dioxide breaks down during the decontamination phase, the concentration can be increased by further injection of gas.

tions, peroxide is used for pollution control and chemical neutralization, due to its potent oxidizing activity.

Benzoyl peroxide is considered bactericidal and fungicidal, but its activity is slow, based on in vitro investigations. Interestingly, the activity of benzoyl peroxide is enhanced in the presence of lipids (on the skin), and it also breaks down to form benzoic acid, which is itself an antimicrobial agent (see section 3.2). The antimicrobial activity of benzoyl peroxide against *P. acnes* has been particularly well studied, and that against dermatophytes to a lesser extent.

PAA. PAA is considered a more potent biocide than hydrogen peroxide; it is sporicidal, bactericidal, tuberculocidal, virucidal, and fungicidal at low concentrations (<0.35%) at room temperature. The bactericidal and fungicidal activities are rapid, even at concentrations as low as 0.003%. Virucidal activity varies, with the nonenveloped viruses demonstrating the greatest resistance at 0.2%; enveloped viruses can be sensitive to PAA at concentrations as low as 0.001%. As with other biocides, the effects of temperature (Fig. 3.26) and concentration can be significant. For example, a sterility assurance level of 10^{-6} has been demonstrated with PAA in formulation at 1,000 mg/liter and 50°C.

Liquid PAA has some cleaning effects (particularly for lipids and carbohydrates), which have been useful for biofilm remediation or prevention, although this activity is dependent on the product formulation. Further, PAA is not broken down by catalase and peroxidases and demonstrates greater efficacy in the pres-

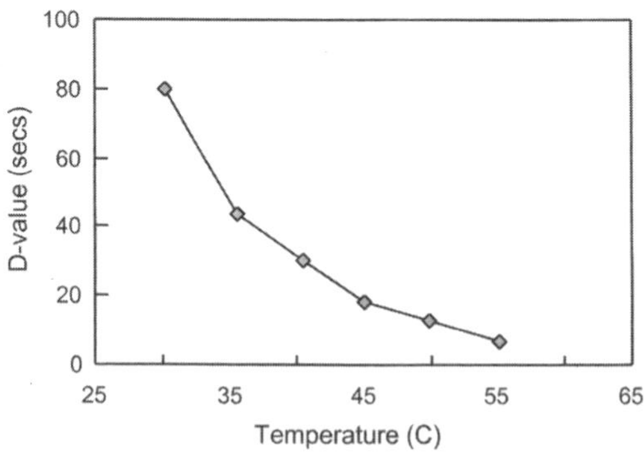

FIGURE 3.26 The effect of temperature on the sporicidal efficacy of PAA. The average *D* value (the time required to kill 1 log unit of test organisms in seconds) was determined for *Geobacillus stearothermophilus* spores at 1,000 mg of PAA/liter in formulation at various test temperatures.

ence of soils. For example, liquid PAA can dissolve inorganic salts, which can be a challenge for other disinfection and sterilization methods, such as steam and ethylene oxide. Some efficacy has been reported against *Cryptosporidium* and *Giardia*, which increases with temperature. Of further note, PAA has been reported to neutralize pyrogens (including endotoxins) and to have some effect against prions, depending on the temperature, concentration, and formulation.

Chlorine dioxide. Chlorine dioxide has a spectrum of activity similar to, if not greater than, that of chlorine or other chlorinated compounds (see section 3.11). It is active over a wider pH (pH 6 to 10, with greater activity at the higher levels) and demonstrates greater activity at increased temperatures. Relatively low concentrations are required for bactericidal and virucidal activities (within 0.2 to 0.7 mg/liter at room temperature and pH 7). Chlorine dioxide has been used as a cleaner, for biofilm control, and as an algicide. Cysticidal activity has been demonstrated against *Giardia*, *Naegleria*, and *Cryptosporidium* in water at ~1 mg/liter. Higher concentrations (1 to 2 mg/liter) are required to ensure sporicidal activity for some applications. Some reports have suggested activity against prions, but this requires confirmation.

Advantages

Ozone. Ozone and other oxidants are potent antimicrobials that are effective at relatively low concentrations. They are environmentally friendly methods for liquid decontamination, as they rapidly break down into oxygen and water; lack of residual taste or odor is an aesthetic advantage over chlorine and bromine. Further, ozone is an efficient agent for taste and odor control in water treatment and can efficiently neutralize algal toxins. Ozone is effective at neutralizing chemical contamination, including cyanides, phenols, some detergents, and metals (e.g., iron). For area decontamination, little or no aeration time is required following ozone exposure, and it has a reasonable safety profile (it is safe to work in an area at 0.1 ppm over a typical 8-h day).

Hydrogen peroxide. Hydrogen peroxide is a potent biocide that is effective at low concentrations against vegetative organisms, with higher concentrations required for sporicidal activity. Hydrogen peroxide is considered environmentally friendly and nontoxic, as it can rapidly degrade into water and oxygen. Peroxide solutions are generally safe for use directly on the skin and other surfaces at 3 to 6%; however, at higher concentrations (35 to 50%), burns and material damage can occur. At concentrations greater than 50% the broad use of peroxide is limited due to safety concerns. Peroxide gas, particularly when maintained below the condensation point at a given temperature, demonstrates wide material compatibility for low-temperature fumigation and sterilization; applications include use on electronic equipment and other sensitive materials that cannot withstand liquid treatments. Fumigation with peroxide is more rapid and safer than traditional formaldehyde methods, and reports have also suggested chemical neutralization activity (e.g., of chemical-warfare agents, such as VX [$C_{11}H_{26}NO_2PS$] gas and bacterial toxins). The recommended safety level for a typical 8-h workday is 1 ppm of peroxide gas. With a sufficient concentration of the biocide, peroxide can demonstrate antimicrobial efficacy in the presence of organic or inorganic soil loads.

Benzoyl peroxide has been successful as a treatment for skin-associated infections, particularly acne vulgaris, due to its keratinolytic (exfoliative) activity, drying of the skin (with reduced production of sebum), and good lipid solubility; *P. acnes* is generally found deep within the skin, and benzoyl peroxide is considered more penetrating than other antiseptic biocides.

PAA. PAA provides broad-spectrum activity at relatively low concentrations. It also decomposes into safe, nontoxic by-products (a low concentration of acetic acid and water) but has the added advantages over hydrogen peroxide of being free from decomposition by peroxidases and having greater activity in the presence of organic and inorganic soils. There have been no reports of development of resistance, presumably due to its rapid breakdown in the environment, and it is not considered carcinogenic. PAA is compatible with stainless steel and other surfaces; however, material compatibility is dependent on the biocide formulation and application.

Chlorine dioxide. Chlorine dioxide is a potent biocide at relatively low concentrations and even in the presence of soils at sufficient concentrations. It is often preferred over chlorine for water disinfection, due to the lack of taste and odor at typical concentrations. There are no known health effects at the concentrations typically used in water, and it is not considered carcinogenic or mutagenic. Chlorine dioxide reacts with and neutralizes many harmful or undesirable chemicals (including phenols and aldehydes) and, unlike chlorine, does not react to form THMs or chloramine derivatives. For applications in the gaseous phase, it can be detected at harmful concentrations (>0.1 ppm) and provides rapid fumigation in comparison to formaldehyde. Unlike hydrogen peroxide gas, with concerns about condensation, chlorine dioxide can tolerate a greater range of temperatures. The biocide degrades into nontoxic residues, although it is recommended that chlorine dioxide be neutralized prior to release into the environment.

Disadvantages

Ozone. Ozone's restricted material compatibility is probably its greatest disadvantage, as it can be corrosive on surfaces. Similar profiles have been described for mixed-oxidant systems. Corrosion-resistant materials can be treated, including high-quality stainless steel, titanium, ceramics, and some polymers; however, even in these cases, damage can occur, such as premature rusting of stainless steel. Rust (FeO_2) forms upon exposure of iron (e.g., on stainless steel surfaces) to ozone. Maintenance of higher concentrations of ozone is required for sporicidal activity, which is also more aggressive on surfaces and requires longer cycle times. For fumigation applications, the requirement for humidification may also be restrictive, and as for other gaseous peroxygens, applications that contain adsorptive or proteinaceous materials require special consideration, due to neutralization of the active agent. Finally, ozone is an irritant to mucous membranes and can cause significant damage to tissues at the concentrations typically used.

Hydrogen peroxide. Hydrogen peroxide can cause bleaching of surfaces, including colored anodized aluminum. Contact with various surfaces, such as organic materials, cellulosic materials (e.g., paper or wood), brass, copper, and iron, can cause the rapid degradation of peroxide. Direct exposure to high concentrations can cause skin burns and, particularly in gaseous form, irritation and damage to mucous membranes. For applications in the gaseous phase, liquids cannot be disinfected or sterilized. High concentrations of liquid peroxide can pose a risk of explosion on contact with certain surfaces (e.g., when contaminated with solvents).

Benzoyl peroxide has low solubility and is considered unstable, which is an important consideration for optimal formulation of the biocide. The major disadvantage in its use as an antiseptic is skin irritancy, including itching and burning in some applications (depending on the concentration and formulation of the biocide). Allergic reactions and some concerns about toxicity (due to absorption into the blood and breakdown to benzoic acid) have been reported. At the concentrations typically used, benzoyl peroxide is an eye and respiratory irritant.

PAA. Concentrated PAA has a strong pungent odor, which can be irritating to the eyes, mucous membranes, and respiratory system. Direct exposure at high concentrations, which should be avoided and is not believed to have long-term effects, can also cause nausea.

Adequate ventilation is required in areas where high concentrations of PAA are stored or used in open applications. PAA should be stored in vented containers to prevent explosion, due to the build up of oxygen on degradation. Material compatibility is a concern, particularly on copper, brass, aluminum, and some plastics; these effects can be minimized by correct formulation of the biocide. PAA also causes burns to the skin at >3% and damage to the eyes at >0.3%. PAA is unstable (e.g., 35% solutions decrease by 0.4% per month at room temperature), and controls should be in place to ensure that adequate concentrations are present for the given application.

Chlorine dioxide. Chlorine dioxide needs to be generated on site and is short-lived. Many of the chemicals used for its generation may also offer some safety concerns and should be controlled. For liquid applications, care should be taken to ensure that prepared solutions are at the required concentration for their intended use. There remains some controversy regarding the health effects of chlorite and chlorate by-products in the use of chlorine dioxide. It can be explosive at 7 to 8% in air; therefore, care should be taken to control its manufacture in large-volume applications. The recommended safety level is 0.1 ppm, above which it is a respiratory, eye, and mucous membrane irritant; at higher concentrations (e.g., 19 ppm), exposure can be lethal. The biocide is light sensitive, and therefore, applications are best conducted in the dark. Chlorine dioxide can be corrosive to certain metals (including copper and brass) and plastics (e.g., polycarbonate and polyurethane), depending on the application. Bleaching of colored surfaces may also be observed. Liquid chlorine dioxide is often considered more corrosive, particularly due to the various acids involved in generation processes. Breakdown products (especially chlorine gas) contribute to the observed incompatibility and can be minimized by reducing the concentration used and the formulation effects (in liquid) and by performing fumigation under darkness. For fumigation processes, humidity needs to be maintained above 65% for efficacy, and a fine white powder may remain on surfaces, but it is not considered toxic. As for other oxidizing-agent-based processes, standing liquids cannot be decontaminated and efficacy can be limited on cellulosics (e.g., paper) or other absorptive materials.

Modes of Action

Ozone. Ozone causes oxidation of external and internal cellular components. As a strong oxidizing agent, ozone has been shown to cause enzyme inactivation and cell wall and membrane damage. Direct effects (degradation) on viral nucleic acids and polypeptides have also been reported. These effects are thought to be primarily due to direct interaction with ozone itself, particularly in water applications at acidic pH, although the indirect production of other unstable reactive species (including the hydroxyl and peroxyl free radicals) may play a greater role at alkaline pH. These effects may also explain the requirement for high humidity (or the presence of water) during area fumigation applications.

Hydrogen peroxide. Similar to other peroxygens, the antimicrobial effect is directly due to hydrogen peroxide on the microbial surface, in combination with the presence of short-lived breakdown products, such as the superoxide and hydroxyl radicals. The increased presence and production of these radicals may be responsible for the greater antimicrobial efficacy observed with gaseous peroxide. These effects culminate in the oxidation of key cellular components, including lipids, proteins, and nucleic acids, causing cell death. The effects on proteins may be particularly important, with observed removal of proteins from spore coats and direct breakage of peptide bonds. It has been proposed that exposed protein sulfhydryl groups and fatty acid double bonds are particularly targeted.

The mode of action of benzoyl peroxide is linked to its oxidizing activity and the production of hydroxyl and other radicals. In addition, the biocide degrades to give benzoic acid, which is itself an antimicrobial acid biocide (see section 3.2).

PAA. The mode of action of PAA is similar to that of hydrogen peroxide and is primarily due to direct effects on microbial surfaces and indirectly to the production of short-lived radicals, particularly the hydroxyl radical. Specific effects on bacterial cell walls and membrane permeability and on viral capsids have been studied. PAA has been shown to denature and degrade proteins and enzymes, particularly by disrupting sulfhydryl (-SH) and sulfur (S-S) bonds. Effects on nucleic acids, including DNA and RNA strand breakage, have been observed and are particularly important in antiviral efficacy.

Chlorine dioxide. The chlorine dioxide molecule is a reactive radical, reacting with surfaces on contact. Thus, the main mode of action is believed to be disruption of cell walls and membranes and microbial surfaces, which culminates in cell death or loss of infectivity. Specifically, it reacts with amino acids (particularly tryptophan, cysteine, and tyrosine) to cause loss of protein and enzyme structure and function. Direct reaction with fatty acids has been reported. Little or no effect was observed on nucleic acids (DNA and RNA), although it is clear that their synthesis is inhibited (presumably due to protein inhibition); these results are in contrast to the specific effects on nucleic acids observed with chlorine and chlorine-releasing agents (see section 3.11).

3.14 PHENOLICS

Types. Phenolics are essentially a class of alcohol compounds with one or more hydroxyl (-OH) groups attached to an aromatic hydrocarbon ring. A wide variety of phenolics are used for disinfection, preservation, and antisepsis (Table 3.6). The traditional range of phenolics, including phenol, cresols, and xylenols, were first identified by fractionation from coal or tar. Subsequently, many of these and alternative phenolic compounds ("non-coal-tar" phenols) were synthetically produced and investigated, which included modification by halogenation (e.g., chlorination or nitrification) and condensation (e.g., with aldehydes or ketones to give bisphenols).

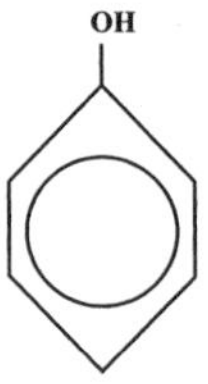

Phenol 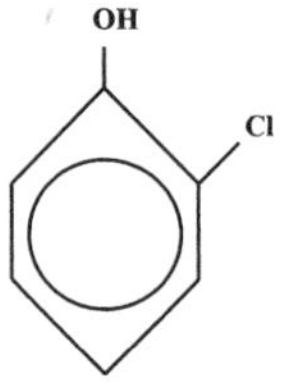   2-chlorophenol 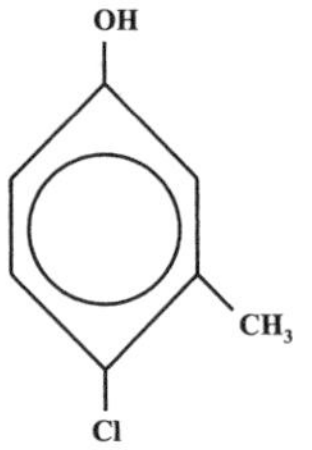   Chlorocresol

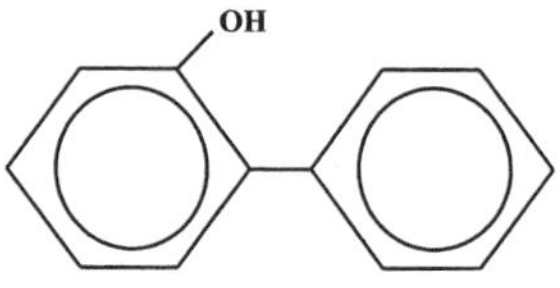

O-phenylphenol 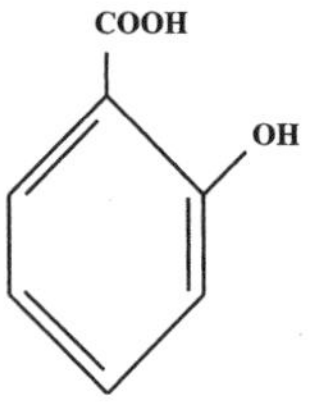   Salicylic Acid

Applications. Phenolics and their derivatives are an important class of compounds that are widely used. In addition to their antimicrobial properties, phenolic compounds are also

TABLE 3.6 Various types of phenolic compounds

Coal tar
Phenol
Cresols
Xylenols
Naphthols

Non-coal tar
2-Phenylphenol
4-Hexylresorcinol

Halogenated phenols
4-Chloro-3,5-dimethylphenol (chloroxylenol; PCMX)
4-Nitrophenol
2-Chlorophenol
Chlorocresol

Bisphenols
Triclosan
Hexachlorophene
Fenichlor

Other phenol derivatives
2,3-Diaminophenol
Salicylic acid
8-Hydroxyquinoline

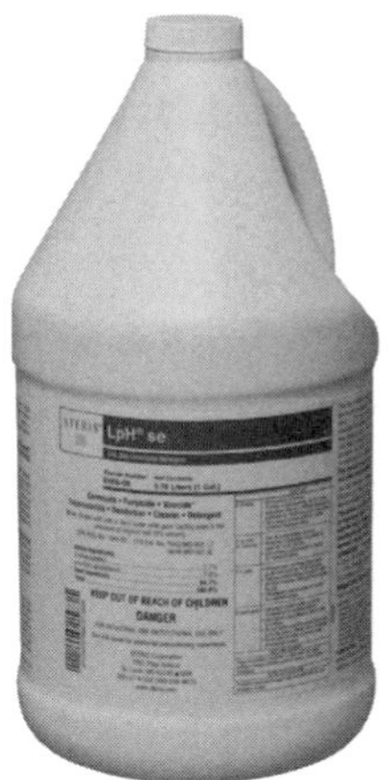

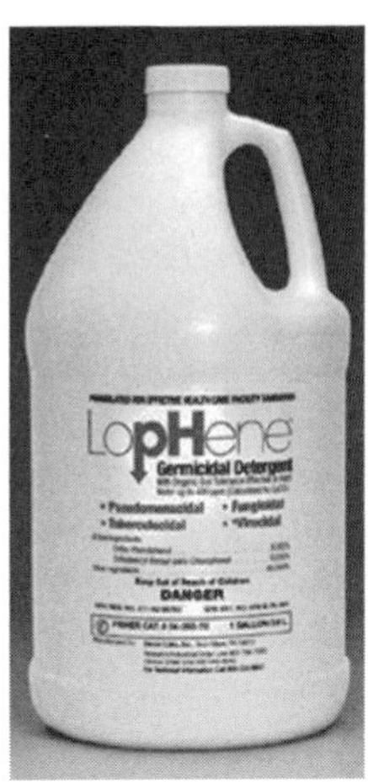

FIGURE 3.27 Phenolic-based disinfectants. Both are formulation concentrates (which are diluted in water prior to use).

used as pain killers (e.g., acetylsalicylic acid, or aspirin) and herbicides and in the manufacture of resins and synthetic fibers. Phenolic compounds have long been used for their antiseptic, disinfectant, and preservative properties. Phenol itself, despite its irritation to the skin, was successfully used during pioneering antiseptic surgical procedures by Joseph Lister (1827–1912). The phenolics most widely used on the skin today are the bisphenols (hexachlorophene and triclosan), chloroxylenol (commonly known as PCMX [*p*-chloro-*m*-xylenol]), and salicylic acid, which are further discussed as antiseptics (see section 3.15 and chapter 4). Chloroxylenol has also been widely used as a preservative and in surface disinfectants. Phenol is still used in antiseptic ointments and sprays at lower concentrations in combination with other biocides (such as chlorhexidine [see section 3.8]). Due to their insolubility in water, phenolics are combined (or formulated) with soaps, oils, or synthetic anionic detergents for solubilization. Soaps and surfactants are molecules that change the properties of a liquid at its surface or interface by breaking the surface tension. In both cases, they consist of a water-soluble ("ionic," "polar," or hydrophilic) part and a long-chain water-insoluble ("nonpolar," or hydrophobic) part. They aid in phenol solubilization by micelle formation, where the phenolic is solubilized in the central hydrophobic region (see section 1.4.6). Formulation effects, therefore, play a key role in the optimization of phenolic activity, so that it is available for antimicrobial activity, as well as remaining soluble (e.g., when diluted in water in concentrated disinfectants). Most phenolic disinfectant formulations contain two or more phenolic types, due to synergistic attributes, including efficacy. Phenolics are widely used as broad-spectrum, intermediate-level disinfectants for general surface disinfection, including walls and floors (Fig. 3.27).

For some applications (such as clean-room disinfection), formulations are provided sterilized (by filtration or radiation) to reduce the risk of spore contamination; phenols are sporistatic but not sporicidal. Phenolics are also used at low concentrations as preservatives, due to broad-spectrum inhibition at relatively low concentrations. Notably, phenol itself has been used in a method to standardize the resistance of bacterial and fungal cultures used for disinfection efficacy studies; the AOAC International phenol coefficient test exposes a test culture to a known concentration of phenol to determine its intrinsic resistance. Some bisphenols (particularly triclosan) have been successfully integrated into various polymers, including fabrics and surfaces such as cutting boards and toothbrushes, to provide some residual antimicrobial activity.

Spectrum of Activity. Most phenolics demonstrate rapid activity against bacteria (gram positive and gram negative), fungi, and viruses. In general, phenolics are more effective against gram-positive than gram-negative bacteria. Rapid tuberculocidal activity has also been demonstrated. The activity varies considerably depending on the phenol type and its formulation; specific attention should be paid to the label claims on a product and the test methods used to verify the activity. Most formulations contain two or more phenolics, which provide a broader range of activity. In general, the more lipophilic the phenolic, the more activity is observed against lipophilic (enveloped) viruses and the less activity is noted against hydrophilic (nonenveloped) viruses. Similar conclusions can be drawn for mycobacteria, presumably due to their lipophilic cell wall structure. Many of the bisphenols used as antiseptics have slow activity against gram-negative bacteria, which can be enhanced in formulation by the addition of EDTA or other chelating agents, which increase the permeability of the biocides through the cell wall. Bisphenols are rapidly effective against gram-positive bacteria but demonstrate little activity against fungi and mycobacteria. Phenolics are sporistatic, with little or no sporicidal activity. Although they are not generally considered effective against prions, it is interesting that certain types of phenols in formulation have been shown to be effective, although the exact mode of action remains to be determined.

Advantages. Phenolics are widely used as broad-spectrum disinfectants and antiseptics. Most disinfectant formulations have broad-spectrum activities as intermediate-level disinfectants, including tuberculocidal activity. Phenolics are able to tolerate the presence of interfering substances, such as organic and inorganic soil loads, which is of particular importance in the direct cleanup of soils, including blood spills in hospitals. In combination with detergents, phenolics can therefore combine cleaning and disinfection. They have an "institutional" aromatic odor, which may be useful for odor control. As antiseptics, they demonstrate rapid activity against gram-positive bacteria on the skin, with some substantive activity (remaining on the skin following washing). Although irritation varies depending on the active agent, triclosan is generally nonirritating and has been described as inhibiting inflammation. Salicylic acid has good fungicidal and virucidal activities that, combined with its depilatory (or surface skin layer removal) effects, are useful in the treatment of persistent skin infections, such as warts. In contrast, phenolic disinfectants are generally labeled as irritants and are considered relatively toxic. Residual activity on a surface following application can be an advantage in certain situations. Most of the widely used phenolics today are biodegradable, including *o*-phenylphenol and *o*-benzyl-*p*-chlorophenol.

Disadvantages. Most phenolics are considered irritants to the eyes and skin and can be toxic. They are generally contraindicated for use on food contact surfaces. The presence of residues may be a concern in other industrial applications due to cross-contamination and necessitate postuse surface rinsing. Restricted use in health care nurseries has been recommended in some countries due to reported adverse reactions in neonates, although this may have been related to improper use of the product. The often strong odors characteristic of phenolic disinfectants may be undesirable in certain facilities, although newer phenolics often have little associated odor. Phenolics have little or no activity against bacterial spores, which may limit certain applications, but as disinfectants, they are generally considered more efficacious than alternative QAC-based formulations (see section 3.16). Phenolics, depending on the formulation, can be corrosive to certain plastic and rubber surfaces with extended use. Increased tolerance of some phenolics has been reported in some bacteria, although the significance of this has been debated. It is interesting that more triclosan-tolerant strains of *E. coli* and *Pseudomonas* also demonstrated resistance to isoniazid, which is an antibiotic used to treat mycobacterial infections; this has led to speculation concerning the promotion of antibiotic resistance in the environment due to the use of biocides (see sections 3.15 and 8.7.2).

Modes of Action. The antibacterial effects of phenols have been well studied. Phenols are general cellular poisons but have also been shown to have cell membrane-active properties. The hydroxyl (-OH) group is very reactive and forms hydrogen bonds with macromolecules, particularly with proteins. Very low concentrations (in the part-per-million range) of phenolics result in bacteriostatic activity due to inactivation of essential membrane enzyme functions and increased cell wall permeability.

Phenols induce progressive leakage of intracellular constituents, including the release of potassium ions, the first indication of membrane damage. Specific, rapid cell lysis has been shown for actively growing cultures of gram-negative (*E. coli*) and gram-positive (*Staphylococcus* and *Streptococcus*) bacteria, which appeared to be independent of cellular autolytic enzymes. Cytoplasmic leakage has also been shown with bisphenols, including fenticlor and triclosan. Fentichlor and triclosan also affected the metabolic activities of *S. aureus* and *E. coli*, including reports of disruption of cell membrane activities, leading to an increase in permeability to protons with a consequent dissipation of the proton motive force and an uncoupling of oxidative phosphorylation. Similar effects have been observed with other phenolics, including chlorocresol. Actively growing bacterial cultures appear to be more sensitive, which may indicate a specific target during cell division and separation. Recent research into the mode of action of triclosan and similar bisphenols, such as hexachlorophene, has identified specific interactions and disruption of key metabolic processes, including lipid biosynthesis. These studies have shown specific interactions with enzymes involved with lipid biosynthesis; in particular, triclosan forms a complex with the fatty acid synthesis enzyme enoyl reductase and its cofactor NAD^+, which causes a conformational change and precipitation of the complex. Triclosan has also been shown to inhibit the activities of other enzymes and to intercalate into the phospholipid membrane, which can lead to disruption of its structure and functions in bacteria and fungi. Further consideration of the mode of action of the bisphenols is given in section 3.15. At higher concentrations, phenols have multiple effects on the cell wall (e.g., lipid disruption), cell membrane, and cytoplasmic components. They include the coagulation of cytoplasmic constituents, which causes irreversible cellular damage.

The mode of action against other microorganisms has been less well studied. Phenolics possess antifungal and antiviral properties. Similar to their antibacterial action, their antifungal action probably involves damage to the plasma membrane, resulting in leakage of intracellular constituents and other effects, as described for bacteria. Little is known about the specific effects on viruses, but some studies with bacteriophages have shown no effect on phage DNA and some effects on the capsid proteins. Enveloped viruses are more susceptible, presumably due to coagulating effects on the surface proteins and membrane disruption.

3.15 ANTISEPTIC PHENOLICS

Types. Various phenolics (see section 3.14) have been widely used as effective antiseptics, and they are specifically discussed in this section. They can be subdivided and considered as bisphenols, halophenols, and the organic acid salicylic acid.

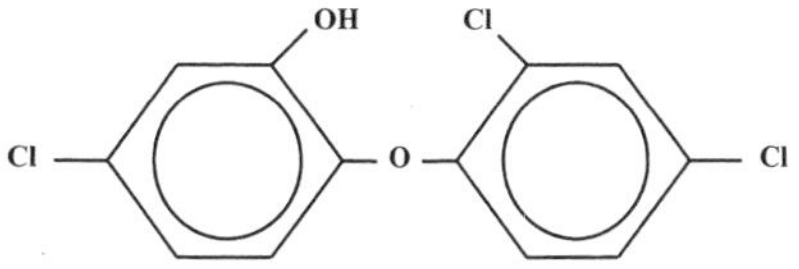

OH Cl
Cl O Cl

Triclosan

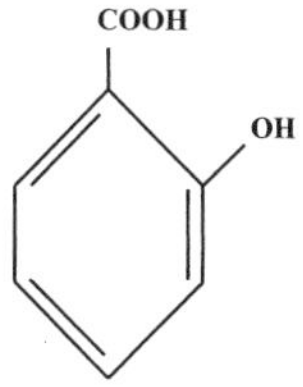

COOH OH OH
CH_3 CH_3
Cl

Salicylic Acid

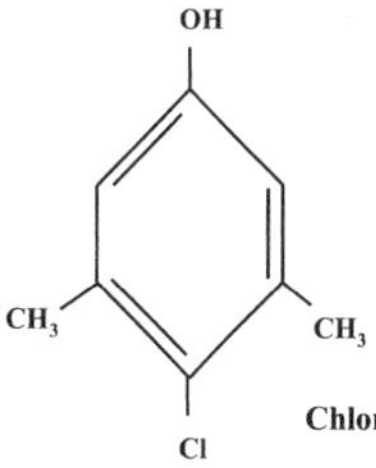

Chloroxylenol

The bisphenols are hydroxyhalogenated derivatives of two phenolic groups connected by various bridges (Fig. 3.28). They are formed from a condensation of a phenol with an aldehyde or a ketone.

In general, they exhibit broad-spectrum efficacy against bacteria and fungi but have little activity against *P. aeruginosa* and molds, and they are sporistatic to bacterial spores. Triclosan (2,4,4′-trichloro-2′-hydroxydiphenyl ether; Irgasan DP 300) and hexachlorophene (hexachlorophane; 2-2′-dihydroxy-3,5,6,3′,5′,6′-hexachloro-diphenylmethane) are the most

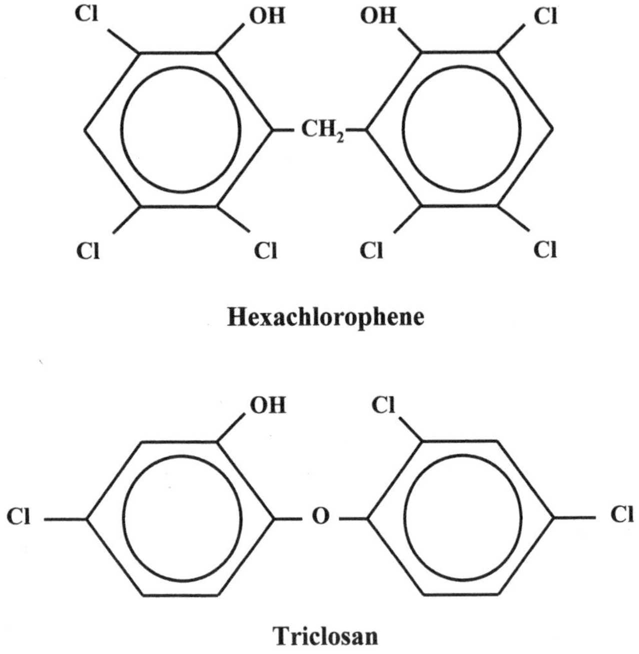

Hexachlorophene

Triclosan

FIGURE 3.28 Typical bisphenolic structures.

widely used biocides in this group, especially in antiseptic soaps and hand rinses. Both compounds have been shown to have cumulative and persistent effects on the skin. Triclosan is a diphenyl ether and is one of the most common biocides used in antiseptics due to its reasonable spectrum of activity and mildness to the skin. Hexachlorophene is a further chlorinated bisphenol and was one of the first widely used as an antiseptic, but it is now less used due to toxicity concerns. Other bisphenols have been described, including fenticlor, but they are not widely used.

Halophenols are used as both antiseptics and disinfectants (see section 3.14). The most widely used as an antiseptic is chloroxylenol. Chloroxylenol has been particularly used in soap-based hand washes, for both high-risk and general-use applications. Formulation of the biocide is particularly important to enhance its broad-spectrum activity, especially against some gram-negative strains, such as *Pseudomonas*.

Salicylic acid (or *o*-hydroxybenzoic acid) is an organic carboxylic acid. In addition to its antiseptic and preservative use, salicylic acid has had limited use as an anti-inflammatory agent, but it is also modified by various chemical reactions to make acetylsalicylic acid (aspirin) and other topical agents used in liniments and tinctures. Salicylic acid is often found in synergistic formulations with a variety of other agents, including isopropanol, sulfur, sodium thiosulfate, and the structurally similar benzoic acid.

Applications. The bisphenols have been widely used in various antimicrobial soaps. Hexachlorophene is now used only for restricted applications, while triclosan had become widely used. Hexachlorophene was typically used in antimicrobial hand and skin washes, including specific applications in wound cleaning, surgical scrubs, and antimicrobial powders. Concentrations of the biocide ranged up to 3%, but with the identification of significant toxicity concerns, its use is now restricted in most countries, usually under prescription. Hexachlorophene has also been used as an effective preservative in cosmetics (at typical concentrations of ~0.1%). Triclosan is widely used in antimicrobial soaps, including professional (surgical scrubs and routine hand washes) and household use. Over the last 10 years, there has been a proliferation of antimicrobial soaps, lotions, cleaners, and shampoos, many of which are based on triclosan for their mode of action. These products vary significantly in antimicrobial activity; in most countries, the antimicrobial claims for these products are not regulated. Applications have included soaps, lotions, deodorants, gels, and antiacne washes. Typical concentrations range from 0.1 to 2%, with higher concentrations used in higher-risk applications. In some cases, triclosan has been combined with other antimicrobials (such as alcohols) to provide persistent activity on the skin over time; this is a particular benefit for the use of triclosan as a deodorant and as an odor control wash. Triclosan is particularly suited for use as an antiseptic due to its lack of toxicity or irritation to the skin and mucous membranes. Other applications have included mouth rinses and antibacterial toothpastes; these formulations may often include other active agents, such as zinc citrate and sodium fluoride, for the treatment of gingivitis and periodontitis. Triclosan has also been used as a preservative in cosmetics and other products, although usually in combination with other biocides. Due to the thermal and chemical stability of the biocide, triclosan has been integrated into various plastics and fabrics as proposed antibacterial surfaces. In a particularly interesting recent finding, triclosan has also been recommended therapeutically as an antiparasitic agent, with efficacy reported against *Plasmodium falciparum*, *Toxoplasma gondii*, and *Trypanosoma brucei*. These reports have led to the investigation of alternative drugs in the treatment of diseases such as malaria and toxoplasmosis.

Chloroxylenol has been used in a variety of antimicrobial soaps, including surgical scrubs, preoperative preparations, and hand washes. Other applications have included shampoos and medicated powders. Chloroxylenol may also be used at lower bacteriostatic and fungistatic concentrations as an effective preservative, especially in antiseptics and cosmetics, but also in a variety of other products, such as paints, textiles, and polishes. Formulations are often in combination with other phenolic compounds, including pine oils, terpineols, and alcohols. Typical concentrations vary from 0.5 to 4%.

Salicylic acid is primarily a skin exfoliant due to its keratinolytic activity. This, combined with antibacterial and antifungal activities, has made it a popular biocide in the treatment of skin disorders, such as acne, seborrheic dermatitis (dandruff), and psoriasis. Other formulations are specifically used for the treatment of viral infections, such as skin warts, caused by papillomaviruses. Although the antimicrobial activity is a benefit in diseases like psoriasis, which are prone to bacterial and fungal infections, many of these applications are used particularly for surface skin layer removal rather than for antimicrobial benefits. As an example, psoriasis is a nonspecific, chronic, but noncontagious skin disease which benefits from exfoliation of dead skin layers. Similarly, the use of higher concentrations of salicylic acid-based formulations directly on warts allows the removal of the wart and stimulates the host immune response to target the papillomavirus infection. Also, the presence of the biocide prevents viral replication and infection. Acne is a complicated disease of the skin, but salicylic acid allows the combined effects of skin pore cleaning and unblocking and antibacterial activity against bacteria implicated in acne. A variety of products are available, including general-use shampoos, soaps, and gels and targeted-use paints, drop medications, and plasters (which release the active agent over time). Other applications include antimicrobial toothpastes and mouthwashes. Concentrations vary depending on the application. Generally, concentrations from 1 to 6% (usually 1 to 2%) are used for acne or psoriasis applications over wider application areas. An example of a traditional preparation is Whitfield's ointment, containing 6% benzoic acid and 3% salicylic acid. Higher concentrations, ranging from 10 to 17% for paints and 20 to 50% in plasters, are also used for limited application areas. Salicylic acid has also been used at lower concentrations (0.04 to

0.5%) as a preservative, particularly in acidic foods, as it has an optimum pH range from 4 to 6. Due to toxic restrictions, salicylic acid is less used as a preservative, and only at lower concentrations (<0.06%).

Antimicrobial Activity. The bisphenols are rapidly effective against gram-positive bacteria and most gram-negative bacteria. They are much less effective against *Pseudomonas* and other pseudomonads, but the activity can be dramatically increased by many formulation effects. An example is synergism with chelating agents (e.g., EDTA), which destabilize the gram-negative cell wall by chelating metal ions, allowing the biocide to contact more sensitive cell membrane and intracellular targets. Hexachlorophene is particularly active against gram-positive bacteria, including pathogenic and antibiotic-resistant *Staphylococcus* strains (such as methicillin-resistant *S. aureus*). For this reason, hexachlorophene was widely used to prevent wound infections. Some activity is observed against gram-negative bacteria, but little effect has been reported against mycobacteria, fungi, and viruses. Triclosan shows a wider spectrum of activity than hexachlorophene, with particularly rapid activity against gram-positive bacteria, including *Staphylococcus* species, which are prevalent on the skin. For example, many staphylococci are sensitive to inhibitory concentrations as low as 0.1 μg/ml, although higher concentrations (>10 μg/ml) are generally required for bactericidal activity. Triclosan is also active against gram-negative bacteria and yeasts; it has generally poorer activity against some enveloped viruses, some pseudomonads, and fungi. The lack of appreciable activity of triclosan itself against pseudomonads has allowed its use in selective media for pseudomonas isolation. The overall antimicrobial activity of triclosan-containing antiseptics can be particularly enhanced by formulation effects; the biocide alone, as present when integrated into plastics and other materials, has little sustainable antimicrobial activity. Recent studies have shown activity against many parasites, including *P. falciparum*, *T. gondii*, and *T. brucei*; triclosan or similar bisphenols have been recommended as potent inhibitors of blood-borne parasites. Reports have also suggested that, in addition to its antibacterial properties, triclosan may have anti-inflammatory activity.

Chloroxylenol demonstrates good bacteriocidal activity against gram-positive and gram-negative bacteria. Some gram-negative bacteria, particularly *P. aeruginosa* and other pseudomonads, can demonstrate higher resistance to the biocide alone. Chloroxylenol is also effective against a wide range of fungi, particularly yeasts, with some molds (including *Penicillium* and *Mucor*) demonstrating higher tolerance of the active agent. Efficacy against pseudomonads and molds can be dramatically increased by various formulation effects; therefore, chloroxylenol-based products can vary significantly in antimicrobial activities and claims. For example, similar to other phenolics, the efficacy against *Pseudomonas* can be potentiated by the presence of EDTA or other chelating agents, due to their removal of metal ions from the cell wall structure, which causes destabilization. These formulation effects can also enhance the activity of the biocide against mycobacteria and viruses. Due to disruption of lipid envelopes, chloroxylenol formulations may also be effective against enveloped viruses, but little activity has been reported against nonenveloped viruses. Chloroxylenol is a stable biocide; it demonstrates good skin penetration and can remain persistent on the skin for a number of hours following application to provide a further bacteriostatic and fungistatic barrier.

Salicylic acid at lower concentrations is an effective bacteriostatic and fungistatic agent. Higher concentrations are also bactericidal and fungicidal. Most studies have focused on microorganisms that are associated with skin acne, including *Propionibacterium, Corynebacterium*, and *Pityrosporum*. Fungicidal activity has been described against yeasts and dermatophytes, including species that cause tinea. Some antiparasitic activity has also been reported. Low concentrations inhibit viral infection and replication, although the antiviral activity of salicylic acid has not been well studied.

Advantages. The bisphenols have potent activity against gram-positive and, in formulation, gram-negative bacteria and fungi. They are very stable and persistent biocides on the skin and can afford bacteriostatic and fungistatic activity following application of the product over an extended period. They can be easily formulated with a variety of soaps and detergents. The bisphenols also retain significant activity despite the presence of organic soils. These advantages make them popular for antiseptic applications. Triclosan, in particular, can penetrate into and through the skin but has shown no toxic, allergenic, or mutagenic effects after extensive investigation and prolonged clinical use. Despite its persistence on the skin, it has not been shown to cause irritation (which, when observed, may more likely be due to other constituents of the antiseptic formulation than to the biocide itself). Its stability and activity are also somewhat preserved in the presence of organic soil and excessive heat, which has allowed the use of triclosan as an integrated antimicrobial barrier in textiles and plastics.

Chloroxylenol is a nontoxic biocide at the concentrations typically used. It is mild to the skin, and despite its ability to penetrate into the skin, it has rarely been shown to be sensitizing or irritating. Chloroxylenol demonstrates good bactericidal and fungicidal activity, particularly against gram-positive bacteria. It is a stable biocide and is persistent on the skin, remaining antimicrobial for some time (up to hours) following application.

Salicylic acid is a mild biocide for topical use with few or no side effects reported at the concentrations or in the applications typically used. The biocide is an effective exfoliant, which aids in dead-skin removal and also allows penetration of the active agent into the lower skin layers. It is effective against most common bacterial and fungal skin pathogens.

Disadvantages. The bisphenols demonstrate a restrictive spectrum of activity, are not effective against pseudomonads (unless enhanced by formulation effects), and are incompatible with nonionic surfactants. Their relative stability also means that they may be biocumulative or ecocumulative in some cases, particularly with hexachlorophene. Hexachlorophene has been shown to be toxic to humans and animals, presumably due to its increased halogenation in comparison to triclosan. Neurologic effects were initially highlighted in the bathing of patients with burns and wounds and were verified in animal studies. Hexachlorophene is absorbed through the skin but is particularly contraindicated for those with broken skin and for the treatment of mucous membranes. The use of hexachlorophene is restricted in most countries, particularly with neonates; for example, in the United States, it can be used only by prescription and under strict regulation. Although triclosan is also stable and is absorbed through the skin, there is no evidence of toxicity or mutagenicity despite extensive studies and clinical use. It has, however, been found at detectable levels in the environment, including in foods, which has raised some concerns over its potential ecological effects; this has been particularly highlighted with the recent demonstration at low levels of triclosan of the potential promotion of cross-resistance to antibiotics (see section 8.7.2).

Lower doses of salicylic acid can cause some skin irritation, particularly if combined with other antiseptics, such as alcohol, acids, and peroxides. The biocide can cause slight stinging and is not generally recommended for use on broken skin, wounds, or mucous membranes. Specific inactivation of other common topical agents has been reported, including calcipotriene, which is commonly used for treatment of psoriasis. High concentrations are considered toxic to humans and animals and can lead to "salicylism," a syndrome that includes gastrointestinal irritation, dizziness, and ringing in the ears. These effects are usually characteristic of overdosing with the biocide.

Chloroxylenol demonstrates a narrower range of antimicrobial activity than other biocides commonly used in antiseptics; although these effects can be enhanced by formulation, products can also vary considerably in antimicrobial activity on the skin or other applications. The activities of chloroxylenol products are highly dependent on formulation attributes. Persistent activity on the skin can be neutralized in the presence of nonionic surfactants, which can be present in some soaps and cleaners.

Mode of Action

Triclosan. Over the last few years, triclosan has become one of the most studied biocides for its mode of action. It is clear that triclosan has some specific effects on some proteins at low concentrations and further nonspecific effects, typical of other phenolics, at higher concentrations. Earlier studies showed that the primary effects of triclosan are on the cytoplasmic membrane. In studies with *E. coli*, triclosan at subinhibitory concentrations inhibited the uptake of essential nutrients, while at higher, bactericidal concentrations, it caused the rapid release of cellular components and subsequent cell death. Other investigations have highlighted the importance of fatty acid biosynthesis as a target for triclosan. Studies with a divalent-ion-dependent *E. coli* triclosan mutant that exhibited a 10-fold greater triclosan MIC than a wild-type strain showed no significant differences in total envelope protein profiles but did show significant differences in envelope fatty acids. Specifically, a prominent 14:1 fatty acid was absent in the resistant strain, along with minor differences in other fatty acid species. It was proposed that in these mutants the divalent ions and fatty acids may adsorb and limit the permeability of triclosan to its site of action. Minor changes in fatty acid profiles were also found in gram-positive (*S. aureus*) isolates that had elevated triclosan MICs but not minimum bactericidal concentrations. The recent investigation of *E. coli* triclosan-tolerant mutants, which demonstrated increased MICs of triclosan in vitro, identified a specific enzyme target for triclosan: enoyl-acyl carrier protein reductases. Enoyl reductases are involved in type II fatty-acid-synthetic processes. Type II fatty acid synthase systems in bacteria use a dissociated group of enzymes (in contrast to mammalian type I synthases, which use a multienzymatic polypeptide complex) for the synthesis of fatty acids; this involves the cyclic addition of two carbon units to a growing fatty acid chain. Enoyl reductases catalyze the last stage in this elongation cycle, which is dependent on the presence of the cofactor NADH or NADPH. The cofactors are used as electron carriers during the reaction and vary between bacterial types; for example, NADH is specifically used by *E. coli* and *Bacillus subtilis*, while NADPH has been identified in *S. aureus*. The typical reaction is shown in Fig. 3.29.

Triclosan has been shown to specifically interact with the substrate binding site (particularly tyrosine residues) on the enzyme, simulating the enzyme's natural substrate. It also interacts with the nicotinamide ring of the cofactor, which allows the tighter, irreversible binding of the biocide. These interactions are noncovalent and are formed by hydrogen bonding, van der Waals forces, and other hydrophobic interactions. Inhibition of enoyl reductases is a key target, as they play a role in controlling the rate of fatty acid biosynthesis. The effect is referred to as a "slow, tight interaction" whereby the initial reversible interaction causes a conformation change in the protein-coenzyme structure over time, leading to irreversible complex formation. These effects remove the enzyme from its key role in fatty acid biosynthesis and also cause complex precipitation. Similar yet distinct effects are observed with the antibiotic isoniazid, the diazoborines, and the bisphenolic hexachlorophene. Isoniazid and the diazoborines form covalent bonds with the cofactors at the enzyme active site, while hexachlorophene forms noncovalent interactions similar to those of triclosan but does not form the irreversible complex with the enzyme cofactor (Fig. 3.29). Although both biocides bind to the same active site, the effect of hexachlorophene appears to be reversible, does not induce a conformational change, and is not as significant for the overall mode of action. It has been suggested that the ether linkage in triclosan (Fig. 3.28) allows greater flexibility of the biocide to permit greater interaction with the cofactor and the conformational changes observed. Binding

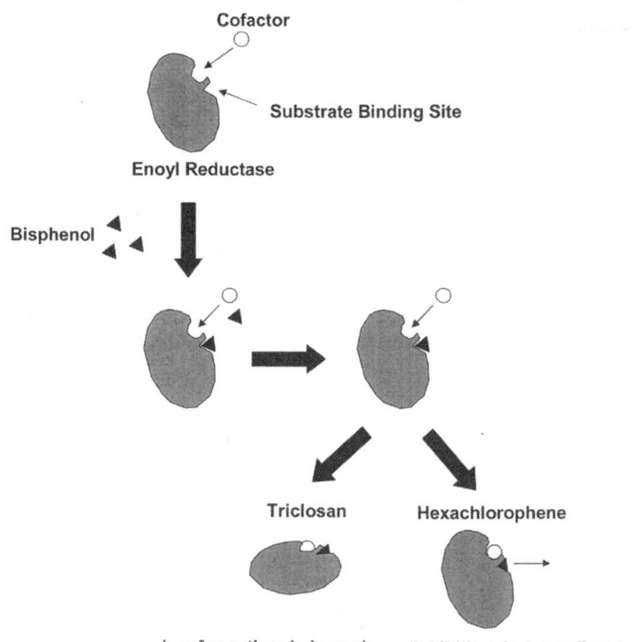

FIGURE 3.29 The modes of action of triclosan and hexachlorophene against enoyl reductases.

of triclosan to enoyl reductases has been observed in gram-positive (*S. aureus*) and gram-negative (*E. coli*, *P. aeruginosa*, and *Haemophilus influenzae*) bacteria, including *Mycobacterium smegmatis* and *Mycobacterium tuberculosis*. The effect of triclosan at lower concentrations on enoyl reductases clearly plays an important role in its mode of action; however, other specific and nonspecific interactions have been observed. Many examples have also been reported in the literature. Overexpression of glucosamine-6-phosphate aminotransferase (which is involved in the biosynthesis of various amino sugar-containing macromolecules) also showed increased resistance to triclosan in *E. coli*, but not to other biocides, such as hexachlorophene or antibiotics. Direct inhibition of other enzymes, including various transferases, has been reported in vitro.

Triclosan inhibition of type II synthases (in chloroplasts and mitochondria) in plants and parasites has also been observed, although in the cases of *Trypanosoma* and *Plasmodium* investigations, fatty acid elongation by enoyl reductases was not specifically inhibited; in these cases, the overall activity appeared to be due to nonspecific disruption of the subcellular membrane structure, which disrupted the overall fatty acid biosynthetic pathway. The effect of triclosan on the phospholipid membrane has been specifically investigated in bacteria; studies have shown that the hydrophobic biocide can integrate into the upper region of the membrane via its hydroxyl group, which causes membrane disruption and loss of various functions (including catabolic and anabolic processes) and integrity. These studies confirm that triclosan has multiple effects on key proteins and the cell membrane, which have cumulative effects and contribute to bactericidal and fungicidal activities.

Hexachlorophene appears to have a mode of action similar to yet distinct from that of triclosan. Initial studies of *Bacillus megaterium* showed that the primary action of hexachlorophene was inhibition of the membrane-bound part of the electron transport chain and that the other effects noted above are secondary and occur only at high concentrations. It also induces leakage, causes protoplast lysis, and inhibits respiration. Hexachlorophene disrupts the proton motive force on the surfaces of bacteria, with dramatic effects on structure, motility, and oxidation and phosphorylation. These effects are typical of those observed with other phenols, including bisphenols. The threshold concentration for the bactericidal activity of hexachlorophene is 10 μg/ml over a wide range of temperatures, including as low at 0°C. As the concentration was increased, cytological changes were observed at 30 μg/ml with maximal cytoplasmic leakage at 50 μg/ml. Hexachlorophene clearly causes protein and enzyme inhibition (both membrane associated and cytoplasmic) at lower concentrations, with macromolecule precipitation and membrane disruption at higher concentrations. It is interesting that hexachlorophene, similar to triclosan, has also been shown to specifically interact with bacterial enoyl-acyl carrier protein reductases, but in a reversible reaction (Fig. 3.29). Specific inhibition of other enzymes, including esterases and dehydrogenases, has been observed.

Chloroxylenol. The mode of action of chloroxylenol has been little studied, despite its widespread use over many years. Because of its phenolic nature, it is expected to have similar effects on surface proteins and microbial membranes, leading to enzyme inactivation, structure disruption, and loss of viability (see section 3.14).

Salicylic acid. Similar to other phenolics, the primary targets of salicylic acid, on the basis of the limited studies performed, are surface and intracellular proteins. The effects on proteins lead to cell wall and membrane damage, as well as inactivation of key membrane enzymes (see section 3.14). Specific interference with porins in the cell walls of gram-negative bacteria has been reported, leading to reduced uptake; paradoxically, this has also been reported to cause decreased antibiotic uptake and increased tolerance of the antibiotic (see section 8.3.4).

3.16 QACs AND OTHER SURFACTANTS

Types. Surfactants (or "surface-active agents") are a group of compounds with the unique property of having hydrophobic ("water-repelling"; nonpolar, or lipophilic) and hydrophilic ("water-attracting"; polar, or lipophilic) portions (Fig. 3.30). They are referred to as "surface acting," as they interact with a liquid

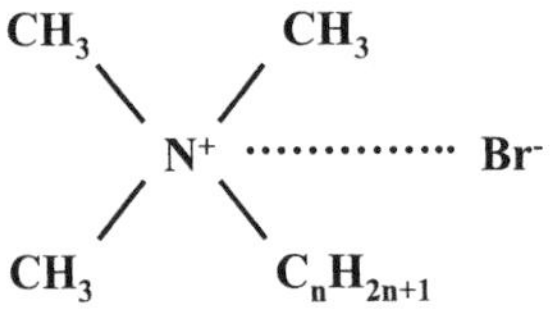

CH_3 CH_3 N^+ Br^- CH_3 C_nH_{2n+1}

Cetrimide

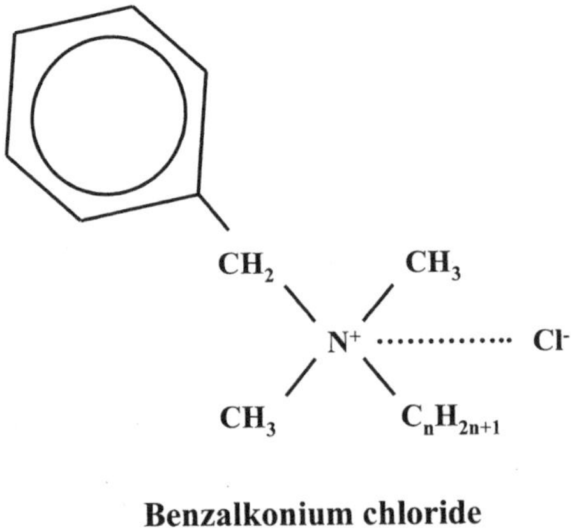

CH_2 CH_3 N^+ Cl^- CH_3 C_nH_{2n+1}

Benzalkonium chloride

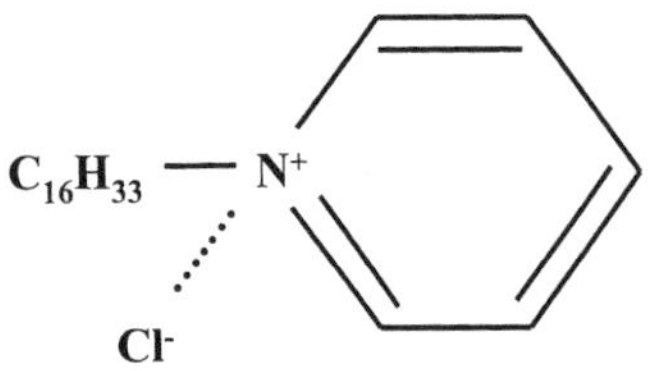

$C_{16}H_{33}$ — N^+ Cl^-

Cetylpyridinium chloride

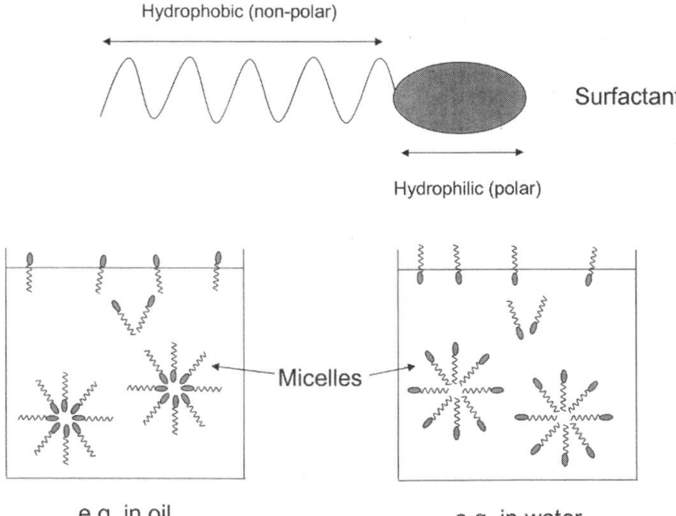

FIGURE 3.30 Basic surfactant and micelle structures.

(such as water) surface to reduce the surface tension and also form micelles, allowing dispersion in the liquid. Taking water as an example, the hydrophilic portion of the surfactant molecule is soluble at the water surface, with the hydrophobic end repelled from the surface; the resulting reduction in surface tension allows greater dispersion of water across a surface. Dispersion also occurs in the water by micelle formation, with the hydrophobic ends interacting to repel the hydrophilic ends (Fig. 3.30). Surfactants can therefore be useful as foaming agents (liquid-gas interactions), emulsifiers (liquid-liquid interactions, for example, for mixing oil in water), or dispersants (liquid-solid interactions, for example, dispersion of a water-insoluble solid). Surfactants can be classified based on their overall charges (Table 3.7).

These classes vary in their observed antimicrobial activities and detergencies. Detergency is the ability to act as a cleaning agent, which is associated with the ability to remove and solubilize soil from a surface. For example, anionic and nonionic surfactants have little or no intrinsic antimicrobial activity but are widely used as cleaners, in formulations, and to enhance the activities of other biocides. Amphoteric surfactants have increased in use due to improved antimicrobial activity in combination with good detergency. From an antimicrobial perspective, cationic surfactants, particularly the QACs, are the most widely used.

TABLE 3.7 Classification of surfactants

Surfactant type	Antimicrobial efficacy	Detergency	Charge[a] (pH above pK_a)	Examples
Cationic	+++	+	+	Benzalkonium chloride, cetrimide
Anionic	+/−	+++	−	Sodium or potassium fatty acid salts ("soaps"), sodium lauryl sulfate
Nonionic	−	+++	Neutral	Polysorbates (Tweens), nonoxynol-9
Amphoteric	+++	++	+/−/neutral	Betaine, alkyldimethyl oxide

[a]Depending on pH.

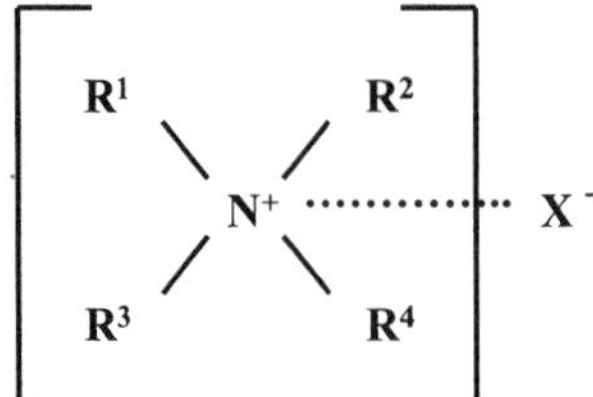

FIGURE 3.31 The basic structure of QACs.

The basic QAC structure is shown in Fig. 3.31. The cation (positively charged) portion consists of a central nitrogen with four attached groups, which can contain a variety of structures and is the functional part of the molecule. The anion (negatively charged) portion (X^-) is usually chlorine (Cl^-) or bromine (Br^-) and is linked to the nitrogen to form the QAC salt. QACs can be further classified based on their structures (e.g., the anion or the nature of the associated [R] groups, which can include the number of nitrogens, the degree of saturation, branching, and the presence of aromatic groups) or as developed generations. For example, benzalkonium chloride is a first-generation QAC, including an aromatic ring, two methyl (CH_3) groups, and a long-chain ethyl (CH_2^- CH_3)/methyl chain, which can vary in length from C_{12} to C_{16} (e.g., 40% C_{12}, 50% C_{14}, and 10% C_{16}). Further QAC generations were synthesized to improve antimicrobial activity (including synergism between QAC mixtures), detergency, and toxicity. The full names of QACs are often descriptive of their structures. Examples are hexadecyltrimethylammonium bromide (also known as CTAB, or cetrimide), alkylbenzyldimethylammonium chloride (also known as benzalkonium chloride, or BKC), and hexadecylpyridinium chloride (also known as cetylpyridinium chloride, or CPC).

Applications. Nonionic and anionic surfactants can be used as preservatives but find their primary applications as cleaners, enhancing the efficacies of other active agents (including phenols and QACs), and as formulants (dispersants, emulsifiers, foaming agents, etc.). Anionic and amphoteric surfactants have been used as antimicrobials for food and beverage applications, as surface or direct food sanitizers, and as general surface disinfectants, particularly in combination with cleaning. Amphoterics have also been used as antiseptics, particularly in combination with other biocides (such as chlorhexidine, also a surfactant [discussed in section 3.8]). QACs are extensively used as household, industrial, and health care general surface disinfectants (Fig. 3.32).

QACs are often used for food surface disinfection, as many formulations do not require posttreatment rinsing with water. They can be used as direct "spray-and-wipe" applications for tabletops, walls, floors, etc., or indirectly, by fogging within a room. Due to their lack of sporicidal activity, certain products are provided sterilized (by radiation or filtration) for cleanroom or isolator applications. QACs are not widely used for critical medical- or veterinary-device disinfection but can be considered for noncritical devices. Antiseptic applications include skin and mucous membrane bioburden reduction, for example, for wound cleansing and as mouthwashes for the control of dental plaque. In addition to disinfection, QAC formulations are used for their cleaning and deodorization attributes. Other application include as preserv-

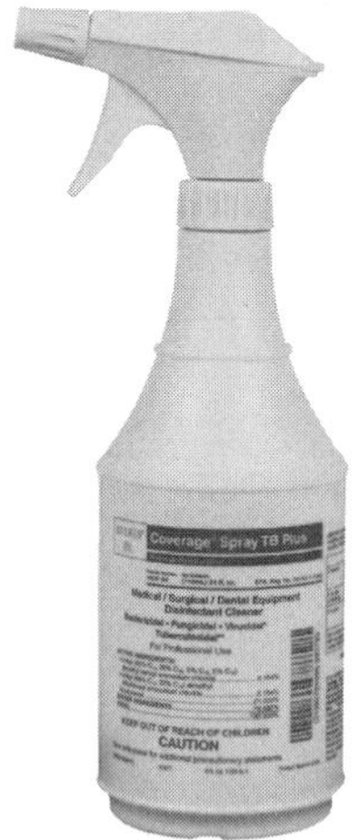

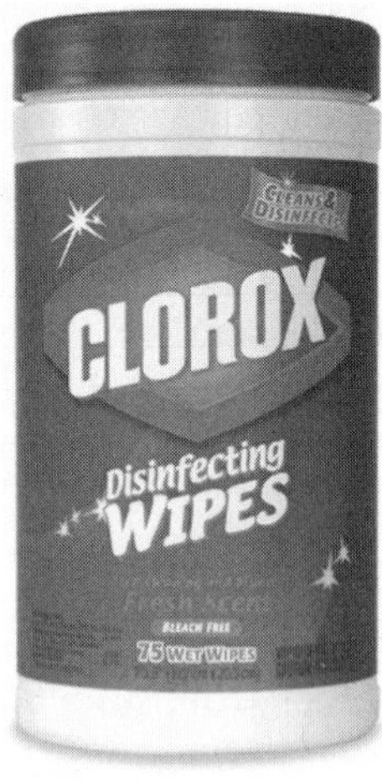

FIGURE 3.32 QAC-based disinfectants. A ready-to-use spray formulation and an example of QAC-impregnated wipes are shown. Photo of container of wipes courtesy of The Clorox Sales Company.

atives (e.g., in paints, contact lens solutions, and cosmetics), fabric or laundry deodorization or softening, hair conditioning, and pool or pond treatment for control of algae and slime. Biologically active QACs include vitamin B and acetylcholine (a neurotransmitter).

Antimicrobial Efficacy. Nonionic and, in particular, anionic surfactants can demonstrate some bactericidal activity but are generally considered useful inhibitory agents, which can include bacteriostatic, fungistatic, and sporistatic activities; they are not considered further as biocidal agents in their own right. Amphoteric surfactants have good bactericidal (including gram-positive and gram-negative bacteria) activity at low concentrations, with greater resistance observed for some pseudomonads, mycobacteria, and fungi (which can be improved by formulation effects). They are generally considered effective against enveloped, but not nonenveloped, viruses. QACs vary in their antimicrobial activities depending on the type and formulation. In general, they are bacteriostatic, fungistatic, tuberculostatic, sporistatic, and algistatic at very low concentrations (<500 μg/ml), with gram-positive bacteria particularly sensitive (<10 μg/ml). Higher concentrations (>1 mg/ml) are generally required for broad bactericidal, algicidal, and fungicidal activities. Although effective against enveloped viruses (including human immunodeficiency virus and hepatitis B virus), QACs are not generally effective against nonenveloped viruses or, indeed, mycobacteria; activity can also be improved by formulation effects, including the addition of nonionic surfactants and synergism between QAC types. QACs are not considered sporicidal, although some activity has been observed at higher concentrations and temperatures. They are sporistatic and inhibit the outgrowth of spores, but not the actual germination processes.

Advantages. Surfactants provide excellent cleaning ability, which, in the case of QACs and some amphoteric surfactants, can be combined with disinfection. They are also essential components of formulations such as antimicrobials and cosmetics, including as preservatives and emulsifiers. As sanitizers and disinfectants, they are also considered to be gentle (noncorrosive and nonstaining) on surfaces and do not require to be rinsed off following application. It should be noted that this may be considered an advantage, not only for ease of use, but also because it allows residual antimicrobial activity on the surface; however, it is also a disadvantage due to the difficulty in removing these residues for some applications (e.g., for pharmaceutical production). QACs, in particular, have the ability to penetrate and solubilize organic soils while retaining efficacy. They have a pleasant, "clean" odor and are regarded as nontoxic under typical conditions of use. They can be used in antiseptics at low concentrations without irritation to skin or mucous membranes.

Disadvantages. Some formulations (e.g., anionic and amphoteric surfactants formulated at acid pHs) can be aggressive on certain material surfaces, such as copper and brass. The antimicrobial efficacy of QACs can be negatively affected in the presence of hard water (if it is a diluted product), fatty materials, and anionic surfactants (including soaps); this varies depending on the QAC type and formulation. Surfactants can be difficult to rinse from critical surfaces and can cause excessive foaming, which may be undesirable. Most surfactants have limited activity against mycobacteria and nonenveloped viruses, which can limit their use for some applications. Higher concentrations of QACs and other surfactants can cause severe irritation to skin and mucous membranes. The presence of low-level residues may allow the selective development of bacterial strains with greater tolerance of QACs over time (e.g., in *Pseudomonas*); intrinsic and acquired resistance mechanisms have been described (see chapter 8).

Mode of Action. The primary targets for surfactants, including QACs, are the bacterial and fungal cell walls and membranes. They quickly adsorb to and penetrate the cell wall, which can disrupt its structure and function. On contact with the cell membrane, they have been shown to react with the membrane lipids and proteins (including enzymes), leading to a cascade of effects, including loss of structure and function and leakage of cytoplasmic material. Direct insertion into the lipid bilayer has been suggested. Further effects on cytoplasmic proteins (including precipitation) and nucleic acids, which culminate in cell death, have also been reported. Direct interaction with viral and spore surface proteins may also cause prevention of growth, loss of function, and disintegration. For example, QAC-based products induced disintegration and morphological changes in human hepatitis B virus, which resulted in loss of infectivity.

3.17 MISCELLANEOUS BIOCIDES OR APPLICATIONS

3.17.1 Pyrithiones

The most widely used pyrithione, primarily for fungicidal activity, is zinc pyrithione (or zinc 2-pyridinethiol *n*-oxide). Chemically, pyrithiones have low solubility in water, but they are relatively stable and also act as chelating agents. They are primarily used as antiseptics in the topical treatment of psoriasis and dermatitis, and also in antidandruff shampoos. They are provided in a variety of product types, including soaps, creams, and sprays. Other applications are as algicides and as preservatives in adhesive coatings and other surface applications. They demonstrate broad-spectrum antimicrobial activity, particularly fungicidal, bactericidal, and algicidal activities. Their fungicidal activity has been especially well studied, particularly against *Pityrosporum ovale* (which is often associated with dandruff), but also against other fungal skin infections, such as the dermatophytes (tinea infections, including various ringworms). They are also effective against bacteria, particularly gram-positive bacteria, and have been used for the treatment of eczema-related infections. Pyrithiones are also not known to be keratinolytic (i.e., breaking down keratin, which is associated with the epidermal skin layers [see section 4.3]). They are not considered to be toxic, although some cases of irritation and allergic reactions have been noted. The mode of action of the pyrithiones is not known but is believed to be related to DNA interactions and disruption of function.

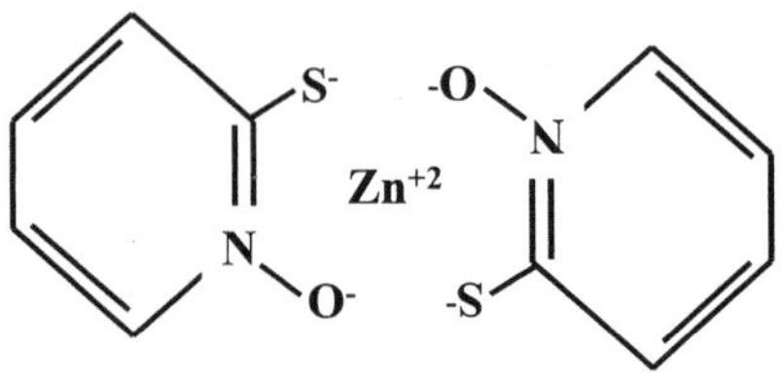

Zinc Pyrithione

3.17.2 Biocides Integrated into Surfaces

Various types of biocides have been successfully used to provide antimicrobial surfaces or surfaces that release the biocide or biocidal activity over time. The most widely used biocides are summarized in Table 3.8. They include metals (e.g., silver- and copper-releasing agents), halogen-releasing agents, biguanides, bisphenols, and QACs.

The biocide can be provided on the surface by a variety of techniques, including simple application to the surface (directly or as a coating), impregnation, incorporation into a polymer or during the polymer formation, and fixing onto the surface. Antimicrobial surfaces have found particular applications on the skin and mucous membranes (e.g., antimicrobial dressings and plasters) and devices that are associated with the skin (e.g., catheters). Catheters and other devices that contact and/or penetrate the skin are considered to be at high risk for contamination and as sources of infection, particularly when they are present for extended periods and with immunocompromised patients. The slow release of biocides from these surfaces can reduce the risk of bacterial or fungal colonization and prevent wound infections. Other applications include the prevention of biofilms on water contact surfaces, in textiles, in water or air filters, and on general surfaces, such as cut-

TABLE 3.8 Various biocides used on antimicrobial surfaces

Biocide	Description	Applications
Silver and silver sulfadiazine	Silver-releasing coatings or impregnated surfaces (e.g., silver zeolites or silver sulfadiazine) (see section 3.12)	Textiles, wound and skin dressings, devices (e.g., catheters), and packaging materials
Copper	Metallic copper or copper alloys used for surfaces and devices; copper-releasing coatings or impregnated surfaces (see section 3.12)	Various industrial (water pipes, food-handling surfaces, etc.) and medical surfaces
Chlorhexidine	Coatings or impregnated surfaces (see section 3.8)	Wound and skin care dressings, dental floss, toothpicks, wipes, and some devices (such as catheters)
Triclosan	Coatings or impregnated surfaces (see section 3.15)	Wound and skin care dressings, but also general surfaces, such as cutting boards and toys
Benzalkonium chloride and other QACs	Hydrogels and other coatings; impregnated plastics and textiles (see section 3.16)	Reduces biofouling and bacterial adherence; wound and skin dressings; catheters
Titanium dioxide	Photocatalytic, releasing active oxygen species on exposure to UV light	Preservative (e.g., paints) and antimicrobial coating on air filters, food preparation surfaces, and medical devices
N-Halamines	Halogen (chlorine or bromine)-releasing agents (see section 3.11); includes monomeric and polymeric compounds	General or food contact surfaces, textiles, water disinfection, and odor control

ting boards, toys, and food-handling surfaces. It should be noted that their overall benefit in reducing the risk of surface and surface-associated contamination depends on the application, the biocide used, and its practical efficacy over time.

Most of the biocides listed in Table 3.8 are discussed in other sections. Further description of titanium dioxide and the *N*-halamines is provided here.

Titanium dioxide (TiO_2, or titania) is the most widely used white pigment in paints, plastics, and paper. Cosmetic applications include use as a sunblock. It can be applied to surfaces, such as air filters, metals, and plastics, as a thin layer. Some applications have also included the inactivation of gram-negative bacteria and viruses in wastewater and the prevention of biofilm formation on water contact surfaces. The chemical is photocatalytic, and on exposure to near-UV (<380-nm) light, it releases active oxygen species, including superoxide ions and hydroxyl radicals (see section 3.13). These active species prevent bacterial and fungal growth and can inactivate microorganisms in contact with the surface over time. The antimicrobial activity is generally slow and is primarily used to inhibit the growth of bacteria and fungi on surfaces. It addition, due to the reactive nature of released oxygen species, organic pollutants and other chemical contaminants are also neutralized. Titanium dioxide surfaces are corrosion resistant and are considered nontoxic.

The *N*-halamines are essentially halogen-releasing agents (see section 3.11). They are nitrogen-containing compounds with anchored chlorine or bromine groups, which are released on contact with microorganisms (Fig. 3.33) (other examples are discussed in section 3.11).

They can be used as water-soluble monomers (e.g., 1-chloro-2,2,5,5-tetramethyl-1,3-imidazolidin-4-one), as preservatives, or in disinfectants, and when integrated into antimicrobial surfaces [e.g., the chlorinated polystyrene hydantoin, poly-1,3-dichloro-5-methyl-5-(4′-vinylphenyl)hydantoin]. Other bromine-based *N*-halamines include PSHB and DBDMH (see section 3.11). Antimicrobial

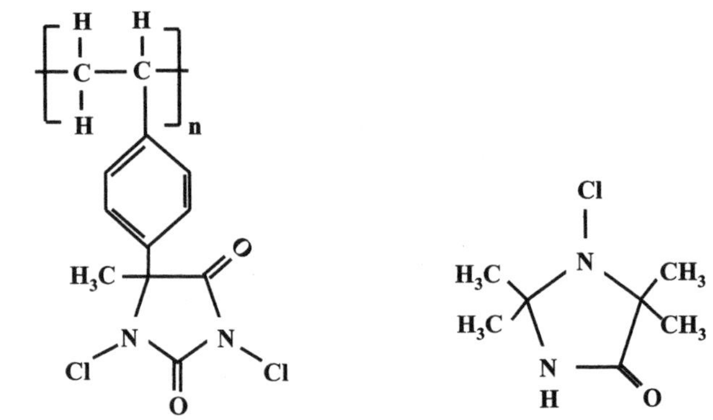

FIGURE 3.33 Examples of chlorine-based *N*-halamines.

polymers can be made by polymerization of the monomers, attachment to an existing plastic polymer, or copolymerization. These polymers are stable and odorless. Applications have included their use on various hard surfaces (medical, dental, and industrial); in textiles, paper, and antimicrobial paints and coatings; and for water disinfection. The choice of *N*-halamine can depend on the application, with slowly releasing compounds used for odor control, biofilm control, and as preservatives, while faster-releasing compounds are used for more immediate activity, such as on general-use surfaces and for water disinfection. A key advantage of these compounds is that, following exhaustion of the antimicrobial activity, the surface can be reactivated by application of a chlorine- or bromine-containing formulation, which is not the case for other biocidal surfaces. *N*-Halamines are broad-spectrum antimicrobials, but their effectiveness varies depending on the type. In general, they are stable over wide pH (pH 4 to 10) and ambient-temperature (4 to 37°C) ranges, with efficacy against bacteria, fungi, viruses, and protozoa (such as *Giardia*). Slow cysticidal and sporicidal activities have been reported in some applications. They also have long functional lives and are considered safer to use than higher liquid concentrations of chlorine and bromine (see section 3.11). Their modes of action are considered to be similar to those described for halogens and other halogen-releasing agents (see section 3.11).

3.17.3 Antimicrobial Enzymes, Proteins, or Peptides

Various types of naturally occurring antimicrobial peptides or proteins have been identified from microorganisms, insects, plants, and animals. Their primary roles are as part of the hosts' intrinsic defenses or immune systems against various types of fungi and bacteria and certain viruses. In general, they have limited applications, as they demonstrate restricted spectra of activity, but they have been utilized in some instances as biocides. For the purpose of this discussion, they are considered antimicrobial enzymes and peptides (Table 3.9).

Lysozyme is one of the most widely studied enzymes; it specifically degrades bacterial peptidoglycan by hydrolysis of the β-1,4 glucosidic linkages between *N*-acetylmuramic acid and *N*-acetylglucosamine (Fig. 3.34).

Due to its specific mode of action, lysozyme is bacteriostatic or bactericidal only against bacteria that contain peptidoglycan, and then predominantly against gram-positive bacteria; genetic modification of the enzyme has allowed the isolation of enzymes with greater penetration of and activity against the gram-negative cell wall. Lysozyme has been used as a preserva-

TABLE 3.9 Various types of proteins, peptides, and enzymes used as biocides

Type	Description	Application(s)
Antimicrobial enzymes		
Lysozyme	Limited activity against some gram-positive and gram-negative bacteria; some investigations have attempted to alter the structure of the enzyme to allow greater activity against gram-negative bacteria.	Limited to bactericidal and bacteriostatic activity; pharmaceutical (eye drops and lozenges) and food (preservative in cheese and wine) applications
Chitinases	Fungistatic and fungicidal activity against chitin-containing fungi	Limited to fungistatic and fungicidal activity; primarily agricultural applications
Proteases	Endopeptidases, such as keratinases, proteinase K, and other thermostable proteases	Proposed activity against prions
Antimicrobial peptides		
Aprotinin	Polypeptide serine protease inhibitor with some activity against bacteria	Some potential industrial applications as a preservative; used therapeutically to reduce bleeding
Nisin	Isolated from *Lactococcus lactis*; particularly active against gram-positive bacteria; sporistatic	Food preservative
Magainins	Isolated from *Xenopus laevis*; bactericidal, fungicidal; some activity against protozoa	Developing applications, including treatment of impetigo

tive in pharmaceutical and food applications, such as eye drops, antibacterial lozenges, wines, and dairy products, the last specifically to limit spoilage by lactic acid bacteria. In a similar manner, other enzymes have been used specifically against fungal cell walls. The most widely studied are the chitinases. Chitin is a major polysaccharide component of many fungal cell walls, associated with the inner cell membrane (see section 1.3.3.2). Chitin is degraded by various chitinases by hydrolysis of the glycosidic bonds within the polysaccharide. This weakens the cell wall structure and eventually causes cell lysis. Proposed agricultural applications have included prevention of fungal growth on plants and biopesticidal activity. Other antifungal proteins are glucanases and chitin-binding peptides, which also have fungistatic activities.

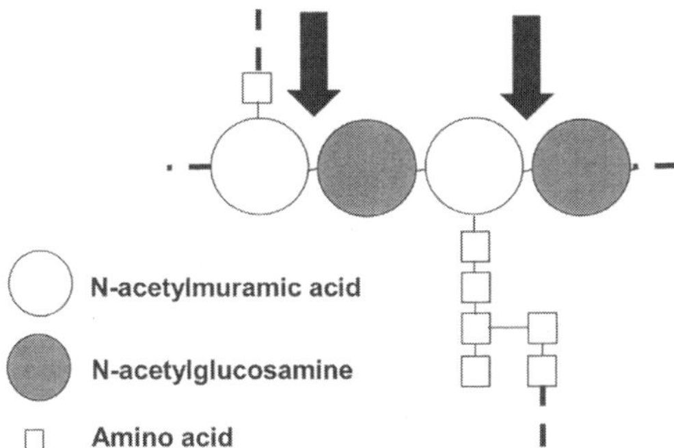

FIGURE 3.34 The enzymatic activity of lysozyme. The structure of peptidoglycan (see section 1.3.4.1) is cleaved at the glycosidic bonds between *N*-acetylmuramic acid and *N*-acetylglucosamine in the polymer.

Prions are unique infectious agents that are composed exclusively of protein and do not appear to have an associated nucleic acid (see section 1.3.6). Although prions have been characterized as having high resistance to proteases, some reports have suggested the use of various endopeptidases to degrade them over time. These include thermoresistant proteases, such as keratinases, although these reports need to be verified for practical use as prion inactivation methods.

Various types of antimicrobial peptides have been isolated (some examples are given in Table 3.9). They are typically cationic peptides of various lengths but with a high proportion of basic amino acids (such as lysine and arginine). Their hydrophobic nature appears to be associated with their antimicrobial activity, by affinity with the surfaces of microorganisms and insertion into cell membranes. In addition to cell membrane structure disruption, other negatively charged macromolecules (like DNA and some proteins) may also be affected. They also appear to have limited spectra of activity, and few practical applications have been described. For example, nisin is particularly active against gram-positive bacteria and has also been shown to be sporistatic (e.g., against *Clostridium botulinum* spores). The primary application for nisin has been as a natural preservative in heat-processed and low-pH foods. Nisin is regarded as safe to use but has little or no effect on gram-negative bacteria, yeasts, molds, or other microorganisms; however, synergy has been observed with other biocide preservatives, lysozyme, and chelating agents. The magainins are another group of antimicrobial peptides, isolated from the frog species *Xenopus laevis*, and have been shown to have activities against bacteria, fungi, and protozoa. They range in length from 21 to 27 amino acids and have α-helical, hydrophobic structures. They have also been shown to disrupt lipid bilayers, leading to disruption of cell permeability, and to bind to lipopolysaccharide (see section 1.3.4.1). Proposed applications have included the treatment of skin infections, such as impetigo.

FURTHER READING

Ascenzi, J. M. 1996. *Handbook of Disinfectants and Antiseptics*. Marcel Dekker, New York, N.Y.

Block, S. S. 1991. *Disinfection, Sterilization, and Preservation*, 4th ed. Lea & Febiger, Philadelphia, Pa.

Block, S. S. 2001. *Disinfection, Sterilization, and Preservation*, 5th ed. Lippincott Williams & Wilkins, Philadelphia, Pa.

Hoffman, P. N., C. Bradley, and G. A. J. Ayliffe. 2004. *Disinfection in Healthcare*, 3rd ed. Blackwell Publishing Ltd., Malden, Mass.

Izadpanah, A., and R. L. Gallo. 2005. Antimicrobial peptides. *J. Am. Acad. Dermatol.* **52:**381–390.

McDonnell, G., and A. D. Russell. 1999. Antiseptics and disinfectants: activity, action and resistance. *Clin. Microbiol. Rev.* **12:**147–179.

Russell, A. D., W. B. Hugo, and G. A. J. Ayliffe. 1992. *Principles and Practice of Disinfection, Preservation and Sterilization*, 2nd ed. Blackwell Science, Cambridge, Mass.

ANTISEPTICS AND ANTISEPSIS

4

4.1 INTRODUCTION

Antiseptics can be defined as biocidal products that destroy or inhibit the growth of microorganisms in or on living tissue, e.g., on the skin. In theory any biocide or biocidal process could be used on the skin or mucous membranes, although only a limited number are widely used. Living tissues are more sensitive to damage than hard surfaces; therefore, the requirements for the safe use of antiseptics restrict the choice to those that have limited or no toxicity. Antiseptics can include a variety of formulations and preparations, such as antimicrobial hand washes, surgical scrubs, preoperative preparations, ointments, creams, tinctures, mouthwashes, and toothpastes. Overall, antiseptics should demonstrate the following characteristics

- A wide spectrum of biocidal activity, particularly against bacteria, fungi, and viruses
- Rapid biocidal activity
- Little or no damage, irritation, or toxicity to the tissue
- Little or no absorption into the body
- If possible and applicable, some persistent biocidal (or biostatic) activity (many biocides used in antiseptics remain on the skin following washing or application, allowing continuing biocidal and growth-inhibitory action or cumulative activity over time)

4.2 SOME DEFINITIONS SPECIFIC TO ANTISEPTICS

Antimicrobial soap: A soap- or detergent-based formulation that contains one or more antiseptic agents at concentrations necessary to inhibit or kill microorganisms.

Antisepsis: Destruction or inhibition of microorganisms in or on living tissue, e.g., on the skin or mucous membranes. Antiseptics are biocidal products used for antisepsis. They include washes (which contain soaps or other detergents and are used with water) and rubs (which are applied directly to the skin with no washing, e.g., tinctures and alcohols).

Antiseptic hand washes or hand rubs for health care workers: Antiseptics that are fast acting, with minimal irritation, and designed for frequent use on the skin, particularly for the reduction of transient microorganisms. They are widely available for regular use, particularly in health care facilities. They are also known as hygienic hand disinfectants, which may have persistence.

Persistence: The ability of a biocide to demonstrate continued antimicrobial activity on the skin following application of an antiseptic product for an extended time to prevent or inhibit the growth of microorganisms.

Plain (or "bland") soap: A soap- or detergent-based formulation that does not contain specific biocides, except for the purpose of product preservation.

Preoperative preparation: An antiseptic, preferably with persistent activity, to reduce the number of microorganisms on the skin at the site of surgical intervention. Preoperative preparations are used for the localized antisepsis of a patient's skin prior to surgical incision.

Substantivity (residual activity): The ability of a biocide to bind to the skin, thereby maintaining a chemical presence on the surface, or to increase levels through cumulative effects.

Surgical scrub: An antiseptic, preferably with persistent activity, used to reduce the number of microorganisms on intact skin prior to surgery. Surgical scrubs are used by surgical staff on their hands and forearms prior to a procedure. They are sometimes referred to as surgical hand disinfectants.

Wound: Any break in the skin caused by injury or surgical intervention.

4.3 THE STRUCTURE OF SKIN

The skin is the largest human organ, consisting of approximately one-sixth of typical body weight. It has a variety of functions, including temperature regulation, energy storage, and acting as a barrier and protection against water loss, various microorganisms, chemicals (including biocides), and radiation (e.g., UV light). The skin has a complex structure consisting of three layers: the outer epidermis, the dermis, and the innermost subcutaneous layer (Fig. 4.1).

The epidermis is the outermost layer and can itself be further divided into various layers,

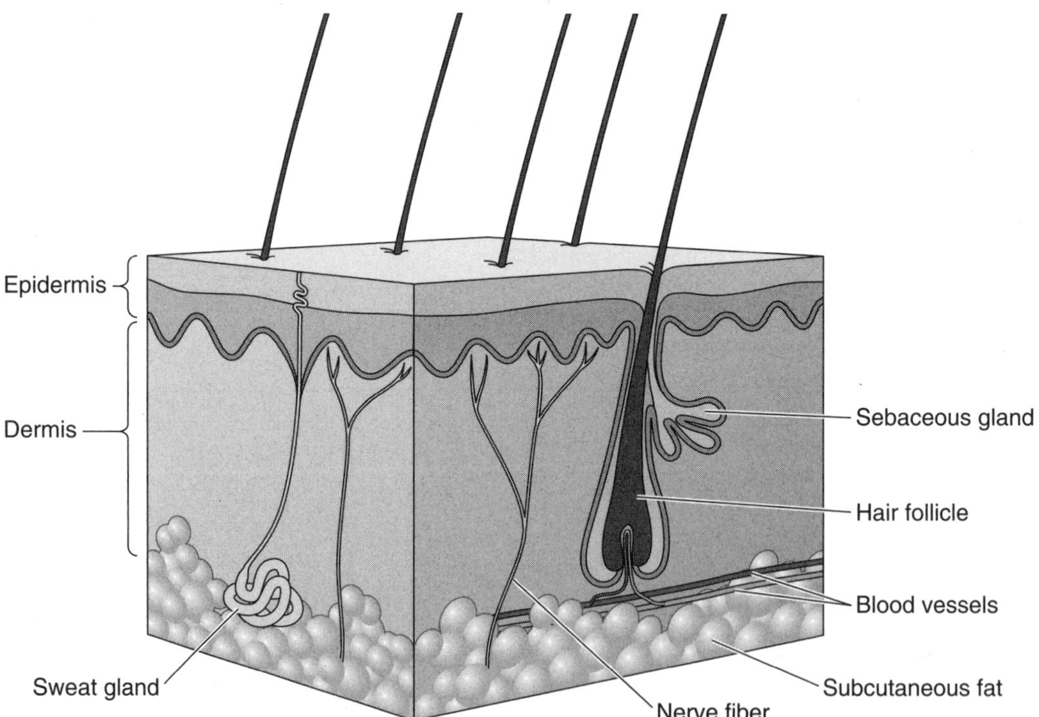

FIGURE 4.1 Cross section of skin structure. Illustration by Patrick Lane, ScEYEnce Studios.

from an innermost layer (stratum basale) of actively multiplying skin cells (keratinocytes) to the outer layer (stratum corneum) of dead, flattened cells held together by various skin lipids, which are constantly released from the surface and replaced by new cells from the lower epidermal layers. The keratinocytes, which produce keratin as they develop into the skin surface layers, are the most prominent cell type in the epidermis. Another cell type associated with the epidermis, particularly the lower layers, is the melanocytes, which produce the dark pigment, melanin, that gives the skin a tanned color as a protective mechanism on exposure to UV light. The epidermal cells are separated from the lower dermis layer by a basement membrane and are dependent on the dermis for nutrients and oxygen. The dermis largely consists of fibroblast cells, which produce collagen and elastin to give flexibility and strength to the skin. The dermis also contains various glands (like sebaceous glands), blood and lymph vessels, hair follicles, muscle cells, and nerve endings. Finally, the subcutaneous layer (or subcutis) is composed of larger blood and nerve vessels and sweat glands, with specific fat storage cells known as adipose cells.

4.4 SKIN MICROBIOLOGY

The overall structure and constituents of the skin, including its thickness, pH, temperature, wetness, density of hair, and distribution of secretory glands, vary across the body. The variety of microorganisms found on the skin also varies, depending on these and other environmental factors. Overall, the microbiological ecology of the skin is complicated and varies in type and population from site to site and from individual to individual. Skin floras have traditionally been considered as two types: resident and transient floras. Resident floras are considered to be permanently found growing on the skin or a given skin area; typical residents include various types of *Corynebacterium*, *Propionibacterium*, *Staphylococcus* (coagulase-negative staphylococci, like *Staphylococcus epidermidis*), and *Micrococcus*. In general, drier areas of the skin (like the hands) have a larger population of gram-positive cocci, including *S. epidermidis* and *Micrococcus* species, while those areas associated with greater moisture or the presence of sebum (increased oil content) have more prominent populations of the diphtheroid gram-positive rods, like *Corynebacterium* and *Propionibacterium* species. Gram-negative bacteria (including *Klebsiella*, *Escherichia*, and *Enterobacter*), as well as various types of fungi (particularly *Candida* species), are found to a lesser extent. Transient residents of the skin are described as being short-lived or simply carried on the skin but are not consistently identified as resident flora in most individuals. Transient populations vary considerably and include bacteria, yeasts, fungi, viruses, and other microorganisms. Many of these can be pathogenic to the skin, particularly within wounds, or can be transmitted from various surfaces and between individuals. Antiseptics are used to reduce the presence and transfer of resident and transient microbes on the skin and mucous membranes; many are also used to reduce the risk or treat the presence of various skin infections, including wound infections. Various types of infections of intact skin and wounds are listed in Table 4.1. Some of the most common wound or surgical site infections are caused by *Staphylococcus aureus* (including methicillin-resistant strains), coagulase-negative staphylococci, *Enterococcus*, *Escherichia coli*, *Enterobacter*, and *Candida albicans*. There is some correlation between the site of the wound and the associated pathogen; for example, gram-negative bacteria are often associated with intestinal and urological wounds or surgical site infections, as they are often found at high concentrations in those regions of the body.

4.5 ANTISEPTIC APPLICATIONS

Antiseptic applications are considered here as routine skin hygiene, skin treatment prior to surgical intervention, treatment of skin or wound infections, treatment of mucous mem-

TABLE 4.1 Common or notable infections of the skin

Microorganism	Comments
Intact-skin infections	
Streptococcus pyogenes	Impetigo, an infection of the epidermis, particularly in children (also caused by *S. aureus*). Some virulent strains can cause significant damage to the skin, as in the case of necrotizing fasciitis ("flesh-eating bacteria").
Staphylococcus aureus	Boils and carbuncles, such as infections of hair follicles and sebaceous glands
Propionibacterium acnes	Associated with acne
Treponema pallidum	Syphilis, a sexually transmitted disease with lesions in the genital region and other areas of the skin
Herpes simplex virus	Cold sores
Varicella-zoster virus	Chickenpox and shingles
Papillomaviruses	Common and other types of warts
Dermatophytes (*Trichophyton, Microsporum,* and *Epidermophyton* species)	Fungal infections of keratinized tissues, including skin, nails, and hair. Diseases are referred to as "tinea" or "ringworm," including tinea unguium (nail ringworm), tinea corporis (body ringworm), and tinea pedis (athlete's foot).
Leishmania species	Cutaneous leishmaniasis, with skin ulceration on the face and limbs
Onchocerca volvulus	Infects the skin subcutaneous layer but can also lead to complications like "river blindness"
Wound or surgical site infections	
Staphylococcus aureus	The most prevalent cause of infections in wounds (~15 to 20%)
Coagulase-negative staphylococci, including *S. epidermidis*	Often associated with bite wounds and catheter-associated infections
Enterococcus species	Opportunistic wound infections, including burn contamination with *E. faecalis*
Clostridium species	*C. perfringens* causes gas gangrene, and *C. tetani* causes tetanus, both associated with deep-wound infections
Escherichia coli	The most common gram-negative bacterium associated with wound infections
Pseudomonas aeruginosa	Opportunistic infections in burns; difficult to treat due to intrinsic antibiotic/biocidal resistance
Candida albicans	The most common fungus isolated from wounds, particularly burn infections

branes, and biocide-impregnated materials used for antiseptic applications. Some examples of the various types of antiseptic products are shown in Fig. 4.2. Examples of various guidelines and standards that describe the types and uses of antiseptics are given in Table 4.2.

4.5.1 Routine Skin Hygiene

Skin, particularly hand, hygiene is often cited as an important step in reducing the potential of microbial cross-contamination from surfaces to individuals and between individuals. Washing with plain soap can remove a certain amount of transient and surface-resident flora associated with the surface epidermal layers, as well as contaminated soils, like dirt and blood, by mechanical action alone; however, in some studies, it has been suggested that washing with plain soap alone may increase the shedding of bacteria. The use of antimicrobial hand washes and hand rubs can provide a greater reduction of microorganisms on the skin. This is particularly important in high-risk situations, for example, in hospitals, surgeries, and other health care facilities, as well as in food handling and preparation. It should be remembered that the purpose of antiseptics is to reduce the level of contamination; although antiseptics can vary considerably in antimicrobial activity on the skin, they do not completely remove all

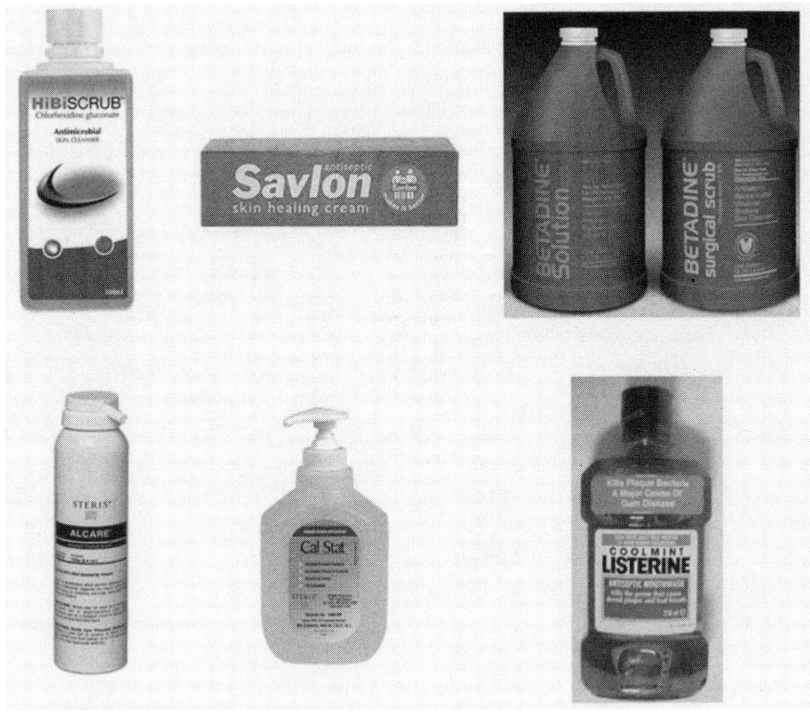

FIGURE 4.2 Examples of various types of antiseptic products.

transient and resident microorganisms (see section 4.4). There are many reports of cross-transmission by pathogens from contaminated hands in these situations, and studies have shown that the use of antiseptics can reduce the risk of transmission; their effects vary from formulation to formulation, despite the presence of similar concentrations of various biocides.

TABLE 4.2 Examples of various guidelines and standards on the use and application of antiseptics

Reference[a]	Title	Summary
APIC (1995)	*Guidelines for Handwashing and Hand Antisepsis in Health Care Settings*	Guidelines on the types and use of antiseptics in health care settings
CDC HICPAC (2002)	*Hand Hygiene in Healthcare Settings*	Guidelines on hand washing and hand antisepsis in health care settings, including recommendations to promote improved hand hygiene practices and to reduce transmission of pathogenic microorganisms
HC Infection Control Guideline	*Hand Washing, Cleaning, Disinfection and Sterilization in Health Care*	General guidelines on hand washing and hand antisepsis in health care settings
EN 1499	*Chemical Disinfectants and Antiseptics. Hygienic Handwash. Test Method and Requirements (Phase 2/Step 2)*	Test method for demonstrating the efficacy of an antiseptic hand wash
EN 14885	*Chemical Disinfectants and Antiseptics. Application of European Standards for Chemical Disinfectants and Antiseptics*	Guideline on the testing of chemical disinfectants and antiseptics

[a]APIC, Association for Professionals in Infection Control and Epidemiology; CDC HICPAC, Centers for Disease Control and Prevention, Healthcare Infection Control Practices Advisory Committee; HC, Health Canada; EN, European Standard (Norm).

Hand washes include a range of biocides, usually in soap- or detergent-based formulations, such as chlorhexidine, triclosan, chloroxylenol, triclocarban, essential oils (particularly tea tree oil), benzalkonium chloride, and some iodophors. An example of these products is the hand washes that are used by personnel in health care facilities for routine washing of the hands; the most widely used biocides in these products are chlorhexidine, triclosan, and chloroxylenol. Various antibacterial soaps have become popular for general household use (particularly those with triclosan, triclocarban, and essential oils) and are particularly recommended in the handling of food or in food preparation facilities or for those caring for small children or immunocompromised patients. The efficacies of these products can vary significantly, depending on the concentration of the biocide and its formulation, as well as the correct use of the product (washing time, adequate coverage, etc.). Examples are the use of emollients (like oils and creams), which are used to soften and sooth the skin by reducing water loss and to improve the aesthetics of the formulation. Hand rubs (or hand rinses) include various types of alcohols (in particular, ethanol, isopropanol, and *n*-propanol) at various concentrations, which are applied to the skin without water and rubbed into the skin until they evaporate. Alcohols are probably the most widely used antiseptic biocides. Unlike some hand washes (Table 4.3) (see section 4.6.2), they are rapidly effective, but once evaporated, they do not provide any persistent (or residual) activity (which may be desired). The efficacy of alcohols can be increased by decreasing the evaporation rate on the skin by using various emollients or thickening agents, which can also reduce the drying effects associated with alcohol use; alternatively, lower concentrations of other biocides (e.g., 0.5% chlorhexidine in 70% ethanol or preservatives) can be formulated into the hand rub to provide residual activity following alcohol evaporation. In these and other cases, the antimicrobial activity can be increased due to synergy between the biocides within the products.

4.5.2 Pretreatment of Skin Prior to Surgical Intervention

Preoperative preparation of the patient's skin is considered an important action before surgical

TABLE 4.3 Examples of biocides most widely used as skin antiseptics and washes[a]

Biocide(s)	Antimicrobial activity	Typical concn (%)	See section:	Persistence	Reported toxicity
Alcohols, including ethanol, isopropanol, and *n*-propanol	Bactericidal, fungicidal, virucidal, tuberculocidal	60–92	3.5	None	Skin drying and some irritancy
Chlorhexidine	Bactericidal, fungistatic, tuberculocidal, some virucidal activity	0.5–4	3.8	Yes	Keratitis, irritancy, and ototoxicity reported
Iodine and iodophors	Bactericidal, fungicidal, virucidal, tuberculocidal	0.5–10 (iodophors) 2–5 (iodine in tinctures)	3.11	Some	Irritation and some toxicity reported
Chloroxylenol	Bactericidal (depending on formulation), fungistatic, some virucidal activity	0.5–4	3.15	Yes	Not reported
Triclosan	Bactericidal (depending on formulation), fungistatic, tuberculostatic	0.1–2	3.15	Yes	Not reported

[a]It should be remembered that the characteristics of these biocides vary depending on the antiseptic formulation in which they are used.

intervention to reduce the introduction of potential pathogens during surgery and the risk of surgical site infections. These products are also used before the introduction of catheters or needles. In most cases, the skin in the area is initially cleaned and then treated with an antiseptic. The most widely used biocides include alcohols (e.g., in wipes at 60 to 90%), iodine tinctures or iodophors (e.g., povidone-iodine [PVPI] solutions or scrubs at 7.5 to 10%), and chlorhexidine (usually at higher concentrations, typically 2 to 4%). Chlorhexidine, iodophors, and other routine antiseptics are also used for preoperative bathing or showering, although the significance of preoperative bathing in reducing the risk of postoperative infections is not known. In some cases, various impregnated films or barriers, which allow slow release of the biocide over time, are applied to the surgical site; examples are chlorhexidine, triclosan, and silver, and they have found particular application in the prevention of indwelling skin catheter-related infections (for further discussion, see section 4.5.5).

In an application similar to preoperative preparations, surgical hand scrubs and rubs are used to reduce the transient and resident populations of microorganisms on the hands and forearms of surgery personnel. The rationale behind their use is the frequent occurrence of glove damage or tears during surgery or, in particular, cases where gloves are not used. Typical surgical scrubs are conducted for up to 5 min and include washing with chlorhexidine (1 to 4%) or iodophor-containing antiseptics or repeated application and rubbing of alcohol antiseptics for the same length of time. Other biocides, like triclosan, hexachlorophene, and chloroxylenol, are also used as surgical scrubs. The residual microstatic activities of biocides like chlorhexidine and, to a lesser extent, iodophors are considered important in reducing the growth of bacteria under gloves during surgical procedures. Specific surgical rub formulations that include alcohols and iodine are also used. Recommended exposure times of surgical scrub or rub application vary, depending on the product formulation and country-specific efficacy requirements.

4.5.3 Treatment of Skin or Wound Infections

It is common to use a variety of antibiotics and other anti-infectives to treat skin or wound infections, particularly if the infection is present in the deeper layers of the skin (see section 4.3). Despite this, various biocides are often used for localized applications to prevent skin infections, to clean and treat wounds (particularly over large surfaces, as in the case of burns), or to treat skin surface infections.

In these cases, the objective is similar to that for other antiseptics, i.e., to reduce the microbial population in a wound or skin surface infection without significant damage to the tissue or interference with the healing process. A typical application would be in cases of eczema, which is inflammation of the skin leading to itching, scaling, and blistering and making the skin prone to infections; the use of biocides can be helpful in reducing the risk of or treating various infections that can occur under these and similar conditions. The most common causes of wound infections are gram-positive cocci, including *Staphylococcus* and *Enterococcus*, although gram-negative bacteria and some yeasts are also frequently implicated (Table 4.1). Older applications to control these infections included mercuric chloride (and other mercury compounds), diamidines, acridines, and some dyes. Most of these biocides are not widely used today, and in the case of mercury, this is primarily due to risks of toxicity, poisoning, or other adverse effects. Antimicrobial dyes (like crystal violet) are still used, but primarily on animals for various wound treatments. Hydrogen peroxide solutions (ranging from 3 to 6%) or cream formulations (typically in the 1 to 3% range for the treatment of ulcers or pressure sore infections) are widely used for cleaning infected wounds; they are also used to prevent infections following injury to the skin. Among the antimicrobial heavy metals, silver (for example, silver nitrate solutions [see section 3.12]) is used for topical treatments and has also found some application integrated into wound dressing and catheter materials to prevent or control infections (especially in burn patients). Some biocides are specifically used to treat infections of intact skin (Table 4.4). Various phenolics have been used for wound treatment and are provided in creams, ointments, dusting powders, and liquid formulations. They include hexachlorophene (e.g., 0.33% dusting powder, in particular, to treat or prevent neonatal staphylococcal infections), triclosan (e.g., washes at 0.5 to 2%), and 2,4,6-trichlorophenol. Some essential oils have been recommended, especially in the treatment of *S. aureus* infections, although their actual benefits remain inconclusive. Iodine tinctures have become less used due to irritation issues and have been mostly replaced by iodophors. Typically, antiseptics with PVPI for wound applications are provided at <5% (e.g., 2.5% powders, sprays, and solutions), in contrast to the higher concentrations used for preoperative surgical scrub preparations for intact skin, due to irritation and wound tissue damage. Other halogen solutions, including 1% sodium

TABLE 4.4 Miscellaneous biocides used as antiseptics and their applications

Biocide	Antimicrobial activity	See section:	Applications and comments
Antimicrobial dyes, e.g., acridines and crystal violet	Bactericidal, fungistatic, virucidal (enveloped viruses), algistatic, some protozoal activity	3.7	Wound and wound dressing (human, animals, and fish) Mucous membrane infections Various fungal infections, e.g., tinea
Anilides, e.g., triclocarban	Bactericidal, fungistatic	3.6	Preservative, deodorant, and antimicrobial soaps
Boric acid	Bactericidal, fungicidal, virucidal	3.2	Suppositories for the treatment of vaginal yeast and viral infections
Diamidines, e.g., propamidine and dibromopropamidine	Bactericidal, fungicidal, amebicidal, some protozoal activity	3.9	Wound or skin infections Eye infections
Metals, e.g., silver, silver sulfadiazine, and mercury	Bactericidal, fungicidal, algicidal, virucidal (enveloped viruses)	3.12	Burn, wound, and mucous membrane infections Preservative Antimicrobial dressings
QACs, e.g., benzalkonium chloride and cetrimide	Bactericidal, fungicidal, sporostatic, virucidal (enveloped viruses), algistatic	3.16	Skin and mucous membrane washes Shampoos Treatment of seborrhea and psoriasis Mouth rinses
Salicylic acid	Bactericidal, fungicidal	3.15	Exfoliant (keratinolytic) Wart removal Acne and other skin infections (e.g., associated with psoriasis and dermatitis), as shampoos, gels, washes, and integrated plasters or swabs
Hydrogen peroxide	Bactericidal, fungicidal, virucidal, mycobactericidal, some sporicidal activity	3.13	Preservative Wound and wound infection treatment
Benzoyl peroxide	Bactericidal, in particular, studied against *P. acnes*	3.13	Acne control
Chlorine dioxide	Bactericidal, fungicidal, virucidal	3.13	Mastitis control Preoperative preparations
Essential oils, e.g., tea tree oil and thymol	Bactericidal, fungistatic (some fungicidal), some virucidal activity (enveloped viruses)	3.10	Mouthwashes Antimicrobial hand and face washes Acne treatment
Pyrithiones, e.g., zinc pyrithione	Bactericidal, fungicidal, algicidal	3.17.1	Treatment of psoriasis and dermatitis, as skin washes, sprays, or creams Antidandruff shampoo

hypochlorite and 5% chloramines, are used to a much lesser extent, primarily as wound cleaners. Chlorhexidine is also used in various dusting powders, creams, and solutions ranging in concentration from 0.05 to 1%; some formulations are provided as a synergistic mixture with chlorhexidine, for example, 0.015% with 0.5% cetrimide (a quaternary ammonium compound [QAC] [see section 3.16]) for wound applications. Other surfactants (including QACs) are frequently used at relatively low concentrations as wound-cleaning solutions. Further examples of synergistic formulations are mixtures of various acids, like salicylic acid, benzoic acid, and maleic acid. Some reports, although limited, have suggested the benefit of using UV (specifically, the UV-C wavelength range [see section 2.4]) for wound treatments at dosage levels in the 100- to 300-mW/cm^2/s range; radiation has not found widespread use in antiseptic applications.

The treatment of infections of intact skin with biocides is often limited to those that are associated with the surface skin layers and that have not spread to deeper layers, which are inaccessible to biocidal penetration. Examples are the use of antiseptic skin washes to control bacterial infections like cellulitis, erythema, impetigo, and acne. They include triclosan, chlorhexidine, iodophors, some essential oils, salicylic acid, and QACs. In the case of boils and carbuncles, moist heat is often used to help drain the infections, followed by an antiseptic ointment to aid wound healing. Similar biocide-based washes, mouthwashes (particularly chlorhexidine), lozenges, or suppositories (e.g., boric acid) are recommended in the treatment of candidiasis, which is often associated with various mucous membranes, particularly in immunocompromised patients. Medicated shampoos, skin washes, and localized skin applications have been useful in controlling the spread of various fungal dermatophytes (tinea) and other fungal infections (Table 4.1). Virus infections causing cold sores, warts, or other skin eruptions are a particular challenge to biocide penetration. Salicylic acid and/or lactic acids (either as liquids or in impregnated patches) are used to soften the skin to allow the removal of warts over time, although typical application times are a number of weeks; in the case of salicylic acid, this is primarily due to its keratinolytic activity, allowing the breakdown of surface skin layers over time. Warts are also conveniently removed by cryotherapy: localized freezing with liquid nitrogen and allowing the wart to flake off following treatment. Common biocides used to treat acne, which is associated with *Propionibacterium acnes* and other bacteria on the skin, are salicylic acid, triclosan, hydrogen peroxide, and benzoyl peroxide. Most other viral and parasitic skin infections are treated with specific antiviral or antiparasitic drugs.

4.5.4 Treatment of Oral and Other Mucous Membranes

A similar range of biocides are used for the treatment of more sensitive oral and other (including urogenital) mucous membranes. They are used to treat specific infections or as a prophylaxis, for example, oral mouth rinses in the treatment of gingivitis, ulcers, and throat infections and prior to oral surgery. Mouth rinses can include various formulations with QACs (like cetylpyridinium bromide, cetrimide, and dequalinium chloride), chlorhexidine, hydrogen peroxide, essential oils, and PVPI (1% with 8% alcohol). For example, a widely used essential-oil-based formulation uses thymol (0.06%), eucalyptol (0.09%), and menthol (0.045) in combination with methyl salicylate.

Some, including low-concentration hydrogen peroxide solutions and chlorhexidine, have also been used directly on the eye. Antibacterial toothpastes can include triclosan, zinc chloride, fluoride, and chlorhexidine, although there are mixed reports concerning the benefit of antibacterial toothpastes in reducing periodontal diseases. Urinary or genital tract infections, including those by bacterial, fungal, and viral pathogens, can be treated with products such as hexamine, silver nitrate, boric acid, chlorhexidine, octenidine, phenols, and QACs; these products include rinses, suppositories, and creams.

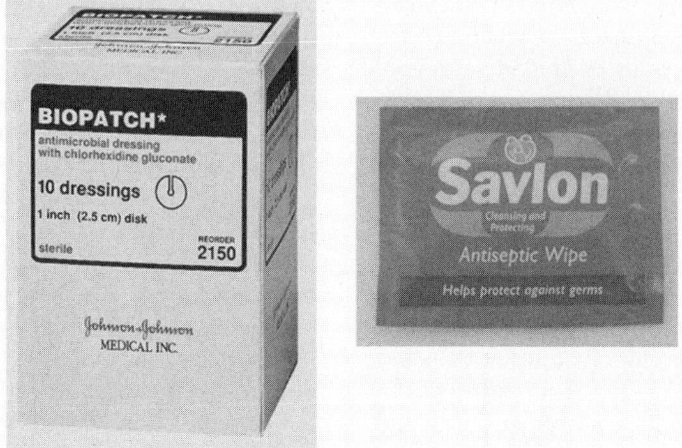

FIGURE 4.3 Examples of biocide-impregnated materials for skin application.

4.5.5 Material-Integrated Applications

Various polymers, textiles, and other materials have been successfully impregnated with biocides (see section 3.17.2). They include medical devices, like catheters and needles, that can remain in contact with the skin or mucous membranes and bandages, dressings, and patches that are used on the skin or wounds over extended periods (Fig. 4.3).

Other applications include surgical drapes and gowns that could contact the skin during surgical procedures. Biocides that have been successfully integrated into these materials and polymers for use in contact with the skin or mucous membranes include triclosan, silver, silver sulfadiazine, and chlorhexidine. These and other biocides have been used for other hard-surface applications (see chapter 3). Some applications have shown some success in reducing the rate of wound and/or indwelling medical device infections. Antimicrobial surfaces have been developed by incorporation directly into the polymer or by impregnation or coating of various materials and surfaces. In some cases, they release the biocide over time into the area associated with the device or material, while in others, they remain an intrinsic part of the surface to prevent the attachment and growth of bacteria and fungi.

4.6 BIOCIDES USED AS ANTISEPTICS

4.6.1 General Considerations

Antiseptics should provide a spectrum of activity, considering the various transient and resident microbial populations that can be present on the skin and mucous membranes or associated with skin or wound infections (see section 4.4). With the exception of some specific therapeutic applications, emphasis has primarily been on the antibacterial or bacteriostatic properties of these products, with some investigation of their effects on fungi (particularly *C. albicans*) and viruses. Although the biocide itself has a known spectrum of antimicrobial activity, its formulation into antiseptic products must optimize not only its effectiveness but also its compatibility with the skin or mucous membrane (the effects of formulation are discussed in section 1.4.6). Examples of these effects in antiseptics include the following:

- The use of chelating agents (e.g., EDTA) with triclosan to improve the penetration of the biocide into the cell walls of gram-negative bacteria
- The formulation of iodophors as iodine-releasing agents in comparison to the use

of high concentrations of iodine in tinctures, which are more irritating

- The formulation of lower concentrations of alcohols (60 to 70% in the presence of other agents that reduce the evaporation rates of the alcohols and allow them to remain on the skin longer) to minimize drying and irritation of the skin over multiple uses

For these and other reasons, the antimicrobial efficacies of antiseptics (similar to disinfectant formulations) can vary significantly, even in the presence of similar concentrations of the biocide. The efficacy is dependent on the use of the product. In some cases, routine hand washes or rinses should provide rapid activity within the typical amount of time used to apply the product, which is generally within the range of 5 to 20 s. An important variable is the correct use of the products, not only for the recommended exposure time, but also to ensure coverage (e.g., over the hands, between fingers, and under the nails) and adequate rinsing (when required). In other cases, as with preoperative preparations and surgical scrubs or rubs, much longer times are generally recommended (~2 to 5 min), and given their professional use, it can be easier to ensure compliance with minimum exposure times and proper application of the product. The condition of the skin can also affect the activity of a product, due to variations in soiling (e.g., blood or various foods), the pH of the skin, the microbial load, etc. Finally, when used with hand washes, the quality of the water (for example, water hardness and the presence of inactivating substances, like phosphates, chlorine, and other inorganic ions) can also limit the activity of the biocidal formulation on the skin.

Irritation associated with the use of an antiseptic is also an important consideration. Similar to the biocidal effects discussed above, the irritation observed with a product can be based on the biocide (type, concentration, pH, etc.), various formulations, excipients (like the choice of surfactants), individual sensitivity, and the use of the product. Formulation residuals remaining on the skin due to inadequate rinsing are often associated with irritation and can be further exacerbated with extended use of gloves. An increase in sweating under the gloves can itself lead to loss of moisture, drying, cracking, and allergic reactions (most commonly associated with the use of latex gloves). Most of the commonly used biocides are considered nontoxic, but in some cases, allergic reactions have been reported, and certain restrictions are recommended; for example, chlorhexidine infusion into the ear is not recommended due to reports of ototoxicity; allergic and toxic effects have been reported with the use of iodine (although these reports are generally associated with tinctures and less so with iodophors), and in a notable extreme case, the use of hexachlorophene is contraindicated for use on broken skin due to neurotoxicity risks. In contrast, some interesting reports have suggested that triclosan (and some other phenolics used on the skin) may inhibit histamine-induced inflammation of the skin and mucous membranes.

Persistence of the biocide on the skin following washing or application is considered an advantage and is associated with a strong affinity for the skin. Persistence has been observed with various biocides, including chlorhexidine, triclosan, hexachlorophene, antimicrobial metals and dyes, essential oils, chloroxylenol, and, to some extent, iodophors. The benefit of persistence is believed to be inhibition of the growth of bacteria and fungi on the skin, particularly for high-risk applications, like preoperative preparations and surgical scrubs and rubs. The persistence of chlorhexidine, in particular, has been studied in some detail. Chlorhexidine has affinity for the skin and is predominantly found associated with the outermost layers of the epidermis, with little or no significant penetration further into the skin (Fig. 4.4). The stratum corneum is a particular barrier to penetration, although at high concentrations and with damaged skin, the biocide can be found to penetrate to the dermal skin layers.

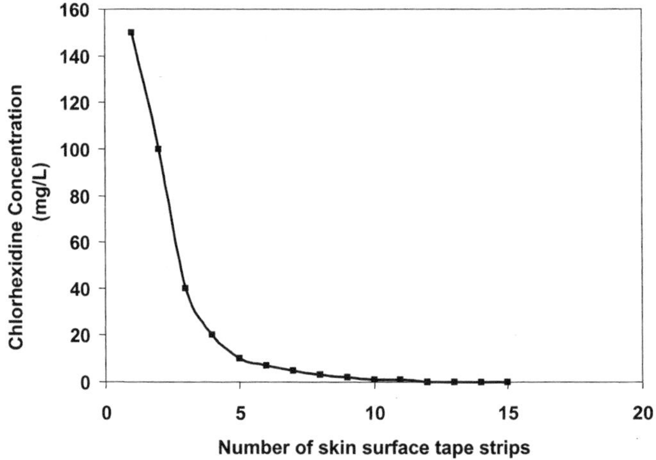

FIGURE 4.4 A representation of the penetration of chlorhexidine into the skin epidermis. The concentration of residual activity varies, depending on the formulation and application of the antiseptic. In this case, residual activity was present following washing with a 4% chlorhexidine formulation. The concentration can be determined by removing various layers of the epidermis by tape stripping (using adhesive tape to remove various layers) or by histologically removing layers by sectioning, followed by chlorhexidine extraction and determination.

Persistent activity can be achieved by direct application (e.g., 0.5% chlorhexidine in alcohol rubs or encapsulated applications) and by single washes with higher concentrations (2 to 4%) of chlorhexidine-containing products or multiple applications of lower-concentration formulations (0.5 to 2% washes). The persistent concentration is generally sufficient to inhibit the growth of most gram-positive bacteria, including *S. aureus* (with a typical inhibitory concentration in the 0.2- to 8-mg/liter range), some gram-negative bacteria, and fungi. However, as chlorhexidine is a cationic surfactant (see section 3.8), this activity can be neutralized by various factors, including the presence of inorganic anions (like phosphates and chlorides) in water and organic soils, organic anions (like soaps), and other detergents and lotions that contain either anionic or certain nonionic surfactants. Similar neutralizing effects have been found with other persistent biocides on the skin.

Overall, there is no perfect antiseptic for all applications, and the choice of the biocide and/or product to be used will vary depending on:

- The application (intact or broken skin, high or low risk of cross-contamination, presence of water, etc.)
- The extent and type of contamination (presence of soils, mechanical removal, microbial load, types of microorganism[s], etc.)
- The spectrum of antimicrobial activity (bactericidal, fungicidal, or virucidal)
- Previous reports of irritation, toxicity, and/or allergic reactions (skin condition, personnel history, label warnings, and restrictions)

4.6.2 Major Types of Biocides in Antiseptic Skin Washes and Rinses

The most commonly used biocides in antiseptic washes and rinses are summarized in Table 4.3. These biocides have been discussed in some detail in chapter 3 and are only briefly discussed in this section with respect to their antiseptic uses.

Alcohols, including ethanol, isopropanol, and *n*-propanol, are widely used as antiseptics, the last primarily in Europe (see section 3.5). They are provided as various hand rinse formulations or as impregnated wipes, and also in combination with other biocides, like chlorhexidine. They are also used at lower, nonbiocidal concentrations in other formulations. In general, they have rapid antimicrobial activity over relatively short exposure times at typical antiseptic concentrations ranging from 60 to 92%, with optimal activity generally around the 70% range. Most alcohol antiseptic formulations contain emollients and other excipients to reduce the drying effects often associated with the use of alcohols on the skin and to decrease the evaporation rate, allowing lower concentrations of alcohol (60 to 65%) to be used. Alcohols demonstrate broad-spectrum antimicrobial activity, with the notable exception of having no appreciable effects on bacterial spores (although they are sporostatic). They are rapidly effective against bacteria, including mycobacteria, and against fungi, with mixed reports in the literature regarding their efficacy against viruses and fungal spores. Enveloped viruses are rapidly sensitive, with various activities described for nonenveloped viruses. As they are used as hand rubs they have the advantage of not requiring the presence of water for application, but this is also a disadvantage in the case of the presence of soil. Although they can be used to treat wounds, particularly small abrasions, they sting in contact with damaged skin; despite widespread use, alcohols have rarely been associated with any toxic effects, but care should be taken to avoid contact with the eyes at the concentrations typically used. Alcohols are flammable and should be stored according to the manufacturer's instructions.

Chlorhexidine is a bisbiguanide used both as a preventative and as a therapeutic antiseptic (see section 3.8). It is used in various salt forms, particularly gluconate, acetate, or hydrochloride salts, but also in combination with other biocides, like QACs (e.g., cetrimide) and alcohols. Chlorhexidine is one of the most widely used and accepted biocides in high-risk hand washes or rinses, including as preoperative preparations and surgical scrubs.

Furthermore, it is used as a biocide impregnated into various surfaces for release over time into the skin and for treating mucous membrane infections, including as oral rinses for the treatment of minor infections, mouth ulcers, and gingivitis. Chlorhexidine is also used for direct instillation into the eye at concentrations of $<0.1\%$; higher concentrations are considered damaging to the eye tissue. Formulations of the biocide can vary considerably; an important consideration is pH, with optimal activity at pH 5.5 to 7.0, as well incompatibility with various anionic and nonionic substances. For example, lotions containing anionic surfactants neutralize residual chlorhexidine concentrations on the skin. In general, formulations demonstrate broad antibacterial activity, with particularly rapid activity against some gram-positive bacteria, including staphylococci, as well as gram-negative bacteria. Chlorhexidine is bactericidal at low concentrations, with the highest MICs reported for strains of *Providencia stuartii*. In general, higher bactericidal concentrations have been reported against gram-negative bacteria, including pseudomonads. At relatively low concentrations, chlorhexidine is also mycobacteriostatic and fungistatic, although its fungicidal effects can be improved in formulation, particularly against *Candida* species, which are often associated with skin and membrane infections. As the primary mode of action of chlorhexidine is considered to be disruption of the lipid membrane (see section 3.8), virucidal activity against enveloped viruses has been reported, but little or no effect has been observed against nonenveloped viruses. Chlorhexidine also demonstrates residual activity on the skin, providing some protection against microbial growth over time. One of the main reasons for the wide acceptance of chlorhexidine as an antiseptic is the limited reports of adverse effects and toxicity. It is considered nontoxic, with little adsorption into the skin. Many studies have confirmed limited or no toxicity, carcinogenicity, or irritancy, although some cases of irritancy may be related to other formulation effects and some cases of allergic reactions have been reported; despite this, higher concentrations of chlorhexidine cause eye damage and ototoxicity. Other biguanides have been used as antiseptics, including alexidine and octenidine (see section 3.8).

Iodine is a halogen (see section 3.11). Various alcoholic and aqueous iodine solutions have been used, although the most effective are the various tinctures of iodine in alcohol, which are predominantly used as preoperative preparations (directly or in various swabs or gauzes) and to a lesser extent for wound applications or general hand washes. This is primarily due to toxicity, irritation, and staining disadvantages with higher concentrations of iodine in solution. These have all but been replaced by the use of various iodine-releasing agents, like the iodophors, particularly PVPI. They have the advantage of greater solubility for formulation and release of active (or "free") iodine over time and as required and therefore are less irritating and damaging to the skin, depending on the concentration used. The chemistry of iodine in solution is complicated, with two species primarily associated with antimicrobial activity (free iodine [I_2] and hypoiodous acid [HOI]). Therefore, the activity of an iodophor solution is dependent on the actual concentrations of these species released over time. For example, a freshly prepared 10% PVPI solution contains approximately 1% available iodine (with respect to the total capacity of the iodine reservoir of the iodophor) and releases free iodine in the 0.5- to 5-mg/liter range for antimicrobial activity; however, as the equilibrium between bound and available iodine is disrupted, for example, by dilution or biocidal use, the iodophor will release further iodine for antimicrobial activity. Iodophors are provided as various solutions, powders (for wound applications), and lotions.

Depending on the free-iodine concentrations, iodophors can be used for routine and high-risk applications, including surgical scrubs and preoperative preparations. Unlike tinctures, they are generally associated with low toxicity and little irritation, even in wounds, and are nonstaining, depending on the concentrations used over time; however, allergic and toxic effects, including absorption into the blood, have been reported. As an oxidizing agent (see section 3.11), iodine has been shown to have broad-spectrum antimicrobial activity, including bactericidal, fungicidal, virucidal, and mycobactericidal activities, with some sporicidal and protozoal activity over time. As it readily reacts with organic soils, the presence of these soils can inhibit penetration to target microorganisms but can be compensated for by the further release of iodine in the case of the iodophors. As for other biocides, various formulation effects affect the activity and shelf life of the antiseptic.

Chloroxylenol (or parachlorometaxylenol) is a phenolic biocide used as a skin antiseptic wash and, in some cases, as a surgical scrub and preoperative preparation (see section 3.15). Typical antiseptic concentrations range from 0.5 to 4%. It is also used in medicated shampoos and as a medicated powder for wound applications. Its antimicrobial activity is limited in comparison to those of other antiseptic biocides, with particular bactericidal activity against gram-positive and gram-negative bacteria. Formulation also plays an important role in optimizing its efficacy against some gram-negative bacteria, like *Pseudomonas*; yeasts; molds; and enveloped viruses. Chloroxylenol is mycobacteriostatic and sporistatic, but no activity has been reported against nonenveloped viruses. It also has a good safety profile, despite penetration into the epidermis and persistence on the skin, and is considered to have low or no toxicity and little irritancy. In some cases, allergic contact dermatitis has been reported. Similar to chlorhexidine, residual concentrations on the skin can be neutralized by various chemicals, including nonionic surfactants.

Triclosan is a diphenyl ether (see discussion of bisphenols in section 3.15) and has an antimicrobial profile similar to that of chloroxylenol, with rapid activity against gram-positive bacteria and yeasts, less activity against gram-negative bacteria, and limited activity against fungi and viruses. Formulation also plays an important role in optimizing the activity of triclosan on the skin, including combination with low concentrations of EDTA and other chelating agents to improve penetration into gram-negative bacteria, fungi, and some yeasts. Overall, triclosan has limited activity against molds, but it is fungistatic at relatively low concentrations. Triclosan is used in a variety of antiseptic hand washes, ranging from 0.1 to 2%; its primary use is for routine and frequent hand or body washing, although some formulations have been used as hand washes for health care personnel and as surgical scrubs.

Lower concentrations of triclosan are used for odor control in various body washes and deodorants, due to its bacteriostatic activity at low concentrations. Other applications include shampoos and lotions and integration into various dressings and bandages for release over time onto the skin. Triclosan has demonstrated some residual activity on the skin, although it is due to a different type of binding than a cationic molecule, such as chlorhexidine. Triclosan-containing antiseptics have shown particular clinical use for the control of staphylococcal (*S. aureus*, including methicillin-resistant *S. aureus*) carriage on the skin. Although these results may be primarily due to the potent activity against these bacteria, it should also be considered that triclosan products have good compliance rates in use due to their low irritation. Triclosan is generally nonallergenic and nonmutagenic and has a good safety profile; some reports have suggested that the biocide may also inhibit histamine-induced inflammation on the skin and mucous membranes. Concerns have been raised about the use of triclosan (and chlorhexidine) due to the development of bacterial resistance (or, more correctly, reduced susceptibility or increased tolerance) to low concentrations of the biocide and cross-resistance to some antibiotics (see sections 3.15 and 8.7.2); the overall significance of these reports is considered minimal, due to both the concentrations typically used and the broad sites of action on the microorganisms, but they require further investigation. A similar bisphenol used as an antiseptic is hexachlorophene (see section 3.15), which has a similar range of activity and greater persistence and penetration into the skin; however, confirmed reports of neurotoxicity have led to the limited use of this biocide as an antiseptic, and its use is recommended only on intact skin.

4.6.3 Other Antiseptic Biocides

A variety of other biocides are used as antiseptics. A summary of these is given in Table 4.4.

FURTHER READING

Ascenzi, J. M. 1996. *Handbook of Disinfectants and Antiseptics*. Marcel Dekker, New York, N.Y.

Block, S. S. 1991. *Disinfection, Sterilization, and Preservation*, 4th ed. Lea & Febiger, Philadelphia, Pa.

Block, S. S. 2001. *Disinfection, Sterilization, and Preservation*, 5th ed. Lippincott Williams & Wilkins, Philadelphia, Pa.

Boyce, J. M., and D. Pittet. 2002. Guideline for hand hygiene in health-care settings. Recommendations of the Healthcare Infection Control Practices Advisory Committee and the HICPAC/SHEA/APIC/IDSA Hand Hygiene Task Force. *Morb. Mortal. Wkly. Rep.* **51:**1–48.

Olmsted, R. N. 1996. *APIC Infection Control and Applied Epidemiology: Principles and Practice*. Mosby, St. Louis, Mo.

Russell, A. D., W. B. Hugo, and G. A. J. Ayliffe. 1992. *Principles and Practice of Disinfection, Preservation and Sterilization*, 2nd ed. Blackwell Science, Cambridge, Mass.

Wilson, M. 2005. *Microbial Inhabitants of Humans: Their Ecology and Role in Health and Disease*. Cambridge University Press, New York, N.Y.

World Health Organization. May 4, 2005. *WHO Guidelines for Hand Hygiene in Health Care*. World Health Organization, Geneva, Switzerland. [Online.] http://www.who.int/.

PHYSICAL STERILIZATION

5

5.1 INTRODUCTION

In chapter 2, the various physical disinfection methods were described. The basic concepts behind these methods also apply to physical sterilization techniques. Sterilization is a defined process used to render a surface or product free from viable organisms, including bacterial spores. The methods of sterilization discussed in this chapter are the most widely used physical sterilization techniques and include the use of moist heat, dry heat, and radiation. Heat-based methods have previously been discussed as physical disinfection methods (see section 2.2). Moist-heat (steam) processes, based on the application of steam under pressure, are the most widely used methods of heat-based sterilization and are considered the most reliable. High-temperature dry-heat sterilization methods are also used for particular applications, including the incineration of contaminated waste products and materials. Low-temperature but equally reliable alternatives for physical sterilization include the high-energy ionizing-radiation methods (such as X rays, γ rays, and electron beams [E beams]), although they are used primarily for industrial applications. (For an introduction to radiation, see section 2.4.) This chapter also includes a discussion of some of the developing methods of physical sterilization, including plasma, pulsed light, supercritical fluids, and pulsed electric fields, that have been successfully used for some applications.

5.2 STEAM STERILIZATION

5.2.1 An Introduction to Steam Sterilization

High-temperature steam (or steam under pressure) is the most widely used sterilization method. Steam is simply a gas that is produced by the heating of water and therefore can be explained by the gas laws that consider four variables: volume, temperature, pressure, and the amount of gas.

1. Boyle's law describes the relationship between pressure (*P*) and volume (*V*) at a constant temperature and amount of gas, where as the pressure rises, the volume of steam decreases, and

$$P_1 = P_2V_2$$

2. Charles' law describes the relationship between temperature (*T*) and volume (*V*) at a constant pressure and amount of gas, where as the temperature increases, the pressure increases, and

$$\frac{V_1}{T_1} = \frac{V_2}{T_2}$$

3. Combining equations 1 and 2, the combined gas law is given as

$$\frac{P_1 V_1}{T_1} = \frac{P_2 V_2}{T_1 T_2}$$

Therefore, if we consider the introduction of a given amount of steam into a fixed volume, the temperature of the steam can be varied by changing the pressure. At atmospheric pressure (~101.3 kPa; 14.7 lb in^{-2}; 1 bar; 760 mm Hg [or torr] at sea level), water boils to produce vapor (steam) at 100°C. If the pressure is increased, the boiling temperature of water also increases, and high sterilization temperatures can be achieved. Equally, as the pressure is decreased (e.g., by pulling a vacuum), the temperature at which steam forms decreases; this is referred to as "low-temperature" steam, which is used in other sterilization and disinfection methods. The relationship between the steam temperature and pressure is shown in Fig. 5.1.

At each point along the line, the steam quality is referred to as being "saturated," which is optimal for steam sterilization processes. Under these conditions, steam contains as much water as possible prior to condensation and is therefore considered "dry." At a given point, if the temperature is lowered (for example, where the steam meets a cold surface), water will condense and also heat the surface. Excessive condensation should be avoided, as it restricts the penetration of steam. At the same point, if the temperature is increased, the steam becomes "superheated," or essentially drier (more like dry air), which is less effective for sterilization.

Types. Steam sterilization is performed in controlled vessels (known as autoclaves, steam sterilizers, or pressure vessels) that are capable of safely withstanding the pressures required for sterilization (Fig. 5.2).

Efficient air removal is essential to ensure steam sterilization, as air prevents the penetration of steam and leaves cold spots within the chamber/load that will not be adequately sterilized. All autoclaves are designed for the removal of air from the vessel and its load and can therefore be classified based on the mechanisms of air removal.

Upward-Displacement Autoclaves. Upward-displacement autoclaves are generally small laboratory autoclaves—a typical example is a pressure cooker (Fig. 5.3). Water is placed at the base of the vessel and heated (e.g., by an electric heater or on a burner) to produce steam. As the steam rises, air and steam are expelled from the vessel under pressure through a safety valve on the lid for a given time, and then the valve is closed. The vessel is heated during the steriliza-

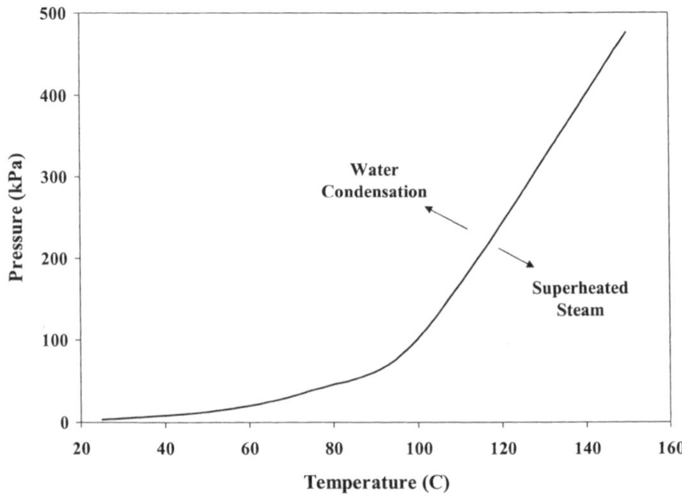

FIGURE 5.1 The relationship between saturated steam temperature and pressure.

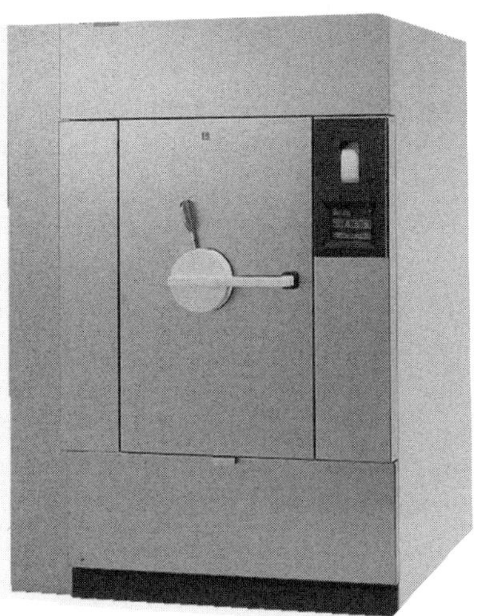

FIGURE 5.2 A steam sterilizer. Sterilizers are available in a variety of sizes and shapes, depending on the application. In addition, the steam sterilization process can be conducted as an intrinsic process of some manufacturing/industrial equipment, which can be routinely sterilized without being disassembled.

tion time and then allowed to cool before being opened. These designs can be effective for simple devices but are less reliable for efficient air removal with complex loads.

Downward-Displacement Autoclaves. Downward (or gravity)-displacement steam sterilizers vary in size from small bench-top models to large laboratory, industrial, or hospital autoclaves. They are widely used for liquid and surface sterilization (of devices, cages, vessels, etc.). They are generally not recommended to be used for porous materials (foodstuffs, towels, etc.) due to limited efficiency of air removal. A simplified design is shown in Fig. 5.4. The pressure vessel is usually jacketed to allow preheating of the load prior to sterilization (or cooling after sterilization); preheating can be achieved electrically or by using steam. Steam is then slowly introduced into the top of a pressure vessel and passes through a water separator and baffle. The water separator provides a tortuous path for the removal of a significant amount of water that may be carried in the incoming steam. Further, the separator/baffle reduces the velocity of steam entering the chamber to reduce mixing with the air, which would result in inefficient air removal. Steam is less dense (lighter) than air and initially fills the chamber from the top; then, the mass of steam pushes down through the chamber to force (displace) the air out through a valve at the base of the chamber. Correct control and design of the autoclave optimizes the removal of air from the chamber. When the required temperature and pressure are achieved, the incoming steam is shut off and the load is held for the given sterilization time. The temperature is controlled at the coldest point in the chamber, which is at the base of the chamber in the drain line. Following the required sterilization time, air is introduced into the chamber, and the contents are allowed to cool (generally to below 80°C).

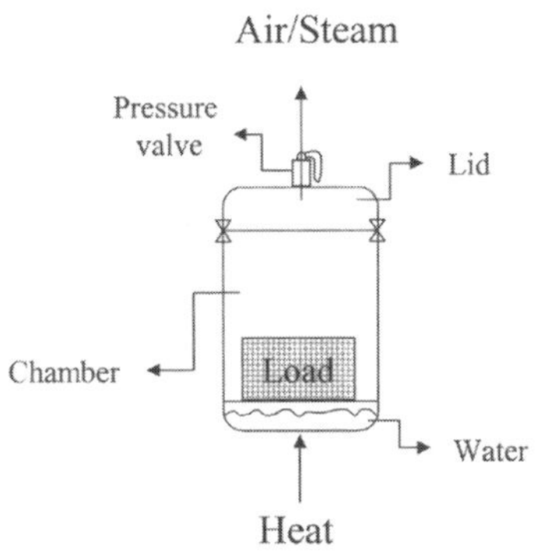

Air/Steam
Pressure valve
Lid
Chamber
Load
Water
Heat

FIGURE 5.3 The basic design of an upward-displacement steam sterilizer.

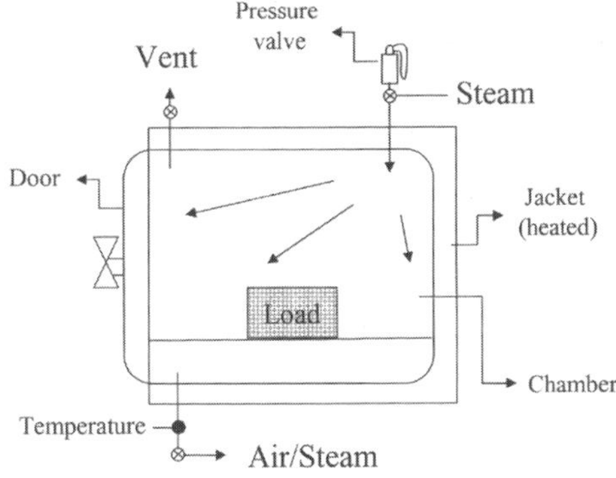

FIGURE 5.4 The basic design of a downward-displacement steam sterilizer.

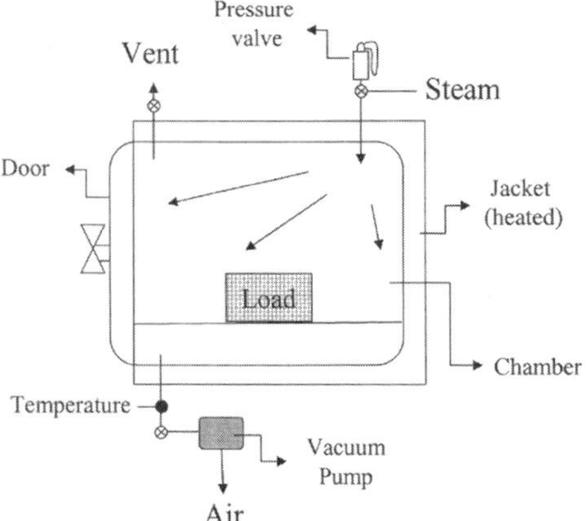

FIGURE 5.5 The basic design of a prevacuum steam sterilizer.

Vacuum and Pressure-Pulsing Autoclaves. A variety of designs and sizes of vacuum and pressure-pulsing autoclaves are available for porous and nonporous loads. Porous loads include fabrics, towels, and certain wrapped plastic items, which can trap air, limiting the penetration of steam. The simplest systems use a vacuum pump to draw air out of the chamber ("pulling a vacuum") (Fig. 5.5).

The lower the pressure (or "deeper" the vacuum), the greater the air removal from the chamber and its contents. Following evacuation, steam is introduced to heat the load and is placed under positive pressure to reach the desired sterilization temperature for the required time; the chamber is then vented to atmospheric pressure to cool (a typical cycle is shown in Fig. 5.6). The load can be more rapidly cooled by pulling a vacuum following sterilization. Steam can be pulsed into the chamber to aid in the removal of air and to allow even penetration of steam through the load (Fig. 5.6).

These active pulsing cycles are generally more efficient and include the following.

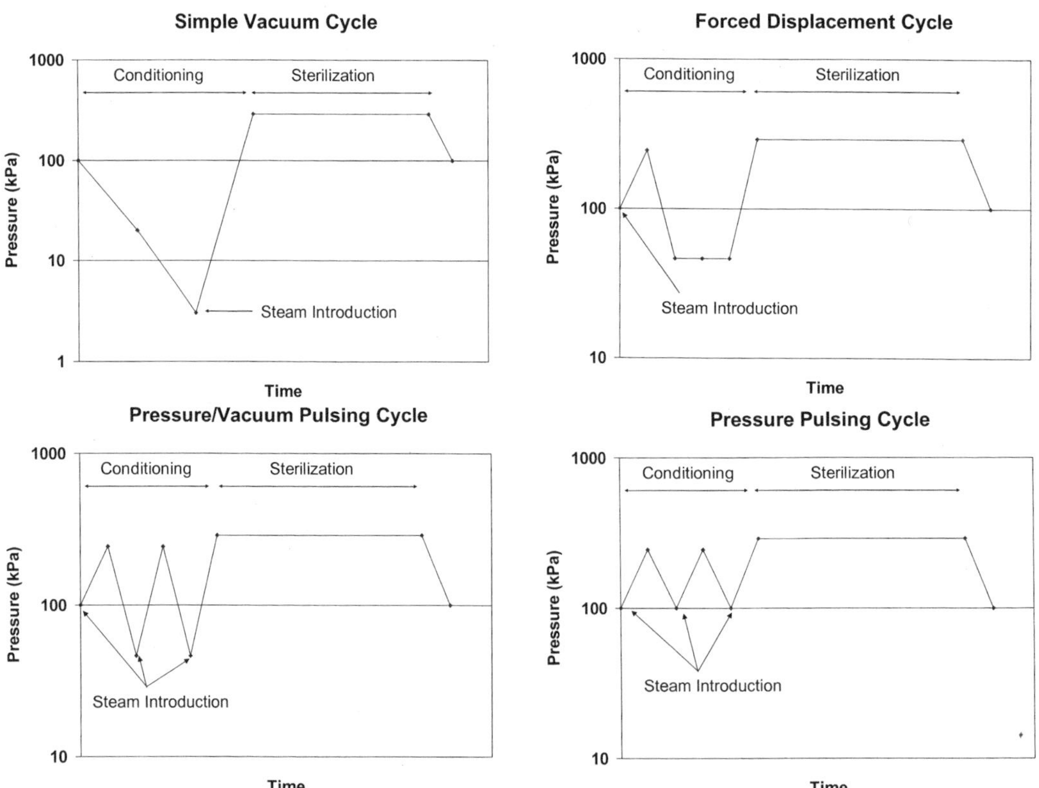

FIGURE 5.6 Typical steam sterilization cycles, showing different mechanisms of air removal and load conditioning prior to sterilization.

1. Forced displacement. Steam is introduced into the chamber under pressure and is continually provided as a vacuum is pulled, followed by an increase in pressure to the desired set point for sterilization. Air removal and heating to the sterilization temperature are referred to as conditioning.

2. Pressure-vacuum pulsing. Steam is introduced into the chamber under pressure, and the air-steam mixture is evacuated by pulling a vacuum. These pulses can be repeated to optimize air removal and load heating.

3. Pressure pulsing. Pressure pulsing is similar to pressure-vacuum pulsing, but the chamber is evacuated to atmospheric (or above atmospheric) pressure.

5.2.2 Factors That Affect Steam Sterilization

When considering steam sterilization, it is important to understand the factors that can affect the efficiency of steam sterilization processes.

1. Air removal. It is important to remove air and other noncondensable gases (gases that do not condense under the conditions of steam sterilization) from the chamber and load. Since air cannot condense under conditions of steam sterilization, it impedes the penetration of steam. For prevacuum-based processes, it is particularly important that the chamber be airtight, which can be confirmed by performing a leak test before sterilization or by conducting other periodic tests to confirm the efficient removal of air. The most common method is referred to as a Bowie-Dick test (Fig. 5.7). This test can be used to measure the efficiency of mechanical air removal and leak detection in a prevacuum sterilizer.

2. Water content. Optimal sterilization is achieved with saturated steam, which is dependent on the temperature and pressure (Fig. 5.1). As the steam becomes wetter (or supersaturated), condensation forms, which can limit the steam penetration into a load. Exces-

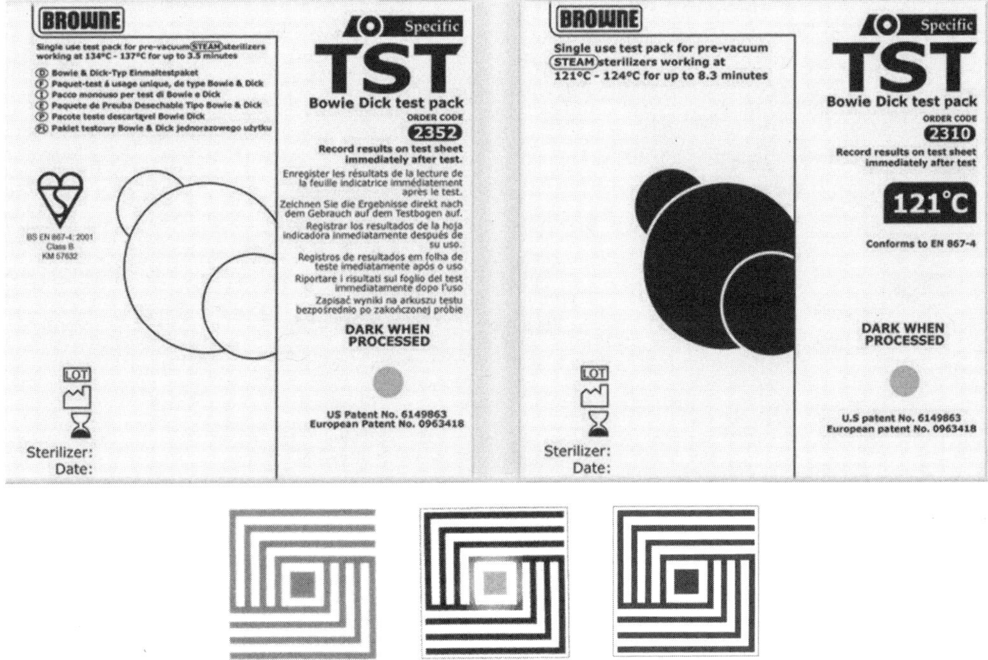

FIGURE 5.7 The Bowie-Dick test, a method of testing the steam penetration and air removal capabilities of a vacuum sterilizer. Single-use test packs are shown at the top; they consist of a chemical indicator at the center of the test pack, which changes color on exposure to the correct combination of time, temperature, and steam. An unused indicator and one failing and one passing chemical indicator results are shown from left to right at the bottom.

sive wetness can also leave the load difficult to handle and prone to recontamination. In these cases, drying is recommended. Conversely, as steam becomes drier (defined as superheated, where the water vapor temperature is higher than the boiling point of water at the corresponding pressure), it is less effective for sterilization.

3. Steam purity. The purity of steam is determined by the quality of water from which it is made and can also be affected during the transfer of the steam to the autoclave. Many water contaminants can be carried over in steam and deposited onto surfaces, including devices being sterilized, packaging materials, pipe work, and the autoclave itself. These can have toxic effects and can cause significant damage to surfaces. The most common contaminants and their effects are shown in Table 5.1.

TABLE 5.1 Common steam contaminants and their effects

Contaminant	Effect
Organic materials	
Pyrogens (e.g., bacterial endotoxins)	Pyrogenic reactions (fever)
Amines	Toxicity
Particulate materials	Discoloration of packaging materials
Inorganic materials	
Toxic metals (e.g., cadmium, lead, mercury)	Cumulative poisons
Alkaline earth metals(e.g., calcium, magnesium)	Hardness (calcium carbonate) deposits
Iron	Corrosion (iron oxide)
Chlorides	Corrosion

Because the quality of water can vary significantly, it may be necessary to pretreat the water, control the generation of steam, and protect its quality during distribution. Examples of pretreatment systems are given in Fig. 5.8.

For certain applications, the steam is required to be "clean," which may be defined as steam whose condensate meets criteria for water quality equal to those for water for injection (WFI). WFI has limits for organic and inorganic contaminants that have been shown to be safe when injected directly into the bloodstream (e.g., as used for the preparation of dried parenterals or drugs for injection). These requirements are defined in various pharmacopoeias used worldwide (e.g., the United States Pharmacopeia and the European Pharmacopoeia) (Table 5.2).

Applications. Steam sterilizers can range in size from small bench-top sterilizers to large chamber sterilizers, depending on their use and applications.

A variety of steam sterilization cycles may be used, depending on the application. Essentially, any combination of temperature and time that

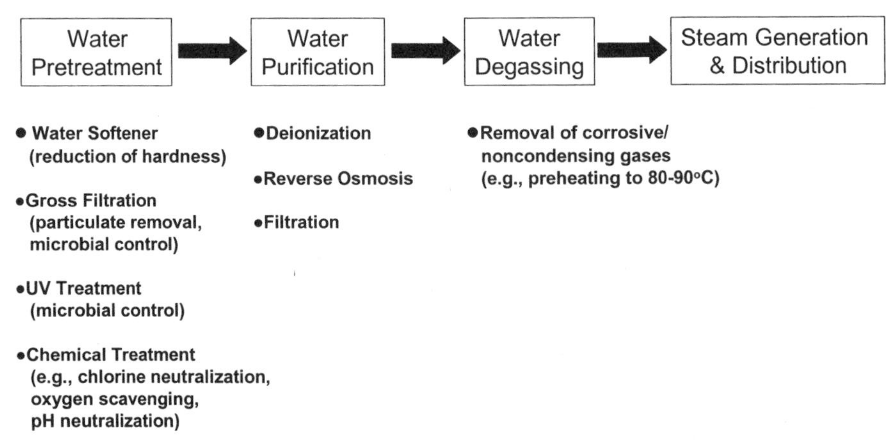

FIGURE 5.8 Typical water pretreatment systems for the production of steam.

TABLE 5.2 Typical qualities of WFI and "clean" steam[a]

Property	Value		
	European Pharmacopoeia (EP 4)	*U.S. Pharmacopeia* (USP27-NF 22)	EN 285 *Steam Condensate*[b]
Characteristics	Clear, colorless, odorless, and tasteless		Colorless, clear, no sediment
pH	5.0–7.0	5.0–7.0	5.0–7.0
Oxidizable substances	Below detection	Below detection	Below detection
Chlorides	<1 mg/liter		<1 mg/liter
Nitrates	<0.2 mg/liter		<0.2 mg/liter
Sulfates	<1 mg/liter		<1 mg/liter
Ammonium	<0.2 mg/liter		<0.2 mg/liter
Calcium, magnesium	<2 mg/liter, <1 mg/liter		<2 mg/liter, <1 mg/liter
Heavy metals[c]	<0.1 mg/liter		<0.1 mg/liter
TOC[d]		<500 ppb	
Conductivity	<1.1 μS/cm (20°C)	<1.3 μS/cm (25°C)	<3 μS/cm (20°C)
Endotoxin[e]	<0.25 EU/ml	<0.25 EU/ml	<0.25 EU/ml

[a]The permitted levels are based on methods described in the respective guidelines.
[b]"Clean steam" (2002). EN, European Standard (Norm).
[c]Heavy metals include iron, cadmium, and lead.
[d]TOC, total organic carbon.
[e]EU, endotoxin unit.

has been demonstrated to provide the necessary microbial reduction and has been validated for the appropriate purpose can be applied. Some of the more typical overkill steam sterilization cycles are given in Table 5.3.

Steam is widely used for reusable-device sterilization in medical, dental, and veterinary facilities. Reusable devices are generally cleaned, wrapped in steam-penetrable and microbe-retentive material (paper, plastic, or fabric), and sterilized. The sterilization cycle includes the removal of air (as described above), a minimum exposure time within a minimum range of temperatures, and evacuation. Some cycles can be followed by an extended drying cycle. Drying is essential to prevent recontamination of or damage to the material on subsequent storage and depends on the nature and size of the load. In some applications, rapid "flash" sterilization cycles are used, typically at 132 to 135°C for 3 to 10 min in a prevacuum sterilizer (depending on the load). These cycles are primarily used in emergency situations, where a specific device is required immediately for a surgical procedure and may have been unavailable or inadvertently contaminated during the procedure. In general, nonporous materials and nonlumened devices required shorter cycle times, as air can be efficiently removed from these loads; longer times are required for porous (e.g., textiles, like gowns, towels, and dressings) and lumened devices. So-called porous-load cycles are designed to optimize air removal from porous loads or lumened devices. Gravity drain cycles are recommended for use with liquids and generally up to 121°C; as for any steam sterilization process, care should be taken in the design of liquid cycles to ensure even temperature distribution and to prevent boiling over of the product during heating or

TABLE 5.3 Typical steam sterilization cycles

Temp (°C)	Time (min)
115	>30
121	>15
126	>10
132	>4
134	>3

cooling. Other loads can be conveniently sterilized by steam as long as they can withstand the required temperature for the required time, including single-use manufactured devices, water, liquid media, liquid and solid wastes (including infectious materials), containers, utensils, and vials.

Steam sterilization is also used for routine vessel decontamination, including manufacturing equipment, freeze-dryers, and aseptic filling lines. It should also be noted that as steam can be generated at higher temperatures and pressures for sterilization, some processes can use the same principle to allow liquids (including water) to be sterilized. As shown in Fig. 5.1, if water is heated and maintained at a pressure above the saturation line, the water will remain in the liquid stage and can be held at that temperature for the required sterilization time. These systems have been described for water and wastewater treatment. Steam production and condensation (by distillation processes) is the preferred method for the production of high-quality/sterile water, including water for cleaning and WFI, which is used during the manufacturing and use of pharmaceutical products (e.g., dilution and injection of sterile and nonsterile drugs). Steam (particularly low-temperature steam) is used as an effective humidification and heating process, which is an essential part of other sterilization processes, including those using ethylene oxide, formaldehyde, and some oxidizing agents (like ozone and chlorine dioxide).

Examples of various standards and guidelines for steam sterilization applications are given in Table 5.4.

Spectrum of Activity. The spectrum of activity of heat is discussed in section 2.2. Steam sterilization is widely regarded as having rapid, broad-spectrum activity. The efficacy of steam

TABLE 5.4 Examples of standards and guidelines for steam sterilization applications

Reference[a]	Title	Summary
EN 285	*Sterilization. Steam Sterilizers. Large Sterilizers*	Specifies design requirements and tests for large steam sterilizers primarily used in health care or commercially
EN 764	*Pressure Equipment—Terminology and Symbols—Pressure, Temperature, Volume*	Definitions and requirements for pressure equipment used for steam sterilization
ISO 11134	*Sterilization of Health Care Products—Requirements for Validation and Routine Control—Industrial Moist Heat Sterilization*	Specifies requirements for the use of moist heat in the sterilization process, including development, validation, and routine control of the sterilization process
ISO 17665	*Sterilization of Health Care Products—Requirements for the Development, Validation and Routine Control of a Sterilization Process for Medical Devices—Moist Heat*	Specifies requirements for the use of moist heat in sterilization process, including development, validation, and routine control of the sterilization process
AAMI TIR 13	*Principles of Industrial Moist Heat Sterilization*	Guidance on steam sterilization for industrial processes
HTM 2010	*Sterilization*	Guidance on the design, installation, and operation of sterilizers, including steam, formaldehyde, and ethylene oxide
HTM 2031	*Clean Steam for Sterilization*	Guideline on the quality of steam for sterilization
PDA Technical Report 1	*Moist Heat Sterilization in Autoclaves: Cycle Development, Validation and Routine Operation*	Guidance of the development and validation of steam sterilization cycles in industrial applications

[a]EN, European Norm; ISO, International Standards Organization; AAMI, Association for the Advancement of Medical Instrumentation; HTM, Health Technical Memorandum (United Kingdom); PDA, Parenteral Drug Association.

against bacteria, fungi, viruses, protozoa, and spores has been well described. *Geobacillus stearothermophilus* spores are widely regarded at the organisms most resistant to steam sterilization and are therefore used to confirm and validate steam sterilization processes. These may include the use of liquid suspensions or standard inoculated materials (like biological indicators) or direct inoculation onto the surfaces being sterilized. The efficacy of steam against *G. stearothermophilus* spores depends on the intrinsic resistance of the spore crop preparation and the exposure temperature/time. The intrinsic resistance of spores varies depending on a number of factors, including age and growth conditions, which are discussed in more detail in section 8.3.11. At a given intrinsic resistance (known as the *D* reference), there is a linear relationship between the exposure temperature and the average *D* value, as discussed in section 2.2. The *D* value is defined as the time (in minutes or seconds) at a given temperature required to kill 1 log unit (or 90%) of a given microbial population; a *D* reference is usually given at 121°C (D_{121C}). The *Z* value, the temperature change required to change the *D* value by a factor of 10, can also be determined for the spore population. The *D* and *Z* values for a given spore population can be determined by exposing the spores to various temperatures for various times. These reference values are usually provided by the spore or biological indicator (section 1.4.2.3) manufacturer and are determined in tightly controlled pressure vessels known at BIER vessels. Therefore, at a typical *Z* value of 10°C for a given spore population and a determined *D* reference of 1 min at 121°C, the predicted log reductions at various temperatures can be calculated and graphed (Fig. 5.9).

Using this graph as a reference, for any given temperature, the minimum sterilization time can be determined based on the log reduction required. For most steam sterilization processes, where overkill is desired, a minimum 12-log-unit reduction is recommended to give a sterility assurance level of 10^{-6}. With the example in Fig. 5.9, a 12-log-unit reduction may be achieved at 131°C for 72 s (6 s × 12 = 72 s) or at 141°C for 7.2 s (0.6 s × 12 = 7.2 s). It can therefore be appreciated that for typical steam sterilization processes, the contact temperatures and times have an appreciable safety factor built into them; an example is device sterilization cycles at 134°C for >3 min, which can be esti-

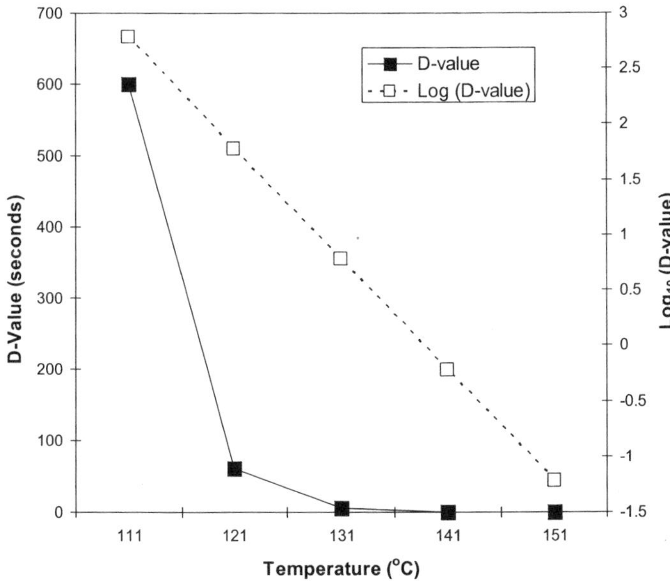

FIGURE 5.9 Effect of temperature on the lethality of a *G. stearothermophilus* spore population with a D_{121C} of 1 min and a *Z* value of 10°C.

mated from Fig. 5.9 to provide a minimum reduction of ~60 log units for the organism most resistant to steam, which does not include any additional lethality due to the rise and subsequent decrease in temperature during the conditioning and cool-down phases of the cycle.

Organic and inorganic soils can prevent the penetration of steam. Particular examples are lipid materials, which can repel water molecules, and, to a greater extent, salt crystals, which can form around microorganisms on drying and delay steam access. Practical examples of inorganic salts that can protect microorganisms are calcium carbonate (which can precipitate from hard water, for example, on rinsing following a cleaning process) and iron oxide (which can form as red-brown deposits or rust on a surface). As for any disinfection or sterilization process, it is therefore important that the surface be clean to ensure optimum efficacy; for wastes or other soiled materials, extended sterilization times are usually adopted to ensure adequate penetration and exposure.

Prion decontamination requires special considerations. Although the exact nature of the infectious agent in transmissible spongiform encephalopathies (see section 1.3.6) is unknown, it is widely accepted to be proteinaceous in nature and is termed a prion, to denote an infectious protein. In experiments, steam sterilization has been shown to significantly reduce the infectivities of prion preparations, but residual infectivity has been identified in many of these investigations. This may be due to the use of grossly soiled preparations (i.e., brain homogenates) in these experiments and incomplete accessibility of steam to the infectious particles. In cases of known or suspected transmissible spongiform encephalopathy disease, extended steam sterilization cycles are widely recommended (Table 5.5), although in most cases, critical devices known to be contaminated are not reused and are discarded or incinerated.

In some of these cases, steam sterilization has been shown to be more effective when the material is kept hydrated by immersion in water or sodium hydroxide (1 to 2 N NaOH). The use of NaOH may cause damage to the sterilizer, due to the production of hydroxide aerosols, which can damage the pressure chamber or associated seals and pipe work, as well as posing safety risks in the handling of high concentrations of hydroxide. Special applications have been described for the high-temperature/high-pressure liquid sterilization of devices and materials (including whole animals) with 1 to 2 N NaOH in specifically designed pressure vessels.

TABLE 5.5 Typical steam sterilization cycles recommended for TSE-associated decontamination[a]

Sterilizer type	Process	Comments
Gravity displacement	Immerse in 1 N NaOH and autoclave at 121°C for 30 min Immerse in 1 N NaOH for 1 h; remove, place into water, and autoclave at 121°C for 1 h Immerse in 1 N NaOH for 1 h; remove, rinse in water, remove, and autoclave at 121°C for 1 h Immerse in water and autoclave at 134°C for 18 min 121–132°C for ≥1 h	Can cause damage to the autoclave. NaOH treatment can be replaced with 2–2.5% sodium hypochlorite. Devices should be resistant to chemical treatment.
Porous load	Immerse in 1 N NaOH for 1 h; remove, rinse in water, remove, and autoclave at 134°C for 1 h 134°C for ≥18 min	NaOH treatment can be replaced with 2–2.5% sodium hypochlorite. Devices should be resistant to chemical treatment.

[a]Note that the treatment devices are recleaned and sterilized according to normal practices. TSE, transmissible spongiform encephalopathy.

Advantages. Steam sterilization processes are generally considered the most reliable and efficient for the sterilization of liquids and materials, including devices. They demonstrate broad-spectrum antimicrobial activity and have a significant safety factor built into them to ensure lethality. The processes are flexible and predictable, depending on the required temperature, contact time, and minimum log reduction. The apparatus is economical, widely available, and easy to use, and running costs are low. Materials can be sterilized within packaging for subsequent storage or sterile handling, which is particularly important for critical surgical devices.

Disadvantages. Steam sterilization is not suitable for temperature- or pressure-sensitive materials or devices. In some cases, despite their resistance to heat, some materials may demonstrate stress cracking or other effects after single or repeated steam sterilization and drying cycles. Care should also be taken to ensure that materials have effectively cooled down before handling them; in some cases, the cooling down time is a disadvantage, for example, in large vessels used in manufacturing facilities. The success of steam penetration is dependent on the optimal removal of trapped air or other noncondensable gases. For this reason, specific steam sterilization cycles are recommended for porous loads (including fabrics and towels) and devices that have long internal channels, or lumens. Unlike dry heat, steam is not effective against endotoxins. Endotoxins are released from the cell walls of gram-negative bacteria (see section 1.3.7) and can be present in water or released at high concentrations from these organisms following cell death from steam. In some critical applications, it may be important to control the level of endotoxin on a surface (e.g., some critical devices) or in water or steam (for example, in the production of WFI). Like all other sterilization methods, the presence of organic or, particularly, inorganic soils can retard the penetration of steam. The quality of the steam should be controlled and is often underestimated; the presence of chlorine (which can promote rusting) and hardness or heavy metals (which can lead to scaling and deposits on surfaces) in steam can lead to surface damage (corrosion) or unwanted deposits. This is a particular concern in the industrial sterilization of critical devices but is a growing concern in hospitals due to device damage.

Mode of Action. Steam, as a source of heat, has multiple effects on the viability of microorganisms, which are discussed in section 2.2. An initial increase in temperature causes the denaturation of proteins, nucleic acids, and lipids. This is rapidly followed by the coagulation of protein and other components to cause cell death. Higher temperatures are required to penetrate the multiple protective layers of bacterial spores, which are primarily responsible for their intrinsic resistance to heat; it should also be noted that the presence of dipicolinic acid and calcium in the spores is considered to play a role in protecting proteins in the inner core against heat damage (this is discussed further in section 8.3.11).

5.3 DRY-HEAT STERILIZATION

Types. "Dry" heat may be defined as hot air or, more specifically, as heat at humidity levels of less than 100% (in contrast to saturated steam). Dry-heat sterilization methods include sterilization ovens and incineration. Incineration is essentially burning to ashes, which can be performed by passing material through a naked flame (for example, in microbiological manipulations by flaming) or in much larger scale applications in kilns or furnaces. Typical incineration temperatures are maintained at 800 to 1,300°C, with the required time dependent on the size and nature of the incinerator load. Dry-heat sterilizers (Fig. 5.10) are simple designs consisting of an oven chamber to hold the load, which is fed with electrically heated air. Monitoring of the temperature within the chamber is important to ensure that the correct sterilization temperatures are attained and maintained during the exposure cycle. Most modern sterilizer

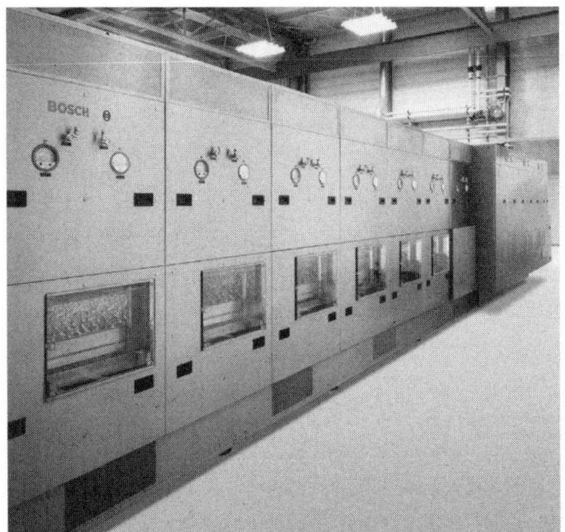

FIGURE 5.10 An industrial dry-heat sterilizer, which is used for depyrogenation. Courtesy of Bosch.

ovens contain fans to ensure equal air temperature distribution and are maintained at a slight positive pressure during sterilization. Typical dry-air sterilization cycles include conditioning to the specified temperature, sterilization, and cooling to <80°C. Sterilization temperatures (>160°C) are much higher and exposure times longer than for moist heat, as air is a less efficient conductor of heat than steam. Following sterilization, ambient air is introduced through a HEPA filter and circulated through the load for cooling. Typical dry-air sterilization hold conditions include the following:

160°C for 120 min
170°C for 60 min
180°C for 30 min
190°C for 6 min

Applications. Incineration is used for the disposal of medical, veterinary, and industrial wastes, including needles, sharps, plastics, and other contaminated materials. Wastes are usually reduced to <10% of the original volume. Dry-heat sterilizers are rarely used for sterilization of reusable surgical devices but can be used for decontamination of heat-resistant materials, including laboratory glassware (Fig. 5.10). Industrial and laboratory applications include the sterilization of powders and water-insoluble materials, such as oils, fats, and ointments; essentially, dry heat is used for materials that cannot be sterilized by moist heat due to risks of moisture damage or lack of penetration. Dry heat is also an effective depyrogenation method (e.g., 180°C for 4 h) for glassware and other heat-resistant surfaces.

Spectrum of Activity. The antimicrobial activity of dry heat is less understood than that of moist heat but is regarded as being rapidly effective against vegetative organisms, including bacteria, molds, yeasts, and protozoa. As with moist heat, enveloped viruses are sensitive to dry heat at ~60°C, but some nonenveloped viruses (including parvoviruses) have been shown to survive temperatures up to 100°C. The activity of dry heat varies depending on the test matrix (for example, dried salts and proteins can protect organisms from heat penetration), the test microbial populations, surface inoculation, humidity, etc. Bacterial spores are considered the most resistant to dry heat (Table 5.6), with *Bacillus subtilis* subsp. *niger* (now known as *Bacillus atrophaeus*) used as a biological indicator for the purposes of sterilization efficacy validation and monitoring. As with moist heat, the exposure time for sterilization is inversely proportional to the temperature, i.e., lower temperatures require longer exposure times.

Dry heat is not considered effective against prions but is widely used for the reduction of endotoxins or other pyrogens (depyrogenation).

TABLE 5.6 Examples of bacterial-spore resistance to dry heat at 160°C

Bacterial species	Avg *D* value (min)[a]
Clostridium sporogenes	1.0
B. atrophaeus	1.8
Bacillus megaterium	0.1
Bacillus cereus	0.05
Geobacillus stearothermophilus	1.5

[a]*D* values can vary significantly, depending on the spore preparation and test methods.

Advantages. Dry-heat sterilization is less expensive than steam processes, is easy to perform, and demonstrates broad-spectrum efficacy. It is a useful process for the sterilization of moisture-sensitive but heat-resistant surfaces (like some metals and glass), liquids (oils and ointments), and solids (powders). Dry heat is considered more penetrating than moist heat over time. For some materials, dry heat is preferred, due to lack of corrosion. Incineration is a useful method for the sterilization and management of waste materials. Dry heat is an effective depyrogenation method.

Disadvantages. Dry heat cannot be used for many widely used rubbers, plastics, and other temperature-sensitive materials. It is clear that liquids cannot be sterilized. Higher temperatures and longer cycle times (including attaining and maintaining sterilizing and cooling temperatures) are required in comparison to other sterilization processes. This can lead to material damage, despite general heat resistance (e.g., stress cracking, warping, and burning).

Hot air rises within the chamber, which may lead to stratification of heat distribution. Therefore, adequate air circulation is required to ensure that the sterilization temperature is attained in all areas of the load; it is particularly important that the chamber not be overloaded, which could hinder heat distribution. Care should be taken to ensure that loads have been allowed to cool sufficiently prior to handling them.

Incineration emissions are the subject of increased regulatory control due to the production of toxic by-products, like dioxins and furans (which are biocumulative and stable in the environment) and chlorine monoxide.

Mode of Action. The mode of action of dry heat is often considered separate from that of moist heat, not only due to the effects of temperature, but also due to oxidation of (removal of electrons from) cellular and viral particle components. This leads to loss of structure and function of biomolecules, including protein, lipids, and nucleic acid. It is clear that during conditioning and sterilization exposure, dry heat causes any water content in the surrounding environment (e.g., humidity) or intracellular water to heat and eventually boil, which also causes effects similar to those of moist-heat sterilization, including protein degradation and precipitation of cellular components. The water contents of air and heat-resistant spores play a role in the observed activity of dry heat, with greater resistance seen at humidity levels between 20 and 40% (Fig. 5.11). Further, the ultimate removal of water also causes loss of biomolecular function and structure. Dry heat causes rapid loss of outer viral envelopes and disintegration of viral particles. The mode of action against pyrogens (including lipopolysaccharides) is unknown.

5.4 RADIATION STERILIZATION

Types. As discussed in section 2.4, radiation is energy in the form of particles or electromagnetic waves. For radiation sterilization, only high-energy or ionizing-radiation sources are utilized, due to their greater penetration and antimicrobial efficacy. Ionizing radiation has sufficient energy to cause the release of electrons from target atoms in a given compound, which leads to the loss of essential structure and function, which is vital to cell or viral survival. The most widely used ionizing-radiation types

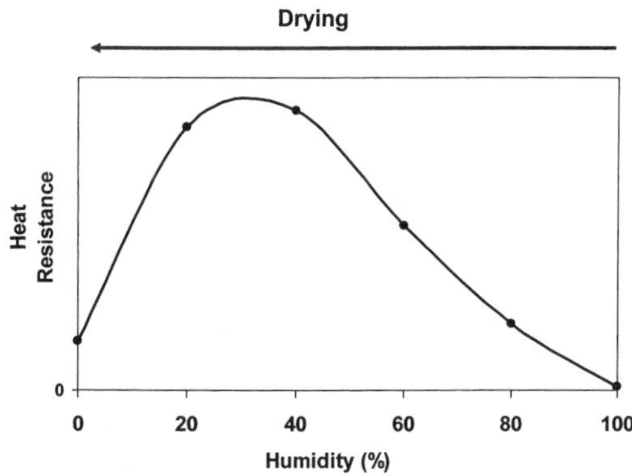

FIGURE 5.11 Representative effects of humidity/water content on the dry-heat resistance of bacterial spores.

are γ radiation, X rays, and electron (or "E") beams. γ radiation and X rays are electromagnetic radiation, which is light waves consisting of photons, which have no mass or electric charge and travel at the speed of light in a wavelike pattern (see section 2.4). γ radiation, the higher-energy source, causes the release of electrons from the atomic nucleus, while X rays have sufficient energy to cause the release of electrons orbiting the nucleus. Other forms of electromagnetic radiation are mostly used for disinfection purposes, including UV, infrared radiation, and microwaves (see section 2.4). An E beam is a source of particle radiation consisting of beams of electrons (or β radiation) that are accelerated to improve their penetration. Like X rays, E-beam particles have sufficient energy to cause the release of orbiting electrons of the target atoms.

γ radiation is energy in the form of electromagnetic waves (high-energy photons) that are released on the decay of isotopes (or radionucleotides), like ^{60}Co, ^{137}Cs, and ^{192}Ir. Isotopes are unstable atoms that have an overall positive or negative nuclear charge, due to an imbalance in the ratio of neutrons (uncharged) to protons (positively charged) in their nuclei (see section 2.4). An example is an isotope of cobalt, ^{60}Co. Elemental cobalt (^{59}Co) is a naturally occurring metal with an atomic number of 27 (i.e., the number of protons or electrons in each atom is 27). ^{60}Co is manufactured by reacting ^{59}Co with neutrons produced from a nuclear reactor, with a subsequent increase in atomic mass (59 to 60). Over time, isotopes spontaneously break down from a higher to a lower energy state in a process called radioactive decay (Fig. 5.12).

Radioactive decay proceeds at a predictable rate over time. This rate is specific to the type of isotope and is expressed as its half-life. The half-life is the time required for the radioactive activity to decrease by one-half of its initial value. ^{60}Co, as an example, has a half-life of ~5.3 years and decays to nonradioactive ^{60}Ni (elemental nickel). ^{137}Cs has a much longer half-life of ~30 years and decays in a similar fashion to give ^{137}Ba. Radioactive decay causes the release of energy in the form of radiation as streaming particles (α or β radiation) or electromagnetic waves (for example, γ radiation). ^{60}Co, ^{137}Cs, and ^{192}Ir are all γ-radiation emitters, but they are not pure γ emitters. As shown in Fig. 5.12, ^{60}Co decays on release of β and γ radiation. During this process, the excess neutrons decay to give a proton and the release of electrons (β particles). The conversion into an additional proton gives rise to a new element. Due to the lack of significant penetration of β particles, the main source of antimicrobial efficacy during sterilization with ^{60}Co is due to γ radiation alone. γ radiation has extremely short wavelengths ($<10^{-11}$), is a high-energy source (at $>2 \times 10^{-14}$ J), and is therefore highly penetrating and rapidly biocidal. Different isotopes decay to release γ radiation at different wavelengths and energy ranges, with ^{60}Co (at 1.17 and 1.3 MeV) more efficient and penetrating than ^{137}Cs (at 0.67 MeV) for sterilization processes.

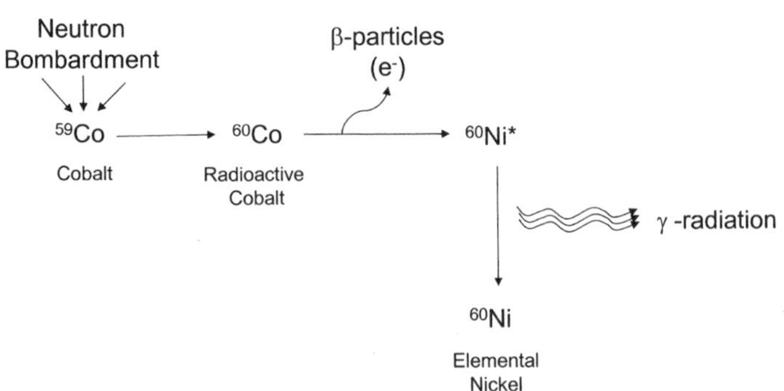

FIGURE 5.12 Generation and decay of ^{60}Co.

X rays are another high-energy form of electromagnetic radiation in the nanometer wavelength range (~10^{-8} to 10^{-11} m). X rays, therefore, have less energy than γ radiation and can be absorbed by many large (or heavy) atoms, as they have greater energy differences between the orbiting electrons in their atomic structures; it is this difference between the absorption of bone, which contains high concentrations of calcium, and smaller atoms present in skin and soft tissues that allows the use of X rays for the visualization of bone structure. Some isotopes (e.g., ^{170}Tl) spontaneously release X rays on decay, but they are generally not used for biocidal processes. X rays are normally artificially generated by the collision of high-speed electrons with a solid metal target (Fig. 5.13).

Typical generators consist of a cathode and an anode in a glass vacuum tube. The cathode is a simple filament, which is heated to cause the release of electrons (e^-). These electrons, at high speed and negatively charged, are attracted to the positively charged anode, which is made of a heavy metal, like tungsten or lead. The choice of metal dictates the frequency of the X rays produced X rays can be generated by two processes as the high-energy electrons approach and collide with the anode metal. The first is referred to as "brehmsstrahlung," in which the electrons are slowed down as they approach the positively charged metal nuclei, causing the release of X rays (Fig. 5.13A). The second process is related to direct interaction with orbiting electrons in the atom structure. It should be remembered that electrons are organized around a given nucleus at various energy levels, known as orbits. When highly energized electrons from the cathode source collide with the metal atoms, they specifically cause the low-energy electrons orbiting close to the nucleus to be expelled (Fig. 5.13B). This is compensated for by the transition of higher-energy orbiting electrons to the lower energy levels, with the subsequent release of energy in the form of photons in the X-ray wavelength range. As these reactions cause the release of heat, X-ray generators are usually cooled (for example, in oil baths) and are contained within a lead shield, which prevents the release of X rays except through a designated window in a controlled manner. X rays are exceptionally biocidal and penetrating, the extent of which depends on the wavelength range produced.

Electrons, or β-particle radiation, are extremely reactive but generally lack sufficient penetration for most sterilization processes. However, electrons produced from a source can be focused and accelerated in electric or magnetic fields to give a more effective high-energy beam for sterilization processes, known as an electron beam, or E beam. These beams are typically within the 1- to 10-MeV range. E beams are produced and accelerated in a variety of machines, known as accelerators (Fig. 5.14). Accelerators can be either linear or circular and vary in design.

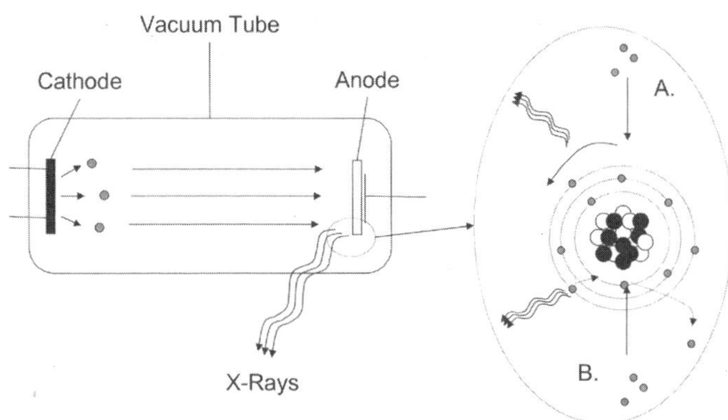

FIGURE 5.13 The generation of X rays. Electrons are shown being generated from the cathode and reacting with atoms at the anode to produce electrons via two mechanisms discussed in the text (brehmsstrahlung [A] and direct collision [B]).

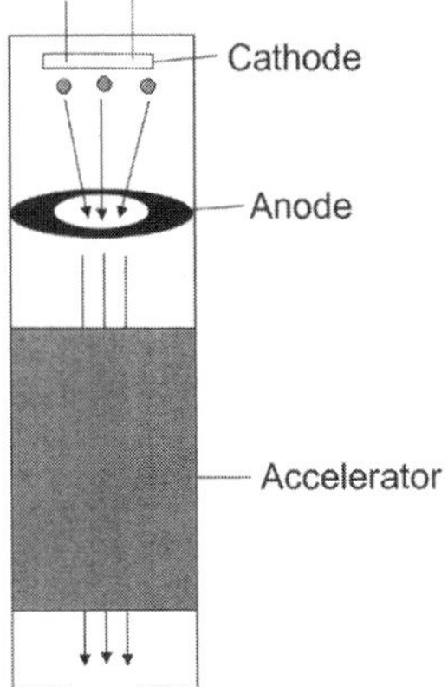

FIGURE 5.14 A simplified linear high-energy E-beam generator.

Electrons are produced in an apparatus known as an electron gun, in a process similar to that described for the generation of X rays. Electrons are generated under vacuum by heating a cathode, for example, by the pulsing or continuous application of an electric current. The cathode is made of a thermionic material, such as a metal, like tungsten, or mixed oxides, which release electrons when heated. The electrons are then attracted to but at the same time deflected from an anode under an electromagnetic field, which focuses the beam into an accelerator. The accelerator uses an electric field to increase the speed of the electrons, depending on the required energy level. Low- or medium-energy accelerators (at <5 MeV) use a high voltage to generate a steady electric field, while high-energy accelerators (at 5 to 10 MeV) use radio frequencies or microwave energy. In general, the longer the accelerator, the greater the energy of the β-beam. The electron beam can then be controlled under a magnetic field to allow direct application to a given target product.

Applications. Ionizing-radiation sources can be used for a variety of disinfection and sterilization processes, including devices, foods (such as pasteurization and insect deinfestation), cosmetics, water, wastewater, and air/gas applications. Sterilization can be routinely achieved for pharmaceutical products, including ointments, liquids and dry materials, and prepackaged devices or garments. A list of typical materials that are sterilized or otherwise treated with radiation is given in Table 5.7.

The usual dose applied in each case depends on the load and the required level of biocidal activity. In all radiation processes, the sterilization efficacy can be verified by the absorbed radiation dose, or dosimetrically. Radiation exposure is expressed as the amount of the absorbed dose (or energy) applied to a load and is expressed in grays. Typical dose ranges for radiation processes are given in Table 5.8.

A variety of dosimeters are used to measure the absorbed dose, including calorimeters and spectrophotometers. Calorimeters monitor the rise in temperature in the load, which is related to the absorbed dose; for example, a 10-kGy dose raises the temperature of water by 2.4°C. Spectrophotometric methods monitor the

TABLE 5.7 Materials disinfected and/or sterilized by radiation

Liquids
Alcohol wipes
Sterile disinfectants
Cements
Water
Serum
Proteins and enzymes
Lubrication gels
Foods
Fruits and vegetables
Meats and poultry
Prepackaged meals
Spices and other dried foods
Devices
Pacemakers
Orthopedic and other implants
Surgical sutures
Needles and syringes
Other materials
Petri plates and other plasticware
Test tubes
Cotton balls
Gloves and gowns
Bandages
Bottles and other liquid containers

TABLE 5.8 Typical doses of radiation for biocidal applications

Typical radiation absorbed doses (kGy)[a]	Applications
<1	Surface modification, deinfestation, food preservation
1–10	Disinfection, pasteurization
10–100	Food, medical device sterilization

[a]1 Gy = 100 rads; 1 kGy = 0.1 megarad.

change in optical density of radiosensitive dyes as an indicator of the radiation dose.

γ rays and X rays are preferred for denser materials, including for food processing and other similarly dense loads, as they are more penetrating than E beams. These applications include the sterilization of solid and liquid pharmaceutical products, ointments, and raw materials. E-beam applications can be limited, depending on the energy level, but are most efficient for surface sterilization. The efficiency of E-beam radiation is more dependent on the product load density, size, orientation, and packaging. X-ray and E-beam applications are in general more flexible, as they can be conveniently turned off when not in use, unlike the isotopes used as γ-radiation sources. Radiation sources may also be used to initiate chemical reactions, like polymerization and physical and chemical material modifications (e.g., cross-linking to increase rigidity) and to cause the breakdown of unwanted chemical and organic contaminants, like benzene and toluene. X rays and γ radiation are used for a variety of medical applications, such as visualization of internal structures and cancer therapy.

A given load is exposed to γ radiation in an irradiator, which can be designed for continuous-duty or batch-type applications (Fig. 5.15). The radiation source is usually stored under water and raised for exposure, generally over a few minutes (Fig. 5.16). The exposure chamber, similar to other irradiator chambers, is shielded by concrete (typically up to 10 feet thick) to prevent worker exposure. The conveyor system can be designed to allow

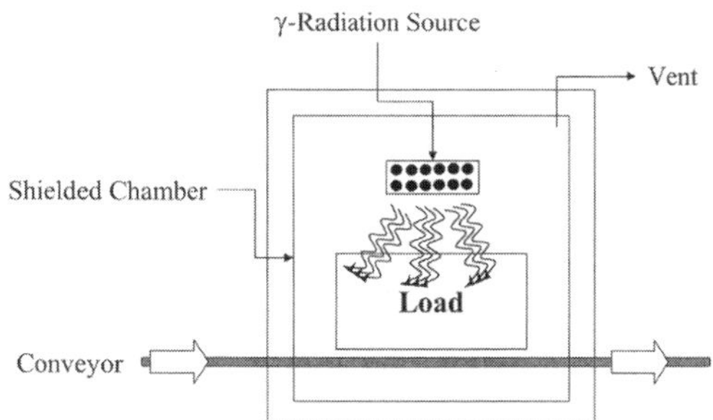

FIGURE 5.15 A typical γ-irradiator sterilizer.

rotation of the load around the source to ensure adequate penetration of the product. It is important that sterilization cycles be specifically developed for each load type, with consideration of the load density, the method of conveyance, and the minimum exposure time required for the process. Following cycle development, only the exposure time and age of the radiation source need to be controlled.

A radiation dose of 25 kGy (or 2.5 megarads) of absorbed energy is generally considered sufficient for γ sterilization in a typical process.

X rays or E beams may be applied to a load in a similar fashion. Processes can be performed as a single batch or, more commonly, as a continuous-duty process, in which the product

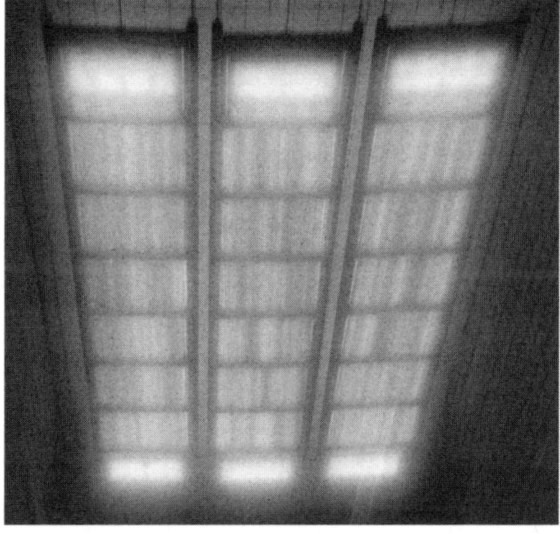

FIGURE 5.16 A typical exposure rack containing ^{60}Co as a γ-radiation source within a γ-irradiator sterilizer.

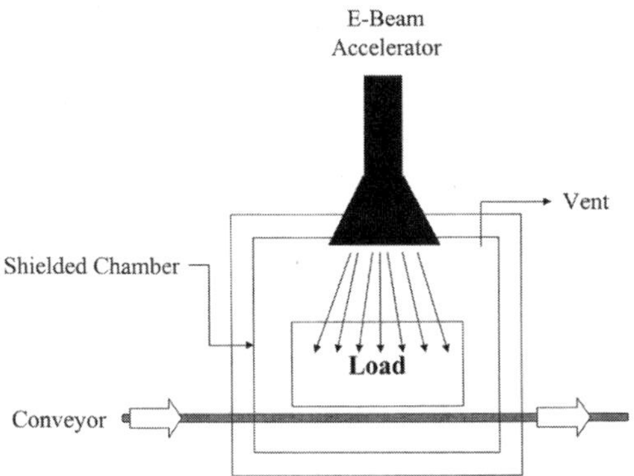

FIGURE 5.17 A typical E-beam sterilizer. An X-ray sterilizer may be in a similar orientation, with an X-ray source as an alternative to the E-beam accelerator.

on a conveyor belt is passed through the beam (Fig. 5.17). E beams may be applied in a single direction (as shown in Fig. 5.17) or in multiple directions to increase load penetration. Another application is in pharmaceutical production, e.g., integrated into aseptic filling lines. In general, radiation sterilization processes are rapid, requiring no preconditioning, exposure times of a few seconds, and minimal aeration times. During the process, activated species, like ozone and radicals, can be formed; they are short-lived and are vented from the chamber.

Examples of various standards and guidelines for radiation sterilization applications are given in Table 5.9.

Spectrum of Activity. When radiation is applied to a load, antimicrobial effects can be direct and indirect. Directly, radiation can cause a variety of biochemical effects, with the primary target being nucleic acids, particularly DNA. Indirect effects are caused by the production of free radicals, ozone, and other short-lived and reactive species, which have significant antimicrobial effects but can also increase damage to surfaces. For this reason, an increase in oxygen tension in a load can result in a greater production of free radicals and other oxygenated species. In general, bacterial spores are the most resistant to radiation, with *Bacillus pumilus* spores often used in the development and verification of sterilization cycles. During development, it is important to understand the bioburden that is normally present in a load, as protective effects, including the presence of carbohydrates, proteins, and other compounds, can affect the response to radiation of a microbial population. This may be the reason for variation in reports of microbial resistance to radiation; for example, many viruses

TABLE 5.9 Examples of standards and guidelines for radiation sterilization applications

Reference[a]	Title	Summary
ISO 11137-1	*Sterilization of Health Care Products—Requirements for the Development, Validation and Routine Control of a Sterilization Process for Medical Devices—Radiation—Part 1: Requirements*	Specifies requirements for the development, validation, and routine control of a radiation sterilization process for medical devices, including γ, E beam, and X ray
ISO 11137-2	*Sterilization of Health Care Products—Radiation—Part 2: Establishing the Sterilization Dose*	Guidance on the radiation dose required for sterilization
AAMI ST32	*Guidelines for Gamma Radiation Sterilization*	General guidelines on the use of γ radiation for sterilization
EN 552	*Sterilization of Medical Devices. Validation and Routine Control of Sterilization by Irradiation*	Specifies requirements for the development, validation, and routine control of a radiation sterilization process
PDA Technical Report 11	*Sterilization of Parenterals by Gamma Radiation*	Guidance on the development and validation of γ-sterilization processes for drug manufacturing

[a]EN, European Norm; AAMI, Association for the Advancement of Medical Instrumentation; ISO, International Standards Organization; PDA, Parenteral Drug Association.

can appear resistant due to the presence of growth media used to culture them. In general, gram-positive bacteria are more resistant than gram-negative bacteria. Some bacterial strains, including *Deinococcus radiodurans* (see section 8.3.9) and *Salmonella enterica* serovar Typhimurium, have greater intrinsic resistance, predominantly due to active repair mechanisms that can reverse the damage to DNA under suboptimal exposure conditions. This is an important consideration for some viruses, whose nucleic acids can remain infectious despite capsid or envelope damage; in some cases, damage to the virus structure can reduce infectivity, but specific damage to the nucleic acid is more likely the primary antiviral activity of radiation.

Advantages. The greatest advantage of radiation sterilization methods is reliability. These processes are essentially "cold," and they do not require preconditioning for heat or humidity, nor do they require postprocess aeration, as they are chemical and residue free. It is important to note that products are exposed to radiation ("irradiated") but are not themselves made "radioactive." Products can be packaged in a variety of materials and orientations, including final packaging, and exposure times are short (from a few seconds to a few minutes, generally). X rays and γ radiation are significantly more penetrating than E beams. E-beam and X-ray machines are generally lower in cost than γ irradiators, with X rays requiring less energy; X rays generally cause a smaller rise in temperature and, with γ radiation, provide a more uniform dose to a load.

Disadvantages. Radiation use has been limited due to cost and safety considerations. The risks associated with accidental exposure to radiation need to be tightly controlled, which requires significant capital investment within a facility. It is for this reason that radiation sterilization is not widely used and is generally restricted to specific facilities that provide contract sterilization. It is also necessary to ensure that all portions of a given load are contacted by the radiation to ensure adequate contact time and dose; this can be a particular concern with low-dose E-beam exposure. In the cases of γ radiation and the use of isotopes, there may be concerns regarding the disposal of radioactive waste, which requires specific handling and control. The bombardment of materials, particularly plastic polymers, foods, and biological materials, with radiation may also cause them to become brittle or have other negative effects. For example, γ radiation is incompatible with polyvinyl chloride, polytetrafluoroethylene and acetyl, depending on the dose. E beams can also cause damage to plastics (like polypropylene) and some resins. Overall, materials that require special consideration for radiation sterilization include polyethylene, silicon rubber, polypropylene, and Teflon. These effects can be due to cross-linking and/or chain breakage. It is therefore necessary during cycle development to minimize the radiation dose required for sterilization that is applied to a load. As the application of radiation also causes a rise in temperature, further consideration should be given to ensuring that the load does not overheat, which could cause damage to temperature-sensitive materials. Other effects include discoloration, unpleasant odor, changes in taste, and accelerated aging of materials. These effects may restrict applications with drugs, foodstuffs, or other materials.

Mode of Action. Radiation causes electron disruption (ionization) in the atoms of molecules that are essential for metabolism and survival. This causes direct disruption of structural and functional molecules, including lipids, proteins, and nucleic acids. An example of this is the fact that radiation processes are less effective at lower temperatures, presumably due to low metabolic rates. Radiation has been specifically shown to cause mutations in DNA that lead to cell death. Indirectly, the production of free radicals occurs due to the absorption of energy by water and oxygen in the target organism, leading to the production of free radicals, including OH^-, H^+, and other reactive species. These free radicals also react with surface and internal structures, leading to a variety of oxidative and reducing effects that can also culminate in cell death.

5.5 FILTRATION

Filtration methods can be used for sterilization of gas (such as air) and liquids, including water. These methods and applications are discussed in section 2.5.

5.6 DEVELOPING METHODS

5.6.1 Plasma

There are three traditional states of matter: liquid, gas, and solids. Plasma may be considered the "fourth" state, in which the molecules of a gas are excited to become a plasma when the gas atoms lose their electrons to give a highly excited mixture of charged nuclei and free electrons. A true plasma is actually considered to consist of positively and negatively charged particles in approximately equal concentrations. Plasmas can be generated by the application of sufficient energy, in the form of heat or an electromagnetic field, to a gas. If we take the example of water, when it is at its lowest energy state it forms a solid, or ice. As energy (in the form of heat) is applied to ice, it becomes a liquid (water), and with further absorption, it boils to produce a gas (steam). A plasma can be subsequently formed by further energy absorption by the gas, which fragments the gas atoms and molecules to produce negative ions, positive ions, electrons, and other short-lived reactive species. An example of the reactive species formed in an oxygen plasma is shown in Fig. 5.18.

It should be remembered that an atom of any element consists of a central nucleus (made up of positively charged protons and neutrons, which have no charge) that is surrounded by negatively charged and paired electrons, which are organized in defined orbits (or orbitals),

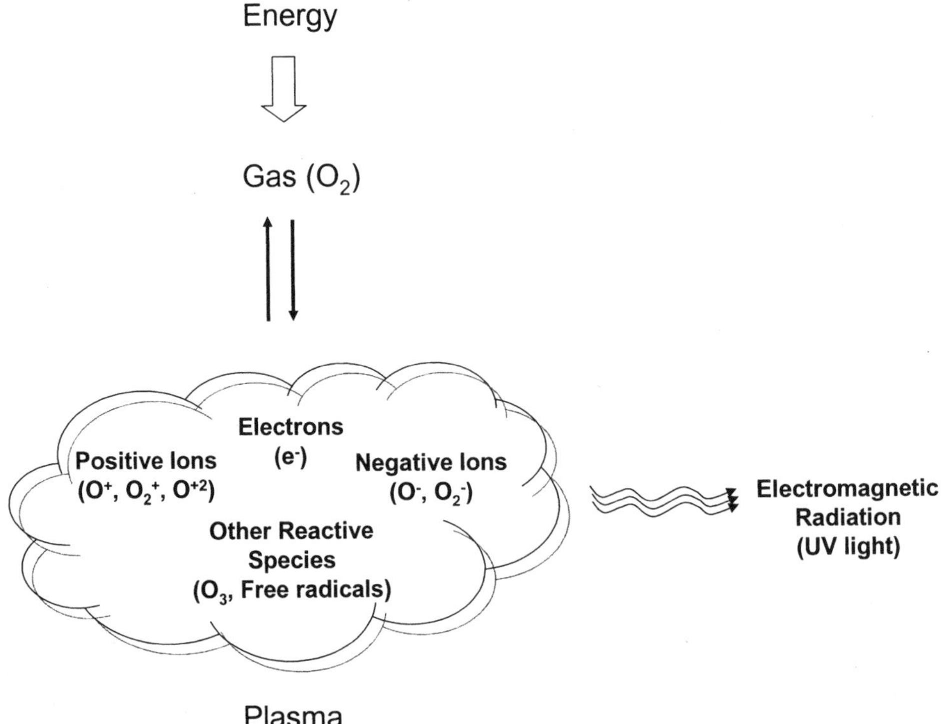

FIGURE 5.18 Example of plasma generation with oxygen gas (O_2).

depending on their energy levels. In this state, each atom is balanced, with an overall neutral charge produced by an equal number of electrons and protons. As energy is applied to the atoms/molecules in a gas, the molecules and atoms fragment to produce positive ions (as they now have a higher number of protons) and free, negatively charged electrons. In some cases, the electrons react with other atoms, thereby gaining an overall negative charge (negative ions). Further unstable species are also generated, including ozone (in the case of oxygen and air plasmas) and other free radicals. The other free radicals that are formed include the hydroxyl radical (·OH); they are reactive in that they have unpaired electrons in their outermost orbitals and therefore bind with electrons from other molecules to produce a chain reaction of electron loss and gain. These species are all highly reactive, causing electron gain and loss from atoms and molecules that they contact. Therefore, on exposure to microorganisms, a variety of effects occur, which cause structural and functional damage to cell components (including protein, lipids, and nucleic acids), leading to cell death. Further, with the excitation of electrons between atom orbitals, as they return to their natural states, they give off energy in the form of heat or photons, for example, within the UV wavelength range (~100 to 350 nm). This also contributes to antimicrobial activity (see section 2.4). When the energy source applied to the gas is turned off, the various species rapidly recombine into lower-energy, stable forms.

A variety of plasmas can be produced, which are usually named after the gas used to create them, e.g., oxygen or neon plasma. Many gases have been used for plasma generation, including oxygen, hydrogen peroxide, peracetic acid, aldehydes (like formaldehyde), and halogens. As discussed above, plasmas are generated by the application of heat or electromagnetic radiation. Heat is generally not used due to the very high temperatures and pressures required for the generation of plasmas (e.g., up to 3,000°C). Lower-temperature plasmas are usually produced in a gas under vacuum with the application of microwaves or high-energy radio frequencies. These plasmas are usually generated under deep vacuums (0.001 to 0.15 kPa) and at low temperatures (30 to 50°C).

Applications for plasma have included liquid waste disposal, water disinfection, and surface and air disinfection. Plasmas are used in sterilization processes, particularly in combination with hydrogen peroxide (see section 6.5) and peracetic acid (see section 6.6.3). They are used for device and material sterilization in health care and industrial applications. In some cases, the plasma is generated using the gas within a given chamber (for example, hydrogen peroxide), while in others, the plasma can be created in a separate chamber and introduced into the sterilization chamber. Plasmas have also been described for the generation of ozone and other reactive species from oxygen, which can then be applied to surfaces. Applications under vacuum are limited due to the need for treatment within a defined chamber. More recent applications have involved plasma production at room temperature and at atmospheric (or slightly negative or positive) pressure by dielectric barrier discharge. This is achieved by the passage of a gas through a pair of electrodes, which are covered by a dielectric material (or simply an insulating or nonconductive material, like quartz glass plates), which prevents arcing when a current is applied. A similar method is used for the production of ozone by corona discharge (see section 3.13). In addition to gases, energy or plasmas can be applied to liquids, including water, which can also cause similar atom or molecule dissociation; although these may not be considered true plasmas, they are similar to the generation of electrolyzed or activated water (see section 6.6.2).

In general, plasmas demonstrate broad-spectrum antimicrobial activity due to the production of many reactive species; not surprisingly, bacterial spores (particularly aerobic spores, including *Bacillus* and *Geobacillus*) demonstrate the greatest resistance, with longer exposure times required for activity. The potency of the plasma depends on the vacuum applied and the gas used to generate the plasma.

They are, however, short-lived, which means they should be generated and applied close to the surfaces to be treated; for these reasons, they are nonpenetrating. Antimicrobial processes of plasmas are generally rapid due to their reactive nature and the fact that little or no residue remains on surfaces following treatment and simple aeration. Due to their reactive nature, plasmas can be damaging to various metal and plastic surfaces (plasmas are actually used industrially for surface modification).

Although the exact modes of action of plasmas are unknown, the various reactive species in a typical plasma react with various surfaces and, potentially, internal proteins, lipids, and other essential molecules. The addition or removal of surface electrons leads to the destabilization of these structures, which causes loss of structure and function of microbial systems.

5.6.2 Pulsed Light

Pulsed-light applications use short, intense pulses of "white" light for the disinfection and/or sterilization of surfaces. The white light includes wavelengths spanning the near-UV–visible–infrared range (~200 to 1,500 nm), although the exact wavelengths used for various applications vary depending on the lamps used in different systems (see section 2.4). Therefore, applications use a range of light-emitting lamps, for example, quartz tubes filled with xenon under vacuum, and some specifically use pulsed light just within the UV range. Although normal white light (sunlight) is generally not effective, the intensity of the light is significantly increased to give a higher energy range (0.01 to 50 J/cm^2), which is rapidly microbicidal. This is achieved by short bursts of a high-voltage/high-current electrical field to the lamp. The light is applied to a surface by short-duration pulses, with each pulse consisting of a number (typically 1 to 20) of short flashes of light, each only a fraction of a second long. The number of pulses varies depending on the application and desired microbial reduction. Various lamps can be assembled within a treatment chamber or tunnel to provide simultaneous or sequential pulses (an example of a chamber system is shown in Fig. 5.19). The process can be controlled by monitoring the dosage applied, particularly the specific UV output of the pulses, and a water cooling system is provided to prevent overheating of the lamps.

Overall, the technology is not currently widely used. Applications include food and food-packaging material disinfection and sterilization. Foods include fruits, eggs, cheeses, and seafood, primarily to extend their shelf life and to reduce the presence of food-associated pathogens on food surfaces. Other applications are treatment of clear liquids (water, vaccines, and biopharmaceuticals) and limited sterilization of medical devices and packaging (particularly transparent) materials. Pharmaceutical investigations have included the use of pulsed light in blow-fill-seal aseptic-manufacturing applications.

Pulsed light demonstrates rapid, broad-spectrum activity. Although test results vary, depending on the lamps used and the doses applied, the technology has been shown to be bactericidal, fungicidal (against yeasts and molds), virucidal, sporicidal, and cysticidal. There are mixed reports regarding the relative resistances of various microorganisms, including high resistance of vegetative fungi and fungal spores (in particular, *Aspergillus niger*) and viruses (for example, poliovirus and other nonenveloped viruses); however, these results may be

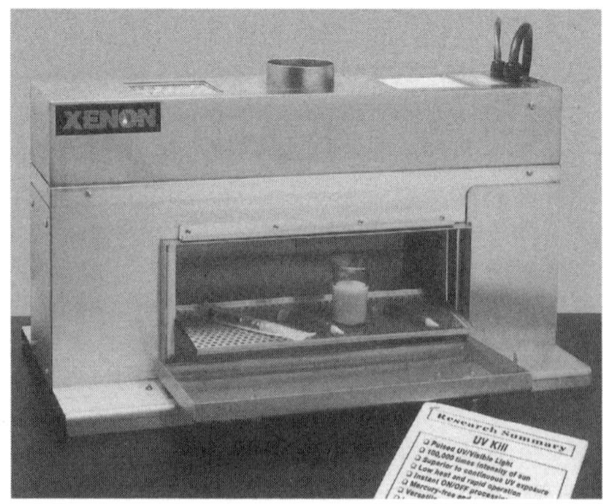

FIGURE 5.19 An example of a pulsed-light sterilizer. Courtesy of Xenon Corporation.

related to the test method used (the presence of soil, distribution of inocula, etc.). Pulsed light is considered sensitive (showing reduced activity) to the presence of contaminating soils, is not considered very penetrating (e.g., in the presence of high concentrations of microorganisms or into adsorptive materials), and is only effective in direct contact with surfaces. Despite these concerns about reproducibility and reliability, the technology has many advantages. There are no process residuals (an important consideration in food and pharmaceutical uses), minimal utility requirements, rapid cycle times, and good material compatibility (similar to other nonionizing-radiation methods [see section 2.4]). In food and liquid applications, the technology has been shown to extend the shelf lives of products and to cause minimal increases in temperature during treatments; however, some reports have found the technology to induce undesirable products in foods due to various photochemical/photothermal reactions. Applications can require high power consumption, and ozone is likely to be produced during a typical cycle (which should be monitored as a safety risk). Only exposed surfaces can be treated, with further limitations for opaque, colored, or irregular surfaces.

The modes of action of pulsed light are considered similar to those described for nonionizing radiation, with the major target being the nucleic acids, particularly DNA (see section 2.4). Chemical modifications to the DNA (including dimers and other photoproducts) have been described, as well as DNA strand breakage (presumably associated with the higher energy levels applied in comparison to normal UV/infrared applications). Other effects have been reported against proteins, lipid membranes, and other cellular components, which may be due to direct effects of the light energy or localized production of ozone and other reactive species.

5.6.3 Supercritical Fluids

Substances can exist in three essential states (solid, liquid, or gas), depending on the temperature and pressure (for example, see the discussion on steam in section 5.2). However, when the substance is above a certain "critical" temperature and pressure, it demonstrates the properties of both a liquid and a gas and is referred to as "supercritical" (Fig. 5.20).

These properties include reduced surface tension of the liquid (similar to the effects of surfactants used in liquids [see section 3.16]) but with the ability of the liquid to dissolve a contaminating substance maintained. For example, supercritical carbon dioxide (CO_2) has been particularly used, as it has a relatively low critical temperature (~31°C) at a critical pressure of ~7,300 kPa and is considered

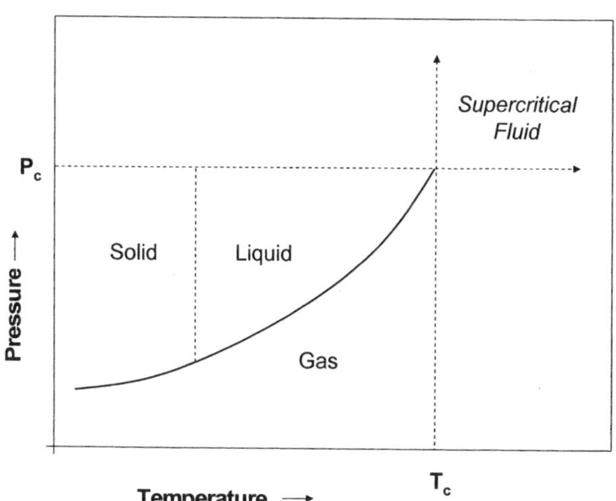

FIGURE 5.20 The relationship between solid, liquid, gas, and supercritical fluid states for a substance. As the temperature and pressure increase, the substance can exist in each state. Above the critical temperature (*Tc*) and pressure (*Pc*), the substance demonstrates combined properties of a liquid and gas and is known as a supercritical fluid.

safe (nontoxic/nonflammable); however, it should be noted that these pressures are relatively high (considering that atmospheric pressure is ~100 kPa and typical steam sterilization cycles are at pressures in the range of 200 to 300 kPa), which has restricted the use of supercritical fluids in general cleaning and disinfection applications.

Supercritical fluids have been particularly used for extraction and purification of various chemicals, including oils, fragrances, pigments, and lipids. They have also been used for precision cleaning of intricate or complex materials in industrial applications, like the removal of lubricants, lipids, and adhesives from laser system components, ceramics, and nuclear seals. In a typical application, the component is exposed in an extraction vessel at the given temperature and pressure to supercritical CO_2, which dissolves the soil, and the CO_2 is then passed through a second, "separating" vessel at a reduced pressure to allow the removal of the soil. In these cases, cleaning is limited to the removal of hydrophobic materials, like oils and other organics, but not particles or salts. Some studies have shown slow bactericidal, fungicidal, and sporicidal activity with supercritical CO_2. Associated applications include the pasteurization of thermolabile liquids, such as foods, blood products, and pharmaceutical preparations. The mode of action appears to be diffusion into the cell and direct alteration of intracellular pH, as no direct disruption of the cell wall has been observed; however, lipid extraction or disruption may also be expected to occur and to contribute to the antimicrobial activity. The spectrum of activity and optimal process requirements have not been investigated in detail.

Advantages of supercritical fluids are that they are "dry" processes with good cleaning activity, they require relatively short exposure times (5 to 15 min) for precision applications, and they have low operating costs. In contrast, the equipment costs are high and they have little activity on hydrophilic contaminants, but the primary disadvantage is the requirement for high pressures and the associated safety risks. Supercritical CO_2 is compatible with most metals but can be incompatible with certain plastics and elastomers. Reports of antimicrobial activity are varied and limited.

5.6.4 Pulsed Electric Fields

The pulsing of an electric field through a bacterial or fungal culture demonstrates some antimicrobial activity. These simple processes apply an electric pulse in the 1- to 20-kV/cm range across a liquid, such as water, juice, a dairy product, or a salt solution. This method is used as a laboratory technique for the introduction of molecules (e.g., plasmid DNA) into a cell in a process known as electroporation. Microscopic investigations of the phenomenon have shown that the specific effect of the application of the electric field is thinning (compression) of the membrane, leading to pore formation and leaking of the cytoplasm. These effects can be initially reversible but over time cause cell death, depending on the duration and strength of the electrical field. Synergy in application of the field has been noted, with an increase in temperature with supercritical fluids, ozonation, hydrogen peroxide, and other biocides; in many of these cases, this is probably due to increased penetration into the already-damaged cells. Studies have primarily focused on vegetative bacteria and yeasts. Considering the mode of action, the efficacies against spores and nonenveloped viruses are considered to be limited. Although some reports on the synergistic application of this method indicate that it could be used for disinfection purposes, it would seem unlikely to be used as a true sterilization technique.

FURTHER READING

Association for the Advancement of Medical Instrumentation. 2005. *Sterilization. Part 1: Sterilization in Health Care Facilities.* Association for the Advancement of Medical Instrumentation, Arlington, Va.

Association for the Advancement of Medical Instrumentation. 2005. *Sterilization. Part 2: Sterilization Equipment.* Association for the Advancement of Medical Instrumentation, Arlington, Va.

Association for the Advancement of Medical Instrumentation. 2005. *Sterilization. Part 3: Indus-*

trial Process Control. Association for the Advancement of Medical Instrumentation, Arlington, Va.

Block, S. S. 1991. *Disinfection, Sterilization, and Preservation,* 4th ed. Lea & Febiger, Philadelphia, Pa.

Block, S. S. 2001. *Disinfection, Sterilization, and Preservation,* 5th ed. Lippincott Williams & Wilkins, Philadelphia, Pa.

Fraise, A. P., P. A. Lambert, and J.-Y. Maillard. 2004. *Russell, Hugo & Ayliffe's Principles and Practice of Disinfection, Preservation & Sterilization,* 4th ed. Blackwell Science Ltd., Malden, Mass.

Meltzer, T. H., and M. W. Jornitz. 2006. *Pharmaceutical Filtration: the Management of Organism Removal.* PDA, Bethesda, Md.

Moisan, M., J. Barbeau, S. Moreau, J. Pelletier, M. Tabrizian, and L. H. Yahia. 2001. Low-temperature sterilization using gas plasmas: a review of the experiments and an analysis of the inactivation mechanisms. *Int. J. Pharm.* **226:**1-21.

Russell, A. D., W. B. Hugo, and G. A. J. Ayliffe. 1992. *Principles and Practice of Disinfection, Preservation & Sterilization,* 2nd ed. Blackwell Science, Cambridge, Mass.

Wallen, R. D., R. May, K. Rieger, J. M. Holloway, and W. H. Cover. 2001. Sterilization of a new medical device using broad-spectrum pulsed light. *Biomed. Instrum. Technol.* **35:**323-330.

CHEMICAL STERILIZATION

6

6.1 INTRODUCTION

Theoretically, any biocide with demonstrated broad-spectrum antimicrobial activity, particularly those with sporicidal activity, could be developed for use in a sterilization process. It is important to remember that the fact that a given process is sporicidal does not necessarily mean that sterilization can be achieved (see section 1.4.3 for discussion). Sterilization is a validated process that ensures that a surface or product is free from viable microorganisms, and evidence should be provided to support such a designation of a process. Examples of the requirements for validation are given in the international standard for the sterilization of health care products (ISO 14937, *Sterilization of Health Care Products—General Requirements for Characterization of a Sterilizing Agent and the Development, Validation, and Routine Control of a Sterilization Process for Medical Devices*). Although this standard has been designed for use specifically with health care applications, it specifies the minimum requirements for any sterilization process, including the following:

- Characterization of the biocidal agent(s), including safety, antimicrobial efficacy, and the effects of materials
- Characterization of the sterilization process and any delivery equipment
- Definition of the sterilization process for a given application
- Definition of the product to be sterilized within the process
- Validation of the sterilization process for its intended use

Despite the wide variety of chemical biocides (see chapter 3), only a limited number have actually been developed for use in sterilization processes. They include the epoxides (particularly ethylene oxide [EO]), formaldehyde, hydrogen peroxide-based systems, and other oxidizing-agent-based liquid and gaseous processes. These systems are primarily used as alternatives to physical sterilization methods, particularly due to material compatibility concerns, for example, as alternatives to steam for the sterilization of temperature-sensitive materials.

6.2 EPOXIDES

Types. EO (also called ETO or oxirane) is widely used as an intermediate in a variety of chemical-manufacturing processes, including those for the production of some solvents and surfactants. At ambient temperature and atmospheric pressure, it is a colorless gas with a slightly sweet, aromatic odor. EO is a flamma-

$O<(CH_2)(CH_2)$ — **Ethylene Oxide**

$O<(CH(CH_3))(CH_2)$ — **Propylene Oxide**

ble, explosive chemical in the presence of as little as 3% air, which has restricted its use to tightly sealed, enclosed environments where the risk of flammable mixtures has been controlled. EO is produced industrially by oxidation of ethylene with air and oxygen and can then be provided as a 100% liquid in compressed-gas cylinders (Fig. 6.1) or as a mixture with inert chemicals, like carbon dioxide or fluoridated hydrocarbons (8 to 10% EO, 90 to 92% carrier), known as EO gas blends.

Propylene oxide was used in the past for food and equipment decontamination but is now limited in its applications. Examples include its use for sterilization of some lubricants and as an alternative to methyl bromide (see section 3.11) for food applications. Propylene oxide is also a colorless, flammable gas but is considered less toxic than EO. Its antimicrobial effect is less, requiring higher concentrations for sterilization (800 to 2,000 mg/liter), which can be difficult to achieve. Propylene oxide breaks down into propylene glycol, which is innocuous and is itself used as a food preservative; toxic residues, including propylene chlorohydrin, can form on reaction with certain salts. The longer cycle times required and the safety concerns have restricted the use of propylene oxide, and it is not considered further here.

Applications. As a reactive antimicrobial, EO has been widely used for low-temperature equipment (including device) sterilization, as well as decontamination (including deinfestation) of dried-food and pharmaceutical products. EO is one of the most widely used products for industrial sterilization, particularly for temperature-sensitive medical devices or other materials. Due to its penetration capabilities, EO is successfully used for the fumigation of paper, fabrics, wood, and leather products. Area fumigation applications have been described, but they have been limited and are not generally used. EO processes are used for effective low-temperature medical-device sterilization in hospitals, but they require careful monitoring and adequate ventilation to reduce the risk of gas exposure, even at low concentrations. EO is particularly effective for porous materials and devices containing long lumens due to its penetration capabilities. EO is widely used for industrial and contract sterilization of

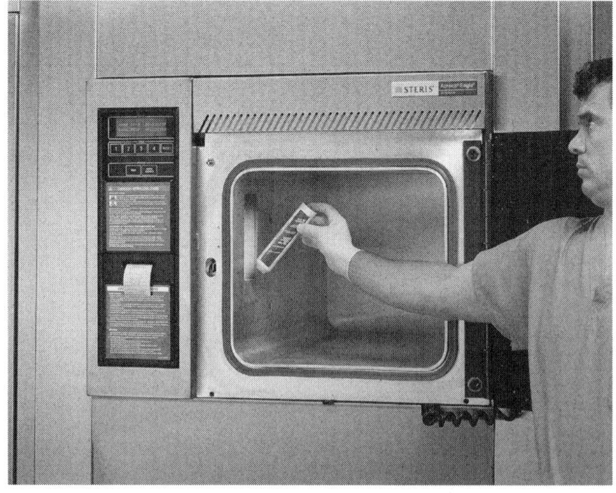

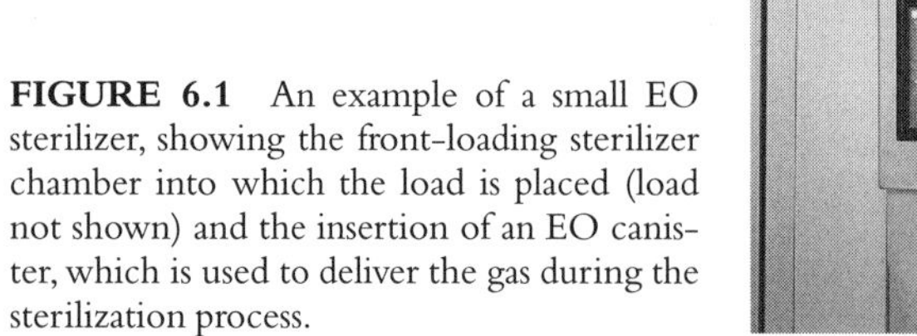

FIGURE 6.1 An example of a small EO sterilizer, showing the front-loading sterilizer chamber into which the load is placed (load not shown) and the insertion of an EO canister, which is used to deliver the gas during the sterilization process.

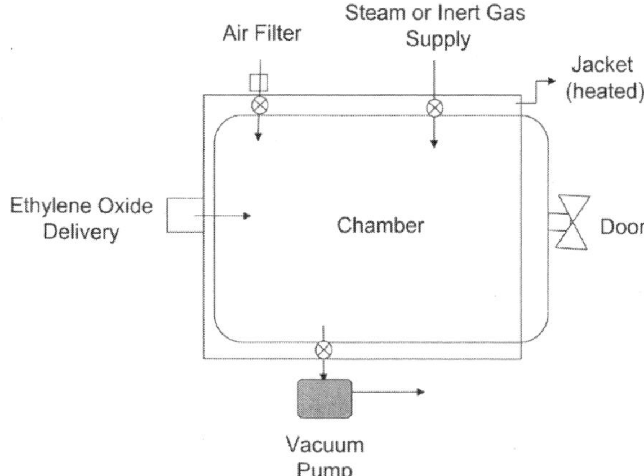

FIGURE 6.2 A typical EO sterilizer.

devices and other materials. A typical EO sterilizer design is shown in Fig. 6.2. Sterilizers can vary in size from small bench-top units to larger industrial-size chambers.

The important variables to ensure efficient sterilization with EO are air removal, temperature, EO concentration, humidity, and time. They are controlled during a typical sterilization process, which includes conditioning, sterilization, and aeration phases (Fig. 6.3).

As for other sterilization processes, the load should be adequately conditioned before sterilization. For EO treatment, this involves heating the load to the desired sterilization temperature and humidifying the load, usually to >40% relative humidity. Preconditioning may be conducted outside of the actual sterilization chamber, which is common for large-scale applications. It is also essential that the air be adequately removed, not only due to the explosive risk (with EO at ≥3% air), but also because air can inhibit the penetration of the biocide and humidity, which are both required for sterilization. The simplest method is by pulling a vacuum and then controlling the introduction of low-temperature steam. Steam is generated at 100°C, but by controlling the pressure within the chamber, the steam can be maintained at a lower temperature (for further discussion, see section 5.2); this allows the load to humidify and rapidly heat up to the desired temperature for sterilization. In some cases, where the load to be sterilized is sensitive to the vacuum levels required, air removal can also be achieved by using an inert-gas (e.g., nitrogen) injection to dilute and replace the air. Following conditioning, typical sterilization conditions are main-

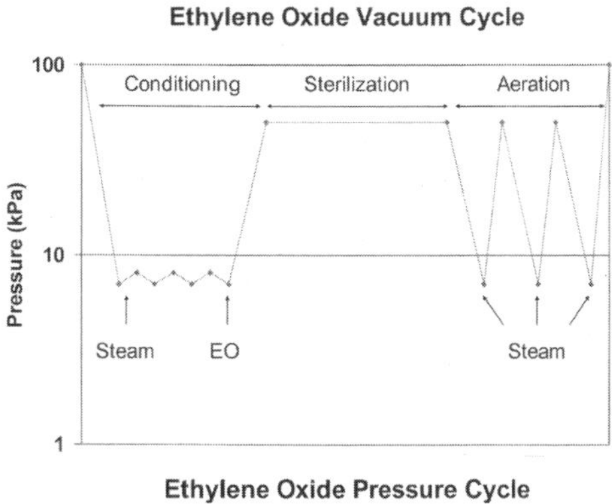

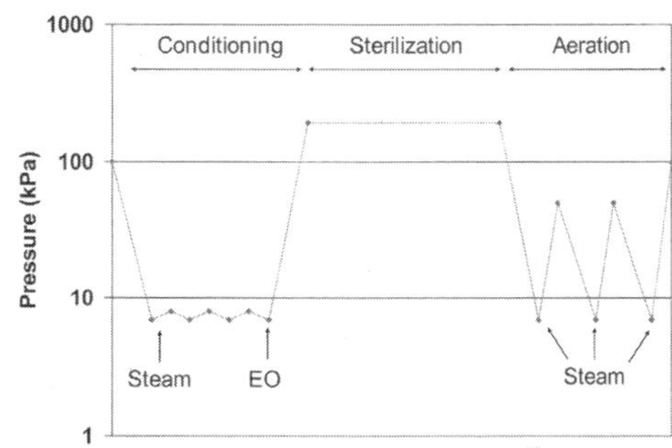

FIGURE 6.3 Typical EO sterilization processes. Vacuum processes (top), in which sterilization is conducted at pressures below atmospheric pressure, are generally applied with 100% EO, while pressurized cycles (bottom), in which sterilization is conducted above atmospheric pressure, use EO mixtures.

TABLE 6.1 Typical ethylene oxide sterilization process conditions, based on FDA-approved cycles for hospital sterilizer applications[a]

Ethylene oxide source	Concn (mg/liter)	Relative humidity (%)	Temp (°C)	Exposure time (h)
100% EO	700–900	50–80	37–38	4–4.5
100% EO	700–900	50–80	55	1
EO-HCFC	550–650	30–70	38	5–6
EO-HCFC	550–650	30–70	55	2
EO-CO_2	350–450	30–80	55	7.5

[a]Note that cycle times do not include extended aeration, which may be required for some porous-load applications.

tained at 400 to 1,200 mg of EO/liter, 40 to 80% relative humidity, and 30 to 70°C, where higher temperatures and concentrations are considered more efficient. Recent efforts have been made to reduce the overall cycle time by reducing the EO concentration to 400 to 450 mg/liter, which can minimize the required aeration time to remove residuals; in general, little benefit in terms of efficacy has been reported at concentrations of >800 mg/liter. Typical conditions for EO sterilization cycles are given in Table 6.1.

EO has a boiling point of approximately 11°C at atmospheric pressure (101.35 kPa), below which it is a liquid; therefore, pure EO is provided as a liquid within a pressurized canister. The gas can be simply produced by passing the liquid (within the canister) over a heated surface under vacuum, for example, at 1.3 kPa and 66°C. Under these conditions, the load can be held under subatmospheric pressure during sterilization. Alternatively, EO gas mixtures (including hydrochlorofluorocarbons [HCFCs] or CO_2 and provided within gas canisters) are required to be put under pressure (28 lb/in^2) to ensure an adequate concentration of EO within the load (Fig. 6.3). Circulation fans can also be used to increase dispersion in the chamber. Following exposure, EO is exhausted from the chamber through a system to remove the gas. This can be achieved by passing the gas through a catalytic converter, an acid scrubber, or another abater system. The EO is broken down into carbon dioxide and water. Residual EO within the chamber can be further actively removed by pulsing ("washing") the chamber with steam or nitrogen gas in a series of vacuum pulses. Despite aeration of the chamber, it is common for extended aeration of the load by heating over time (e.g., 8 to 12 h with dry air at 50 to 60°C, depending on the load type and volume) to be required. This is necessary to remove (also through a catalytic converter) any EO residuals that have been absorbed into various materials and to reduce the presence of other EO residuals that may have formed on reaction with the biocide (e.g., ethylene chlorohydrin). Extended aeration can be conducted in the sterilizer chamber or, more commonly, in a separate chamber or aerator for ≥12 h, depending on the load, with a constant air flow and typically at 50 to 60°C.

Examples of various standards and guidelines for EO sterilization applications are given in Table 6.2.

Spectrum of Activity. Both EO and propylene oxide are broad-spectrum antimicrobials whose spectra include potent activity against bacterial spores. Efficacy has been demonstrated against bacteria, viruses, fungi, and other microorganisms. Activity is very dependent on adequate hydration (or the presence of water), usually between 40 and 80% relative humidity. EO sterilization processes can demonstrate log-linear kinetics under constant conditions of humidity, concentration, and temperature. *Bacillus atrophaeus* (previously known as *Bacillus subtilis* subsp. *niger*) spores are considered the organisms most resistant to EO and are widely used to validate and verify the efficacy of EO sterilization processes. *B. atrophaeus* spores show variable resistance to EO sterilization processes and are usually standardized by determining a *D* reference value at a minimum humidity level and temperature (e.g., at 600 mg

TABLE 6.2 Examples of standards and guidelines for EO sterilization applications

Reference[a]	Title	Summary
ISO 11135	*Sterilization of Health Care Products—Ethylene Oxide—Requirements for the Development, Validation and Routine Control of a Sterilization Process for Medical Devices*	Requirements for the development, validation and routine control of an EO sterilization process for medical devices
ISO 10993–7	*Biological Evaluation of Medical Devices. Ethylene Oxide Sterilization Residuals*	Specifies allowable limits and methods for detection of residual EO and ethylene chlorohydrin on EO-sterilized medical devices
EN 550	*Sterilization of Medical Devices. Validation and Routine Control of Ethylene Oxide Sterilization*	Specifies requirements for the use of EO in sterilization processes, including development, validation, and routine control
EN 1422	*Sterilizers for Medical Purposes. Ethylene Oxide Sterilizers. Requirements and Test Methods*	Guidelines on the design and testing of EO sterilizers
AAMI ST41	*Ethylene oxide Sterilization in Health Care Facilities: Safety and Effectiveness*	Guidelines on the use of EO in health care settings

[a]ISO, International Standards Organization; EN, European Standard (Norm); AAMI, Association for the Advancement of Medical Instrumentation.

of EO/liter, 60% relative humidity, and 54°C) (compare the discussion of steam sterilization in section 5.2). Microbial resistance is significantly increased in the presence of organic and inorganic soils; the presence of inorganic salts can lead to the protection of microorganisms during drying and salt crystal formation; these effects can be minimized by adequate humidification and EO exposure times.

As long as conditioning has been efficient and uniform prior to the sterilization phase, the efficiency of EO sterilization is dependent on the gas concentration, humidity, temperature, and exposure time. Typical sterilization processes are conducted within the 400- to 900-mg/liter EO range, with a typical increase in activity observed as the concentration is increased to ~700 mg/liter and with little substantial benefit observed at higher concentrations (Fig. 6.4).

Greater sporicidal efficacy has also been shown at higher temperatures, typically within the 45 to 65°C range, with restrictions on higher temperatures due to the heat sensitivity of many materials. Lower temperatures are often desired and generally require longer exposure

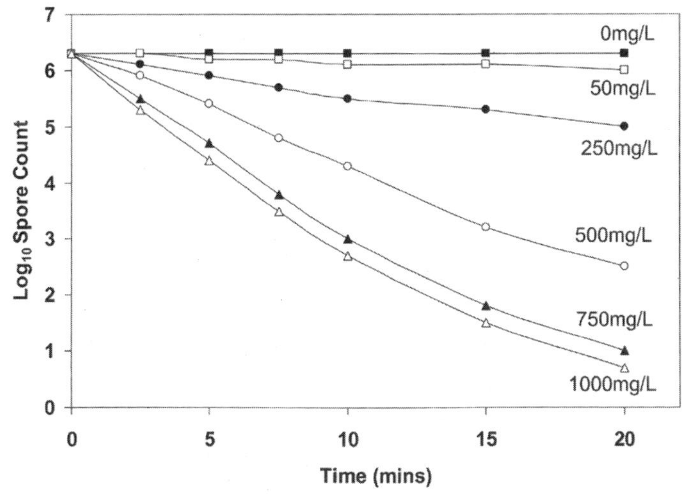

FIGURE 6.4 The sporicidal (*B. atrophaeus*) effects of EO concentrations at 60% relative humidity and 54°C.

times. Optimal and reproducible sporicidal activity is observed within the 30 to 80% relative humidity range, which is important for the demonstration of linear kinetics and acceptable sterility assurance levels (SAL) with EO. Lower humidity levels, including essentially dry conditions at 1% relative humidity, demonstrate initial rapid spore reduction but slow or no further activity. These conditions, which may be due to limited penetration or increased spore resistance in the absence of water, are therefore not acceptable for sterilization processes. Other important considerations, which are not unique to EO, are the presence of organic or inorganic soils, which can prevent the penetration of EO and/or water to shielded microorganisms, and variable activity on various material surfaces, due to differences in EO and/or water absorbance. For example, aluminum, nylon, and paper have greater resistance to penetration than some rubbers, polyester, and stainless steel.

Advantages. EO is a broad-spectrum biocide with high penetrability, including efficacy in porous loads. These attributes have allowed the use of EO for the reliable (although rare) fumigation and sterilization of temperature-sensitive materials, which cannot be treated by steam. Materials for sterilization can be packaged in various plastics or paper wraps, pouches, or containers once there has been adequate penetration of EO and humidity; following sterilization, this allows sterile storage and the maintenance of sterility. EO is a very reactive but relatively stable biocide during typical antimicrobial processes. Despite its stability, EO can be rapidly degraded in the environment. In contrast to other chemical biocides, the active agent itself demonstrates broad material compatibility and is not damaging to plastics, metals, and other materials. This is a particular advantage in the treatment of sensitive materials, including museum artifacts, paperwork, and medical devices, such as reusable flexible endoscopes; however, consideration should also be given to the requirement for adequate humidification, which may cause some damage, and humidity should be controlled to minimize these effects (e.g., the quality of steam [see section 5.2] and minimum humidity levels). Due to increased safety concerns, it is required that EO be monitored and controlled in a given environment to reduce the risk of accidental exposure; sensitive monitoring systems are available for this purpose.

Disadvantages. EO is toxic at relatively low concentrations. The typical recommended daily occupational-safety level is 1 ppm. Short-term exposure can cause irritation to the eyes, skin, and mucous membranes, which can lead to severe damage. Further, EO is sensitizing to the skin and lungs, which can lead to allergic and asthmatic symptoms. The odor level is relatively high at >250 ppm, a level at which EO can be extremely damaging. Nausea and vomiting have been reported in some industrial applications at low concentrations, and concentrations of 800 ppm have been known to be lethal. EO is a listed mutagen, carcinogen, and teratogen (reproductive hazard), which is not surprising, given its reactive nature and mode of action against proteins and nucleic acids. Toxicity concerns have necessitated close monitoring of concentrations in air and, in most cases, the design of dedicated ventilated rooms to house the sterilizer. Other safety concerns are related to the flammability and explosive risks of EO due to its reactivity; the flammability risk is reduced with the use of nonflammable blends of EO. The use of fluorinated hydrocarbons in EO blends has been restricted in favor of 100% EO due to damaging effects on Earth's protective ozone layer. On the other hand, 100% EO (which is stored as a pressurized liquid) can slowly polymerize to form blockages in feed lines and in the sterilization chamber; these effects can be minimized by equipment design and maintenance.

On the cycle development side, care should be taken that the load is adequately humidified to ensure optimal antimicrobial efficacy; this is particularly important in dried loads or in vacuum cycles (which also cause drying), remembering that greater resistance is observed with spores with a lower water content. Overall cycle times also tend to be extended with EO due to the need for adequate aeration to remove residual EO from the load. This has caused a decrease in the use of EO for sterilization of devices and other materials requiring a short turnaround time in hospital applications. Typical aeration times can be up to 10 to 16 h long, particularly in the presence of absorptive materials like rubber and some plastics (e.g., polyvinyl chloride). In addition to toxicity concerns with EO, some toxic breakdown or other residual chemical products can be formed during sterilization. They include EO-based ethers, nonylphenol ethoxylates, and other ethoxylates that are toxic and bioaccumulative. Examples are the reaction of EO with water to form ethylene glycol, which is an eye and skin irritant, and with chlorine (e.g., in polyvinyl chloride) to form ethylene chlorohydrin, which is a suspected mutagen. EO cannot be used for the sterilization of liquids.

Modes of Action. EO is a reactive chemical and is effective by alkylation. As an alkylating agent, it acts to replace any available hydrogen atom within a chemical group (including amino, carboxyl, and hydroxyl groups) with a hydroxylethyl radical. This also leads to cross-linking within and between proteins and nucleic acids. Therefore, most cellular components, including nucleic acids and functional or structural proteins, react with EO to inhibit vital functions, culminating in cell death. Propylene oxide, although less studied, is also an alkylating agent and has a similar mode of action. In both cases, the presence of water for activity is an important consideration. This may be due to a combination of the activities of water to break the epoxide ring to allow reaction with sensitive molecules and to allow penetration of external bacterial-spore layers.

6.3 LTSF

Type and Applications. Formaldehyde (methanal) is a monoaldehyde with a characteristic pungent odor. It is widely used as a biocide in liquid or gaseous form for disinfection, preservation, and sterilization (as discussed in

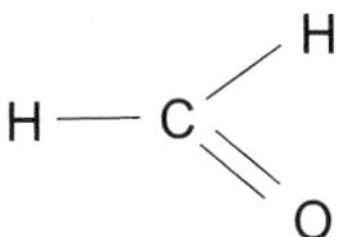

Formaldehyde

section 3.4). Two sterilization methods that use formaldehyde gas can be categorized as low-temperature steam-formaldehyde (LTSF) sterilization, which is discussed further in this section, and high-temperature formaldehyde-alcohol sterilization (see section 6.4).

Formaldehyde gas requires high humidity to be biocidal. The concept of "low-temperature steam" (or steam under vacuum) was introduced in section 5.2, and in LTSF systems, it is used to provide both humidity and temperature control during the sterilization process. A typical sterilizer design is shown in Fig. 6.5.

In some sterilizer designs, a steam supply is not required and the chamber temperature is maintained by using a heated chamber jacket (by conduction). Most modern LTSF systems are programmed with multiple sterilization cycles, which vary in temperature and can range from 50 to 80°C. A typical sterilization process, shown in Fig. 6.6, can be separated into three phases: conditioning, sterilization, and aeration.

Before sterilization, some preheating of the chamber and/or load may be required to prevent water condensation and subsequent loss of

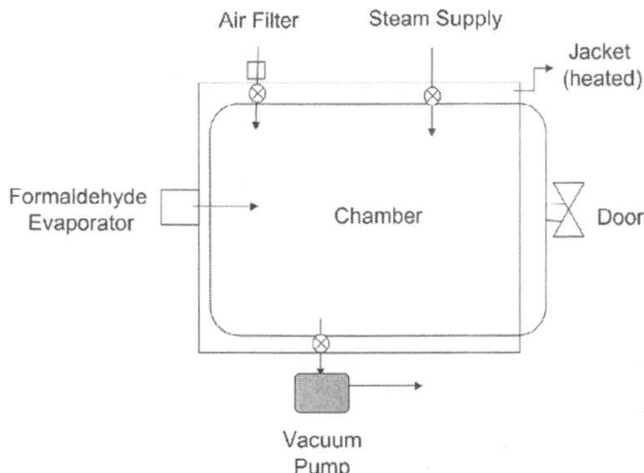

FIGURE 6.5 A representation of a typical LTSF sterilization system.

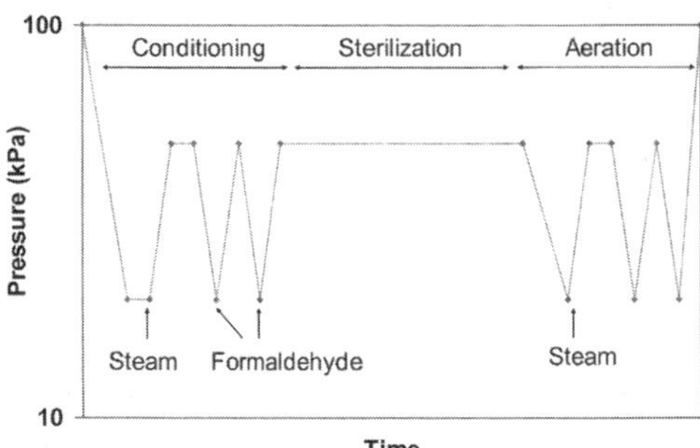

FIGURE 6.6 A typical LTSF sterilization cycle.

formaldehyde gas concentration. It should be noted that condensed water on various surfaces can act to readily dissolve formaldehyde, which can reduce the biocidal gas concentration and reduce the overall efficiency of the process. Air and other noncondensable gases are removed by a series of pulses of drawing a vacuum in the chamber and, in parallel, introducing steam, which heats and adds humidity to the load. By controlling the pressure in the chamber, the temperature of steam under vacuum can be closely controlled, generally in the range of 50 to 80°C. The extent of humidification should also be controlled to prevent the buildup of excess water on surfaces. Vacuum pulses are then repeated, while formaldehyde gas is introduced to equilibrate the load. The gas is generated in a heated evaporator, which is supplied with a formalin solution ranging from 2 to 40% formaldehyde in water (which may also contain a low concentration of methanol to prevent formaldehyde polymerization in storage). When the desired formaldehyde concentration (typically in the 5- to 50-mg/liter range), humidity (75 to 100%), and temperature (50 to 80°C) set points are achieved, the load is considered conditioned and is held under these conditions for a given sterilization time at subatmospheric pressure. During aeration, formaldehyde is removed from the chamber and/or load by a series of vacuum and steam pulses, followed by vacuum and air pulses to cool and dry the load. The formaldehyde residues are condensed, diluted, and discarded down the drain. Postprocess aeration, to remove residues outside of the chamber, may also be required, depending on the load being sterilized (e.g., porous materials or fabrics). Formaldehyde residues can be deabsorbed by heating them over time.

LTSF sterilizer designs and cycle conditions vary from manufacturer to manufacturer. Some systems do not require steam for conditioning but use the temperature-controlled, jacketed walls of the sterilizer chamber alone to heat the load and use the water present during the evaporation of the formalin solution as the source of humidity for the sterilization phase of the cycle. The concentrations of formalin used for different systems also vary from 40% formaldehyde to as low as 2%. Dual-sterilizer designs can be used for high-temperature (steam) and low-temperature (LTSF) sterilization within the same chamber, which is an advantage where space for equipment installation is limited. Other designs can be alternatively used for LTSF or EO sterilization (see section 6.2).

LTSF systems are used for medical, dental, and some industrial sterilization processes. The most widely used application is for sterilization of reusable medical devices in health care facilities (Fig. 6.7). Overall, they are not widely utilized, with particular applications in Scandinavia and some other European countries.

Examples of various standards and guidelines for formaldehyde sterilization applications are given in Table 6.3.

Spectrum of Activity. Under the optimal process conditions of biocide concentration, temperature, and humidity, formaldehyde gas is rapidly biocidal. Formaldehyde sterilization processes are virucidal, bactericidal, mycobactericidal, fungicidal, and sporicidal. The activity of formaldehyde is significantly less effective in the presence of contaminating soil or microbial clumping. Formaldehyde sterilization has been shown to be ineffective against prions. For further discussion of the spectrum of activity of formaldehyde, see section 3.4.

Advantages. Formaldehyde is a broad-spectrum biocide. Recent developments in

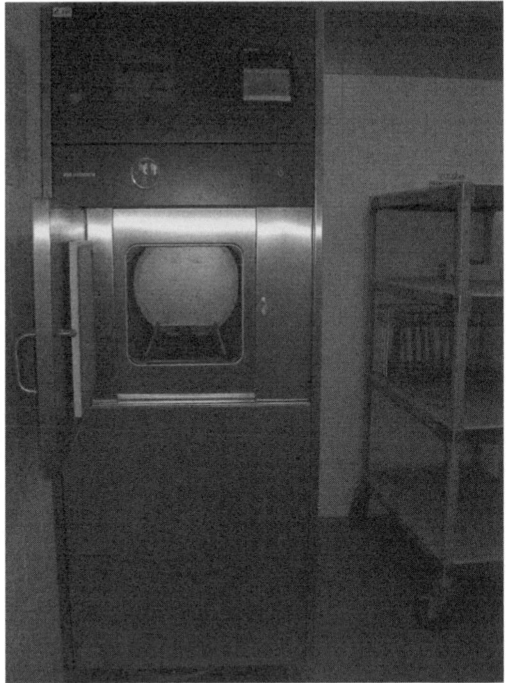

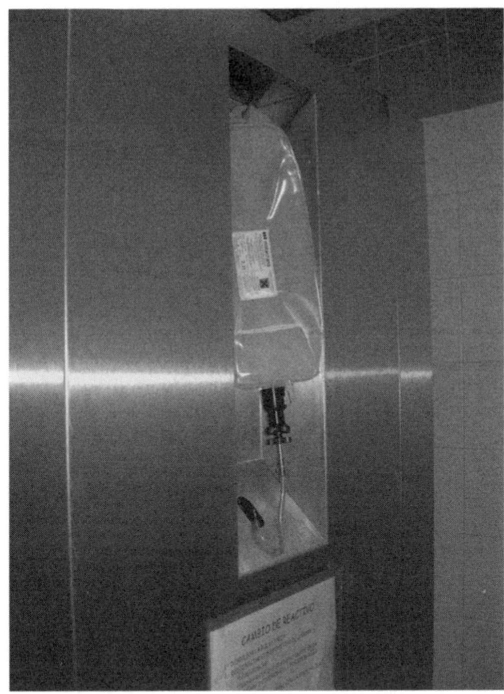

FIGURE 6.7 An LTSF sterilizer. The sterilizer (with the door open) is shown on the left, with the liquid formalin delivery system on the right.

the understanding of formaldehyde sterilization processes and the availability of modern equipment have minimized the disadvantages previously associated with formaldehyde sterilization, particularly the risks of exposure to low levels of the biocide over time. These sterilization systems are generally cost-effective, and some can be used as both low-temperature (LTSF) and high-temperature (steam) sterilizers, which can be an advantage when space is restricted in a facility. Formaldehyde has a good compatibility profile with many plastics and metals, although some processes may be restricted due to temperature conditions (>65°C) which may be incompatible with some plastics and elastomers. Formaldehyde is less stable than EO, breaking down into carbon dioxide and water (typically, a decrease of 2 mg/liter is

TABLE 6.3 Examples of standards and guidelines for LTSF sterilization applications

Reference[a]	Title	Summary
EN 14180	*Sterilizers for Medical Purposes—Low Temperature Steam and Formaldehyde Sterilizers—Requirements and Testing*	Guidelines on the design and testing of LTSF sterilizers
ISO 14937	*Sterilization of Medical Devices—General Requirements for Characterization of Sterilizing Agent and the Development, Validation and Routine Control of a Sterilization Process*	Basic requirements for any sterilization process, including characterization of the sterilizing agent and validation of specific sterilization processes
BS 3970–6	*Sterilizing and Disinfecting Equipment for Medical Products. Specification for Sterilizers Using Low-Temperature Steam with Formaldehyde*	Guidelines on the design and testing of LTSF sterilizers

[a]ISO, International Standards Organization; EN, European Standard (Norm); BS, British Standard.

observed per hour), which is an advantage for more rapid and controlled aeration over time. Further advantages of formaldehyde are discussed in section 3.4.

Disadvantages. As with EO, there remains significant concern about the safe use of formaldehyde gas, which is toxic and irritating and is considered mutagenic and carcinogenic. Adequate equipment design and ventilation can minimize these risks. Formaldehyde can polymerize to form less active paraformaldehyde, which can precipitate onto surfaces. Polymerization can be limited when exposure temperatures are maintained at >65°C. Similarly, tight control of humidity levels between 75 and 100% must be exercised, and care must be taken to avoid steam condensation, which can lead to a loss of process effectiveness. Although formaldehyde breaks down into carbon dioxide and water, the presence of carbon dioxide, like the presence of air, in a load can reduce the penetration of humidity and formaldehyde, which is required for activity. Despite the optimization of the aeration cycles of new LTSF systems, certain types of material (e.g., porous materials and fabrics) can absorb formaldehyde and thus require postprocess aeration in special heated chambers. Formaldehyde penetration into these materials is considered low and can also increase the risk of polymerization. Processes with temperatures of >65°C may be restrictive for some materials (including some polymers and elastomers). LTSF cannot be used for sterilization of liquids.

Mode of Action. Formaldehyde is a cross-linking agent that interacts with and inactivates proteins and nucleic acids (including DNA and RNA). The mode of action is discussed in more detail in sections 3.4 and 7.4.3.

6.4 HIGH-TEMPERATURE FORMALDEHYDE-ALCOHOL

Type and Application. High-temperature formaldehyde-alcohol sterilization is a process that combines the biocidal activities of heat (see section 5.2) with those of formalde-

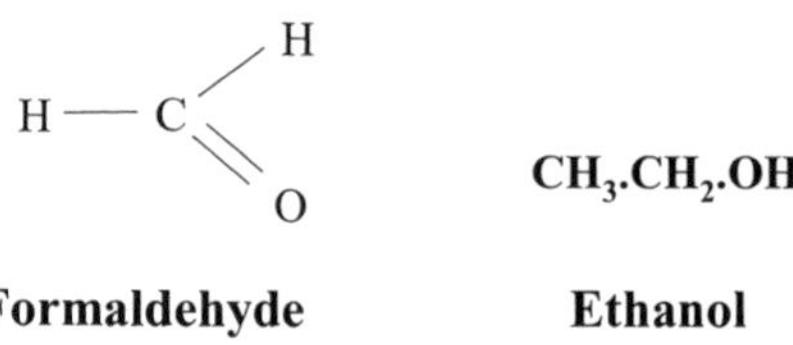

hyde (see section 3.4) and alcohol (see section 3.5). A unique mixture of formaldehyde (0.23%), alcohols (72% ethanol and <4% methanol), and distilled water (known as Vapo-Steril) is vaporized under pressure (138 kPa) by heating it to 132°C in a dedicated sterilizer (e.g., a Harvey Chemiclave).

A typical sterilization cycle includes the chamber warmup, pressurization to 138 kPa and vaporization of the sterilizing agents, exposure for 20 min at 132°C, depressurization, and purging (at 48 kPa) to remove formaldehyde residuals through an emission filter. Older systems may not contain emission filters and should be used under specific venting hoods to reduce noxious and toxic odors. A typical cycle time is ~20 to 40 min, with optional shorter ("flash") cycles with exposure times of 7 min available in some models. Sterilizers are generally small tabletop devices and have had restricted use in dental and medical clinics for reusable-device sterilization.

Spectrum of Activity. The process demonstrates broad-spectrum antimicrobial activity, including rapid sporicidal activity. The antimicrobial activity is primarily due to formaldehyde (see section 3.4) and the high sterilization temperature (132°C) (see section 5.2); the contribution of ethanol (see section 3.5) in synergism with the process may also be significant.

Advantages. As a low-humidity process, high-temperature formaldehyde-alcohol sterilization demonstrates greater material compatibility than steam sterilization, including minimal rusting, corrosion, and staining. No drying phase is required after sterilization, and the process is considered rapid. The process demonstrates broad-spectrum antimicrobial activity.

Disadvantages. The primary disadvantage is due to the toxic nature of formaldehyde, which is a known sensitizer and carcinogen. The risks of toxicity are claimed to be limited with this technology. To minimize exposure, adequate (even dedicated) ventilation is recommended in the use of the sterilizers. Ventilation is also recommended due to the offensive odor of the sterilizing agents. Relatively low exposure limits are proposed (as low as 0.75 ppm for a typical 8-h working day). Short-term exposure to formaldehyde or alcohol also causes damage to the eyes and skin irritation. The sterilizing agent is flammable (due to the presence of alcohol). The sterilizers, in bench-top sizes, have limited capacity and should not be used to sterilize liquids, textiles, nylon, polycarbonate, or sealed containers. Since it is a high-temperature process, temperature-sensitive materials are incompatible with the sterilization process.

Mode of Action. The mode of action of the combination of biocides used in high-temperature formaldehyde-alcohol sterilization has not been specifically investigated. It is considered that the primary mode of action is due to formaldehyde (as a potent aldehyde, which is discussed in section 3.4). The modes of action of heat (see section 2.2) and alcohol (see section 3.5) are also further discussed in other sections.

6.5 HYDROGEN PEROXIDE

Types. Hydrogen peroxide (H_2O_2) is a powerful oxidizing agent with broad-spectrum activity and a good safety profile. Peroxide solutions, or formulations, and gas-based processes are widely used for antisepsis, disinfection, and fumigation (see section 3.13). Although low solution concentrations are required for bactericidal and fungicidal activities, much higher concentrations (generally in the 25 to 60% range) are required for sporicidal activity. These required concentrations have restricted use due to safety and compatibility concerns. In some cases, heated peroxide (30 to 59% solutions in water) has been used for sterilization, and some formulations in combination with other oxidizing agents (e.g., peracetic acid [PAA]) provide rapid sporicidal activity; however, hydrogen peroxide solutions are not generally used in sterilization processes. In contrast, gaseous hydrogen peroxide is rapidly sporicidal at much lower concentrations (>0.1 mg/liter) and is considered significantly less damaging to surfaces. The sporicidal effectiveness depends on the concentration of hydrogen peroxide (Fig. 6.8).

H—O—O—H

Hydrogen Peroxide

Gaseous hydrogen peroxide can be generated by evaporation or vaporization. Evaporation is a slow process in which a peroxide solution is allowed to generate a gas over time

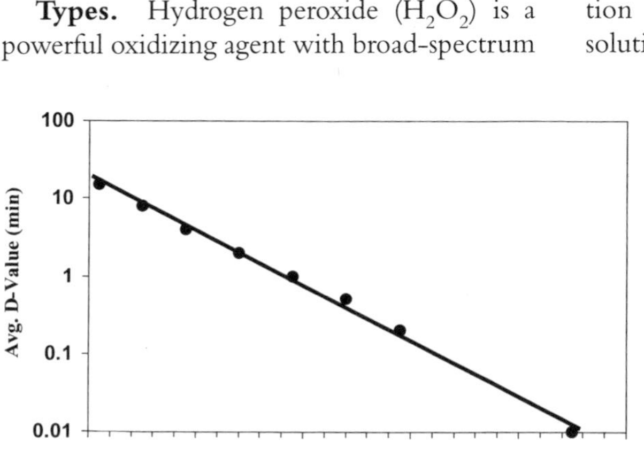

FIGURE 6.8 An example of the effect of the hydrogen peroxide gas concentration on sporicidal activity. Various gas concentrations were tested under atmospheric pressure with *G. stearothermophilus* spores.

in an enclosed environment. This may be enhanced by heating the peroxide solution, but due to the vapor pressure differences between peroxide and water, the final gas mixture at saturation is predominantly water with a relatively low concentration of peroxide, with little practical value. Note that saturation is defined as the point at which the air cannot hold further peroxide or water, which is dependent on the concentration of each gas (water and peroxide vapor) and the temperature. Vaporization instantaneously forms a peroxide-water gas in the same proportions as the starting liquid concentrations. Flash vaporization can be performed by dropping peroxide onto a heated surface (at >100°C), e.g., a simple hot plate, or by passing it through a heated cylinder and introducing the gas into a chamber. Alternatively, the peroxide-water solution is introduced into an evacuated chamber, generally under a deep vacuum (e.g., <1.5 kPa). Low-temperature sterilization processes have been developed with gaseous peroxide alone and in combination with plasma. Plasma may be considered the "fourth" state of matter (with solids, liquids, and gases), in which the molecules of a gas are excited to give a highly excited mixture of charged nuclei and free electrons (see section 5.6.1). A true plasma is considered to consist of positively and negatively charged particles in approximately equal concentrations. Plasmas can be generated by the application of sufficient energy, in the form of temperature or an electromagnetic field, to a gas.

Applications. Liquid-based processes have had limited use, particularly for food applications. Examples are validated processes for the sterilization of containers used in high-speed, aseptic filling lines and consist of 30 to 60% peroxide (minimally food grade) applied to the surface for a given amount of time, which depends on the application. Increased temperature can dramatically decrease the minimum exposure time for the accepted level of sterilization. Peroxide residuals may be removed by rinsing with sterile water or by heating or may be simply tolerated and allowed to contact the contents of the packaging (which can react with the peroxide, causing it to degrade into water and oxygen).

Peroxide gas-based processes have more widespread applications. Atmospheric-pressure processes have been developed for various applications, including as an alternative to the liquid sterilization of aseptic filling lines. A typical high-speed application can use 4.5 mg of hydrogen peroxide/liter at 40 to 45°C directly on a surface for less than a 10-s exposure time and has the further advantage of producing minimal residues. In order to ensure the sterilization of packaged materials (like medical devices), porous materials, or lumened and dead-ended instruments, it is necessary to remove air, similar to the requirement in other sterilization processes, like steam (see section 5.2) or EO (see section 6.2) sterilization. The simplest way to achieve this is by sterilization under vacuum. At least two vacuum-gas peroxide sterilization processes have been developed, which use simple peroxide gas systems or gas in combination with plasma. A typical sterilizer design is shown in Fig. 6.9.

A hydrogen peroxide gas sterilizer consists of an aluminum (or other nonreactive material) chamber capable of withstanding and maintaining pressure levels of <0.02 kPa. The chamber walls may be heated and/or insulated, if required, to maintain the load at a given temperature during the sterilization cycle. The chamber can be evacuated with a vacuum pump, which may have an associated destroyer module capable of degrading the peroxide before it enters the pump or is released into the environment. The chamber may be heated and/or insulated to maintain the load at a given temperature during the process. Liquid hydrogen peroxide is provided in aqueous solution at 35 to 59%, which is either metered at a predetermined volume onto a heated vaporizer and introduced into the chamber or provided in a single-unit-dose cartridge, which is punctured and pulled into the evacuated chamber when required during the process. An air vent (HEPA filtered or similar) is used to vent the chamber during the cycle. The most widely used processes (the

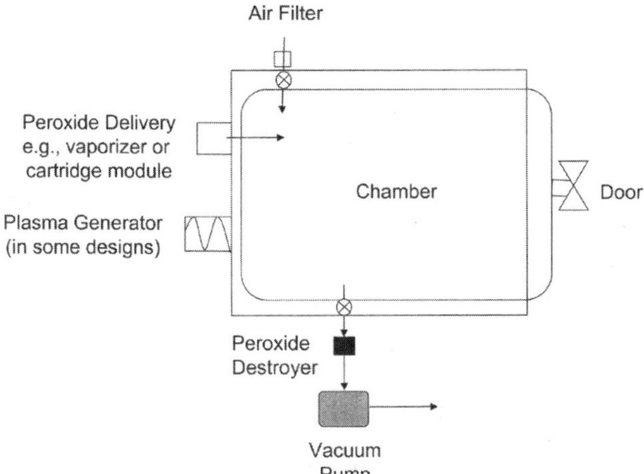

FIGURE 6.9 A typical hydrogen peroxide gas sterilizer.

STERRAD range of sterilizers) contain a plasma generator, which can be activated at various stages during the process (Fig. 6.10).

Typical sterilization processes are shown in Fig. 6.11. Overall, these processes are relatively similar. In both cases, a simple gas cycle comprises multiple phases, including a leak test (not shown), conditioning, sterilization, and aeration. During the leak test, the chamber is held under vacuum for a preset time and pressure is monitored to ensure that the chamber is leak proof. The conditioning phase uses the vacuum system to dry the chamber and load and to condition the load temperature for sterilization (generally in the range of 25 to 55°C). Peroxide gas is then generated from 35 to 59% liquid peroxide in the evacuated chamber by flash vaporization (heating at >100°C) or direct introduction under vacuum and allowed to diffuse. Under some situations, dry air or nitrogen gas may be introduced (which is shown as a rise in pressure in Fig. 6.11) to improve the penetration of the gas. Single or multiple peroxide pulses may be introduced into the chamber, as peroxide will break down over time. The number of peroxide pulses depends on the application (e.g., the device design, materials used for construction, load size, etc.) and the validated process, varying from 1 to 12 pulses under some conditions. Typical peroxide gas concentrations range from 4 to 9 mg/liter, although higher concentrations may be used. Finally, during aeration, the vacuum system is used to rapidly remove peroxide from the chamber and load by a series of vacuum and air pulses. In the plasma-based systems, following exposure to hydrogen peroxide gas, a plasma is created in the chamber. In these applications, the plasma may also be triggered during the conditioning phase, which decreases the conditioning time. The use and

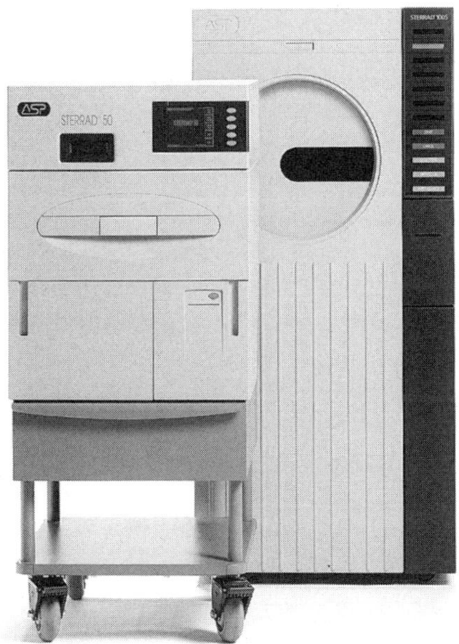

FIGURE 6.10 STERRAD hydrogen peroxide gas-plasma sterilizers. (Reprinted with permission from Advanced Sterilization Products, a Johnson & Johnson company.)

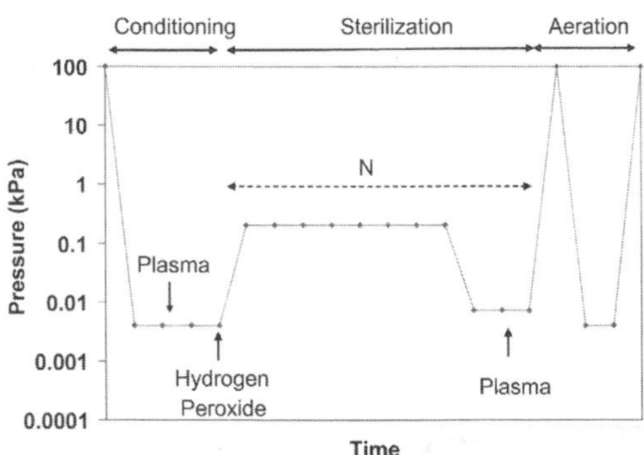

FIGURE 6.11 Typical hydrogen peroxide gas sterilization processes. In the cycle on the right, only single conditioning, sterilization, and aeration pulses, which can vary in number (N) depending on the application, are shown. Similarly, the gas-plasma cycles can have multiple-stage pulses (only a single pulse is shown); for example, the most widely used health care application (the STERRAD 100S) consists of two peroxide injections.

generation of plasmas is considered in section 5.6.1; in these cases, the plasma is produced by applying 400-W radio frequency energy to create an electrical field, which generates the plasma from surrounding peroxide and water molecules. This reaction creates ozone and other radicals (including ·OH and ·OOH) on reaction with residual water and peroxide. These effects may contribute to the overall antimicrobial efficacy, but they also increase the degradation of peroxide, thereby reducing aeration time. In some cycles, the plasma pulse is sufficient to aerate the load, removing the need for subsequent aeration cycles. Following the sterilization phase, the chamber can be aerated by releasing the vacuum, with the introduction of HEPA-filtered air, and single or multiple vacuum pulses can be applied. Developing plasma-peroxide systems have been described that combine these processes during the whole exposure phase, thereby increasing the generation of active oxygenated species. For these processes, no further extended aeration time is required, in contrast to EO sterilization, minimizing the overall time and cost for product availability. Although the cycle times may vary depending on the application, the overall total cycle time can generally be 3 h or less. Other, similar processes have been described in specially constructed exposure containers coupled with the sterilizer peroxide gas generation system to allow the directed, repeated flow of peroxide gas under vacuum through lumens and over the other device surfaces. A previously commercialized example was the AMSCO VHP100 sterilization process for flexible endoscopes and dental devices, which operated at 35 to 49°C and 6 to 8 mg of peroxide/liter for a total cycle time of 30 to 45 min.

Applications include medical-device, material, and equipment sterilization (e.g., freeze-dryer chambers and electron microscopes). A range of hydrogen peroxide-plasma systems (the STERRAD processes) have been widely used for low-temperature sterilization of reusable medical devices in hospitals (Table 6.4 compares these systems). The chamber sizes and sterilization cycles of the systems vary, with cycle times ranging from 45 to 75 min at 45 to 55°C. The applications of some approved systems include the sterilization of lumen instruments, which are a particular challenge for sterilization. The specific uses of the sterilizer and the sterilization cycle vary depending on the device lumen length and diameter and the material used for its construction; for example, they range from ≥1-mm internal lumen diameter and ≥1.5-cm length for stainless steel devices to ≥6-mm

TABLE 6.4 Comparison of STERRAD hydrogen peroxide gas-plasma sterilization systems used in health care applications

Cycle	Conditions			
	STERRAD 100S (100/55)[a]	STERRAD 50 (50/45)	STERRAD 200 (150/75)	STERRAD NX[b] (50/28 or 38)
Conditioning	Vacuum-plasma	Vacuum-plasma	Vacuum-plasma	Vacuum-plasma
Sterilization	Peroxide-plasma 2 gas-plasma pulses	Peroxide-plasma 2 gas-plasma pulses	Peroxide-plasma 2 gas/plasma pulses	Peroxide-plasma 2 gas/plasma pulses
Aeration	None	None	Vacuum hold	None

[a]Chamber size (in liters)/cycle time (in minutes).

[b]Uses the removal of water from the hydrogen peroxide solution to give a higher concentration of 85 to 95% versus 59%.

diameter and ≤31-cm lumen length for some plastic (polyethylene or polytetrafluoroethylene [PTFE]) lumens. In some cases, as for longer lumened devices like endoscopes, a booster device can be used; it contains a volume of 59% liquid hydrogen peroxide, attaches externally to the device lumen, and is vaporized during the sterilization cycle to allow the vapor to flow through the lumen.

Overall, cycle times are dramatically shorter than those of alternative gas sterilization processes, particularly EO sterilizers. Similar peroxide gas or gas-plasma systems are used for industrial-device and material sterilization, with cycles specific to the given application. These cycles can range from 0.1 to 10 mg of peroxide/liter and from 4 to 80°C, although most temperature-sensitive materials are sterilized at <65°C. Hydrogen peroxide gas systems cannot be used for textile or liquid sterilization.

Spectrum of Activity. The broad-spectrum efficacy of hydrogen peroxide is discussed in section 3.13. *Geobacillus stearothermophilus* spores are generally accepted as being the organisms most resistant to gaseous peroxide, with *B. atrophaeus* spores more resistant to liquid peroxide. Either test organism can be used to validate and confirm the antimicrobial efficacy of hydrogen peroxide (including gas-plasma) sterilization processes. Limited biocide penetration is seen with gas atmospheric or liquid processes, with applications generally limited to direct application to exposed surfaces. Hydrogen peroxide is more penetrating under vacuum conditions, due to the removal of air. Vacuum-based cycles demonstrate broad-spectrum antimicrobial activity, with a minimum SAL of 10^{-6} or as required by the process. Gaseous peroxide has been confirmed to be effective against adult and dormant stages of *Cryptosporidium*, *Giardia*, and *Acanthamoeba* spp. and nematodes (*Enterobius*, *Caenorhabditis*, and *Sphacia* spp.). Studies of the efficacy of hydrogen peroxide gas-vacuum cycles against prions have shown mixed results; multiple gas-plasma cycles were required to show a reduction in prion infectivity, in comparison to single hydrogen peroxide gas cycles. Gaseous peroxide also reduces surface contamination with endotoxins and protein exotoxins.

Advantages. Hydrogen peroxide is a broad-spectrum antimicrobial with a good environmental profile (see section 3.13). Liquid peroxide is easy to use, but preferred applications with gas use less peroxide and demonstrate greater material compatibility, including with electrical equipment. Peroxide gas also rapidly breaks down into water and oxygen in the environment. Low-temperature sterilization cycles are rapid in comparison to alternative gas processes (e.g., EO, which takes ~12 h, depending on the application) or, in some cases, steam (e.g., sterilization of larger equipment due to the time required for the equipment to cool down). The ability to sterilize at low temperatures is clearly a benefit in the reprocessing of temperature-sensitive devices and materials. An advantage over steam is that peroxide gas has also been shown under certain conditions to have activity against endotoxins, which are not readily degraded by steam. Synergistic processes with plasma may provide greater efficacy and shorter aeration times, particularly for certain porous plastic materials. Low- and high-concentration peroxide gas sensors can be used to monitor sterilization processes and to detect gas leaks at low concentrations if they are present in a given environment. Peroxide sterilizers have minimal utility requirements (electricity only) in comparison to steam or EO sterilizers.

Disadvantages. Certain materials absorb and break down peroxide, which can lead to inefficient sterilization processes and/or longer aeration times. In general, peroxide (particularly the gaseous form) is not suitable for the sterilization of large amounts of cellulosics or other protein-based materials. For liquid applications, higher concentrations are required, which can pose some safety and handling risks. Also, peroxide residues should be removed by rinsing with water or by dry heat; this is an important consideration in high-speed food-packaging lines, where residuals can lead to spoilage. Although these effects are less of a concern in gaseous processes, some aeration may be required, depending on the material type. Highly absorbent or porous loads require special cycle development to ensure adequate sterilization, due to residuals. Hydrogen peroxide gas is less stable and therefore less penetrating than EO. With gaseous sterilization, only certain synthetic packaging materials or containers that allow the penetration of peroxide (e.g., one- or two-sided Tyvek packaging) can be used; paper packaging cannot be used, which may increase costs. Peroxide gas causes bleaching (or dulling) of colored anodized aluminum; although the plasma process itself does not damage surfaces, the generation of active radicals on reaction with water and peroxide residues can be damaging to some surfaces over time. Widely used solutions of 35 and 59% peroxide cause burns on the skin with direct contact, although these risks have been reduced with the design of single-use, noncontact delivery systems. Low-concentration gas leaks cause short-term health effects, which subside on evacuation of the area. Higher concentrations pose a greater risk, due to inhalation and lung damage. Peroxide vapor cannot be used to sterilize liquids.

Mode of Action. The modes of action of liquid and gaseous hydrogen peroxide, powerful oxidizing agents, are discussed in section 3.13 and in further detail in section 7.4.2.

6.6 OTHER OXIDIZING-AGENT-BASED PROCESSES

This section discusses other oxidizing-agent-based sterilization processes that have been described or that are widely used. They include some specific applications with hydrogen peroxide, chlorine dioxide, PAA, and mixed oxidants (see section 3.13). It should be remembered that although all of these active agents can be sporicidal, their use in sterilization processes is somewhat limited. A sterilization process is required to be validated (and, in some countries, approved) to render a product free from viable microorganisms. In a typical process, the rate of microbiological death can be expressed as an exponential function to be able to give a probability of survival. A key component of this is the demonstration of a SAL (typically at 10^{-6}), which is described in more detail in sections 1.4.3 and 6.1. Processes that have involved the demonstration of a SAL in some applications are discussed further in this section.

6.6.1 Liquid PAA

The most widely used liquid sterilization process is a system for low-temperature sterilization of reusable, immersible medical devices, like flexible endoscopes (the SYSTEM 1 process [Fig. 6.12]).

The process is conducted in a tabletop, compact machine in combination with a single-use cartridge (STERIS 20) containing the sterilant concentrate of liquid PAA, separated from a dry mixture of surfactants, buffers, anticorrosives, and surfactants. During the process, the devices

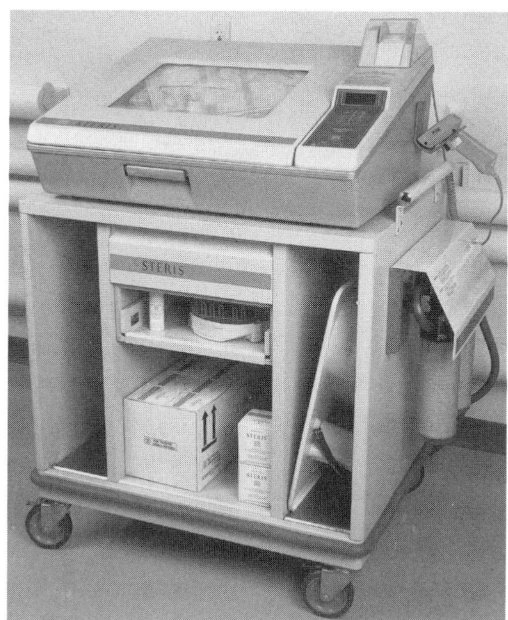

FIGURE 6.12 A SYSTEM 1 processor with STERIS 20 sterilant. (Reprinted with permission of STERIS Corporation.)

and components of the cartridge are immersed in water and automatically mixed. Connectors are also supplied and validated to ensure the flow of sterilant through specific device designs and/or lumens. The sterilization portion of the cycle lasts 12 min at 50 to 56°C and is followed by four water rinses, provided through a 0.2-μm sterile water filter, for a total cycle time of ~30 min. The sporicidal activity of PAA can be dramatically increased at higher temperatures, up to 55 to 60°C, but this also causes a decrease in the half-life of peroxide (see section 3.13 for a discussion). For example, an average *G. stearothermophilus* spore *D* value for the STERIS 20 formulation at 30°C is ~1.4 min, compared to <10 s at 55°C. The sterilant is allowed to contact internal surfaces, including an integral sterile water filter, during sterilization. Following sterilization and rinsing, devices are used directly. The advantages of the system include a rapid cycle time, broad-spectrum antimicrobial activity (including a validated SAL of at least 10^{-6}, biofilm removal, efficacy against *Cryptosporidium* and *Giardia*, endotoxin reduction, and some activity against prions), residual-soil removal, and lack of toxic residues. Disadvantages include no sterile packaging or storage (devices should be used directly following processing) and, for lumened instruments, the need for all channels to be confirmed as being clear of blockages prior to processing (as part of precleaning). The system requires potable or better microbial-quality water for processing. Further consideration of PAA as a biocide is provided in section 3.13.

6.6.2 Electrolyzed Water

Types. A developing technology is the use of electrolyzed water for sanitization, disinfection, and liquid sterilization applications. These processes are based on the electrolysis of water, i.e., the passage of tap water with a small concentration of a salt (for example, 0.1 to 0.5% NaCl or KCl) or other electrically conductive agents added through an electrolysis device (Fig. 6.13).

A variety of generator designs have been described, but they operate on similar principles. A generator consists of an electrolytic cell, with an anode and a cathode separated by an ion-permeable membrane (Fig. 6.13A). The membranes can be charged (e.g., an ion-exchange resin) or uncharged, consisting of some porous structure (e.g., ceramic filters). When a voltage is applied to the electrodes, the water ions that are present are separated based on their respective charges into a reduced, or alkaline (pH 9 to 13), solution at the cathode (referred to as a catholyte) and an oxidized, or acidic (pH 2.3 to 4), solution at the anode (the anolyte), separated by the membrane (Fig. 6.13B). In some designs, in addition to the application of a voltage to the chamber, other forms of energy may be applied. They include electromagnetic radiation sources within the radio frequency and microwave wavelength ranges (see section 2.4), which also act to charge the feed water, with the formation of free radicals and other active species. The anolyte has a

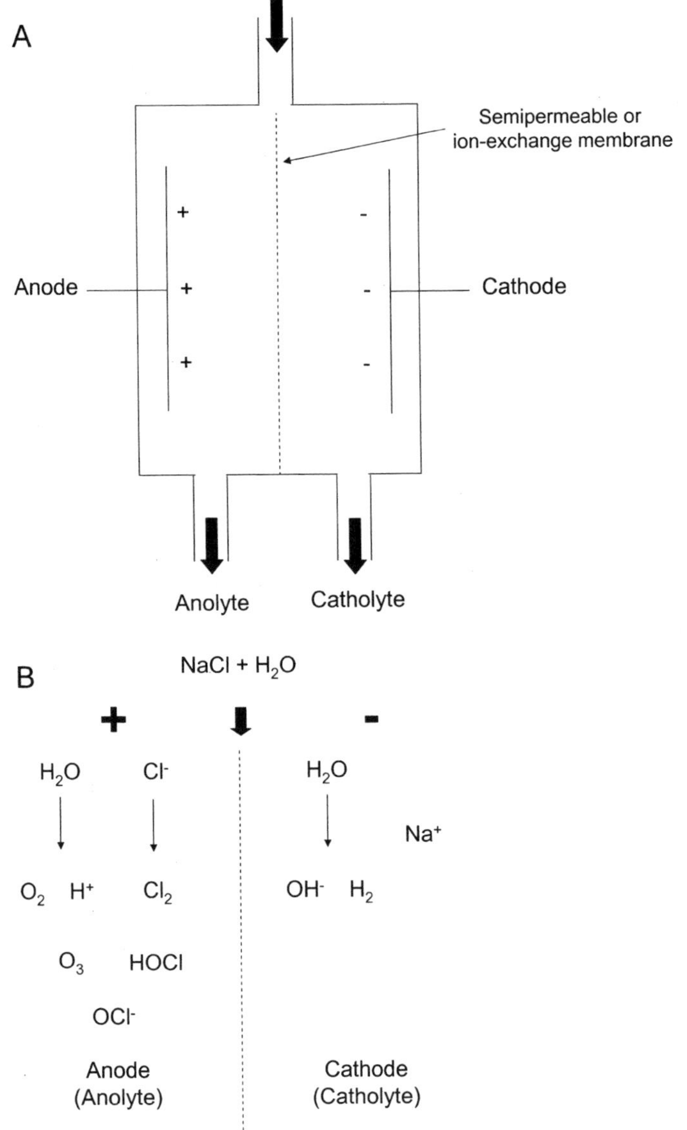

FIGURE 6.13 Electrolyzed water. (A) A typical electrolyzed-water generator. (B) Generation of electrolyzed water, with a simple depiction of the active species formed.

high oxidizing potential, with an oxidation-reduction potential (which is measured by an electrode and an electronic meter) of ~1,100 mV, and is highly antimicrobial. The antimicrobial effect is primarily due to the generation of available chlorine, mostly hypochlorous acid (for further discussion of the chemistry and antimicrobial effects of chlorine, see section 3.11). Anolytes can therefore have a slight or negligible chlorine odor. Other oxygenated and antimicrobial species may also be formed, including dissolved oxygen, ozone, and superoxide radicals (see section 3.13), which also contribute to the overall microbicidal efficacy of the anolyte. Generators can be sized to be able to produce electrolyzed water at the required volumes, e.g., up to 12,000 liters/h or higher. The anolyte itself is essentially sterilized, as it is rapidly effective against bacteria, fungi, viruses, and waterborne parasites, with slower efficacy against spores (including bacterial spores) over time. The anolyte can also be directly applied to surfaces for disinfection and sterilization applications. The solution is not stable and is therefore generated on site and not stored for long periods. In addition to the direct use of the anolyte, it can be combined with a portion of the catholyte (for neutralization or pH adjustment) or used in combination as part of a cleaning-disinfection process. An electrolyzed-water process is used by the Sterilox Maxigen system, in which the pH is controlled to between 5.75 and 6.75 by recirculating a portion of the catholyte into the anode chamber to give a typical range of 180 to 220 mg of available free chlorine/liter at pH 5 to 7. In this case, the pH, temperature, conductivity, and water flow rate of the generation system are tightly controlled to ensure consistent quality. The system requires potable feed water (at <100 CFU/ml with a hardness level of <30 mg/liter as $CaCO_3$) and has a constant capacity of 200 liters of disinfectant water/h and 750 liters of rinse water/h, which is recommended after disinfection. Corrosion inhibitors may be added to the water generator to improve the material compatibility of the anolyte. Water generated from this system is used for medical-device-reprocessing applications. Similar systems have been developed for other applications. Some systems recommend the use of other salts or minerals (e.g., organic acids, like ascorbic acid and gallic acid) during the generation process to control the pH or to remove available free chlorine, which can be overaggressive for some surface applications. In all cases, the antimicrobial solution produced can be referred to as "oxidized," "superoxidized," or "activated" water.

In addition to the use of the anolyte for antimicrobial purposes, the catholyte, a strong alkaline solution that is mostly composed of metal hydroxides, has been found to have excellent cleaning abilities. Alkaline solutions are particularly used for the removal and breakdown of proteins on surfaces.

Applications. Electrolyzed-water generators can be used to sanitize, disinfect, and, in some cases, sterilize water for various applications, including drinking water, wastewater, or other feed water applications (e.g., rinsing). In addition to their antimicrobial activity, systems have been used for odor control. The use for routine water line disinfection is of particular interest, due to the ability of electrolyzed water to remove biofilms and to disinfect surfaces contaminated with them (including *Legionella* and *Pseudomonas* control) (see section 8.3.8 for a detailed discussion of biofilms). Applications have included the use of electrolyzed water for surface rinsing following a chemical disinfection process to remove residues of the disinfection chemistry. The anolyte can also be used as a hard-surface disinfectant and may not require any rinsing postdisinfection due to the short-lived nature of the active species. Surfaces disinfected have included those in food contact, veterinary, industrial, dental, and medical applications. For example, electrolyzed-water systems have been recommended and are used for chemical disinfection of temperature-sensitive devices, including flexible endoscopes. Examples of such systems for these applications are the Sterilox generators (Fig. 6.14).

In these systems, the water generator can be located as a central supply unit that is plumbed with multiple washer-disinfectors in a facility. Electrolyzed water can be generated and stored for up to 24 h before use. The sporicidal disinfectant anolyte is rapidly antimicrobial, within a claimed typical exposure time of 5 to 10 min. Some applications have described the use of electrolyzed water at controlled temperatures (up to 50 to 60°C) for greater sporicidal activity. Some combined cleaning-disinfection applications (e.g., for routine decontamination of dialysis systems, dental units, or other systems containing reusable water or fluid lines) involve the refrigerated storage of the anolyte for up to 14 days and direct use of the low-pH (<3) anolyte for device reprocessing. Systems have been described that use normal water for precleaning of surfaces, cleaning with the catholyte for 2 to 3 min, rinsing (to remove residual

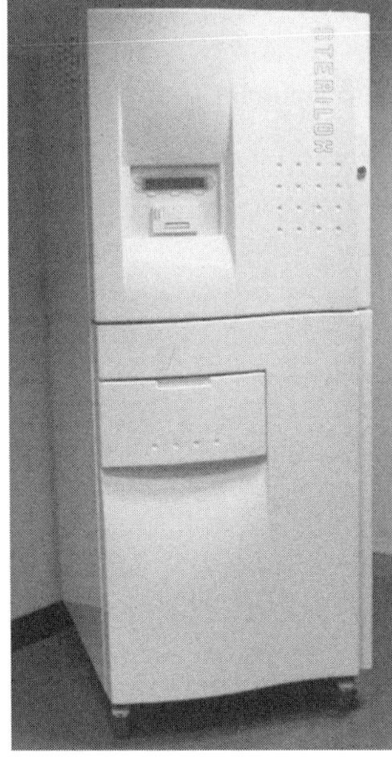

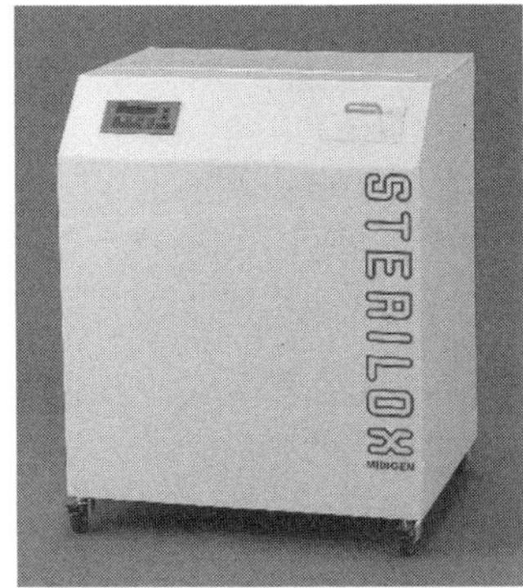

FIGURE 6.14 Examples of electrolyzed-water generators. Courtesy of Sterilox Technologies.

catholyte), and disinfection with the anolyte for the required level of antimicrobial efficacy (generally 5 to 15 min). In these applications, the anolyte can remain in situ (as a preservative) until the next use of the device or the system can be flushed with air to remove residual anolyte; under some conditions of use, no further rinsing is required due to the low concentrations of biocidal species and the fact that they are generally short-lived, posing no toxic risk on subsequent reuse of the system.

Electrolyzed-water systems have been reported to be under development for a wider range of applications. These include the economical production of drinking water, wound or skin rinsing (as a nontoxic antiseptic), food rinsing and disinfection (e.g., of tofu and fruits), and horticulture.

Spectrum of Activity. Given the range of antimicrobial effects observed with anolytes, it is not surprising that they are rapidly bactericidal and fungicidal. Rapid efficacy has been reported in both low-pH (<3) and mid-pH (5 to 7) ranges against gram-positive and -negative bacteria, molds, yeasts, and mycobacteria. Virucidal efficacy has been confirmed against enveloped (including hepatitis B virus) and nonenveloped viruses. Typical exposure conditions for anolytes for efficacy against these organisms are 100 to 250 mg of available free chlorine/liter for 2 min. Lower levels (as low as 100-mg/liter chlorine solutions) have been claimed to be effective for the sanitization of cleaned surfaces against vegetative bacteria. Longer exposure times, between 5 and 10 min, or higher concentrations are generally required for sporicidal activity, although SAL have not yet been published for electrolyzed-water solutions. The presence of organic soil dramatically reduces the observed antimicrobial effects. Electrolyzed-water solutions have shown little or no effect against prions, although the reports have been only preliminary in nature.

Advantages. Electrolyzed water (anolyte) demonstrates broad-spectrum antimicrobial, including sporicidal, activity but is also nonirritating and presents minor toxicity concerns. Solutions have not been found to be sensitizing and can be safely disposed of following use or expiration. Obviously, the lower- and higher-pH solutions generated can cause damage on direct exposure to the skin, mucous membranes, and eyes; for generators that mix and control the pH of the water produced, this is less of a concern. In addition to the anolyte biocidal activity, the high-pH catholyte also acts as an excellent cleaner for surfaces, including biofilm removal. Water generators can be economical, with few operational costs (energy and low concentrations of salts and minerals). Electrolyzed water has been shown to react with some undesirable dissolved organic and inorganic water contaminants, causing them to coagulate and/or precipitate; they can then be removed from the water by simple filtration. Some activity has been reported against bacterial toxins and endotoxins, which can be present in water. Further, the anolyte can also cause the breakdown of toxic substances (for example, sulfides) into nontoxic compounds.

Disadvantages. Electrolyzed water can be damaging to some surface materials; for example, it can promote corrosion of metals like stainless steel and damage to polyurethane over multiple applications. In some applications (e.g., flexible endoscopes), it is recommended that the device surface be coated with an oxidation-resistant protective barrier (e.g., of PTFE), which can reduce these effects. Incompatibility with surfaces can be minimized by formulation effects (e.g., the addition of corrosion inhibitors, like phosphates and sulfates), which are added to the anolyte on production, or by controlling the pH to near neutral by the addition of a catholyte. Equally, the catholyte is incompatible with soft metals, including aluminum. The activity and damage to surfaces vary depending on the quality of water used for generation. For example, when the feed water is chlorinated, high levels of chlorinated compounds may be produced, and they can be aggressive on sensitive plastic and metal surfaces. Degassing from generated solutions should be controlled to ensure that they do not accumulate to toxic levels. Further, other compounds may be formed in the anolyte or catholyte that can remain on a surface following disinfection or be harmful when present in treated water. Examples are chlorinated by-products, as discussed in section 3.11. It is therefore recommended that the chloride levels and pH produced be controlled during use of the anolyte for disinfection. Other concerns can be the buildup of deposits on the electrodes and in the generators over time due to scaling, etc., which may be controlled by pretreatment of the water (ranging from water softening to the supply of reverse-osmosis water). These deposits or precipitates may be a concern on subsequent release from the generator, but this can be prevented by filtration.

The antimicrobial effect of anolyte water is dramatically affected by the presence of contaminating soils. It is recommended that surfaces be adequately cleaned before application of the water to ensure the required level of efficacy. Solutions are unstable, and their stability also depends partially on the redox potential and pH; stability times are shorter at higher temperatures.

Mode of Action. Electrolyzed water, given as a mixture of antimicrobial agents, has multiple modes of action on microorganisms. Overall, these active agents (particularly in the anolyte) cause damage to cell wall, membrane, and intracellular components, as well as to the surfaces of spores and viruses. These targets include proteins, lipids, and nucleic acids. Specific effects observed in bacteria include enzyme inactivation, outer and inner membrane structural changes, cytoplasmic leakage, some DNA breakdown, and cell wall damage. pH effects alone (both high- and low-pH solutions) are at a minimum restrictive to the growth of microorganisms but also cause bactericidal and fungicidal loss of structure and function. Vegetative organisms are particularly sensitive due to the delicate balance between the organism and its environment, as dictated by the cell wall-cell membrane structure, including osmotic pressure and the role of porins (see section 8.3.4). In general, bacteria and fungi (depending on the genus and species) show great variability in their abilities to tolerate high or low pH and redox potential effects. In general, pH can range between 4 and 11, with some extremophiles (see sections 8.3.9 and 8.3.10) surviving at the extremes of this range; however, these highly pH-tolerant microorganisms are generally restricted to extreme environments and are not routinely identified in most environments. With a typical pH of <3 for a directly produced anolyte, little resistance of the solution to the multiple effects of pH is expected, although the mode of action of pH-controlled solutions in the pH 5 to 7 range is more primarily due to the presence of available free chlorine, particularly as hypochlorous acid. The modes of action of hypochlorous acid and hypochlorite ions, as major sources of antimicrobial activity, are discussed in section 3.11. In addition, the combined effects of oxygenated species, including ozone (see section 3.13), also contribute to the overall microbicidal activity.

6.6.3 Gaseous PAA

Similar to the hydrogen peroxide gas systems, sterilization processes have been developed based on gaseous PAA and in combination with plasma. PAA is a broad-spectrum antimicrobial at relatively low concentrations and is primarily used in liquid formulation (see section 3.13). PAA gas can be produced by vaporization of liquid PAA-water solutions at 35 to 45%. PAA solutions are supplied in solution with water, hydrogen peroxide, and acetic acid; therefore, vaporization of these solutions can provide a synergistic mixture of acid and peroxide gases. Some sterilization processes, although not currently commercialized, have involved the use of vaporized PAA under vacuum, in cycles similar to those described with hydrogen peroxide (see section 6.5) for reusable- or single-use-medical-device and industrial sterilization applications. Gaseous PAA sterilization processes consist of the vaporization of PAA-water solutions in an evacuated chamber, exposure for the required time, and aeration of the chamber by evacuation through a catalytic converter to break down the gas into water and acetic acid. The water content of the PAA solution can be sufficient to provide the necessary humidity for optimal antimicrobial activity (generally 30 to 80%) or can be supplemented by further humidification (during the conditioning and/or sterilization phases) with low-temperature steam. Exposures may be controlled at ambient temperatures or up to 40 to 50°C; higher temperatures may also cause the rapid breakdown of the gas and loss of efficacy. A proposed sterilization cycle is 10 mg/liter at 45°C for 60 min. Some systems have used plasma generation (see section 5.6.1) during or following PAA gas exposure for sterilization. As in hydrogen peroxide-plasma systems, this causes the production of reactive radicals on reaction with water or PAA and can also aid in rapid aeration of the chamber and load. A PAA-plasma sterilization process (Plazlyte) was described and marketed in the United States for health care and industrial use, but it is no longer commercially available. During the process, the load was treated with PAA gas at 0.5 mg/liter, generated by direct vaporization in an evacuated chamber, followed by the introduction of a low-temperature plasma. The pulses could be repeated for the desired sterilization time, and then the chamber and load would be aerated by repeated vacuum pulse applications. Other processes have included atmospheric-pressure applications (or a slight pressure differential), which allow the directed flow of gaseous PAA through and over the device or load surfaces. This can be achieved by directed flow under pressure or by creating a pressure differential in a two-component container system. Special containers to allow exposure and subsequent sterile storage of a load have been described for these purposes but have not been made commercially available. Similar to hydrogen peroxide gas, gaseous PAA is a broad-spectrum antimicrobial with efficacy at lower concentrations than are required for liquid formulations. PAA demonstrates greater stability and penetration than other gaseous oxidizing agents, with some penetration of paper and porous materials. As with other gaseous sterilization processes, liquids cannot be treated and surfaces should be dry prior to treatment. PAA (an acid and a powerful oxidizing agent) can be corrosive to surfaces.

Although these effects can be minimized in liquid formulation, PAA gas can be aggressive on many polymers and metals (particularly polyurethane and metals like aluminum, brass, and copper). PAA gas is also irritating and sensitizing at low concentrations, with higher concentrations being toxic and damaging to the eyes, skin, and mucous membranes. Care should be taken to ensure that PAA or other toxic residuals that can form on surfaces during sterilization are adequately aerated to remove the risks of adverse reactions, particularly for critical surgical devices.

6.6.4 Ozone

Many systems have been proposed and designed based on the use of ozone in a true low-temperature sterilization process. Ozone has been widely used for drinking water disinfection and area deodorization applications (see section 3.13) and has some key advantages: it can be generated from water, it demonstrates broad-spectrum antimicrobial efficacy, and it rapidly breaks down in the environment into nontoxic residues (water and oxygen). However, although ozone is effective at low concentrations against vegetative bacteria and other pathogens, much higher concentrations are required for sporicidal activity and to allow the development of validated sterilization processes. Some limited applications for food surfaces have been described in which ozone is produced and directly applied to the surfaces for disinfection or sterilization purposes. These processes have been difficult to apply for sterilization of defined loads, including medical devices, due to the higher humidity and ozone concentrations required to achieve the required SAL. Synergistic processes that combine PAA or hydrogen peroxide gas with ozone have also been described but are not in general use. An ozone system has been described for sterilization of rigid endoscopes and accessories (referred to as the STER-O_3-Zone 100), but it has seen little practical application. The devices were placed into a rigid aluminum chamber module, which was directly coupled to an ozone generator. The process consisted of preconditioning the load to a relative humidity of 75 to 95% and sterilization with ozone for 40 to 60 min at 25 to 30°C. The chamber was then aerated by passing residual ozone through a catalytic converter, and the container was used for subsequent sterile storage. A further approved system uses humidified ozone under vacuum for low-temperature sterilization of medical devices (including metals, plastics, and restricted lumened devices) and other industrial applications (Fig. 6.15).

This sterilizer has minimal utility requirements, including high-quality water (which

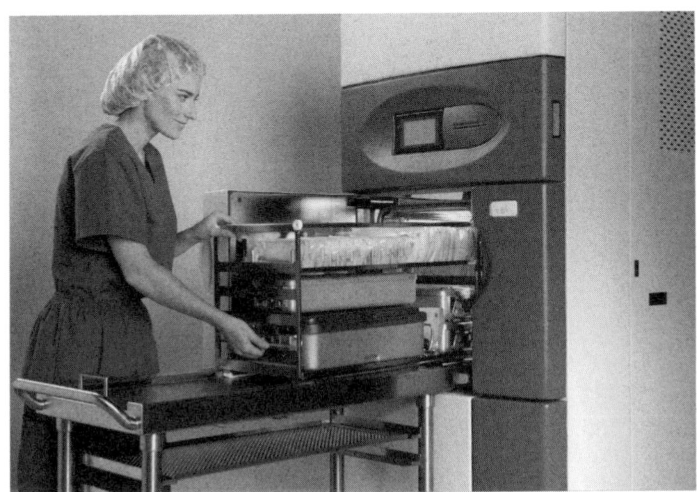

FIGURE 6.15 A 125-liter ozone sterilizer. (Reprinted with permission from TSO_3.)

is provided as prepackaged purified water), medical-grade oxygen, and electricity. The 125-liter sterilizer is a simple design consisting of a chamber, a humidifier, an ozone generator, and a vacuum pump. Similar to other gaseous sterilization methods, the process consists of preconditioning, sterilization, and ventilation phases. During preconditioning, the chamber is evacuated and the load is humidified. The sterilization phase is conducted with two identical stages consisting of evacuation to ~0.01 kPa, humidification, ozone injection, and diffusion. Humidity is controlled at 85 to 100% while avoiding condensation of water and ozone. Antimicrobial efficacy with ozone is claimed to be optimal with the humidity at ~95%. Ozone is generated from medical-grade oxygen by passing it through a corona discharge. The ozone is cooled to prevent decomposition and introduced into the chamber to give an effective dose of 85 mg/liter. Humidified ozone is allowed to diffuse into the load for the required exposure time and evacuated, and the load is exposed to a further sterilization stage. The sterilization temperature is maintained at 30 to 36°C. The chamber is then ventilated by evacuation through an ozone destroyer (a catalytic converter) and then returned to atmospheric pressure to allow access to the load. Approximately 700 to 880 liters of oxygen and a few milliliters of water are used during the process for a typical total cycle time of ~4 h. The ventilation stage is short due to the rapid degradation of ozone, with no requirement for special venting or subsequent aeration. The overall cycle costs are claimed to be low. Humidified ozone is a powerful antimicrobial, but it can also be reactive or damaging to some plastic and metal surfaces over repeated applications. Incompatibility with ozone treatment has previously been observed with aluminum, brass, polyurethanes, and rubber materials. Woven textiles and liquids cannot be reprocessed with ozone.

6.6.5 Chlorine Dioxide

Although not widely commercialized, chlorine dioxide gas-based systems have also been described; they are not dissimilar to the use of EO, ozone, or LTSF. Chlorine dioxide (ClO_2) is a gas at room temperature and, due to its reactive nature, is generated at the site of use (see section 3.13). The sterilization process is performed in an evacuated chamber. A deep vacuum is drawn to <5 kPa, and the load is humidified by the introduction of low-temperature steam. This is important, as humidity should be maintained during the process at >65% for effective ClO_2 activity. ClO_2 can then be generated by a variety of methods (including the use of chlorine gas passed through a column of sodium chlorite) at ~10 to 50 mg/liter and maintained, by the addition of nitrogen gas, at 80 kPa for the desired contact time. Multiple pulses of ClO_2 may be required to ensure the required load penetration and SAL. Sterilization processes have been described at 10 mg/liter, 25 to 30°C, and 70 to 80% relative humidity for up to 1.5 h of total cycle time. A series of vacuum pulses are then used to remove residual ClO_2 (or breakdown products, which include Cl_2 and O_2) from the chamber, usually by passage through a converter column. Aeration times are generally short, due to the rapid breakdown of the gas. Chlorine dioxide is a well-established broad-spectrum antimicrobial, with rapid sporicidal activity. It is a gas that rapidly breaks down on contact with surfaces; therefore, short sterilization cycles could be developed. A key consideration is the development of optimal ClO_2 generation technology to prevent the contamination of the load with chlorine gas (which is destructive to surfaces) and other gases, as well as minimizing the presence of breakdown or generated residuals (including chlorine and NaCl) on critical device surfaces. A further consideration is the fact that chlorine dioxide itself can be damaging to some materials over time, and it has the same restrictions on penetration as other gaseous oxidizing agents, particularly with porous loads. Chlorine dioxide is considered toxic at high concentrations, with a recommended exposure rate of 0.1 ppm over a typical 8-h workday and a short-term exposure safety risk as low as 0.3 ppm for 15 min; gas sensors are available to monitor the presence of the gas in work environments.

FURTHER READING

Association for the Advancement of Medical Instrumentation. 2005. *Sterilization. Part 1: Sterilization in Health Care Facilities.* Association for the Advancement of Medical Instrumentation, Arlington, Va.

Association for the Advancement of Medical Instrumentation. 2005. *Sterilization. Part 2: Sterilization Equipment.* Association for the Advancement of Medical Instrumentation, Arlington, Va.

Association for the Advancement of Medical Instrumentation. 2005. *Sterilization. Part 3: Industrial Process Control.* Association for the Advancement of Medical Instrumentation, Arlington, Va.

Block, S. S. 1991. *Disinfection, Sterilization, and Preservation*, 4th ed. Lea & Febiger, Philadelphia, Pa.

Block, S. S. 2001. *Disinfection, Sterilization, and Preservation*, 5th ed. Lippincott Williams & Wilkins, Philadelphia, Pa.

Booth, A. F. 1999. *Sterilization of Medical Devices.* PDA, Bethesda, Md.

Fraise, A. P., P. A. Lambert, and J.-Y. Maillard. 2004. *Russell, Hugo & Ayliffe's Principles and Practice of Disinfection, Preservation & Sterilization*, 4th ed. Blackwell Science Ltd., Malden, Mass.

Olson, W. P., and F. M. Nordhauser. 1998. *Sterilization of Drugs and Devices: Technologies for the 21st Century.* PDA, Bethesda, Md.

Russell, A. D., W. B. Hugo, and G. A. J. Ayliffe. 1992. *Principles and Practice of Disinfection, Preservation & Sterilization*, 2nd ed. Blackwell Science, Cambridge, Mass.

MECHANISMS OF ACTION

7

7.1 INTRODUCTION

Many compounds and processes have been identified as antimicrobial agents. For the purpose of this review, they are classified as anti-infectives or biocides (see section 1.2). Anti-infectives are substances (or drugs) capable of inhibiting or inactivating microorganisms (particularly pathogens) that are associated with various infections in animals, plants, and humans. The term is used to encompass drugs that act specifically on certain types of microorganisms, including antibacterials (antibiotics), antifungals, antivirals, and antiprotozoal agents. In contrast, biocides are chemical or physical agents that are used on inanimate surfaces or on the skin and mucous membranes. Biocides demonstrate a much wider range of antimicrobial activity than anti-infectives and are used in a wider range of applications. A comparison of the characteristics of anti-infectives and biocides is shown in Table 7.1.

Anti-infectives have been identified and developed for specific use in the control of microbial infections while having limited or no toxic effect on the host. Examples are the antifungal drugs known as azoles and polyenes, which specifically inhibit the biosynthesis or disrupt the structure of ergosterol. Ergosterol is a unique molecule found in many fungal cell membranes (see sections 1.3.3.2 and 8.10) and is distinct from other sterols found in human cell membranes. Specific activity against ergosterol, therefore, allows greater activity against the target fungal infection, with limited damage to the host human cells; however, ergosterol is not found in bacterial cell membranes, and therefore, azoles and polyenes have limited spectra of activity against certain fungi. Similarly, reverse transcriptase (a viral enzyme required for replication) is a unique anti-infective target for retroviruses, including human immunodeficiency virus, as the enzyme is not found in other eukaryotic or prokaryotic cells; equally, anti-infectives that target reverse transcriptases are effective only against those viruses that express those enzymes. Overall, anti-infectives have specific modes of action and limited spectra of activity. Biocides have multiple modes of action and a much broader range of antimicrobial activity; however, their toxic effects have limited their use to surfaces, including inanimate materials and, in a limited number of cases, on the skin or mucous membranes (see chapter 4).

This chapter only briefly considers, for comparison, the modes of activity of various anti-infectives, which are discussed as antibacterials (antibiotics), antivirals, antifungals, and antiprotozoal agents. The modes of action of biocides are discussed under four main classifications,

TABLE 7.1 Comparison of anti-infectives and biocides

Criterion	Description	
	Anti-infectives	Biocides
Spectrum of activity	Generally narrow, e.g., antibiotics effective against vegetative bacteria; can depend on the genus or species	Broad spectrum of activity, depending on the biocide and exposure conditions; can be effective against vegetative (actively metabolizing forms) and "dormant" (including viruses and spores) microbial forms
Effects on humans, animals, plants	Minimal toxicity	Generally toxic
Mechanism of action	Specific to single or, in some cases, a number of targets	Generally multiple targets, including proteins, carbohydrates, nucleic acids, and lipids
Stability	Notably stable to permit uptake and effect at the site of infection	Most unstable in the environment or on contact with organic/inorganic material
Target use	Usually internal to the host, e.g., within the bloodstream or plant structure	Directly on or at the contaminated surface or in liquids
Potentiation ability	Generally none or limited to the presence of the active agent at the correct concentration at the site of infection and susceptibility of the target microorganism	Can be substantially affected by a variety of factors, including concentration, pH, temperature, formulation, state of the biocide, and presence of interfering substances
Potential for development of resistance	High	Limited

based on their primary mechanisms of action: oxidizing agents, cross-linking or coagulating agents, and transfer-of-energy and other structure-disrupting agents. Considerable progress has been made in understanding the mechanisms of action of biocides against bacteria, including vegetative bacteria and endospores. In contrast, studies of their modes of action against fungi, viruses, protozoa, algae, and prions have been limited, and they may be postulated based on known antibacterial mechanisms. As the targets of biocides include one or all of the four major types of macromolecules (proteins, lipids, carbohydrates, and nucleic acids) that make up the range of microbial structures and functions, they are also briefly introduced.

7.2 ANTI-INFECTIVES

Before consideration of the broad-spectrum activities of biocides, some discussion is warranted of the modes of action of specific anti-infectives. Examples are the narrower spectra of activity reported for penicillin, tetracyclines, and some sulfonamides against bacteria, although in some cases, activity has also been demonstrated against some protozoa. In contrast, other antibiotics demonstrate even more restricted spectra of activity; they include the glycopeptides, which are generally effective only against gram-positive bacteria. Many applications using these anti-infectives are restricted by the balance that must be struck between obtaining the minimum concentration of the active agent at the site of infection required for efficacy and also avoiding any adverse effects on the host. Despite this, most antibiotics demonstrate some toxicity or adverse effects; for example, penicillin can cause diarrhea, allergic skin rashes, and, in rare cases, anaphylaxis in some individuals. The narrower spectra of activity of anti-infectives are related to their specific modes of action.

7.2.1 Antibacterials (Antibiotics)

Antibiotics have been indispensable in the treatment and control of bacterial infections

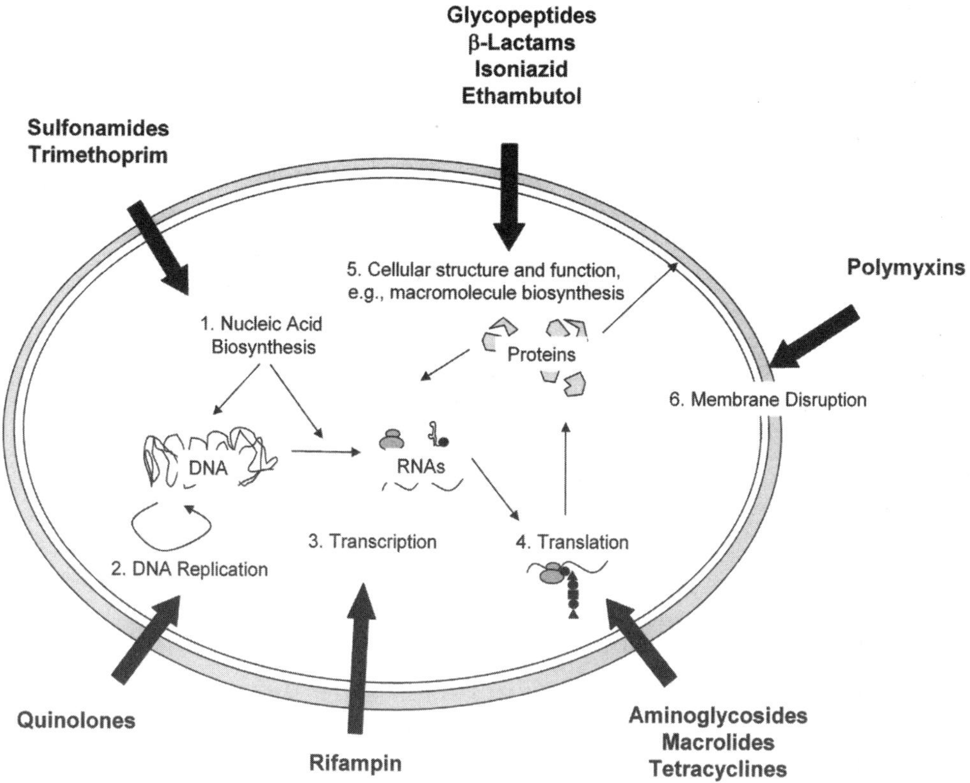

FIGURE 7.1 Primary bacterial targets of key antibiotics.

since their discovery and use in the 20th century. Summaries of some of the major antibiotics and their modes of action are given in Fig. 7.1 and Table 7.2. Many antibiotics specifically interact with certain cellular targets that are involved in key bacterial processes, including DNA replication, transcription, translation, and formation of cell components (Fig. 7.1). They act by specifically binding to ribosomes (which are required for protein biosynthesis), proteins (particularly key enzymes), protein-DNA complexes, and cell wall components (Table 7.2). In addition, some antibiotics specifically interact with the gram-negative cell membrane (e.g., the polymyxins), not unlike the modes of action of some biocides, including surfactants, which disrupt structure and function (see sections 3.16 and 7.4.5).

Given the specific mechanisms of action of antibiotics, it is not surprising, considering their widespread use and often misapplication, that bacterial resistance has developed. Resistance can be a natural attribute of bacteria due to the lack or inaccessibility of a specific target or to other natural resistance mechanisms that they express. Bacteria, originally sensitive to antibiotics, have also demonstrated great resilience in developing acquired resistance through mutations or the acquisition of genetic material (plasmids and transposons; see section 8.7.3). Acquired resistance mechanisms include reduced uptake, drug inactivation, and specific loss or alteration of key cellular targets. Bacterial resistance to antibiotics is a major concern and highlights the importance of the safe and prudent use of antibiotics.

7.2.2 Antifungals

Similar to antibiotics, antifungals specifically target key biosynthetic or structural targets in various fungi (Table 7.3). The structure of ergosterol and its biosynthetic process are

TABLE 7.2 Widely used antibiotics (antibacterials) and their mechanisms of action

Class	Example	Spectrum of activity	Mechanism of action
Aminoglycosides	Streptomycin	Gram-positive and gram-negative bacteria, including *Mycobacterium* spp.	Inhibition of protein synthesis; bind to rRNA to inhibit initiation, cause misreading of mRNA, and prevent translocation
β-Lactams	Penicillin	More effective against gram-positive and gram-negative bacteria, but also some activity against actinomycetes and protozoa (*Treponema* spp.)	Inhibition of cell wall synthesis; bind to enzymes involved in peptidoglycan cross-linking
Chloramphenicol		Inhibitory against gram-positive and gram-negative bacteria including mycoplasmas	Inhibition of protein synthesis; bind to rRNA
Glycopeptides	Vancomycin	Gram-positive bacteria, but not mycobacteria	Inhibition of cell wall biosynthesis; bind to peptidoglycan precursors to prevent cell wall formation
Isoniazid		Mycobacteria	Inhibits mycolic acid biosynthesis in mycobacteria
Macrolides	Erythromycin	Broad spectrum against gram-positive and gram-negative bacteria (generally inhibitory), including *Mycobacterium* spp.	Inhibition of protein synthesis; bind to rRNA
Polymyxins	Polymyxin B	Gram-negative bacteria, including *Pseudomonas* spp.	Cell membrane insertion and disorganization
Quinolones	Ciprofloxacin	Gram-positive and gram-negative bacteria, including *Mycobacterium* and *Mycoplasma* spp.	Inhibit DNA replication by inhibiting DNA gyrase
Sulfonamides	Sulfapyridine	Broad spectrum, including gram-positive and gram-negative bacteria, actinomycetes, and some protozoans (e.g., *Plasmodium* and *Toxoplasma* spp.)	Inhibit nucleotide biosynthesis by binding to bacterium-specific enzymes
Tetracyclines	Tetracycline	Gram-positive and gram-negative bacteria, including *Mycobacterium* spp. and some protozoans (e.g., *Plasmodium* spp.)	Inhibition of protein synthesis; bind to rRNA

important targets for many anti-infectives, which cause disruption of the structure and function of the fungal cell membrane. Most of the important fungal pathogens, including molds (*Aspergillus* spp. and dermatophytes) and yeasts (*Candida* and *Cryptococcus* spp.), contain ergosterol and are generally sensitive to these anti-infectives, although this can naturally vary depending on the species and the specific drug (primarily due to variable accumulation). As with bacteria, fungal resistance can easily develop due to various adaptations, including changes in sterol structure and levels in the cell membrane and in specific enzymes involved in biosynthetic pathways. Other specific antifungal targets are inhibition of 1-3-β-D-glucan and, therefore, cell wall biosynthesis (Table 7.3).

7.2.3 Antivirals

Anti-infectives that target viruses have been identified or specifically developed to inhibit

TABLE 7.3 Widely used antifungal drugs and mechanisms of action

Class	Example	Spectrum of activity	Mechanism of action
Polyenes	Amphotericin B	Broad antifungal, including *Candida, Cryptococcus*, and *Aspergillus* spp.	Disruption of cell membrane synthesis; bind to ergosterol.
Azoles	Ketoconazole	Broad antifungal, including *Candida, Cryptococcus*, and *Aspergillus* spp.	Inhibit ergosterol biosynthesis, required for cell membrane structure
Allylamines	Terbinafine	Dermatophytes, but also other fungi, including *Candida* spp.	Inhibit ergosterol biosynthesis, required for cell membrane structure
Antimetabolites	Flucytosine	Broad antifungal, including *Candida, Cryptococcus*, and *Aspergillus* spp.	Integrate into fungal RNA and inhibit DNA synthesis
Glucan synthesis inhibitors	Caspofungin	Broad antifungal, including *Candida, Cryptococcus*, and *Aspergillus* spp.	Inhibit cell wall synthesis; block synthesis of 1-3-β-D-glucan

key stages in viral infection and replication within cells (Table 7.4). Some antivirals can specifically block viral penetration into target cells, while others inhibit various stages of intracellular virus multiplication. An important class of antiviral drugs, the interferons, primarily act to induce the host immune system to target the viral infection; however, some specific inhibitory effects on virus multiplication, including penetration, virion release, and nucleic acid translation, have been reported.

7.2.4 Antiparasitic Drugs

Various antiparasitic drugs have been widely used for protozoal or helminth infections or as preventative drugs. They have also been shown to be somewhat tolerated by the host and to have specific mechanisms of action (Table 7.5). Some are also well-known antibiotics, including tetracyclines and sulfonamides (see section 7.2.1).

7.3 MACROMOLECULAR STRUCTURE

The basic structures of microorganisms are described in chapter 1. Although they present a variety of different sizes, structures, and arrangements, they are essentially composed of four basic macromolecules, which give them

TABLE 7.4 Widely used antiviral drugs and mechanisms of action

Class	Example	Spectrum of activity	Mechanism of action
Nucleoside analogues	Acyclovir	Herpes simplex viruses	Inhibit genome replication; viral-DNA polymerase inhibition
Virus penetration inhibitors	Amantadine	Influenza viruses	Block a cellular membrane channel, which prevents membrane-virus fusion
Mutagens	Ribavirin	Broad spectrum against RNA viruses, including hepatitis C virus, herpes simplex virus, measles virus, mumps virus	RNA mutagen
Assembly, maturation, release inhibitors	Oseltamivir (Tamiflu)	Influenza virus	Prevention of virus budding from the cell; neuraminidase inhibitors
Cell defense promoters	Alpha, beta, and gamma interferons	Hepatitis B and C viruses	Activation of host cell defense mechanisms

TABLE 7.5 Widely used antiparasitic drugs and mechanisms of action

Class	Example	Spectrum of activity	Mechanism of action
Macrolide endectins	Ivermectin	Arthropods and nematodes	Inhibit a neurotransmitter in the parasite
Benzimidazoles	Mebendazole	Nematodes, cestodes, helminths, and protozoa	Inhibit cytoplasmic functions; bind to microtubules (tubulin)
Pyrazinoisoquinolines	Praziquantel	Nematodes and trematodes	Affects cell membrane permeability and causes tegument disintegration
Tetracyclines	Doxycycline	Protozoa and bacteria	Block protein synthesis
Sulfonamides	Sulfadimethoxine	Protozoa, including *Isospora* spp., and bacteria	Inhibit nucleotide biosynthesis and folic acid synthesis
Quinine-related	Chloroquine	*Plasmodium* spp.	Multiple effects related to malarial parasite infection of red blood cells

structure and function: nucleic acids, proteins, carbohydrates, and lipids. These macromolecules combine to form complex and balanced structures, including cell walls, envelopes, capsids, cell membranes, nucleic acids, and cytoplasmic constituents, which are required for the growth and/or proliferation of the microorganism. Brief descriptions of each of these are given as background for a discussion of the modes of action of biocidal processes.

Macromolecules are all composed of the same major elements: carbon, hydrogen, oxygen, nitrogen, phosphorus, and sulfur. These elements are linked to form the basic building blocks of macromolecules, which are amino acids (proteins); sugars (polysaccharides); fatty acids or, in some cases, phytanes (lipids); and nucleotides (nucleic acids). The linkages between these building blocks can be considered covalent or noncovalent bonds. Covalent bonds are strong bonds between elements and include peptide bonds (in proteins) and glycosidic (in polysaccharides) and phosphodiester (in nucleic acids) bonds. Noncovalent bonds are considered weaker associations but have an essential role in dictating the structures and functions of macromolecules; they include hydrogen bonding, van der Waals forces, and hydrophobic interactions.

Proteins (or polypeptides) are composed of repeating units (or polymers) of amino acids. There are 21 types of amino acid commonly found in microorganisms. The basic amino acid structure is shown in Fig. 7.2. Amino acids are covalently linked by peptide (or amide) bonds to give the primary (or amino acid) structure of the protein.

It is the sequence and types of amino acids present that dictate the structure and function of the protein. This is achieved by folding of the primary sequence to give the protein secondary and tertiary structures. The amino acids interact by hydrogen bonding with adjacent and distant residues in the primary structure to give the secondary structure of the protein, consisting of local formations known as α-helixes and β-sheets. This arrangement allows further interactions between amino acids (by covalent bonding, hydrogen bonding, etc.) to give the protein tertiary structure. In many cases, the tertiary form is the final structural and functional form of the protein; however, in some cases, a quaternary structure is also formed by similar covalent and/or noncovalent interactions between different proteins (or polypeptides) to give a larger functional assembly. Tertiary and quaternary forms can change their conformations as part of their biological functions or relative to various environmental conditions. The functions of proteins can be considered structural and/or enzymatic, and they play essential roles in the growth and survival of microorganisms.

Polysaccharides are also polymers consisting of multiple subunits of monosaccharides (or simple sugars). Sugars have a simple structure consisting of carbon, hydrogen, and oxygen (Fig. 7.3).

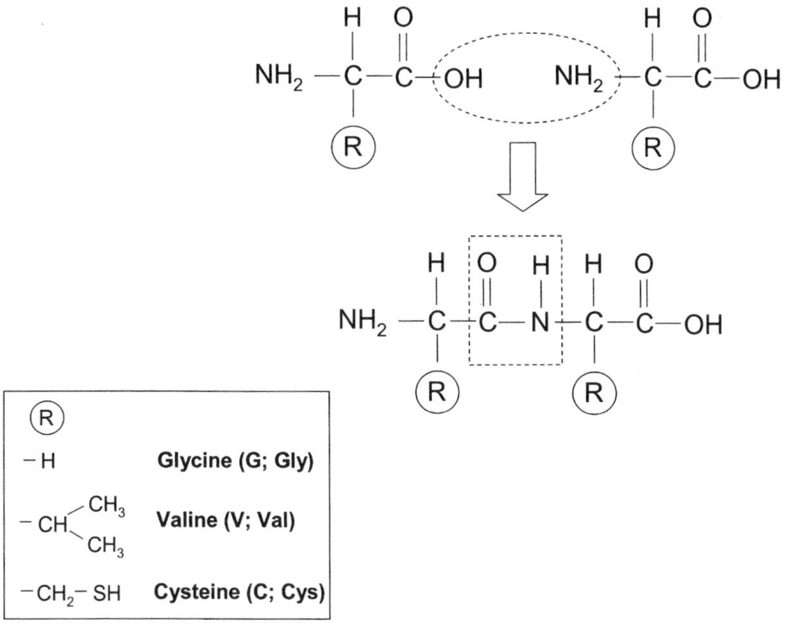

R	
$-H$	**Glycine (G; Gly)**
$-CH(CH_3)_2$	**Valine (V; Val)**
$-CH_2-SH$	**Cysteine (C; Cys)**

FIGURE 7.2 The structures of amino acids and peptide bonding. Representations are shown of two amino acids condensing to form a dipeptide linked by a peptide bond. Examples of the various side groups (R) that define the different amino acids are also shown.

Sugars can be classified according to the number of carbon units, for example, pentoses (five carbon units, like ribose and deoxyribose, which are the building blocks of nucleic acid backbone structures) and hexoses (six carbon units, including glucose). Polysaccharides, such as starch, glycogen, cellulose, and peptidoglycan, are formed by monomeric sugars linked by various types of glycosidic bonds. For example, starch, glycogen, and cellulose are all polymers of glucose but are linked by different glycosidic bonds (Fig. 7.3). Peptidoglycan is a more complex polysaccharide consisting of two repeating sugars, *N*-acetylglucosamine and *N*-acetylmuramic acid, linked by β-1,4 glycosidic bonds to form the glycan chains, which are cross-linked by peptides; peptidoglycan is a major component of bacterial cell walls (see section 1.3.4.1). Polysaccharides play important roles in the structure and energy storage of microorganisms.

Lipids are a structurally diverse group of organic compounds that are typically insoluble in water. They include various types of fats, oils, and waxes. Major components of many microbial lipids are fatty acids, which are long hydrocarbon chains with a hydrophobic and a hydrophilic region (Fig. 7.4).

Fatty acids can be classified based on the number of carbons and the presence or absence of double bonds within the hydrocarbon chain, with those containing double bonds referred to as unsaturated and those without them referred to as saturated (e.g., palmitoleic acid is a $C_{16:1}$ monounsaturated fatty acid, and stearic acid is a C_{18} saturated fatty acid). Simple lipids commonly found in microorganisms include the triglycerides (fats), which are composed of three fatty acids linked by ester bonds to glycerol (a type of alcohol). Lipids that are more complex include phospholipids (which contain a phosphate group) and glycolipids (which are linked to various sugars). Examples of lipid structures are shown in Fig. 7.5. The phospholipids and sterols are important parts of the structures and functions of membranes (e.g., see section 1.3.4.1). Overall, lipids play key roles in microbial structure and as energy reserves.

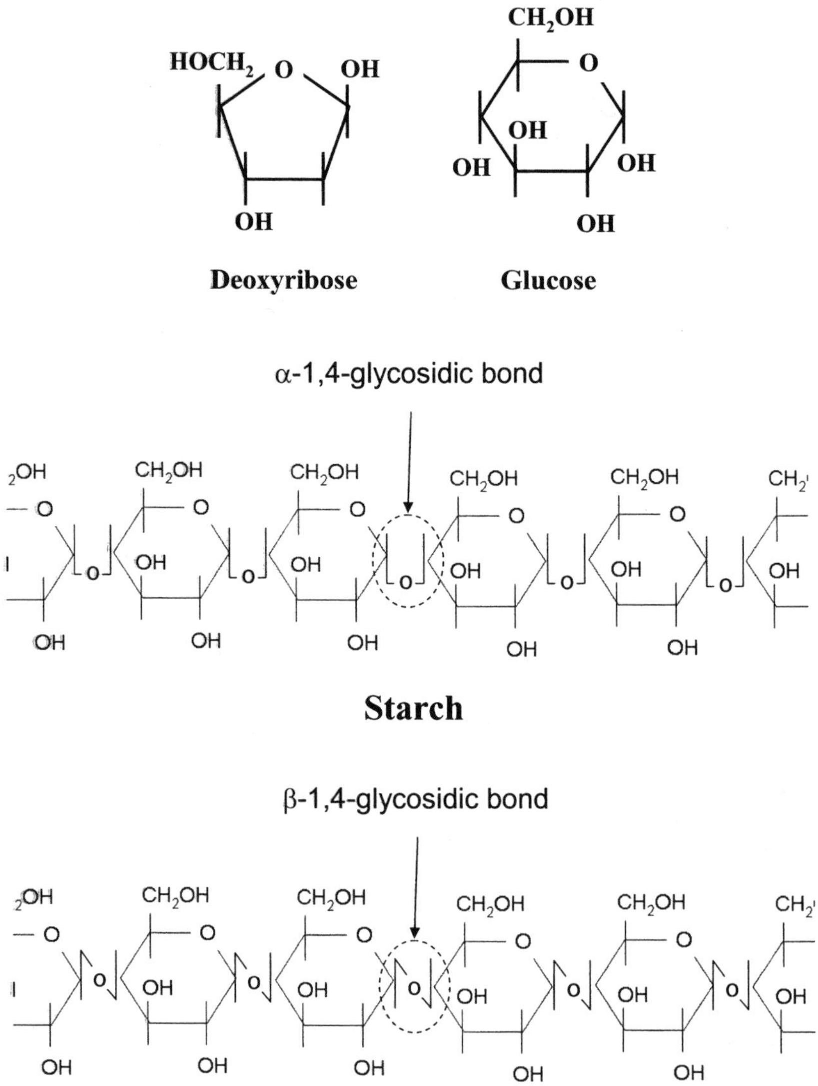

Deoxyribose Glucose

α-1,4-glycosidic bond

Starch

β-1,4-glycosidic bond

Cellulose

FIGURE 7.3 Examples of sugars, polysaccharides, and glycosidic bonds. The polysaccharides shown are both polymers of glucose but vary in the structures of the glycosidic bond linkages.

Nucleic acids are polymers of nucleotides (and therefore are also known as "polynucleotides"), which are molecules consisting of three components: a sugar, a nitrogen-containing base, and a phosphate group (Fig. 7.6). The five carbon sugars can be either ribose or deoxyribose, with attached bases (purines, adenine and guanine, or pyrimidines, thymine, cytosine, and uracil) and phosphate groups.

Polynucleotides are formed by nucleotides covalently linked via their phosphate groups to form sugar-phosphate ("phosphodiester") bonds. Polynucleotides include DNA and RNA, which are the genetic materials found in

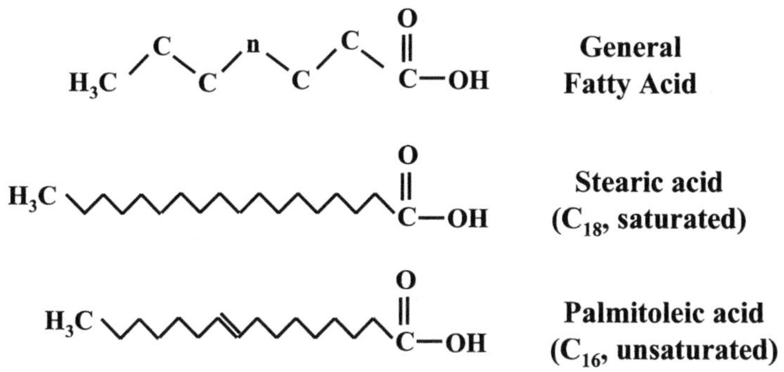

General Fatty Acid

Stearic acid (C_{18}, saturated)

Palmitoleic acid (C_{16}, unsaturated)

FIGURE 7.4 The basic structures of fatty acids. The numbers of carbons in the fatty acid structure can vary, and examples of stearic acid (C_{18}) and palmitoleic acid ($C_{16:1}$) are shown.

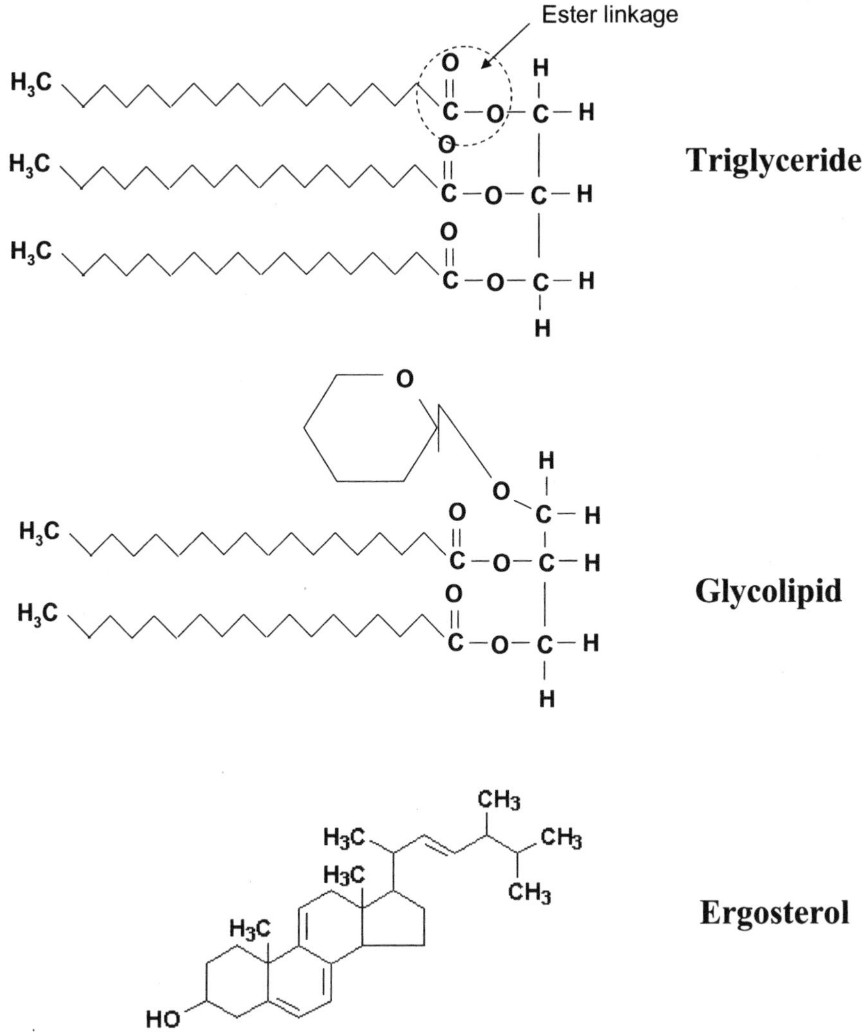

Ester linkage

Triglyceride

Glycolipid

Ergosterol

FIGURE 7.5 Examples of various types of lipids. The general structures of a triglyceride, a glycolipid (with one sugar linked to two fatty acids), and a sterol (ergosterol) are shown.

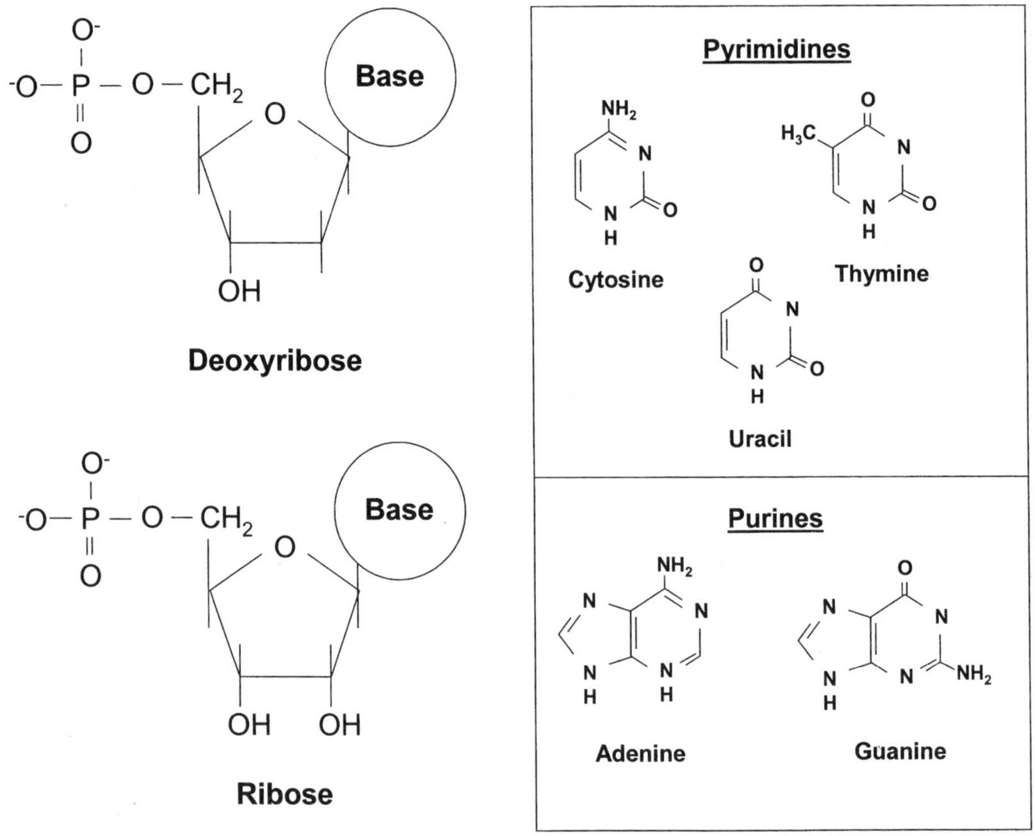

FIGURE 7.6 The basic structures of nucleotides. The structure consists of a sugar (ribose or deoxyribose) linked to a phosphate (only a monophosphate group is illustrated) and various bases (pyrimidines and purines).

microorganisms. DNA is a double-stranded polynucleotide in a double-helix structure and is the inherited material in most organisms (Fig. 7.7). In addition to the covalently linked nucleotides within each DNA strand, the individual bases of the strands are also linked by noncovalent hydrogen bonding between complementary purine and pyrimidine bases (A:T and G:C), which keeps the strands in the double-helix structure. DNA contains only deoxyribose sugars and adenine, guanine, thymine, and cytosine bases; RNA contains ribose sugars and uracil bases instead of thymine. RNA is generally single stranded (e.g., mRNA), although it can assume various secondary structures by folding and base-pairing between complementary sequences (as in the cases of tRNA and rRNA, which are involved in protein translation) (Fig. 7.7). It should be noted that the inherited (genetic) material found in viruses can include double- or single-stranded DNA or RNA (see section 1.3.5). Monomeric nucleotides are also found, and they play important roles in cellular metabolism (e.g., ATP is a source of energy) (Fig. 7.7).

7.4 GENERAL MECHANISMS OF ACTION

7.4.1 Introduction

Unlike the anti-infectives discussed in section 7.2, the antimicrobial effects of most biocides and biocidal processes are generally broad spectrum, with multiple effects on target microorganisms and their associated macromolecules. The following discussion considers the known

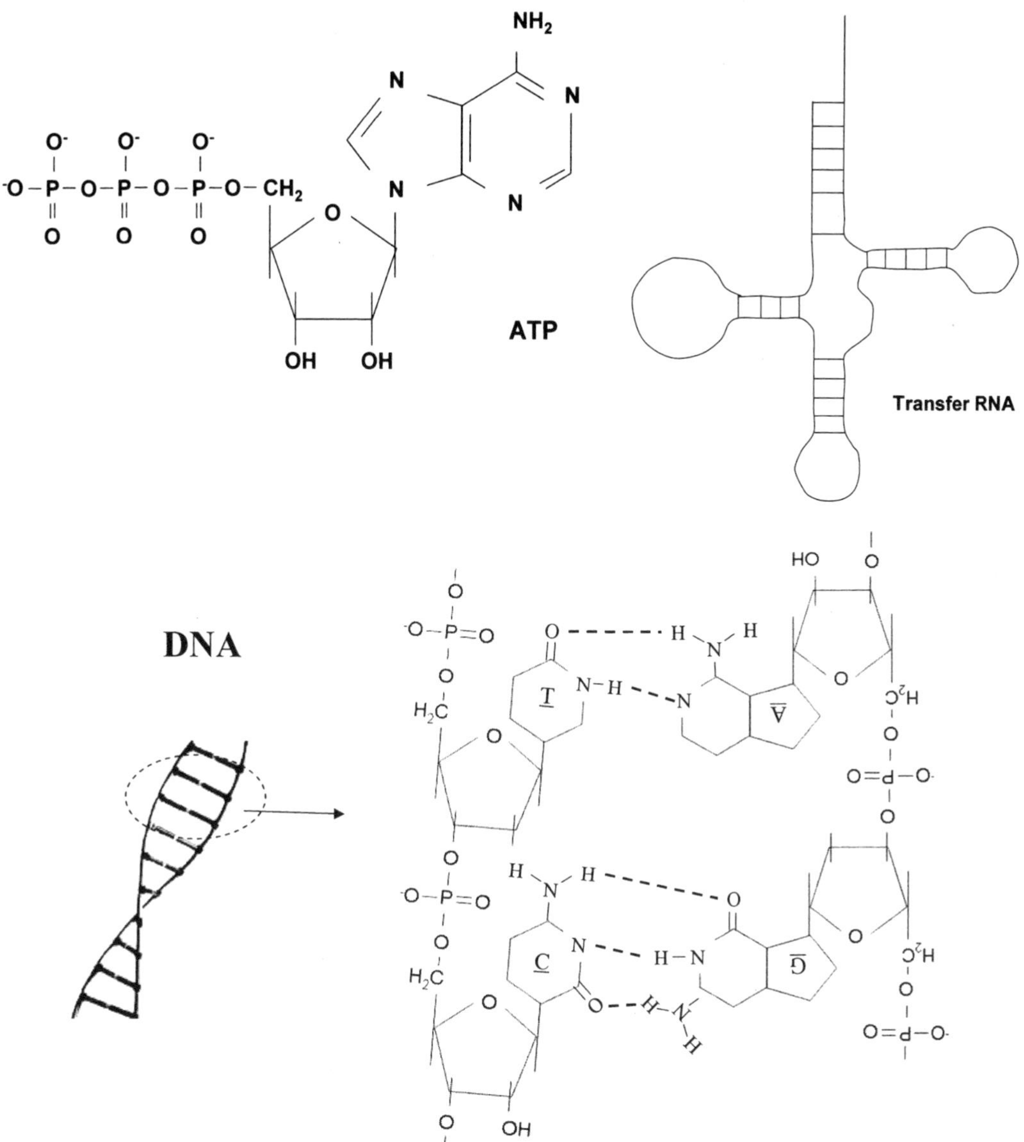

FIGURE 7.7 Nucleotide structures. ATP (top left) is a mononucleotide, while DNA (bottom) and RNA (top right; simple structure shown) are polynucleotides. DNA is a double-stranded polynucleotide (with hydrogen bonding holding the two parallel strands together), while the representation of a tRNA polynucleotide shows single- and double-stranded sections (with hydrogen-bonded bases shown as lines between the strands).

major targets or effects of certain groups of biocides, but in many cases secondary, and in some cases multiple, chemical effects have been observed. The effects of ionizing radiation on a target cell can be taken as an example. It is clear that the major targets of action of radiation are the nucleic acids; however, the reactions of radiation with water, with other cellular molecules, and even with the associated surface on which the microorganism is found also lead to the localized production of free radicals. These radicals include hydroxyl radicals, which are powerful oxidizing agents that have multiple destructive effects on nucleic acids, proteins, lipids, and other molecules. Further, in some cases, specific key targets for some biocides have been identified, and they are known targets for some antibacterial antibiotics (e.g., triclosan, which is discussed in more detail below).

Overall, biocides are microbial poisons, and what is known about their effects on microorganisms is discussed for each active agent in chapters 2 and 3. They are covered in more detail in this section. It is convenient to consider the major modes of action of biocides in four groups: oxidizing agents, transfer-of-energy agents, cross-linking agents, and agents that specifically bind to and disrupt the structures of macromolecules.

7.4.2 Oxidizing Agents

Oxidizing agents remove electrons (oxidation) from a substance, thereby gaining electrons themselves (Table 7.6). Biocides that possess oxidizing-agent ability are widely used and include the halogens (chlorine, bromine, and iodine) and peroxygens (peracetic acid and hydrogen peroxide).

Although the exact modes of action of these biocides are unknown, direct studies of microorganisms have shown some common effects. Further investigations into their specific effects on macromolecules, particularly at lower concentrations of the oxidizing agents, have been done. These studies have focused on the effects of oxidizing agents that have been associated with cell aging and some diseases (particularly those associated with aging) and the associated defense (including repair) mechanisms that can protect the cell from damage. Oxidizing agents are naturally formed in prokaryotic and eukaryotic cells that use oxygen during respiration and/or metabolism. They include hydrogen peroxide and short-lived radicals (like the hydroxyl radical, ·OH, and the superoxide anion radical, O_2^-). The significance of the presence of these reactive species as antimicrobial agents was discussed earlier (see section 3.13). Their specific effects have been found to have four major targets: nucleic acids, lipids, proteins, and carbohydrates.

TABLE 7.6 Biocides with an oxidizing-agent-based mode of action

Halogens and halogen-releasing agents
Iodine
Iodophors, e.g., povidone-iodine
Chlorine
Hypochlorites
Chloramines, e.g., sodium dichlorisocyanurate
Bromine
Bromine-releasing agents, e.g., bronopol
Peroxygens and other forms of oxygen
Hydrogen peroxide
Peracetic acid
Chlorine dioxide
Ozone

Oxidizing agents have dramatic effects on DNA and RNA structures. They readily attack both the nucleotide bases and the sugar-phosphate backbone (Fig. 7.8). These effects cause strand breakage and can also cause reactions between converted bases or sugars and other molecules associated with the nucleic acid, including the formation of adducts. These effects disrupt the functions of polynucleotides, including DNA, RNA, and other, similar nucleotide monomeric structures (such as ATP, which is a source of chemical energy required for cellular activities). Specific effects on polynucleotides not only can lead to mutations, but also disrupt cellular processes, like replication, transcription, and translation, that are required for multiplication and microbial survival.

Specific effects on lipids, particularly the fatty acids associated with the cell membrane, have also been studied. Reactions with oxidizing agents cause changes in structure and degradation into shorter-chain fatty acids. Unsaturated fatty acids, which contain double bonds within long carbon chain structures, are particularly sensitive due to specific reactions at these double bonds. Some of these reactions can lead to the production of other toxic substances, for example, aldehydes, like 4-hydroxyalkenals and malonaldehydes. The reactions cause lipid peroxidation, which can lead to changes in fatty acid structure and degradation into other reac-

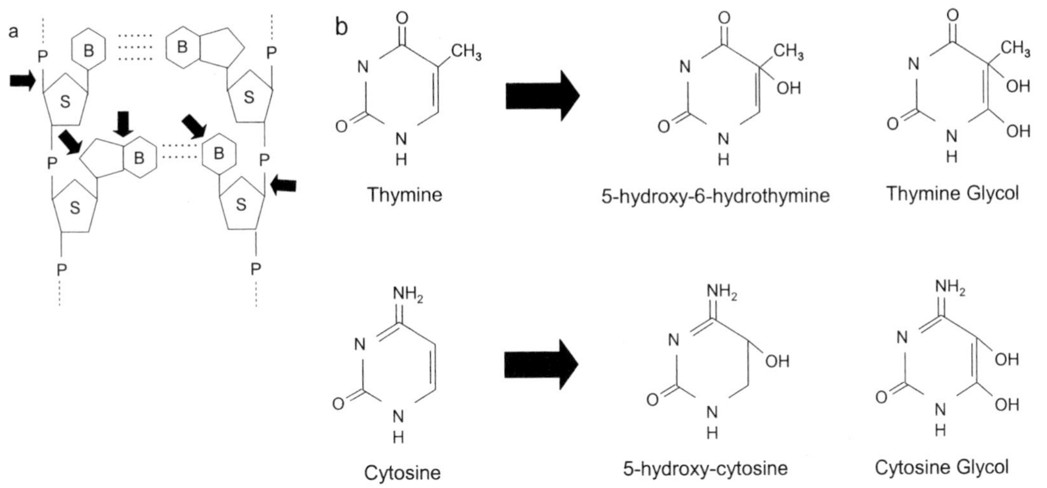

FIGURE 7.8 The major target sites for oxidizing agents on the structure of DNA (a) and, specifically, on the nucleotide bases (b), with examples of the pyrimidine bases thymine and cytosine.

tive agents, which, as radicals themselves, can react with other cellular components, particularly other fatty acids and proteins within cell membranes. The overall effects on the cell membrane are dramatic, especially those leading to a loss in fluidity that disrupts the overall structure and function (including permeability) of the membrane. These include the disruption of embedded proteins, as the membrane increases in hydrophilicity, and ultimately lead to leakage of cytoplasmic constituents as the membrane loses its structure. Given the importance of the cell membrane for a variety of cellular functions, it is clear that these effects have a dramatic impact on the viability of bacteria, fungi, and some enveloped viruses.

Other investigations have focused on the specific reactions of oxidizing agents on amino acids and proteins. For example, the accumulation of protein damage due to oxidizing agents has been observed in certain diseases, including neurodegenerative diseases. As in the discussion of the effects on polynucleotides, oxidizing agents can specifically affect the primary and higher-order (e.g., secondary and tertiary) structures of proteins. Oxidizing agents have multiple effects on proteins, including changes in amino acid structure, peptide bond breakage (leading to protein fragmentation), interruption of metal binding sites (which are required for some catalytic protein functions), and specific reactions with other amino acid bonds (for example, disulfide bonds between cysteine amino acids). These effects cause the loss of enzymatic activities and of protein structure, which are required for their normal functions. As for the primary sequences of proteins, oxidizing agents can specifically modify the side chains of amino acids, which can lead to changes in the amino acid sequence. Notable effects include the formation of carbonyl groups and an increase in acidity. As the primary sequence dictates the folding and overall protein structure, these reactions lead to disruption of the protein structure and therefore loss of function. Some of the specific reactions that have been described are shown in Table 7.7. They can include specific changes in the amino acid structure, as well as the production of reactive side chains that can readily react with other structures to cause cross-linkages.

Notable is the effect of oxidizing agents on the amino acid cysteine. As well as being a normal amino acid in the structures of many proteins, cysteine residues can play an important role in the folding of certain proteins, particularly those that are excreted from the cytoplasm and are associated with the cell wall or cell

TABLE 7.7 Examples of products observed on reaction of oxidizing agents with amino acids

Target amino acid	Product(s) observed
Arginine	Glutamic semialdehyde
Cysteine	Cysteic acid, disulfides
Histidine	Asparagine, aspartic acid
Lysine	2-Aminoadipic semialdehyde
Tyrosine	3,4-Dihydroxyphenylalanine; cross-linkages or adducts between tyrosine residues

membrane. Two cysteine residues within the primary structure of a protein can interact to form disulfide bonds, due to reactions between the sulfurous side chains. These bonds not only play important roles in the overall structures of some proteins, they also play important regulatory roles in the proteins' activities. For example, *Escherichia coli* cells can react to oxidative stress within their environment (as in the case of the presence of oxidizing agents) by a specific response mediated by a transcriptional activator protein (OxyR), which causes the cell to express specific protective and repair mechanisms that can aid the cell in survival. OxyR is specifically activated by the formation of a disulfide bond between two cysteine residues due to the presence of oxidizing agents. This so-called "oxidative response" is discussed in more detail in section 8.3.3 as a specific adaptive response mechanism to increase bacterial resistance to oxidizing-agent damage. While the formation of disulfide bonds is a benefit in this case, the opposite is true in the case of proteins, particularly intracellular proteins, which do not normally contain disulfide linkages between cysteine residues. The effect of the oxidizing agent, which causes the formation of disulfide bonds, leads to the loss of structure and function by many enzymes and proteins, thus also contributing to the overall mode of action.

Some oxidizing agents have also been shown to cause peptide bond breakage. Peptide bonds are covalent bonds that connect amino acids to form peptides and proteins (see section 7.3). These effects are postulated to be due to specific reactions with hydrogen atoms in the amino acids, which become reactive and cause bond disruption. These structures are known cellular targets for proteolysis, including attachment by intracellular proteases, which causes further degradation by the cells' natural enzymatic activities. Further effects can be postulated due to the reaction of these amino acids with other biomolecules, including associated amino acids, which can cause adducts to or within the protein structure. In contrast to the sensitivity of proteins that have been damaged by disruption of peptide bonds by proteases, some of these protein-protein interactions have been proposed to be less sensitive to proteases and to lead to toxic accumulation within the target cell. The subtle difference in these effects may be an important factor in the optimization of oxidizing agent activity on prions, which are proposed infectious proteins. In one case, the optimization of the peptide bond breakage may enhance activity against prions, but in contrast, the increased cross-linking may improve the overall resistance of the entity. These effects may be responsible for the differences observed between oxidizing agents, in combination with other liquid formulation properties or in various states (e.g., liquid or gas), in their activities against prions.

As many proteins have bound metals that are required for their enzymatic activities, for their structures, or for the safe transport of toxic metals (for example, iron) within the cell, the specific disruption of their structures by oxidizing agents causes the release of these metals into or around the microorganism, which can also add to the observed toxic effects. The toxicity of heavy metals is discussed further in section 7.4.5.

Some studies have suggested that certain bacterial and yeast proteins are clearly major targets for the effects of oxidizing agents. For example, studies of *E. coli* have shown specific inactivation of many key bacterial proteins and enzymes associated with essential bacterial metabolic functions. These include glucose metabolism (enolase), protein biosynthesis and folding (e.g., EF-G, an elongation factor involved in protein translation from mRNA, and DnaK, a protein chaperone that is involved in the folding of newly synthesized proteins into their correct secondary structures), and outer membrane structure (e.g., OmpA, a major structural protein in the *E. coli* cell wall). These proteins may not be particularly sensitive to the effects of oxidizing agents, but damage to them clearly has major consequences for cell survival. It is clear that further investigations into the effects of oxidizing agents on cellular targets may identify other key targets in microorganisms that are central to cell survival or pathogenesis.

The exact reactions of oxidizing agents on carbohydrates have been less studied, but overall, reactions similar to those of proteins are expected. Hydrogen atoms are specifically targeted on carbohydrate molecules, leading to reactive species, which are proposed to cause chain breakage (such as glycosidic-bond disruption), polysaccharide breakage, and reactions with other cellular targets. These effects likely contribute to the overall loss of structure and function of key carbohydrate and carbohydrate-linked (e.g., glycoprotein) molecules, as well as disruption of other functions by cross-reactions.

Overall, oxidizing agents have multiple effects on proteins, lipids, carbohydrates, and nucleic acid, which lead to the loss of their structures and functions. Specific effects include changes in structure, breakdown of these macromolecules into smaller constituents, and transformation of structural and functional groups, as well as some effects leading to cross-linking within and between the molecules. These effects culminate in the loss of viability of the microbial target. The effects on vegetative and actively metabolizing microorganisms, including bacteria and fungi, are clearly significant. The overall damage to the structures of spores, cysts, and viruses also appears to cause a loss of viability, presumably due to specific effects on surface proteins and lipids, but also on penetration into the nucleic acid.

7.4.3 Cross-Linking, or Coagulating, Agents

Cross-linking, or coagulating, agents cause specific interactions between macromolecules, particularly proteins and nucleic acids, that lead to loss of structure and function (Table 7.8). Many biocides and biocidal processes can cause the clumping or coagulation of macromolecules at higher concentrations due to their modes of action. Notably, they include some oxidizing agents, which in addition to the oxidation mode of action discussed in section 7.4.2, can also cause the production of aldehydes, leading to cross-linking under certain conditions. These coagulating reactions are also seen with other types of biocides, like quaternary ammonium compounds (QACs), heat, and alcohols. However, some biocides demonstrate specific interactions with macromolecules that suggest a primary mode of action as cross-linking, or coagulation, agents. Of particular note are the aldehydes and alkylating agents, although some discussion of the phenolics and alcohols, which are considered general coagulating biocides, is also appropriate.

TABLE 7.8 Biocides with cross-linking- or coagulation-based modes of action

Aldehydes (cross-linking agents)
Formaldehyde
Glutaraldehyde
Orthophthaldehyde
Alkylating agents (epoxides)
Ethylene oxide
Propylene oxide
Phenolics
Phenols
Cresols
Bisphenols
Alcohols
Ethanol
Isopropanol

Alkylating agents are highly reactive chemical compounds that can react with amino, carboxyl, sulfhydryl, and hydroxyl groups, particularly in protein amino acids or within nucleic acids. "Alkylating" refers to the ability to introduce alkyl (methyl or ethyl) groups into macromolecules. Many alkylating agents are specifically used as anticancer agents (e.g., mitomycin C and cyclophosphamide), as they are toxic to eukaryotic cells. The major mechanism of action of many of these drugs is the DNA molecule, particularly the cross-linking of guanine bases that inhibits the unraveling and separation of DNA, which is required for its replication and transcription. Ethylene oxide is the most widely used alkylating agent for disinfection and sterilization. Ethylene oxide, like other alkylating agents, specifically targets proteins and nucleic acids. Three principal effects of alkylating agents on nucleic acids have been described:

1. They specifically react to guanine (and to a lesser extent adenine) nucleotide bases, which causes the addition of alkyl (or, in the case of ethylene oxide, ethyl) groups (Fig. 7.9). These structural changes can promote cellular repair mechanisms, which can cause DNA strand breakage and can culminate in cell death. Further, the presence of alkyl groups also inhibits the replication and transcription of DNA, as well as causing functional changes to cellular RNA molecules.

2. The presence of alkylated guanine bases can cause mispairing of nucleotide bases in DNA and RNA structures due to pairing with thymine and uracil residues in place of the normal cytosine pairing. Mispairing causes changes in RNA folded structures and may also cause point mutations in DNA over time.

3. The presence of the alkyl groups promotes the formation of cross-linkages between other adjacent nucleotide bases via the terminal hydroxyl group. These cross-linkages can occur within the same or parallel DNA strands or with other associated macromolecules (particularly proteins). The formation of cross-linkages also inhibits DNA and RNA functions, specifically, DNA unwinding and RNA translation.

Overall, these effects on nucleic acids cause mutations, arrest of essential cellular functions (replication, transcription, and translation), and loss of cell viability and viral infectivity.

Similar introductions of alkyl groups are observed in reactions with amino, carboxyl, sulfhydryl, and hydroxyl groups of amino acids (Fig. 7.10).

The alkylation of amino acids disrupts the structures and functions of proteins, including essential enzymes. In addition, similar to the reactions described with nucleic acids, epoxide bridge cross-links can form due to further reactions with adjacent amino acid side chains, which also disrupt protein structures and cause precipitation. Certain exposed amino acids appear to be targeted, including cysteine, histidine, and valine. These are probably key effects in the initial attacks on the surfaces of microorganisms, including dramatic effects on the structures of peptidoglycan and other surface glycans due to cross-linking of peptides that link the polysaccharide chains. Reactions of alkylating agents with other macromolecules

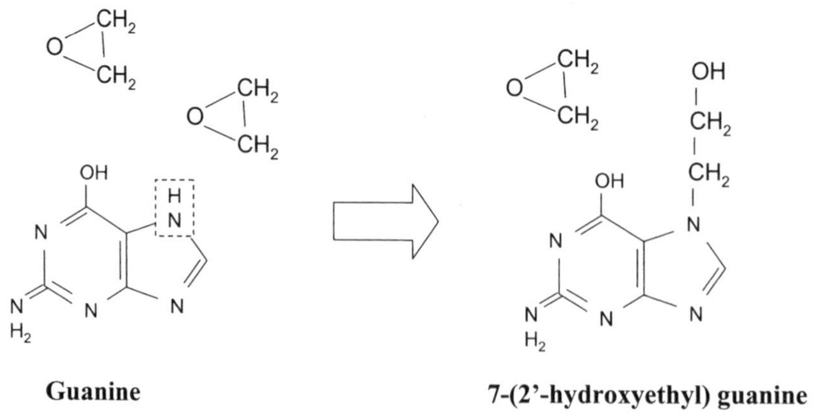

Guanine **7-(2'-hydroxyethyl) guanine**

FIGURE 7.9 Reaction of ethylene oxide with guanine.

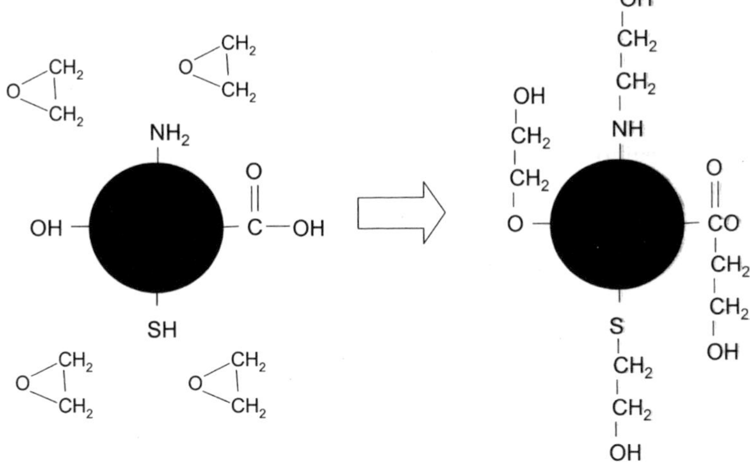

FIGURE 7.10 Reaction of ethylene oxide with amino acid side chains.

most likely occur, but they have not been specifically studied.

Aldehydes are typical cross-linking agents and are widely used for a variety of biochemical and industrial purposes due to their mode of action of fixing materials, including attachment of materials to surfaces (see section 3.4). An example is the use of glutaraldehyde as a fixative to stabilize the structures of cells for electron microscopy analysis. Aldehydes widely used for biocidal purposes include formaldehyde, which is used for fumigation, and glutaraldehyde and orthophthaldehyde, which are used as low-temperature hard-surface disinfectants and sterilants. The primary targets for aldehydes are proteins and, to a lesser extent, other macromolecules, but the mode of action is more specific than that described for alkylating agents. Although aldehydes have dramatic effects on intracellular components and processes, the primary mode of action is on the surfaces of microorganisms and therefore on exposed proteins and peptides, including peptidoglycan.

Aldehydes cause cross-linkages to form between amino acids within or between proteins, specifically, the amine group of lysine or hydroxylysine. Free amine groups, at terminal amino acids within a peptide or protein or as side chains on some amino acids, are particularly sensitive to cross-linking with aldehydes (Fig. 7.11).

The formation of these covalent bonds causes changes in the structures and functions of proteins and enzymes and protein aggregation. Access to lysine or other sensitive amino groups is an important factor in protein susceptibility to cross-linking; clearly, if the amino group is exposed on the protein surface, it will be at greater risk for cross-linking, in contrast to groups that are protected due to protein folding. Further, proteins with a higher proportion of lysine residues are also more susceptible to cross-linking. An example that has been specifically studied is the sensitivity of exposed lysine residues within the capsid proteins on the surfaces of nonenveloped viruses, which appear to be primary targets leading to the loss of viral infectivity. The number and accessibility of lysine residues within a given type of surface protein appear to be important considerations in the sensitivity of nonenveloped viruses to glutaraldehyde. Direct crystallography examination of glutaraldehyde-treated viruses has indicated a loss of capsid flexibility and an increase in surface rigidity, which is proposed to disrupt the release of the viral genome on contact with the host cell. Cross-linking can occur between the nitrogen atoms of free amino groups and other atoms within or adjacent to

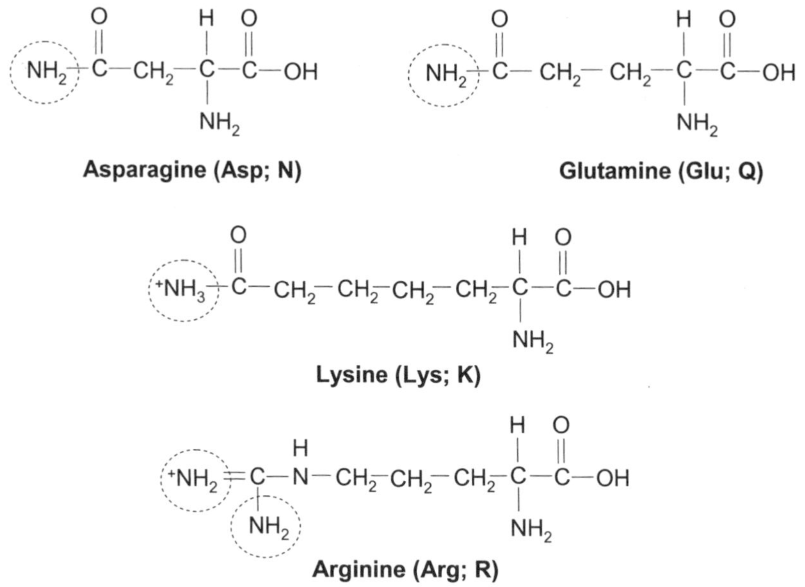

$NH_2-C(=O)-CH_2-CH(NH_2)-C(=O)-OH$

Asparagine (Asp; N)

$NH_2-C(=O)-CH_2-CH_2-CH(NH_2)-C(=O)-OH$

Glutamine (Glu; Q)

$^+NH_3-C(=O)-CH_2-CH_2-CH_2-CH_2-CH(NH_2)-C(=O)-OH$

Lysine (Lys; K)

$^+NH_2=C(NH_2)-NH-CH_2-CH_2-CH_2-CH(NH_2)-C(=O)-OH$

Arginine (Arg; R)

FIGURE 7.11 Amino acids, showing free amine groups (circled), susceptible to cross-linking by aldehydes. The side chain amino group of lysine is particularly sensitive; in addition, other amino groups that are not associated with peptide bonds and therefore are at the ends of proteins and peptides are also susceptible.

the protein; the most common cross-link with formaldehyde is between lysine residues and adjacent peptide bonds to form methylene ($-CH_2-$) bridges (Fig. 7.12).

Reactions with formaldehyde and proteins may also cause the entrapment of associated nucleic acids (intracellularly) and lipids or carbohydrates (at the cell membrane or cell wall); however, reports have suggested that there are no direct effects on the chemical structures of these molecules. The normal functions of the macromolecules are clearly disrupted, which also affects the overall viability of the microorganism.

The glutaraldehyde molecule is more flexible in its cross-linking ability than formalde-

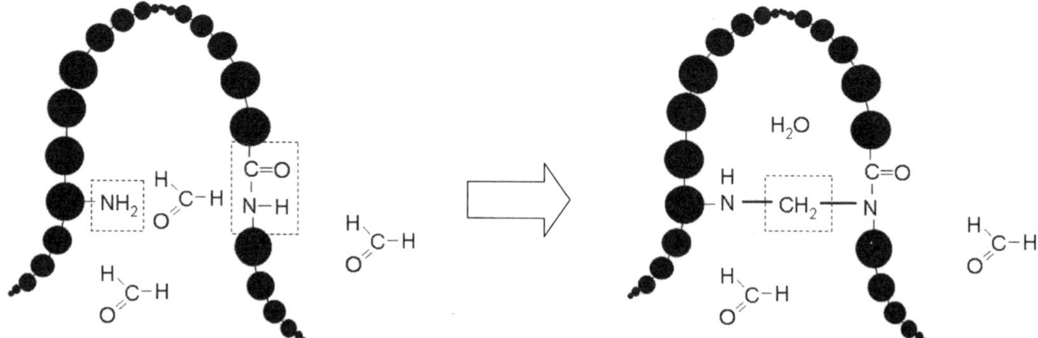

FIGURE 7.12 A typical cross-linking reaction with formaldehyde between a lysine amino acid side chain and an adjacent peptide bond. The sensitive amino group (NH_2) of the lysine residue is shown, as well as the reaction of the N atom of the peptide bond with formaldehyde to form a methylene bridge.

hyde, presumably due to its structure, which consists of three flexible methylene bridges and two terminal aldehyde groups (see section 3.4). This is in contrast to a single aldehyde group in formaldehyde and allows the interaction of the aldehyde groups over a wider access range. In addition to reactions with free glutaraldehyde, aldehyde polymers can also be present and can cross-link amino acids over a greater distance, both with nitrogen atoms within the same protein and with adjacent proteins. At the same time, glutaraldehyde monomers demonstrate greater penetration than aldehyde polymers. In addition to cross-linking free amino groups, glutaraldehyde may also form cross-linkages between other nitrogen atoms within the amino acid structure (Fig. 7.13).

The bactericidal activity of glutaraldehyde has been particularly well studied. Early reports demonstrated the following:

- Strong binding of glutaraldehyde to the outer layers of gram-positive (*Staphylococcus aureus*) and gram-negative (*E. coli*) bacteria
- Inhibition of solute transport in gram-negative bacteria
- Inhibition of the activities of surface and periplasmic enzymes
- Prevention of lysis with other agents, like lysostaphin in *S. aureus* and sodium dodecyl sulfate in *E. coli*
- Increased cell membrane resistance to lysis (in spheroplast and protoplast studies)
- Direct inhibition of RNA, DNA, and protein synthesis

It is clear that the mechanism of action of glutaraldehyde is mainly due to cross-linking within the outer layers of bacterial cells, specifically, with exposed amino groups on the cell surface. These effects cause a dramatic inhibition of the activities of key surface proteins involved in transport into and out of the cell and, directly, on enzyme systems, where access of the substrate to the enzyme is prevented. In studies in which the bacterial cell wall is partially or completely removed to produce spheroplasts or protoplasts, glutaraldehyde appeared to react with the cell membrane proteins to increase the membrane's resistance to lysis when placed in a hypotonic environment; this "tightening," or increase in rigidity, would make the membrane less sensitive to direct disruption. Direct studies of *Micrococcus lysodeikticus* supported this conclusion, as treatment with glutaraldehyde pre-

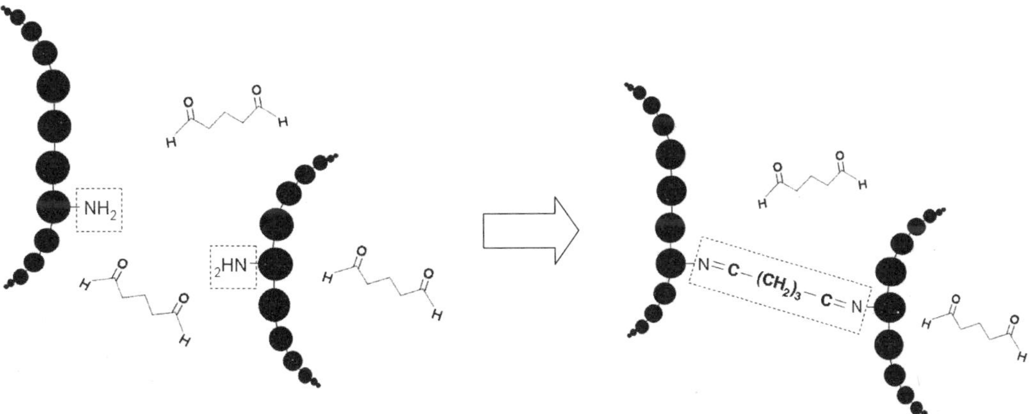

FIGURE 7.13 A typical cross-linked reaction by glutaraldehyde between two amino acids in adjacent proteins. The reactive amino group in each amino acid reacts with the aldehyde group on each end of the glutaraldehyde molecule, leading to the formation of a flexible methylene bridge.

vented the release of some membrane-bound enzymes.

Other studies have investigated the activity of glutaraldehyde against bacterial spores. Clearly, bacterial spores demonstrate greater resistance to aldehydes than vegetative bacteria. This may be related to their sensitivity to and uptake of the biocide or the availability of reactive sites. The bacterial spore presents several sites (including the spore coats) at which interaction with glutaraldehyde is possible, although in contrast to vegetative bacteria, interaction with particular surface sites does not necessarily have an effect on spore inactivation. *E. coli*, *S. aureus*, and vegetative cells of *Bacillus atrophaeus* bind more glutaraldehyde than do resting spores of *B. atrophaeus.* Spores are more susceptible during their development (sporulation) and activation to a vegetative state (germination or outgrowth) (see section 8.3.11). During sporulation, the bacterial cell becomes less susceptible to glutaraldehyde (see section 8.3.11). In contrast, germinating and outgrowing cells reacquire sensitivity. Uptake of glutaraldehyde is greater during germination and outgrowth than with mature spores, but still much less than with vegetative cells. Low concentrations of the glutaraldehyde (0.1%) inhibit germination, in contrast to the typical 2% concentration used for sporicidal activity. Glutaraldehyde clearly exerts an early effect on the germination process. L-Alanine is considered to play an important role during bacterial-spore germination by binding to a specific receptor on the spore coat, which triggers germination and the irreversible loss of the spore's dormant properties. Glutaraldehyde at high concentrations has been shown to inhibit the uptake of radioactive alanine by *B. subtilis* spores via an unknown mechanism, but this is probably the result of a sealing effect of the aldehyde on the cell surface. Direct interaction with the proteinaceous outer spore layers has been described. The resulting cross-linked structure inhibits the germination of the spore and even, as with vegetative bacteria, increases resistance to other sporicidal methods. Low concentrations of glutaraldehyde increase the surface hydrophobicity of spores, which is again indicative of an effect in the outermost regions of the spore; binding seems to be greater under alkaline pH, suggesting that increased surface cross-linking, and not spore penetration, is responsible for increased activity under alkaline conditions.

There are a limited number of studies that have investigated the effects of glutaraldehyde on other microorganisms. A mode of action similar to that against bacteria is expected against fungi, with the fungal cell wall observed to be a major target site, especially the major wall component, chitin, which is analogous to the peptidoglycan found in bacterial cell walls. Glutaraldehyde is also a potent virucidal agent that has effects on viral envelope and capsid proteins, particularly on cross-linking of lysine residues within and between these proteins. These effects are thought to cause loss of structure and reduced viral infectivity. Low concentrations ($<0.1\%$) of alkaline glutaraldehyde were shown to be effective against whole, purified nonenveloped polioviruses, but they had little effect on poliovirus RNA up to 1% at pH 7.2 and only slowly inactivated the nucleic acid at pH 8.3. These results suggest that the major mode of activity against viruses is associated with capsid damage. Viruses do demonstrate various levels of resistance to low concentrations of glutaraldehyde, presumably reflecting major structural differences in the exposed, sensitive amino acid amino group in their external envelope and capsid structures. For example, echoviruses are much more sensitive to glutaraldehyde than polioviruses. It should be noted that, like the differing abilities of aldehydes to form cross-links, which explain their varying effects on bacteria, aldehydes have also shown differences in their abilities to form protein-nucleic acid cross-links in viruses. In studies of viral DNA synthesis in vitro, some aldehydes (including the less used glyoxal, furfural, and acetaldehyde) did not show significant cross-linking abilities and had no effect on the viral DNA synthesis; this was in contrast to inhibition of DNA synthesis observed with aldehydes that did form such cross-links, including glutaraldehyde and formaldehyde.

Overall, aldehydes have similar modes of action, but it is difficult to accurately pinpoint the mechanism(s) responsible for microbial inactivation. Their interactive and cross-linking properties certainly play considerable roles in their activities, but they vary. For example, formaldehyde and, even more so, *o*-phthalaldehyde (OPA) are much slower sporicidal agents than glutaraldehyde, although both glutaraldehyde and OPA are rapidly effective against vegetative bacteria and fungi. The difference between the activities of dialdehydes (glutaraldehyde and OPA) and monoaldehydes (formaldehyde) may be related to the distance between the two aldehyde groups in glutaraldehyde (and possibly in OPA) for optimal interaction between sensitive protein and nucleic acid groups. OPA appears to demonstrate greater penetration through bacterial cell walls and membranes than glutaraldehyde, but as a dialdehyde, it is less cross-reactive than glutaraldehyde. OPA reacts only with the free amino groups at terminal amino acids and at arginine or lysine residues; in contrast, glutaraldehyde reacts with other nitrogen atoms within the amino acid structure. Further, the OPA molecule is structurally less flexible than glutaraldehyde due to the greater rigidity of the benzene ring (see section 3.4) and restrictive interaction with other available amino groups. It is proposed that the greater penetration of OPA through bacterial cell surfaces may be due to differences in the structure of the biocide under different conditions. In hydrophilic environments, which are observed at the external surface of the cell, the biocide may adopt a "locked" structure (1,3-phthalandiol), with unexposed, unreactive aldehyde groups, allowing penetration of the bacterial cell. Under hydrophobic conditions, typical in the cell wall and membrane, the open, active dialdehyde structure is proposed to be prevalent and therefore cross-reactive.

The mode of action of phenolics is discussed briefly in section 3.14. Phenolics particularly target surface and internal proteins. They can physically bind to proteins by a variety of interactions, including covalent binding, hydrogen bonding, and ionic and hydrophobic interactions. These interactions cause the protein, along with other associated macromolecules, to lose its structure (denature), coagulate, and precipitate. Many phenolics are actually used for their protein precipitation and inactivation activities in biochemical and molecular biological manipulations. The reactive form of the phenolic is the free hydroxyl (–OH) group, with other substitutions of groups in the phenol ring having multiple effects that could increase antimicrobial efficacy. For example, certain substitutions either increase or decrease the relative hydrophobicity of the molecule, which can be important in improving the penetration of the phenolic through gram-negative or mycobacterial lipophilic cell walls (see section 1.3.4.1). Others may increase the toxicity of the phenolic molecules. These substitutions can include the addition of alkyl (methyl or ethyl) groups with up to six carbons to improve solubility in lipids without decreasing solubility in water, halogenation (particularly the addition of chlorine atoms, called "chlorophenols"), and nitration (called "nitrophenols"). However, some chemical modifications cause a decrease in antimicrobial activity, as observed with the condensed bisphenols that are particularly effective against gram-positive bacteria but less so against gram-negative bacteria and with little or no activity against mycobacteria.

As the phenolic biocide approaches the microbial surface, it interacts with any available proteins. These effects have been particularly studied in bacteria, with the major targets being the cell wall and membrane proteins. Initial effects are observed on surface or surface-associated proteins, including disruption of energy metabolism, lipid and other macromolecule (e.g., peptidoglycan) synthesis, motility and chemotaxis, and secretion and transport proteins. For example, phenolics at low concentrations (particularly as described for the chlorophenols) have been shown to specifically interfere with the membrane-associated electron transport carrier proteins; these are involved in the generation of electrical energy across the membrane (the proton motive force [PMF]) (see section 8.3.4), which is used for many cellular functions, including ion transport, ATP formation (oxidative phosphorylation), and bacterial motility (chemotaxis and flagellar rotation). These interactions fundamentally change the structure of the bacterial surface, resulting in a rapid increase in cell wall and membrane permeability. The effects on the cell wall allow greater penetration to intracellular constituents and further damage the cell membrane proteins. Most phenolics can diffuse into the membrane, causing disruption of the phospholipids and interaction with embedded proteins. At low concentrations of phenolics, this disruption of the cell membrane rapidly leads to leakage of intracellular components, as the membrane structure is destabilized. Further penetration of the biocide into the cytoplasm also disrupts the structures and functions of proteins and enzymes, which culminates in loss of cellular activities and precipitation of the cytoplasm. Specific effects on proteins and lipid membranes have been studied with bisphenols (which are discussed in section 3.15).

It is likely that similar effects are also seen with other microorganisms, particularly molds and yeasts. Phenolics are not generally effective against bacterial spores, except in some cases with extended incubation, but they have activity against less resistant fungal spores. These effects are considered to be due to direct interaction with surface proteins. Studies have investigated the modes of action against viruses, which vary depending on the viral structure. Some phenolics (including phenol itself, which is rarely if ever used as a biocide anymore due to human toxicity concerns) demonstrated activity against enveloped and nonenveloped viruses; however, other phenolics (including *o*-phenylphenol) are effective only against the more sensitive enveloped viruses. Enveloped viruses are more sensitive to phenolics due to the accessibility of key surface protein and lipid targets that are required for virus infectivity. *o*-Phenylphenol is particularly effective against enveloped viruses due to its greater lipophilicity, which allows it to penetrate the lipid envelope. As with bacteria, halogenated and nitrated phenols are more effective against most viruses. Overall, phenols react with and cause precipitation of viruses due to interaction with surface proteins.

Chemically, phenolics are a class of alcohols. Other alcohols are simple compounds that possess a hydroxyl (–OH) group attached to a hydrocarbon chain. Shorter-chain alcohols, including isopropanol, *n*-propanol, and ethanol, are also widely used and are effective as antiseptics and disinfectants (see section 3.5). Since these alcohols have both water and lipid solubility properties, they can also have rapid effects on surface and membrane-associated proteins. Alcohols cause lipid peroxidation, protein adducts, and lipid and protein denaturation, leading to coagulation and precipitation. As in the reactions described for phenolics, since the hydroxyl group can readily react with proteins to form or break hydrogen bonds, this leads to protein denaturation and coagulation. Alcohols can particularly denature the tertiary structures of proteins by disrupting hydrogen bonding between exposed amino acid side chains; in this reaction, the alcohol reacts with the side chain to form new hydrogen bonds with the amino acid. Direct inhibition of enzyme activity is observed at relatively low concentrations of alcohol (~50% ethanol and 30% isopropanol). Overall, these effects are similar to those observed with phenols. Direct interaction with the various cell membrane, envelope, or specific cell wall lipids also causes membrane hydration, lipid extraction, and disruption of structure and function. These effects play further roles in the rapid antimicrobial activities of alcohols.

7.4.4 Transfer of Energy

Macromolecules are dependent on their structures to perform their various biological functions. Their structures are further dependent on the close interactions of various atoms and molecules, which are sensitive to chemical and physical agents that cause disruption and therefore loss of their specific and associated functions. The transfer of energy, in the form of heat

TABLE 7.9 Biocidal processes with transfer-of-energy-based modes of action

Heat
Moist heat
Dry heat
Nonionizing radiation
UV
Infrared
Microwaves
Ionizing radiation
X rays
γ rays
E beam

or radiation, has a dramatic effect on macromolecular structure (Table 7.9).

Heat is a form of energy that is transferred from one system to another due to differences in their temperatures. It is therefore not surprising, considering the effect of temperature on biological systems, that most common bacteria, fungi, viruses, and parasites are readily inactivated at temperatures of >60°C. Heat can be directly applied in a moist or dry form, both of which are widely used in disinfection and sterilization techniques (see chapters 2 and 5). Heat transfer also plays an important role in the modes of action of radiation methods, particularly the low-energy, nonionizing methods (infrared radiation and microwaves). The effects of heat include the denaturation of nucleic acids, lipids, and proteins; loss of structure and function; and coagulation of proteins and other macromolecules. In particular, as the temperature increases, the molecules present in these structures become more disordered as they absorb heat energy, which disrupts their structures and functions.

Temperature has a dramatic effect on the structures of nucleic acids, particularly DNA and double-stranded RNA molecules (like tRNAs in bacteria and fungi or the nucleic acids in some viral genomes). Temperature denaturation of nucleic acids has been investigated, and it is an important method in molecular biology investigations; for example, heat denaturation is used as part of the cyclic reaction to amplify sections of DNA in PCRs. Double-stranded nucleic acids are formed by hydrogen bonding between two complementary polynucleotide strands. These structures are actually quite resistant to the effects of heat but can be broken at ≥85°C to produce separated (or denatured) strands. The absorption of heat by the linked molecules causes them to vibrate vigorously, leading to disruption of bonding (Fig. 7.14).

Nucleic acid denaturation can be further enhanced under alkaline conditions (pH >11). rRNAs and other RNA molecules have been shown to degrade at relatively low temperatures (45 to 65°C). The rate at which DNA denatures (referred to as its melting temperature) varies depending on its guanine-plus-cytosine content; greater hydrogen bonding (three rather than two hydrogen bonds) (see section 7.3) is observed between these base pairs in comparison to adenine-thymine pairings (or adenine-uracil pairings in RNA molecules). Further, the topology (or rate of supercoiling) of the microbial DNA has also been suggested to cause heat and cold resistance, particularly in some thermophiles. Double-strand polynucleotide denaturation is itself reversible, and if the temperature is lowered, the structure can readily reform. However, at 85°C over time, or at higher temperatures, the polynucleotide strands are further damaged by specific breaks in the phosphodiester linkages between nucleotides in the sugar-phosphate backbone (known as "nicks"), causing nucleic acid fragmentation. Single- and double-strand breaks in the nucleotide backbone structure have also been observed at lower test temperatures. These effects can be repaired in bacteria and fungi but are also recognized by endogenous nucleases, which can lead to further enzymatic degradation; the overall effect on the target microorganism ultimately depends on the extent of damage and the organism's ability to repair that damage. Clearly, viral nucleic acids are particularly sensitive to the effects of heat, as unlike bacteria and fungi, they are unable to repair any such damage.

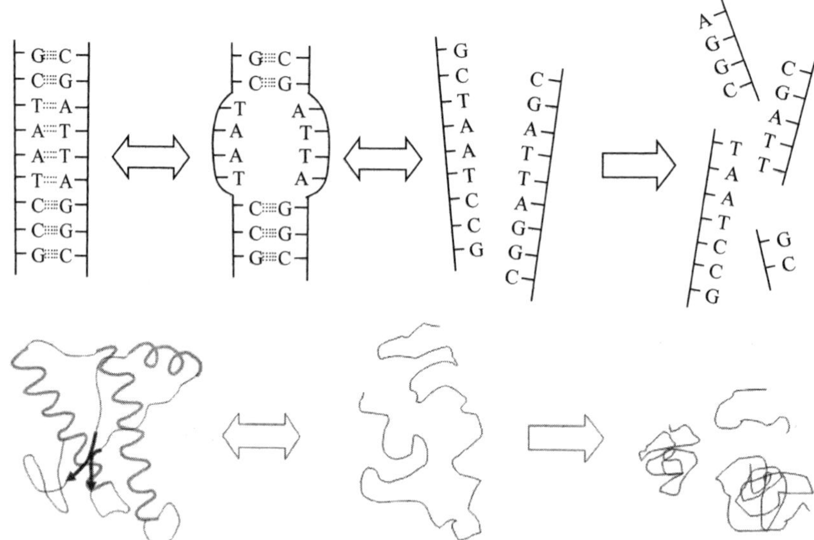

FIGURE 7.14 Heat denaturation of DNA (above) and protein (below). As the temperature rises, the hydrogen bonding between the DNA nucleotides is broken, with adenine-thymine linkages being particularly sensitive. Above 85°C, the strands are further denatured and eventually separate. On cooling, the DNA strands can reanneal, but fragmentation also occurs due to breaks in the sugar-phosphate backbone. Similarly, the noncovalent interactions in proteins are disrupted, causing them to lose their functional structures and assume their primary structures. In some cases, on cooling, the protein may refold to its original structure, but most proteins reassemble into inactive forms and precipitate. Breakage of peptide bonds that link amino acids also occurs, leading to peptide fragmentation.

The enzymatic and structural properties of proteins are also affected by heat (Fig. 7.14). As hydrogen bonding is disrupted in nucleic acid structures, so are similar bonds and other nonpolar hydrophobic interactions in the secondary, tertiary, and quaternary structures of proteins. Increased heat directly affects the various interactions that allow the biological functions of proteins in their tertiary and quaternary forms, including hydrogen bonding, salt bridges, disulfide bonds, and nonpolar interactions. Further denaturation of protein secondary structure also occurs, due to the disruption of α-helices and β-sheets, which are primarily formed by the presence of hydrogen bonds between the amine groups of amino acids. The majority of the resulting protein primary structures do not reform correctly on cooling and therefore precipitate and coagulate. The covalently linked (via peptide bonds) amino acids are more resistant to heat damage, but higher temperatures also cause peptide bond disruption and peptide fragmentation. In addition to the direct effects on amino acid bonds, subtle effects on protein hydration (or the degree of the absence or presence of water) also affect their structures and functions. Water is required for the correct folding and maintenance of protein structure. Water allows the formation (and, at higher temperatures, the disruption) of hydrogen bonds and other interactions, but it also affects the degree of flexibility of the protein structure, which is also important for biological functions. Therefore, as the temperature changes to a colder or hotter environment, the structure of the protein changes, eventually leading to denaturation. Under dry-heat conditions, the water is both removed and heated, which interferes with protein functions prior to the denaturating effects at higher temperatures. The opposite effect is seen initially with the application of moist heat, with increased hydration of the protein structure, but this is quickly followed by denaturation. Specific effects are observed with the hydration of hydrophilic amino acids (including lysine, serine, and aspartic acid), leading to protein denaturation under cold conditions; however, these effects are often reversible, except under freezing conditions, when the formation of ice crystals can disrupt and denature the protein structure. Heat denaturation appears to affect primarily hydrophobic amino acids (including leucine, tyrosine, and valine), causing an increase in the degree of disorder within these molecules. For example, in specific studies with various viruses, differences in their heat stabilities appeared to be due to the various sensitivities of the viral capsid proteins to heat denaturation and precipitation; some were easily denatured at <50°C, while others required higher temperatures. These effects aid protein survival under harsh conditions, as observed in some viruses and hyperthermophilic bacteria (see section 8.3.10). Many proteins from thermophilic bacteria have been found to have greater hydrophobicity and more internal bonding between amino acids, which demonstrates greater resistance to unfolding and denaturation due to heat. Similar effects of hydration and hydrogen bonding have also been observed with various polysaccharide structures: the presence or absence of water affects their flexibility and conformation, and increased heat leads to denaturation and polysaccharide fragmentation. Overall, these effects are similar to the various effects of heat on nucleic acid denaturation, with the disruption of these key macromolecules upon both changes in water interaction and breakdown of the various bonding interactions that are responsible for their biological functions.

Lipids are also affected by extremes of cold or hot temperatures. Heat, as a form of energy, causes the oxidation of fatty acids, particularly unsaturated fatty acids, in which the degree of oxidation increases with the degree of unsaturation. Fatty acid oxidation causes the production of free radicals, which leads to the deterioration and breakdown of their structures. Various reactive breakdown components can be formed, including ketones, alcohols, and aldehydes, which can also react with proteins, causing cross-linking and other reactions. Considering the effects of temperature fluctuations on proteins alone, lipid structures, like membranes, are indirectly affected by the disruption of integrated and associated proteins. The phospholipid membrane structure is also directly affected by the degree of hydration, with colder temperatures leading to less flexibility and membrane fluidity and higher temperatures eventually causing the bilayer to separate. The phospholipid bilayer is held together by hydrophobic interactions (including van der Waals forces), which stabilize the membrane structure; with an increase in temperature, these interactions are disrupted and the membrane changes from a highly ordered structure to disordered states. The effects on the lipid bilayer may play specific roles in the mode of action of heat against microorganisms. This can be proposed, based on the lack of membrane bilayers in some hyperthermophilic bacteria; in these cases, specific lipid monolayers that would not be prone to separation at higher temperatures have been identified. Specific effects on bacterial membranes have been observed, including increased leakage of cytoplasmic constituents as the temperature increases, suggesting membrane disruption. Similar effects are expected on fungal, viral, and parasite lipid structures.

The overall effects of cold or freezing temperatures have been less studied than those of higher temperatures. Clearly, the removal of heat (or energy) also has effects on various macromolecular structures. In general, these effects initially arrest the various functions of enzymes and change the structures and functions of various other proteins, lipids, and nucleic acids. The effects on lipids prevent the correct functioning of various lipid membranes. Overall, cold temperatures appear to be more preservative for microorganisms, which can be revived after repeated cooling and heating cycles; however, single or multiple freeze-thaw cycles cause macromolecules to degrade and bacteria, fungi, and parasites to lyse. The formation of ice crystals, especially large ice crystals formed during slow freezing, plays a role in the disruption of structure and function.

The mode of action of radiation is also due to the direct transfer of energy to target molecules. Radiation is energy in the form of particles or electromagnetic waves (see section 2.4). Their specific modes of action vary depending on the respective energies applied to the target microorganism and can be conveniently considered nonionizing or ionizing radiation effects (Fig. 7.15). The lower-energy sources (including microwaves and infrared and UV light), which cause the excitement of electrons within the atomic structure, are nonionizing. The higher-energy radiation sources (including γ radiation, E beams, and X rays) transfer so much energy to target electrons that they are ejected from the atomic structure, leading to further irreversible destruction of the target molecules.

The energy transmitted by microwaves and infrared radiation is absorbed by macromolecules and causes a rise in heat, and their primary mode of action is believed to parallel those described for heat disinfection and sterilization methods. Direct absorption of radiation by the target molecules also causes destabilization of their structures and functions, particularly due to disruption of hydrogen bonding and other noncovalent interactions. Further absorption of heat by available water molecules also causes the localized production of moist heat, leading to additional disruption of noncovalent and covalent bonds (including peptide and phosphodiester bonds), denaturation, and fragmentation of macromolecules (see section 7.3). Some studies have proposed that low-energy radiation doses may cause direct disruption of covalent bonds, particularly within nucleic acids. Reports of the application of microwave energy have suggested that, despite having sufficient direct energy to break covalent bonds, fragmentation of DNA was observed, in contrast to heating to the same temperature alone. These effects may simply be due to localized higher production of heat within the cell (as microwaves heat from the inside out) in comparison to the application of "external" moist or dry heat to the production of oxygen radicals on reaction with water, which act as oxidizing agents to cause fragmentation (see section 7.4.2). The specific effects on microbial macromolecules are discussed in the consideration of heat.

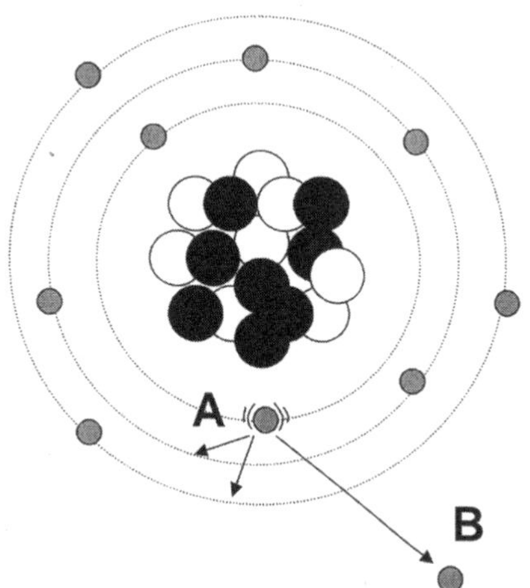

FIGURE 7.15 The effects of ionizing and nonionizing radiation on a target atom. Nonionization (A) causes the excitation of electrons due to absorption of energy, which, if sufficient, will cause electrons to move to a higher, outer energy orbital. In the case of ionization (B), sufficient energy is absorbed to expel the electron from the atom entirely. In both cases, these effects destabilize the individual atoms, the molecules they are part of, and the interactions between those molecules.

Disruption of specific molecular bonding and of molecules themselves is increased as high-energy sources, like UV radiation, are applied. The particular effects of UV on nucleic acids have been well studied, and they are considered its primary microbial targets. Many lines of evidence suggest this; for example, the most effective antimicrobial wavelength for UV is 265 nm, at which DNA and RNA demonstrate maximal absorption. UV not only causes a certain amount of DNA unraveling, due to disruption of hydrogen bonding between nucleotides, it specifically causes photochemical reactions between adjacent pyrimidine bases within the same nucleic acid strand. These reactions lead to the production of cyclobutane pyrimidine dimers, particularly thymine dimers (Fig. 7.16). Other, similar dimers are also observed, but at a lower frequency, including thymine-cytosine

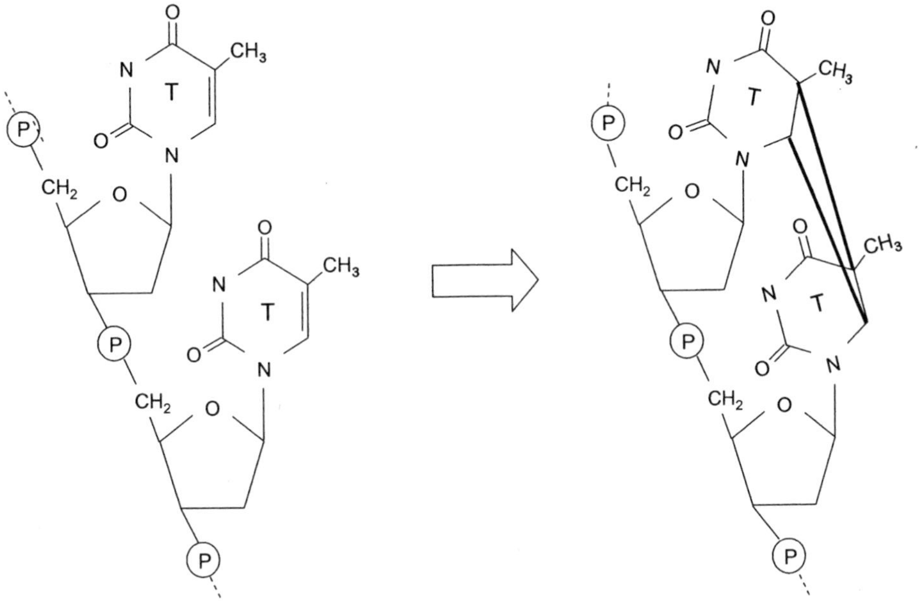

FIGURE 7.16 The production of thymine dimers between adjacent thymine bases in DNA.

and cytosine-cytosine dimers. Further photoreactive products, including thymine radicals (thyminyl and thymyl radicals) and pyrimidones, also contribute to the toxic effects within a microorganism. One such product, 5-thyminyl-5,6-dihydrothymine, has been specifically observed in UV-treated bacterial spores.

Overall, dimer formation causes distortion of nucleic acid structure, limiting the access of key polymerase enzymes and preventing the unraveling of DNA for replication and transcription and RNA-related functions within a target cell. Damage to viral nucleic acid can also prevent its injection on attachment of the virus to a cell, and indeed, its infectivity if introduced into a cell. Other macromolecules are also affected by the presence of UV radiation. The aromatic amino acids within proteins, including tyrosine, tryptophan, and phenylalanine, have been reported to be particularly sensitive to UV. Effects on the structures and functions of cell membranes have also been reported.

The biocidal effects on the transfer of energy to microorganisms are particularly rapid and destructive in the presence of ionizing radiation (see section 5.4). Both direct and indirect effects on macromolecules have been described. As ionizing radiation interacts with various molecules, energy is transferred, depending on the atomic composition and the density of the material. This leads to both excitation and ionization of electrons within the atomic structure to various degrees. The most destructive type of ionizing radiation is the highest-energy source, γ-irradiation. Direct effects on lipids, carbohydrates, nucleic acids, and proteins cause disruption of covalent and noncovalent bonds, leading to rapid loss of structure and precipitation. The resulting charging of atoms and molecules also leads to reactions between adjacent atoms and molecules to cause precipitation. Nucleic acids appear to be the primary targets, particularly due to fragmentation (single- and double-strand breaks). In a study comparing genetically "simple" microorganisms, like viruses, to more complicated organisms with complex and multiple chromosomes (animals and plants), the organisms with greater nucleic acid volume were predictably more sensitive to the effects of ionizing radiation. Further, specific resistance to ionizing radiation has been partly linked to efficient DNA repair mechanisms, which can remediate the effects of radiation damage (this is discussed further in chapter 8). Loss of protein structure and cell membrane damage have also been reported as important effects in the biocidal activities of these radiation methods.

Similar to other biocidal processes, the transfer of energy, in the form of heat or radiation, also causes other secondary or indirect effects on microbial structures and functions. An important example is the localized production of oxidizing and reducing agents due to interactions with water and other chemicals around or within the microorganism. These agents also affect macromolecular structures. In particular, the effects of the oxidizing agents that are produced have been described, including the production of hydrogen peroxide and hydroxyl radicals due to interactions of radiation with water, leading to further damage (see section 7.4.2). The effects of oxidizing agents have been linked to mutagenic effects on DNA. Direct oxidation of proteins and other structures is also believed to play a particular role in the modes of action of dry-heat processes.

TABLE 7.10 Biocides that act by disrupting the structures and functions of macromolecules

Acridines
Proflavine
Aminacrine
Anilides
Triclocarban
Surfactants
QACs
Nonionic/anionic surfactants
Diamidines
Biguanides
Chlorhexidine
Organic acids, esters
Acetic acid
Benzoic acid
Parabens
Metals
Copper
Silver

7.4.5 Other Structure-Disrupting Agents

Various biocides that disrupt the arrangements and functions of macromolecular structures are listed in Table 7.10.

The acridines are typical examples of biocides whose primary mode of action is direct interference with the structures of macromolecules, in this case, double-stranded nucleic acids. Their exact mode of action has been studied in some detail, as acridine derivatives have been proposed as potent chemotherapeutic agents. Acridines have a central fused aromatic ring that has an overall flattened structure, which can easily intercalate between the nucleotide base pairs of a double-stranded nucleic acid structure (see section 3.7) (Fig. 7.17).

The dye, which is positively charged, is initially attracted to the negatively charged DNA molecule and then can slot in between adjacent nucleotide base pairs. This causes a distortion in the DNA structure but also disrupts DNA-enzyme interactions, which are essential for replication and transcription. Further interaction with the DNA and associated proteins further destabilizes and prevents vital functions. Some acridines have been shown to prevent or disrupt the specific interactions of key enzymes, including topoisomerases, which are involved in the supercoiling (or higher-ordered structure) of DNA. The exact interactions with the acridine molecule vary from molecule to molecule. For example, the intercalation of proflavine appears to follow two mechanisms, depending on the biocide concentration and the time. The first mechanism is rapid, intercalating and binding between every 4 or 5 nucleotides; some reports have suggested a greater affinity for adjacent purine residues, which may be simply related to the accessibility of the biocide at these sites. The actual proflavine molecule not only slots into the DNA structure, but the two amine (NH_2) groups form ionic linkages with phosphate residues in the DNA backbone structure. Other parts of the molecule are also held in place by further interactions (particularly van der Waals

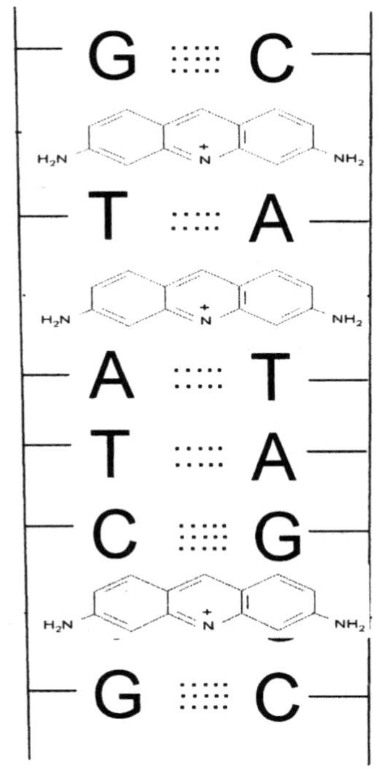

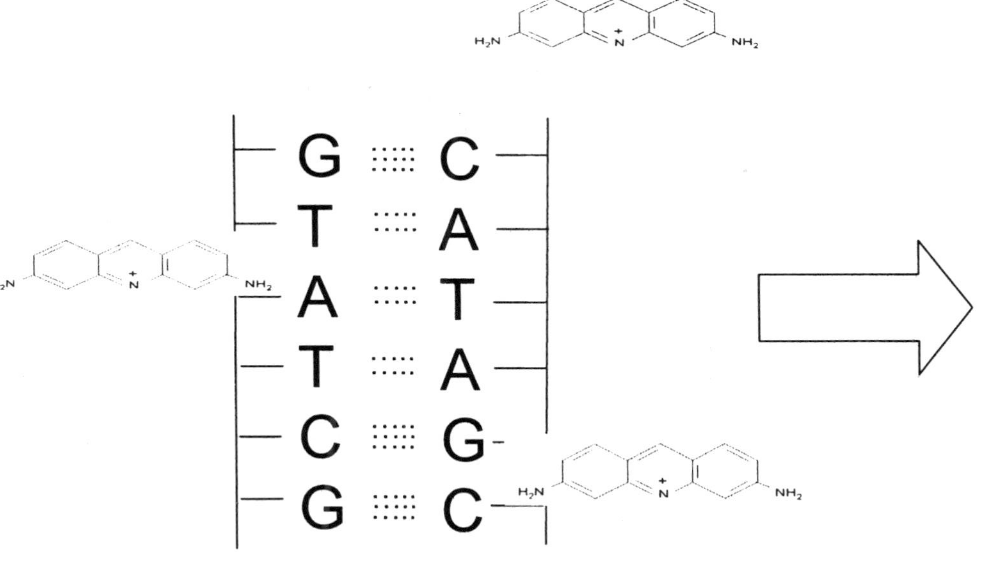

FIGURE 7.17 The mode of action of acridine dyes. The acridine molecule shown (proflavine) intercalates between the nucleotide bases in the DNA molecule, causing disruption of structure and function.

forces) with the purine and pyrimidine rings in the nucleotides. The second mechanism has molecular binding similar to the first, but at a lower rate and intercalating more frequently between all adjacent nucleotides. The acridines are also photosensitive and therefore absorb light energy, causing photochemical reactions. These reactions have specifically been shown to lead to guanine base damage, strand unraveling (due to breaks in hydrogen bonds), single- and double-strand nucleic acid breaks (due to breaking of phosphodiester bonds), and DNA-protein cross-links. These effects are not dissimilar to those of other biocides or biocidal processes described in other sections. Therefore, although the primary effects are due to intercalation, multiple effects, including nucleic acid fragmentation, enzyme inhibition, and surface interactions, also contribute to the mode of action of acridines (see section 3.7).

Further disruption of microbial macromolecular structures has been described with antimicrobial metals. Many metals, including iron, sodium, potassium, and calcium, are required for microbial life, with varied structural and functional roles. Removal of these key metals leads to inhibition of growth, and higher concentrations lead to a variety of toxic effects on the cell. For example, calcium and magnesium play important roles in the structures of the bacterial cell wall and cell membrane. Magnesium is also involved in the stabilization of ribosomes, cell membranes, and nucleic acids, as well as being required for the activities of various enzymes. The activities of chelating agents on bacteria and fungi demonstrate the importance of these divalent ions in their structures and functions. Chelating agents, like EDTA, remove these cations from macromolecules, which can inhibit their activities and cause structural changes. An often-cited example is the effect of EDTA on the gram-negative cell wall structure; EDTA increases the permeability of the cell wall to allow the penetration of other biocides. The general gram-negative cell wall structure differs from that of the gram-positive cell wall, particularly in having an outer membrane that is somewhat similar to the inner, cytoplasmic membrane but that contains lipopolysaccharide (LPS) in addition to phospholipids and integral proteins (see section 1.3.4.1). LPS contains a lipid portion that forms part of the external surface of the outer membrane, which is linked to a polysaccharide portion extending toward the outside of the cell (Fig. 1.15; see section 1.3.7).

Similar to the inner membrane, proteins can be found associated through or at the periplasmic or external surface of the outer membrane. Magnesium ions play an important role in maintaining the integrity of these LPS interactions by interacting with the negatively charged polysaccharide (core) portion. When magnesium is chelated (or removed) from these interactions, it causes disruption and actual release of LPS from the outer membrane structure. This destabilization leads to increased permeability of the outer membrane and disruption of key associated proteins or other functions. It is clear that as divalent cations are required for other functional and structural roles in microorganisms, the effects of chelating agents also disrupt their activities.

The biocidal metals include silver and copper (see section 3.12); others, like mercury and arsenic, are less used due to toxicity concerns but demonstrate similar disruption of structure. As positively charged ions in solution, they all have affinity for negatively charged microbial surfaces. This affinity causes some disruption of the PMF and cell membrane-associated activities, including energy generation and mobility. Surface proteins are particularly targeted by metals. Specific protein binding has been reported with silver, mercury, and other cations, with exposed sulfhydryl groups being particularly sensitive. Sulfhydryl groups, which are present on cysteine amino acids, play an important role in the enzymatic and functional activities of many proteins; for example, sulfhydryl groups are important in the tertiary structures of proteins due to the formation of disulfide bonds to give them the correct folded structure (see section 7.3). Typical reactions reported for metals with sulfhydryl groups are shown in Fig. 7.18. These reactions change not only the

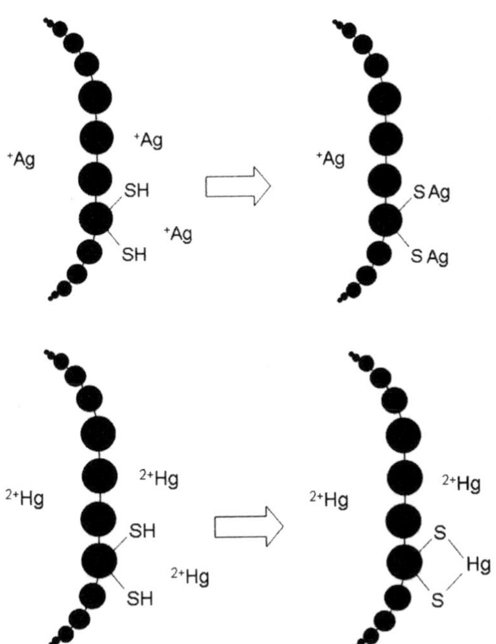

FIGURE 7.18 The reaction of metal ions on exposed sulfhydryl groups on cysteine amino acid within a peptide.

structures of some proteins, but also their activities.

Further specific interactions with nucleic acids, particularly those causing pyrimidine dimers, disrupt the function and structure of DNA, with reports of the prevention of DNA replication. The inhibition of key cytoplasmic enzymes involved in bacterial and fungal respiration may also play a role in the indirect accumulation of reactive oxygen species, which also cause the oxidation of macromolecules. Metals have also been shown to cause structural changes in the cell envelope, with detachment of the bacterial cell membrane from the cell wall.

Many biocides target microbial surfaces, particularly membranes, as a primary mode of action, with a variety of subsequent effects noted due to disruption of membrane structure and functions and associated proteins and enzymes (Fig. 7.19).

Microbial membranes are complex structures consisting of lipids (particularly phospholipid bilayers and, in some archaea, lipid

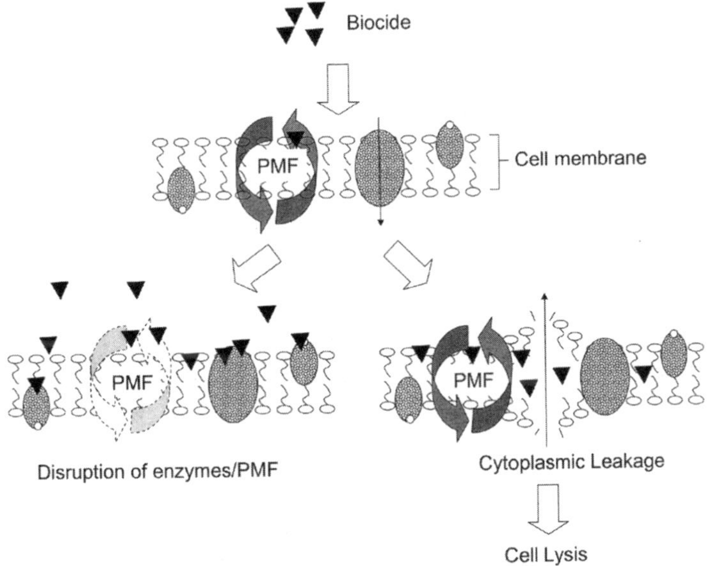

FIGURE 7.19 The effects of biocides on cytoplasmic membranes. The biocide can have subtle effects on membrane functions, including surface- and membrane-associated proteins (involved in substrate transport across the membrane or other enzymatic reactions) and disruption of the PMF. The biocide can also have more drastic effects on the lipid membrane structure, leading to an increase in permeability and cytoplasmic leakage; further damage can eventually lead to cell lysis.

monolayers) and associated proteins (see section 1.3.4). The cytoplasmic membranes of bacteria and fungi provide a permeability barrier against the external environment and to contain the internal cytoplasm. The basic structure consists predominantly of a phospholipid bilayer. The phospholipids are further stabilized by the presence of divalent cations, like Ca^{2+} and Mg^{2+}, but in general it is a fluid structure. Fungi and other eukaryotes may also contain other lipids, like sterols, which can add further stability to the membrane in comparison to bacterial membranes. Membrane and membrane-associated proteins play important roles in cellular processes, including enzymes involved in cell wall biosynthesis, nutrient transport into the cell, export of molecules out of the cell, and energy generation. Key examples of these are the membrane-associated electron transport carrier proteins that are involved in the generation of electrical energy across the membrane that is known as the PMF. As a source of energy, the PMF is required for key cellular processes, including energy (in the form of ATP) synthesis ("oxidative phosphorylation"), active ion transport, and cellular motility and chemotaxis. Similar lipid membrane structures are also seen in the outer membranes of gram-negative bacteria (see section 1.3.4.1) and enveloped viruses (see section 1.3.5). Direct damage to the structures and functions of lipid membranes has been described for various types of active agents. The biocides discussed here have been described as having as their primary mode of action the disruption of the structures and functions of lipid membranes. These membrane-active biocides include surfactants (such as the cationic QACs), the biguanides, organic acids and esters, and anilides. Direct damage to the membrane can cause subtle effects on the protein-related functions, which are observed as enzyme inhibition and disruption of the PMF, including the various associated metabolic processes. More dramatic effects include an increase in permeability, leakage of cytoplasmic materials, and cell lysis (Fig. 7.19).

The surfactants (or "surface-active agents") have been shown to particularly disrupt the structures of bacterial membranes, which leads to leakage of cytoplasmic components. They have two regions in their molecular structures, one a water-repellent (hydrophobic) hydrocarbon group and the other a water-attracting (hydrophilic, or polar) group (see section 3.16). Their overall structure therefore allows them to react with and penetrate into lipid membranes. The most effective are those with a greater positive charge in solution, including the cationics (such as the QACs) and the amphoterics (which have both detergent and antimicrobial attributes). The anionics and nonionics are less effective as microbicides, but they increase the permeability of cell wall and membrane structures and, at higher concentrations, can be biocidal. The QACs have been particularly studied in relation to bacteria (see section 3.16); they have been shown to rapidly adsorb to and penetrate the cell wall and then to react with the membrane lipids and proteins to cause leakage at relatively low concentrations. Indications of cytoplasmic leakage include the extracellular detection of typical intracellular components, such as potassium, inorganic phosphate, amino acids, and even nucleic acids, following treatment with surfactants. It has been known for many years that QACs are membrane-active agents, with target sites predominantly at the cytoplasmic (inner) membrane in bacteria or the plasma membrane in yeasts. The following sequence of events is proposed for microorganisms exposed to cationic agents: (i) adsorption and penetration of the agent into the cell wall; (ii) reaction with the cytoplasmic membrane (lipid or protein), followed by membrane disorganization; (iii) leakage of intracellular low-molecular-weight material; (iv) degradation of proteins and nucleic acids; and (v) cell wall lysis caused by autolytic enzymes. There is thus a loss of structural organization and integrity of the cytoplasmic membrane in bacteria, together with other damaging effects to the bacterial cell. Evidence suggests that the main effects are due to insertion into the lipid bilayer, but direct effects on the protein structure have also been reported. For example, the QAC cetrimide has been shown to interfere with the PMF. The

QACs have been specifically shown to interact with phospholipids, while the anionic surfactants appear to be more active against cell surface proteins. The initial toxic effect of QACs on yeast cells has also been shown to be due to a disorganization of fungal plasma membranes. Similar effects are expected to be responsible for the loss of infectivity observed with enveloped viruses. Further effects on intracellular proteins and nucleic acids culminate in cell lysis. As the diamidines are considered similar to cationic surfactants (see section 3.9), their mode of action is also related to disruption of the cell membrane, leading to inhibition of transport systems and cytoplasmic leakage.

The biguanides and polymeric biguanides demonstrate effects similar to those of QACs, and their interactions with the bacterial and yeast cell membranes have been investigated in some detail. Initial displacement of Ca^{2+} and Mg^{2+} cations that are associated with phospholipids has been observed, followed by direct binding to surface phospholipids and attraction of adjacent molecules to disrupt the membrane structure, leading to cytoplasm leakage. The mode of action of chlorhexidine has been particularly well described in bacteria and yeast. In studies with bacteria, the uptake of chlorhexidine was found to be very rapid in both gram-negative (*E. coli*) and gram-positive (*S. aureus*) bacteria and depended on the biocide concentration and pH. Insertion and interaction with the cell wall were reported to cause damage but were insufficient to induce cell lysis or death. Similar results were observed with yeasts. After passing through the cell wall or outer membrane, presumably by passive diffusion, the biocide subsequently attacks the bacterial cytoplasmic, or inner, membrane or the yeast plasma membrane as the major mode of activity. Direct damage to the semipermeable membrane has been shown to induce leakage of intracellular constituents, but it may be an indirect consequence of further cellular damage and cell death. The exact interactions that affect the structure and function of the cell membrane are not known but appear to involve insertion into the membrane, resulting in disruption. At lower concentrations, chlorhexidine collapses the membrane potential by disruption. The modes of action of alexidine and the polymeric biguanides may differ slightly in the disruption of the cell membrane. Alexidine is more rapidly bactericidal and produces a significantly faster alteration in bactericidal permeability than chlorhexidine. The biocide differs chemically from chlorhexidine in possessing ethylhexyl end groups (see section 3.8). It has been suggested that the nature of the ethylhexyl end group in alexidine, as opposed to the chlorophenol end group in chlorhexidine, may influence the ability of a biguanide to interact with membrane lipids to produce lipid domains in the cytoplasmic membrane. Similarly, polyhexamethylbiguanides cause domain formation of the acidic phospholipids of the cytoplasmic membrane. Permeability changes and altered functions of some membrane-associated enzymes ensue. Membrane damage has also been shown to be the major mode of action of chlorhexidine in other microorganisms, including mycobacteria, protozoa, and enveloped viruses. Other effects are observed at higher biguanide concentrations. For example, high concentrations have been shown to be an inhibitor of both membrane-bound and soluble ATPase, as well as uptake of potassium in *Enterococcus faecalis*; these and other effects on enzymatic and transport protein functions appear to be secondary lethal effects. In bacteria and yeasts, chlorhexidine also penetrates into the cytoplasm of cells. High concentrations of chlorhexidine cause coagulation of intracellular constituents. It has been noted that an initial high rate of cytoplasm leakage rises as the concentration of chlorhexidine increases, but at higher biocide concentrations, leakage is reduced because of the coagulation of the cytosol.

The acids and esters have more subtle effects, as investigated in bacteria and fungi, to disrupt the PMF and therefore associated functions. In the cases of some acids, the change in pH alone is sufficient to disrupt the functions and structures of surface proteins and enzymes and other macromolecules. Therefore, the overall effects appear to disrupt membrane enzymes but without disrupting the overall structure of the membrane, as indicated by the lack of observed leakage. The paraben esters appear to have a greater overall disruptive effect on membrane enzymes than the acids. The more hydrophobic acids and esters are also expected to interact with and disrupt the membrane structure due to integration. The anilides have also been shown to disrupt the PMF across the bacterial surface and to interrupt key membrane functions, including active transport and energy metabolism. Trichlorocarbanilide and trichlorosalicylanide have more specific effects on the cell membrane, as indicated in protoplast (artificial cell wall-free bacteria) experiments. This action is more likely due to direct adsorption and destruction of the semipermeable character of the cytoplasmic membrane. Increased halogenation of anilides appears to cause increased reactions with membrane constituents and an increase in bactericidal activity.

A variety of biocides that cause direct changes in the structures and functions of proteins have been described. They include the effects of oxidizing agents, leading to oxidation; changes in structure and fragmentation; cross-linking of amino acid side chains; transfer of energy, leading to denaturation; and coagulation and disruption of structure, as described above with the interactions of metal ions and surfactants. These effects may also be considered nonspecific protein interactions, although some proteins may be more sensitive to the effects than others, depending on their respective structures and localizations. Until recently, it was widely considered that biocides had more nonspecific modes of action, in contrast to antibiotics and other anti-infective drugs. They included interruption of cellular protein transcription machinery (e.g., the aminoglycosides or chloramphenicol), direct inhibition of specific enzymes (e.g., the quinolones against DNA gyrase), and interference with other functions required for multiplication of the microorganism (e.g., nucleoside analogue inhibitors of viral replication) (see section 7.2.3). Further analysis of the modes of action of some more selective biocides has surprisingly shown preferred inhibition of specific enzymes; these include studies of the modes of action of the bisphenols. Phenols have already been discussed; they target surface and internal proteins by binding to the proteins through a variety of interactions, including covalent binding, hydrogen bonding, and ionic and hydrophobic interactions (see section 7.4.3). These interactions cause proteins, along with other associated macromolecules, to lose their structures (denature), coagulate, and precipitate. At low concentrations, the bisphenols have been shown to specifically inhibit enoyl reductases (see section 3.15). Triclosan interacts with the substrate binding site (particularly tyrosine residues) on the enzyme, simulating the enzyme's natural substrate and the associated nicotinamide ring of the enzyme cofactor (NADH or NADPH), which allows the tighter, irreversible binding of the biocide. X-ray crystallography has shown that these interactions are noncovalent and are formed by hydrogen bonding, van der Waals forces, and other hydrophobic interactions. The enoyl reductases play key roles in the biosynthesis of fatty acids (thus affecting cell membrane structure) and therefore inhibit the growth of bacteria and some protozoa. In the case of triclosan, the interaction is initially reversible but over time causes a conformation change and precipitation of the protein or coenzyme structure that is irreversible. These effects remove the enzyme from its key role in fatty acid biosynthesis and cause complex precipitation. Another bisphenol, hexachlorophene, forms noncovalent interactions comparable to those of triclosan but does not form the irreversible complex with the enzyme cofactor. A similar mode of action has been shown for the antimycobacterial antibiotic isoniazid; however, isoniazid forms covalent bonds with the cofactors at the enzyme active site. Triclosan and hexachlorophene, like other phenols, have been shown to specifically inhibit other enzymes and to affect the structure of the cell membrane. It was therefore not surprising to find that various mutations or overexpression of enoyl reductases in bacteria can increase the MICs of bisphenols, but not necessarily the minimal biocidal concentrations. However, the identification of identical bacterial targets for an antibiotic and a biocide, even at low concentrations, is of some concern, especially if the use of the biocide in the environment could be a factor in the development of cross-resistance to antibiotics that are more restricted in their modes of activity and therapeutic concentrations. The results with bisphenols suggest that this could be the case, although the significance of this continues to be debated (see section 8.7.2).

FURTHER READING

Alberts, B., A. Johnson, J. Lewis, M. Raff, K. Roberts, and P. Walter. 2002. *Molecular Biology of the Cell*, 4th ed. Garland Science, New York, N.Y.

Bedford, J. S., and W. C. Dewey. 2002. Radiation Research Society, 1952–2002. Historical and current highlights in radiation biology: has anything important been learned by irradiating cells? *Radiat. Res.* **158:** 251–291.

Bergamini, C. M., S. Gambetti, A. Dondi, and C. Cervellati. 2004. Oxygen, reactive oxygen species and tissue damage. *Curr. Pharm. Des.* **19:** 1611–1626.

Bryskier, A. (ed.). 2005. *Antimicrobial Agents: Antibacterials and Antifungals*. ASM Press, Washington, D.C.

Dellarco, V. L., W. M. Generoso, G. A. Sega, J. R. Fowle III, and D. Jacobson-Kram. 1990. Review of the mutagenicity of ethylene oxide. *Environ. Mol. Mutagen.* **16:** 85–103.

Denyer, S. P., and W. B. Hugo. 1991. *Mechanisms of Action of Chemical Biocides.* Blackwell Scientific, Cambridge, Mass.

Fraise, A. P., P. A. Lambert, and J.-Y. Maillard. 2004. *Russell, Hugo & Ayliffe's Principles and Practice of Disinfection, Preservation & Sterilization*, 4th ed. Blackwell Science Ltd., Malden, Mass.

Kuhl, N. M., and L. Rensing. 2000. Heat shock effects on cell cycle progression. *Cell. Mol. Life Sci.* **57:** 450–463.

Lindquist, S. 1986. The heat-shock response. *Annu. Rev. Biochem.* **55:** 1151-1191.

Madigan, M. T., J. M. Martinko, and J. Parker. 2003. *Brock Biology of Microorganisms*, 10th ed. Pearson Education, Upper Saddle River, N.J.

Maillard, J.-Y., and A. D. Russell. 1997. Virucidal activity and mechanisms of action of biocides. *Sci. Progr.* **80:**287–315.

Maris, P. 1995. Modes of action of disinfectants. *Rev. Sci. Technol.* **14:**47–55.

McDonnell, G., and A. D. Russell. 1999. Antiseptics and disinfectants: activity, action, and resistance. *Clin. Microbiol. Rev.* **12:**147–179.

Migneault, I., C. Dartiguenave, M. J. Bertrand, and K. C. Waldron. 2004. Glutaraldehyde: behavior in aqueous solution, reaction with proteins, and application to enzyme crosslinking. *Biotechniques* **37:**790–802.

Murray, P. R., E. J. Baron, M. A. Pfaller, F. C. Tenover, and R. H. Yolken (ed.). 2003. *Manual of Clinical Microbiology*, 8th ed. ASM Press, Washington, D.C.

Riley, P. A. 1994. Free radicals in biology: oxidative stress and the effects of ionizing radiation. *Int. J. Radiat. Biol.* **65:**27–33.

Russell, A. D., and I. Chopra. 1996. *Understanding Antibacterial Action and Resistance,* 2nd ed. Ellis Horwood, Hemel Hempstead, England.

MECHANISMS OF MICROBIAL RESISTANCE

8

8.1 INTRODUCTION

Different types of microorganisms vary in their responses to antiseptics, disinfectants, and sterilants. This is hardly surprising, in view of their different cellular structures, compositions, and physiologies (see chapter 1). Traditionally, microbial susceptibility to biocides has been classified based on these differences (Fig. 8.1).

This classification should be used only as a reference for biocidal products and processes; the relative resistances of various microorganisms vary considerably, depending on the biocide itself, the process or application conditions, the formulation effects, and other surface effects (as discussed in sections 1.4.6 and 1.4.7). This chapter discusses the various mechanisms of biocide resistance described in microorganisms. Because diverse types of organisms can react differently, it is convenient to consider bacteria, fungi, viruses, protozoa, and prions separately. Although resistance mechanisms in all of these microorganisms have been identified and described, research has focused on certain bacteria due to their ease of cultivation and manipulation in the laboratory. In contrast, there has been only limited research on viruses and other microorganisms, which are potential areas for further investigation.

8.2 BIOCIDE-MICROORGANISM INTERACTION

Whatever the types of microbial cells (or entities), there is a common sequence of events in their interactions with biocides (Fig. 8.2).

This can be envisaged as (i) interaction of the biocide with the microbial surface, followed by (ii) penetration into the microorganism and (iii) action at the target site(s), which can include the cell wall, the viral envelope and/or capsid, the cell membrane, and the various cytoplasmic or internal constituents. This progression of events depends on the biocide challenge and the target microorganisms.

The biocide should be at a sufficient level (either in intensity or concentration) to interact with and penetrate into the microbial surface. This varies, depending on the biocide type, the product, the process, and the application. Important variables include the mode of action (see chapter 7), concentration, temperature, dose, formulation effects, and environmental conditions. The biocide concentration is an important variable and must at least be at the MIC or, preferably, at the minimum biocidal concentration to have a significant effect. Various formulation effects can assist in the penetration of liquid biocides to and into target cells (as in the case of enhanced triclosan penetration

	Microorganism	Examples
More Resistant	Prions	Scrapie, Creutzfeldt-Jakob disease, chronic wasting disease
	Bacterial spores	*Bacillus, Geobacillus, Clostridium*
	Protozoal oocysts	*Cryptosporidium*
	Helminth eggs	*Ascaris, Enterobius*
	Mycobacteria	*Mycobacterium tuberculosis, M. terrae, M. chelonae*
	Small, nonenveloped viruses	Poliovirus, Parvoviruses, Papillomaviruses
	Protozoal cysts	*Giardia, Acanthamoeba*
	Fungal spores	*Aspergillus, Penicillium*
	Gram-negative bacteria	*Pseudomonas, Providencia, Escherichia*
	Vegetative fungi and algae	*Aspergillus, Trichophyton, Candida, Chlamydomonas*
	Vegetative helminths and protozoa	*Ascaris, Cryptosporidium, Giardia*
	Large, nonenveloped viruses	Adenoviruses, rotaviruses
	Gram-positive bacteria	*Staphylococcus, Streptococcus, Enterococcus*
Less Resistant	Enveloped viruses	HIV, hepatitis B virus, herpes simplex virus

FIGURE 8.1 General microbial resistance to biocides and biocidal processes.

into gram-negative bacteria in the presence of EDTA and other chelating agents) (see section 1.4.6). In addition to direct biocidal-product effects, the presence of interfering substances can limit interactions with microbial surfaces. Two important and often associated variables are the nature of the contaminated surface and the presence of soils. Microorganisms can circumvent the activity of a biocide by protection within a given surface. Examples are the survival of microorganisms on the skin during antisepsis (see chapter 4) and within various surface imperfections (e.g., cracks, crevices, or porous materials) on inanimate surfaces during disinfection and/or sterilization. The surface itself can also be reactive with the biocide, as is the case with cellulose-based materials (e.g., paper) and many chemical biocides, which can also limit the activity on the target microorganisms. Various types of organic and inorganic soils, including blood, serum, water hardness, and the presence of salts, can significantly reduce the penetration of a biocide and interaction with microbial targets; these effects highlight the importance of cleaning, or at least of understanding the extent and effects of soiling present during any biocidal treatment (see section 1.4.8). Other similar interfering effects depend on the nature of the application. For example, the suspension of microorganisms in water can inhibit the penetration of gaseous chemical biocides.

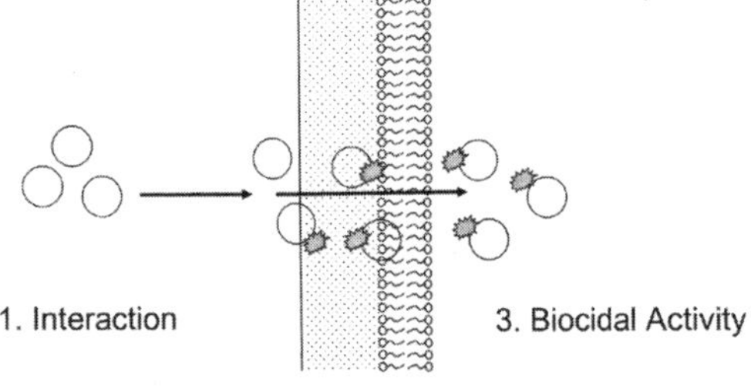

FIGURE 8.2 The initial sequence of events in biocide-microorganism interaction.

The natures and compositions of the different types of microbial surfaces vary from one cell (or entity) to another but can also be altered because of changes in the environment. These alterations are considered in more detail as mechanisms of intrinsic resistance. Biocide interaction at the cell surface itself can produce a significant effect on viability (e.g., with glutaraldehyde, surfactants, and oxidizing agents), but most antimicrobial agents appear to have effects intracellularly. The outermost layers of microbial cells can thus have a significant effect on the microbe's susceptibility (or lack of susceptibility) to biocides. These can range from the relatively sensitive envelopes of enveloped viruses to the highly resistant spore coats associated with endospore structure (see section 1.3 and below). Overall, it is disappointing to note how little is known about the modes of entry of many of these antimicrobial agents into different types of microorganisms.

8.3 INTRINSIC BACTERIAL RESISTANCE MECHANISMS

In recent years, considerable progress has been made in understanding more fully the responses of different types of bacteria (mycobacteria, nonsporulating bacteria, and bacterial spores) to antibacterial agents. Resistance can be either a natural property of an organism (intrinsic) or acquired by mutation or by the acquisition of plasmids (self-replicating extrachromosomal DNA) or transposons (chromosomal or plasmid-integrating transmissible DNA cassettes). Examples of resistance mechanisms are given in Table 8.1.

Mechanisms of intrinsic resistance are described in this section, with further consideration of the various types of bacteria in sections 8.4 to 8.6. The first acquired resistance mechanisms reported were against mercury compounds and other metallic salts, and they are discussed in detail below. In recent years, acquired mechanisms of resistance to other types of biocides have been observed, notably in gram-positive staphylococci, and they are discussed in section 8.7.

8.3.1 General Stationary-Phase Phenomena

Bacteria multiply by binary fission, an asexual reproductive process in which one cell replicates

TABLE 8.1 Examples of intrinsic and acquired mechanisms of resistance to biocides in bacteria

Mechanism	Resistance	Examples
Impermeability	Intrinsic	Bacterial spores, with various layers, act as an efficient barrier to the entry of biocides. Mycobacteria, among all vegetative bacteria, demonstrate notable resistance to biocide penetration due to their unique lipophilic cell wall structure. The outer membrane of gram-negative bacteria may present a more efficient barrier to prevent uptake or penetration of the biocide than that of gram-positive bacteria. Capsules and other extracellular matrices (including biofilm development) can act as effective barriers to biocide penetration.
	Acquired	High glutaraldehyde resistance of some mutant strains of *M. chelonae* is most likely due to decreased uptake by acquired resistance mechanisms. The presence of some plasmids can change the expression of outer membrane proteins in gram-negative bacteria and increase the resistance to biocides like formaldehyde.
Efflux	Intrinsic	Extrusion of the biocide from the cytoplasm due to active efflux mechanism (e.g., with chlorhexidine, antimicrobial dyes, and triclosan)
	Acquired	Plasmids and/or mutations leading to upregulation of efflux mechanisms
Decreased target susceptibility	Acquired	Specific mutations that decrease the affinity of some biocides (e.g., triclosan) to key cellular targets
Inactivation	Intrinsic	Production of enzymes and chemicals that neutralize biocides (e.g., formaldehyde dehydrogenase and peroxidases)
	Acquired	Expression of plasmid-associated enzymes and other proteins in resistance to metals, like mercury, silver, and copper

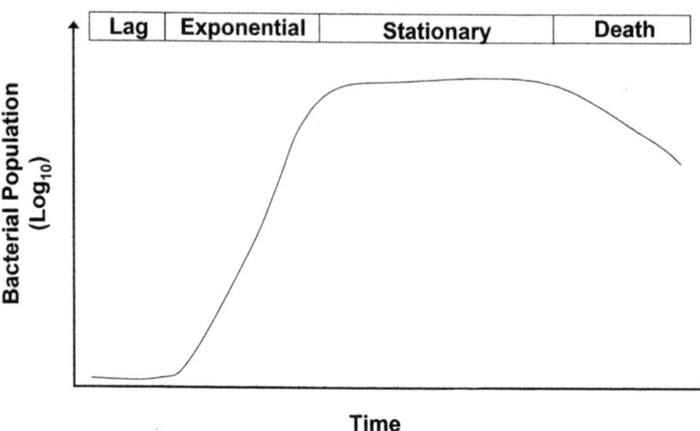

FIGURE 8.3 A typical bacterial growth curve, showing the four phases of growth.

its DNA and separates into two distinct, genetically identical cells. The growth of bacteria in laboratory culture and under optimal environmental conditions follows similar trends, which can be plotted over time (Fig. 8.3).

Four phases can be generally recognized, depending on the environmental conditions. During the initial lag phase, the bacterial cells are actively metabolizing but not multiplying; the length of this stage depends on the nature and type of bacteria present, as well as the presence or absence of various environmental conditions. As the cells begin to multiply by binary fission, a maximal rate will be attained at which the number of bacteria doubles within a given time interval, referred to as the generation time. The actual generation time varies, depending on the bacterial species and growth conditions; under optimal laboratory conditions, *Escherichia coli* strains can demonstrate generation times as short as 15 min, in contrast to the slower-growing *Mycobacterium tuberculosis* (~900 min) and *Treponema pallidum* (~2,000 min). These initial phases of growth are generally the most sensitive to the effects of biocides on the growth and survival of bacteria. Under optimal conditions, where the bacterial culture has a continuous source of nutrients and lacks any inhibitory substance, the bacteria can continue to grow exponentially; however, when nutrients become limiting, toxic by-products of metabolism accumulate, and in the presence of other adverse environmental conditions (including deviations in temperature and the presence of biocides), the bacterial culture enters stationary phase. During this phase, bacteria demonstrate various morphological and physiological response mechanisms to survive in a more competitive environment; many of these responses intrinsically cause an increase in tolerance of biocides and biocidal processes. They include the heat shock and oxidative-stress responses (see section 8.3.3). The length of this phase obviously depends on the severity of the environmental conditions. For example, strains of *E. coli* may survive for up to 3 to 4 days. As adverse conditions continue to develop, the rate of bacterial death (including cell lysis) becomes greater than that of multiplication, with an overall decrease in the bacterial population over time (death phase). In addition to the various physiological cellular responses during the stationary and death phases of growth, some bacterial species can enter more dramatic developmental stages to assume dormant forms of life. These include sporulation (see section 8.3.11) and other low- or nonmetabolizing dormant stages, which allow bacteria to resist adverse conditions. The various stationary-phase responses and the development of dormant forms, which allow bacteria to resist the effects of biocides and biocidal processes, are discussed further below.

8.3.2 Motility and Chemotaxis

Late in the exponential or early in the stationary phase of bacterial growth, many bacteria can adapt specifically to allow them to be motile. The mechanisms include expression of flagella, gliding motility, and chemotaxis. Flagella are thin appendages that are attached to the bacterial surface but freely rotate to allow movement (see section 1.3.4.1). The presence, location on the bacterial surface, and number (single or multitple) of flagella vary. Examples of bacteria that produce flagella are species of *Escherichia, Salmonella*, and *Bacillus*. In comparison, gliding refers to a process of motility on a surface, but in the absence of flagella; the exact mechanism of gliding is not known, but it has been linked to the production of polysaccharide slime. Examples of gliding bacteria are *Myxococcus* and filamentous cyanobacteria. The production of slime or protective capsules also provides an efficient barrier for the penetration of biocides, and they are considered further in section 8.3.7. Nonmotile bacteria also demonstrate the ability to move away from the presence of various chemical agents by chemotaxis. These are considered only indirect mechanisms of biocide tolerance, in that they allow bacteria to relocate to a less adverse environment and permit the circumvention of biocide attack only under limited circumstances.

8.3.3 Stress Responses

During the transition between the exponential and stationary phases of growth, bacteria have been shown to undergo structural and chemical changes in their structures in reaction to the restricted availability of nutrients required for growth. This has been particularly studied in *E. coli*, which demonstrates an overall reduction in cell size, changes in cell structure, increased rigidity of the cell wall peptidoglycan, and changes in the types and lengths of fatty acids in the cell membrane. In general, these cells show increased, although limited, tolerance of biocides due to reduced uptake and decreased cellular metabolism. Initially, this appears to be due to an imbalance in the production of macromolecules and cell division. In some cases, the slowdown in macromolecular synthesis is restricted but cells continue to divide, resulting in a population of smaller cells, which may also include multiple copies of the bacterial DNA molecules in the same cell. With *E. coli*, these smaller cells appear more coccoid than the typical rod-shaped cells (see section 1.3.4.1). These effects become more dramatic as the cells react to the lack of nutrients: the cells continue to become smaller and more compact, which is referred to as "dwarfism." In *E. coli*, this is specifically due to the degradation of parts of the cell membrane and the cell wall (peptidoglycan), but not the outer membrane, with a resulting increase in the size of the periplasmic space. The reduction in size is also observed in other bacteria, although in the case of *Pseudomonas*, sections of the outer membrane are also lost with no subsequent increase in the periplasm size. The components of the outer cell structure that are removed may be used as nutrient sources by the cell but also allow it to assume a more compact structure. Specific changes in the control of fatty acid synthetic and degradative processes have been described. The increased transcription of the *fad* (for *f*atty *a*cid *d*egradative) enzymes in *E. coli* and *Salmonella* allow restricted degradation of the cell membrane-associated and other fatty acids in the cell as carbon sources; however, degradation also appears to be more specific for short- and medium-chain fatty acids, with an observed increase in longer-chain fatty acids in the cell membrane. The increase in longer-chain fatty acids leads to increased hydrophobicity of the membrane and less penetration of some biocides. In combination, these changes in the cell structure and function may allow greater tolerance of the presence of biocides at lower concentrations; this can be significant when the biocide is used at bacteriostatic or preservative concentrations but has little benefit for cell survival under typical disinfection and sterilization conditions.

Bacteria have been shown to have specific responses to various environmental challenges or stresses, particularly during stationary phase, that can also contribute to intrinsic resistance to biocides, either directly or indirectly (Table 8.2). These have been particularly well studied in the gram-negative *E. coli* and the gram-positive *Bacillus atrophaeus*, as they present inter-

TABLE 8.2 Examples of bacterial responses to environmental stress

Environmental stress	Response
Lack of essential nutrients	General nutrient restriction or starvation
Amino acid or other starvation	Stringent response
DNA damage (increase in single-stranded DNA)	SOS response
Increase in heat or presence of biocides that denature proteins (e.g., alcohols)	Heat shock
Changes in pH, acidification	pH or acid tolerance
Presence of reactive oxygen species	Oxidative stress
Changes in osmolarity	Osmotic stress

esting mechanisms of control in the cell. Some of these responses are discussed briefly below as potential mechanisms of intrinsic resistance.

The stringent response is a specific example of a stress response due to a lack of nutrients, particularly amino acid starvation, and is closely linked to the transition of a cell from exponential to stationary growth. In addition to amino acid starvation, the stringent response can also be induced due to fatty acid, carbon, and nitrogen limitations, as well as in response to sublethal UV light. During the response, the level of a nucleotide molecule, guanosine-3′,5′-tetraphosphate, rises in the cell cytoplasm and inhibits the synthesis of rRNA and tRNA. The subsequent restriction of protein synthesis causes a decrease in the various cellular metabolic and structural functions, including cell division and membrane transport, which are typical of transition into stationary phase. The stringent response has been particularly well described in *E. coli* but is also known to be a basic phenomenon in bacteria and fungi, including *Mycobacterium* and *Streptomyces*. In mycobacteria, it is proposed that the stringent response could trigger the developmental adaptation of low-metabolic or dormant stages of growth.

The SOS response has been described in bacteria in response to a variety of environmental factors, including transition to stationary phase, starvation, and the presence of biocides. They are all linked to the detection of DNA damage by the cell. The response can be particularly induced in reaction to low-dose radiation (like UV light) and reactive oxygen species, which both damage DNA by dimer formation and oxidation of susceptible bonds (see sections 7.4.4. and 7.4.2, respectively). DNA damage or the inhibition of DNA replication causes an increase in the presence of single-stranded DNA (ssDNA). A specific bacterial protein, RecA, binds to ssDNA, which activates the protein to promote the autocleavage of LexA, a repressor protein. LexA represses (negatively regulates) the transcription of a variety of genes and the expression of cellular proteins that are involved with DNA repair and inhibition of cell division; cleavage of LexA, therefore, removes the repressor and allows these proteins to be expressed. Inhibition of cell division gives the cell time to repair any damage, mediated by the various DNA repair enzymes. When the level of ssDNA eventually decreases, the process can revert to repression of the SOS genes. The SOS response may afford some intrinsic resistance to biocides and biocidal processes (like radiation) by the inhibition of cell division (lowering the sensitivity of the bacteria), but also by repairing damage, particularly sublethal damage, to the cell.

As discussed in section 7.4.2, various active oxygen species have dramatic effects on the structures and functions of nucleic acids, proteins, and lipids. These oxygen species (including the superoxide ion, hydrogen peroxide, and the hydroxyl radical) are produced during normal cell metabolism, particularly in aerobic or facultative anaerobic bacteria, and need to be controlled to prevent damage within the cell. Bacteria have a variety of enzymatic and nonenzymatic processes that can neutralize these species, and their expression can also offer some advantage as mechanisms for increased

TABLE 8.3 Differences observed in the expression of proteins during the hydrogen peroxide- or superoxide ion-induced oxidative stress response in *E. coli*

Protein or enzyme	H_2O_2 induced[a]	O_2^- induced[a]	Function
Catalases	+	–	Enzymatic degradation of hydrogen peroxide
Superoxide dismutases	±	+	Enzymatic conversion of O_2^-
GroES	+	+	Chaperone[b]
GroEL	–	+	Chaperone
DnaK	+	–	Chaperone

[a]+, induced; –, not induced; ±, sometimes induced.

[b]Chaperones are proteins that assist other proteins to fold correctly to assume their structures and functions.

tolerance of biocides. An increase in the intracellular or extracellular concentrations of oxidants triggers the production of these processes in the "oxidative-stress" response in bacteria. At least two distinct but often overlapping oxidative-stress responses have been described in bacteria as being specifically induced by hydrogen peroxide and the superoxide ion. These responses are usually activated during the stationary phase of growth, when bacteria are generally more resistant to the effects of oxidants. They are considered separate responses, as they demonstrate differences in the enzymatic and nonenzymatic proteins or other antioxidants that are produced during induction; examples of the differences observed in protein expression in these responses are given in Table 8.3. Various response mechanisms have been described, but all of them contribute to the protection of the cell from oxidative damage.

The peroxide stress response is modulated by a specific cellular protein, OxyR. OxyR is both a sensor protein and a transcriptional activator. It is present in an inactive form that is activated by the formation of disulfide bonds between adjacent sulfur groups of cysteine residues in the protein structure, by the same processes by which oxidants damage proteins (see section 7.4.2). Most cytosolic proteins that contain cysteine residues in their sequences are found to be in the reduced (–SH) form, unlike secreted or membrane-associated proteins, which are often in their oxidized form as disulfide (S–S) bonds. Therefore, the presence of oxidants induces the formation of disulfide bonds, with a dramatic effect on the structures and functions of proteins. In the case of OxyR, the formation of disulfide bonds allows the protein to act as an activator to promote the transcription and translation of about 40 proteins associated with the response. This reaction is also reversible when there is a reduction in the presence of oxidants, and the antioxidants expressed during the stress response reverse the effect on OxyR, allowing the cell to return to its nonstressed state (Fig. 8.4).

The superoxide stress response is similarly induced by increasing levels of the superoxide ion and is coordinated by two regulatory proteins, SoxR and SoxS. The response has been particularly well studied in *E. coli*. SoxR is a sensing protein that becomes activated due to

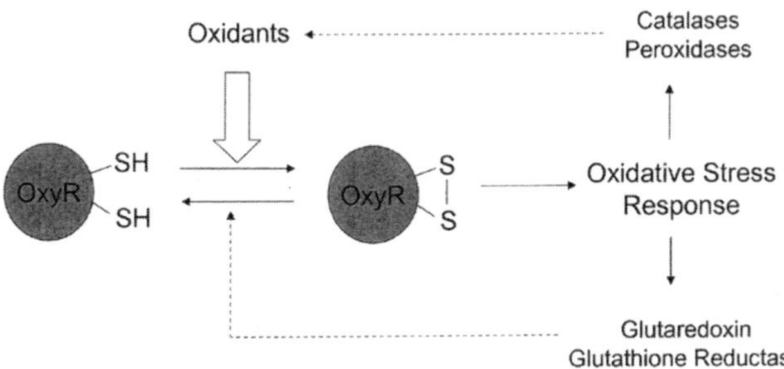

FIGURE 8.4 The activation and deactivation of the OxyR protein, as an activator in the peroxide-induced oxidative-stress response.

oxidation in the presence of the superoxide ion, which stimulates the transcription of SoxS. SoxS is a transcriptional activator protein that directly or indirectly promotes the transcription of about 30 to 40 proteins that are involved in antioxidant, repair, and metabolic functions. The expression of superoxide dismutase, which enzymatically promotes the formation of hydrogen peroxide from available superoxide ions, may also be involved in the activation of the peroxide response in the cell.

In both responses, a variety of enzymatic and nonenzymatic components that counteract the presence of oxidants are expressed. Some examples of enzymatic reactions are given in Fig. 8.5.

The presence of catalases and peroxidases specifically neutralizes hydrogen peroxide. Their expression in various aerobic or facultative anaerobic bacteria has been shown to cause a very marginal increase in their tolerance of the presence of hydrogen peroxide as a biocide, although this depends on the concentration of the biocide present; these effects allow the survival of these bacteria under lower concentrations (generally around the minimum bactericidal concentration [MBC]) of hydrogen peroxide. For example, *B. atrophaeus* was shown to be inhibited by 10 mM hydrogen peroxide during the exponential, but not stationary, phase. The expression of antioxidants (including glutathione, thioredoxin, and the membrane-associated menaquinone) plays a similar role in tolerance of oxidizing agents in bacteria, due to the reaction with the antioxidant and the protection of sensitive macromolecules. Glutathione reacts directly with and neutralizes the various oxidants, as well as reversing the formation of disulfide bonds in proteins (by reduction). Other protective mechanisms expressed during oxidative stress are chaperone proteins, like DnaK and GroEL; chaperones are proteins that assist other proteins to fold correctly to assume their appropriate folded structures and functions and that assist when proteins have been partially denatured to allow them to refold into their normal structures. These proteins also play roles in protecting the cell against sublethal conditions that specifically denature proteins, including heat treatment (as in the heat shock response). Other repair mechanisms expressed are various DNA repair enzymes (endonucleases and exonucleases) and other protein repair enzymes (e.g., for the reduction of disulfide bonds). Differences have been described between the specific oxidative responses in gram-positive and gram-negative bacteria, but with the same overall effect of protecting the cell against damage. These protection mechanisms are seen in not only aerobic, but also anaerobic, bacteria; examples are flavoproteins, which reduce oxygen to form water and superoxide reductases. Similar responses in yeasts have been described. Overall, the oxidative-stress response allows the cell to tolerate some amount of dam-

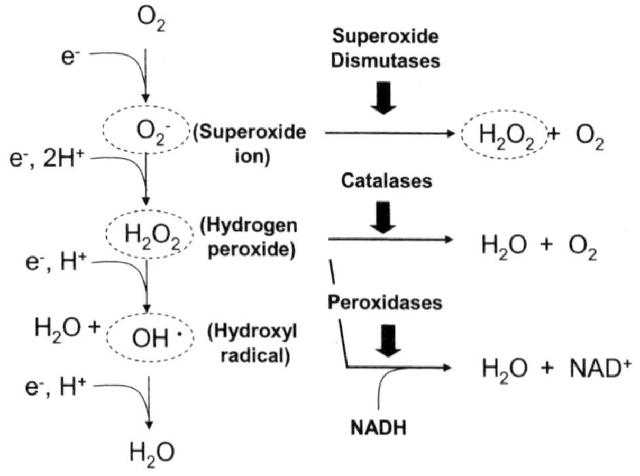

FIGURE 8.5 The functions of various enzymes induced during oxidative stress.

age in the presence of many biocides and biocidal processes, particularly under bacteriostatic and minimal bactericidal conditions.

Another response in *E. coli* and other bacteria is the heat shock response. *E. coli* is a mesophilic organism with an optimum temperature for growth of ~37°C. When the temperature is increased to 42 to 45°C, the bacteria react to shift transcription away from normal housekeeping functions to the production of a series of heat shock proteins (~40 proteins), which aid the cell to survive at these restrictive temperatures. The response has also been shown to be triggered by some biocides, like alcohol, presumably due to a denaturing mode of action, similar to that seen with increased temperature (see section 7.4.4). Many of these proteins, including GroES, GroEL, and DnaK, which are chaperones involved in the correct folding of proteins, are also expressed during other shock or stress responses. The mode of action of heat involves the denaturation and precipitation of proteins; therefore, the presence of chaperones allows the proteins to maintain or resume their correct structures and functions under restrictive conditions. DnaK is also involved in controlling expression of the heat shock response, as it can be reversed as the temperature falls to an optimum level required for growth. Other enzymes that are expressed are proteases (in the cytoplasm, but also in the periplasm, of gram-negative bacteria) that degrade denatured proteins that have lost their structures and functions. The heat shock response allows only partial tolerance of temperature changes in the environment and is thought to have little benefit for the survival of vegetative bacteria under typical disinfection or sterilization conditions.

Other responses to environmental stress have been studied in *E. coli* and other bacteria. They include responses to pH, particularly acid tolerance and osmotic stress. The acid tolerance response demonstrates the expression of up to 50 proteins, including the activation of proton pumps to allow the bacteria to reestablish the normal proton motive force (PMF) and other functions associated with the cell membrane. Up-regulation of the PMF also affects bacterial resistance to certain biocides that have also been shown to disrupt this process (see section 8.3.4). Similar stress responses have been described in *Streptomyces* during particular stages of growth and development, in which the stringent response is coupled to stationary-phase adaptation (the formation of aerial mycelia, leading to spore production) and the production of secondary metabolites (including hydrolytic enzymes and antimicrobial agents).

In conclusion, these responses have evolved in bacteria to allow them to tolerate various environmental stresses experienced during normal growth and survival. Their overall practical contribution to biocidal resistance is minimal, considering the concentrations typically used and the conditions of disinfection and sterilization processes; however, these effects may allow the survival of bacteria under sublethal conditions, where low concentrations are used, and afford them some protection from biocidal effects.

8.3.4 Efflux Mechanisms

A major function of the bacterial membrane is to control the exchange and transport of various chemicals and substances between the cell and its environment. The lipophilicity of the membrane acts as an effective barrier to most compounds. A variety of specific mechanisms have been identified that allow the exchange of materials either into (influx) or out of (efflux) the cell. These can be considered passive diffusion, facilitated diffusion, and active-transport mechanisms (Fig. 8.6).

Passive diffusion is the movement of gases or small, uncharged polar molecules across the membrane driven by a concentration gradient from an area of high to an area of low concentration. Examples are oxygen, ethanol, and water; the passive diffusion of water from a high- to a low-concentration area is known as osmosis. These processes can be facilitated in some cases by membrane-associated transporter proteins—in the case of water (by proteins known as aquaporins), by larger and/or lipophilic molecules. These facilitated processes are still directed by diffusion but can be assisted

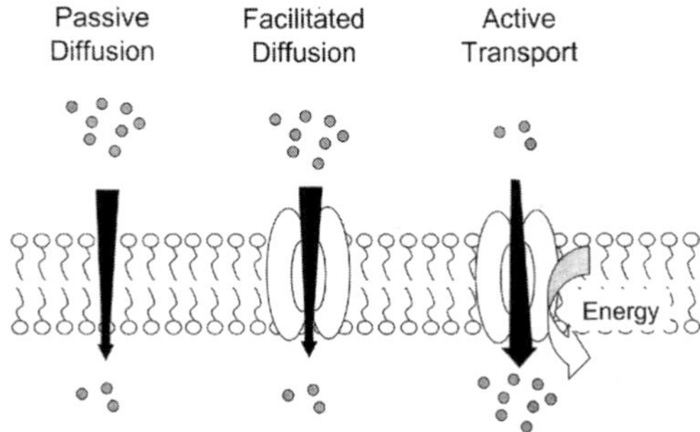

FIGURE 8.6 Transport systems in bacteria across a typical cell membrane.

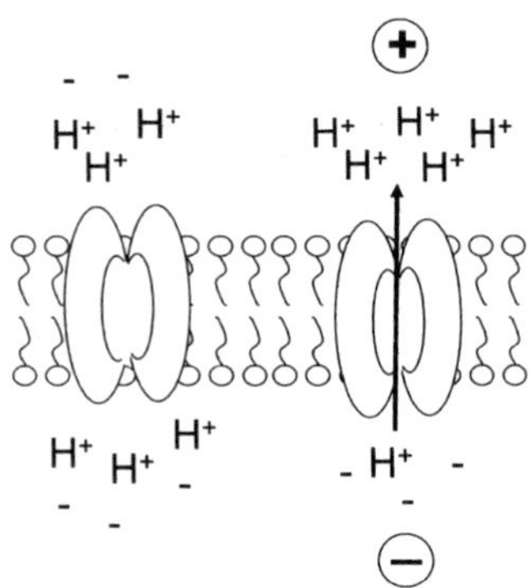

FIGURE 8.7 Establishment of the PMF.

by energy generated from the PMF. In cytoplasmic or membrane-associated electron transport systems, electrons are passed from one carrier to another in a sequence of oxidation-reduction reactions with a simultaneous release of energy. This energy can be used to transport (or pump) protons (H^+) across the cell membrane into the space between the cell membrane and the cell wall. This results in an overall positive charge on the external surface of the membrane and an overall negative charge on the internal surface (Fig. 8.7). This electrochemical gradient is known as the PMF and is used as a source of energy by the cell, specifically, in bacteria, for the synthesis of ATP (or metabolic energy, which is the major source of energy for various cellular processes on hydrolysis to ADP and phosphate), rotation of flagella, and transport of materials across the membrane.

The establishment and maintenance of the PMF becomes important when active transport is considered. Active transport uses energy sources to transport substances against their concentration gradients and is particularly important to consider during the attack of a cell by a biocide at high concentrations from the external environment. Sources of energy include the PMF and the the hydrolysis of ATP or other high-energy compounds. A variety of active transporters have been identified in the influx and efflux of nutrients, ions, and antimicrobial agents. A summary of the major classes is give in Table 8.4.

It is clear that many biocides directly affect these processes by disrupting the cell membrane structure and function, including disruption of the PMF (see section 7.4.5). The prevention of the influx and efflux of various molecules has

TABLE 8.4 Classification of active-transporter systems

Type	Description	Examples
Symporters	Transport of molecules across the membrane in the same direction as another substance; driven by the PMF	Ions (HSO_4^-, HPO_4^-, and H^+), glucose, and some amino acids
Antiporters	Transport of molecules across the membrane in parallel with another substance in the other direction; driven by the PMF	Ions (Na^+ and H^+), glucose, and some amino acids; some antibiotics and biocides
ABC systems	Protein-assisted transfer through the periplasm and active protein-mediated transport through the membrane in an ATP-dependent manner; driven by hydrolysis of ATP	Sugars and amino acids; some antibiotics, chloroquine, some biocides
Group translocation	Substance is chemically modified for unidirectional transport across the membrane	Glucose and other sugars

multiple effects on cell metabolism and survival; however, bacteria have been shown to specifically pump out low concentrations of various biocides, which can reduce the accumulation of the biocide in the cytoplasm. This may be particularly important in cases where the biocide has limited penetration through the cell wall, as in gram-negative bacteria. Active efflux has been shown to be of particular concern in antibiotic resistance in bacteria and has been especially well studied in *E. coli* and *Pseudomonas* species. Many of these efflux systems play significant roles in biocide resistance, as the outer membrane in gram-negative bacteria (particularly *Pseudomonas*) presents a much higher permeability barrier to biocides than the cell walls of gram-positive bacteria, and active-efflux systems can therefore provide an even greater advantage for biocide survival.

For the purpose of this discussion, three major groups of efflux systems have been associated with increased antimicrobial tolerance in both gram-positive and gram-negative bacteria. They include the following:

- The major facilitator superfamily (MFS). For this discussion, this group includes two similar yet distinct families, the small multidrug resistance (SMR) family and the multidrug–toxic-compound extrusion (MATE) family. These families are often considered to be groups of efflux systems separate from the MFS.
- The resistance-nodulation-division (RND) family
- The ATP-binding cassette (ABC) family

Although the exact modes of action of the various efflux systems remain to be elucidated, it is believed that they at least consist of single cytoplasmic membrane proteins that can operate on their own (as is the case in gram-positive bacteria) or, particularly in gram-negative bacteria, in combination with other periplasmic and outer-membrane-associated proteins (Fig. 8.8). The MFS and RND systems consist of a cytoplasmic membrane antiporter protein that uses the PMF as an energy source to drive the biocide out of the cytoplasm in exchange for protons; however, although examples of MFS systems have been shown to require only the cytoplasmic antiporter protein for efflux, the NOD family has been shown to require associated periplasmic and outer membrane components for effective biocide efflux (Fig. 8.8). The ABC family uses ATP as an energy source to pump the active agent out of the cell.

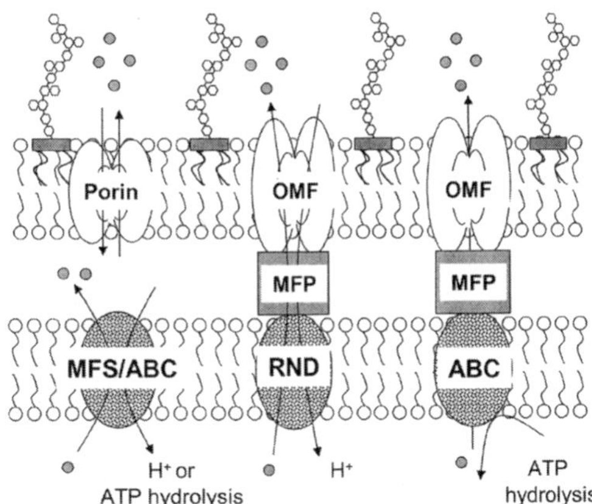

FIGURE 8.8 Summary of the various types of efflux pumps associated with antimicrobial resistance identified in bacteria. A typical gram-negative bacterial cell wall is shown with associated cytoplasmic and outer membranes (see section 1.3.4.1). Note that similar cytoplasmic-membrane-associated efflux pumps (MFS and ABC) have been identified in gram-positive bacteria (which do not have an outer membrane [see section 1.3.4.1]). Efflux is energy dependent, with energy derived from the PMF (antiporter efflux with H^+) or ATP hydrolysis (to ADP plus inorganic phosphate).

The RND-type pumps have been well-studied and identified in gram-negative bacteria, although they have not been identified in mycobacteria. They have been particularly associated with antibiotic and biocide extrusion as mechanisms of multidrug resistance (MDR). They are usually associated as a three-component system consisting of a cytoplasmic-membrane-associated transporter, a periplasm-associated protein (known as a membrane fusion protein [MFP]), and an outer-membrane-associated protein (the outer membrane factor [OMF]). They all use energy from the PMF to pump the compound out of the cell. In many cases, their exact physiological functions are unknown, although they have been linked to controlling divalent metal ion concentrations (CzrAB-OpmD systems in *Pseudomonas aeruginosa*) and solvent (toluene) resistance (the SrpABC and MepABC systems in *Pseudomonas putida*). Solvent resistance in *P. putida* is due to multiple factors. Solvents have been shown to accumulate in and disrupt the structure and function of the cytoplasmic membrane. *P. putida* strains can survive the presence of solvents, like toluene, by varying the structures and types of phospholipids in the cell membrane (with an increase in *trans*-unsaturated fatty acids, which changes the membrane fluidity) and the rate of membrane turnover; by changes in the outer membrane lipopolysaccharide (LPS) and protein composition; and by the presence of normal and inducible efflux pumps. The SrpABC mechanism is a three-component system consisting of a membrane-associated RND pump (SrpB), a periplasmic MFP (SrpA), and an outer membrane OMF (SrpC). This system appears to be inducible by and unique to toluene efflux; in contrast, MepABC allows the efflux of toluene and other compounds, like the β-lactam antibiotics and antimicrobial dyes. It has been suggested that these RND systems may operate in three modes, depending on the type of drug being extruded: the membrane-associated RND pump alone (which drives hydrophilic drugs into the periplasm), the RND pump combined with the periplasmic MFP (to pump out amphiphilic molecules), and the three-component RND-MFP-OMF (for the extrusion of amphiphilic and lipophilic drugs).

The presence or activation of these efflux pump mechanisms can affect the overall influx and concentration of biocides within the cytoplasm and (in gram-negative bacteria) the periplasmic space; however, similar to other physiological responses to biocides, they afford only partial survival at the MIC or MBC of the biocide, which can be an important consideration at preservative or residual levels of the active agent. In some cases, the presence of the biocide has been shown to induce the expression of efflux-related proteins in bacteria, while in others, the efflux pumps are present due to normal vegetative-growth functions. Examples of pumps that have been linked to the efflux of biocides from bacteria are given in Table 8.5. Efflux mechanisms also play a role in acquired resistance to biocides (including both mutation and plasmid-borne mechanisms, which are discussed in section 8.7); the activation or acquisition of efflux mechanisms due to treatment with biocides has been suggested as an important consideration in the development of antibiotic resistance, where increased MICs and MBCs present a greater therapeutic challenge.

TABLE 8.5 Examples of bacterial efflux systems that have been shown to extrude biocides and antibiotics

Efflux protein	Family	Bacterium	Antimicrobials extruded[a]
NorA	MFS	*S. aureus*	Fluoroquinolones, antimicrobial dyes, QACs, tetraphenylphophonium, rhodamine
BmrR	MFS	*B. atrophaeus*	Fluoroquinolones, antimicrobial dyes, QACs, tetraphenylphophonium, rhodamine
LmrA	ABC	*L. lactis*	Fluoroquinolones, acriflavines, antimicrobial dyes
EfrAB	ABC	*E. faecalis*	Fluoroquinolones, acriflavines, antimicrobial dyes
AcrAB-TolC	RND	*E. coli*	β-Lactams, fluoroquinolones, tetracycline, acriplavines, antimicrobial dyes, SDS, pine oil (phenolics), triclosan, chlorhexidine, QACs
MexAB-OprM	RND	*P. aeruginosa*	β-Lactams, fluoroquinolones, acriflavines, triclosan, SDS, toluene, antimicrobial dyes (e.g., crystal violet), QACs
MexCD-OprJ	RND	*P. aeruginosa*	β-lactams, fluoroquinolones, acriflavines, triclosan, SDS, toluene
CzrAB-OpmN	RND	*P. aeruginosa*	Cadmium, zinc

[a]The full spectrum of biocides that may be extruded due to efflux remains to be determined.

8.3.5 Enzymatic and Chemical Protection

Various enzymes and chemicals that allow some tolerance of the presence of biocides have been identified in bacteria and yeast (in addition to those described in the various stress responses in section 8.3.3). In some cases, biocides can actually be used as a carbon source by the microorganism under appropriate conditions, as described for phenols, cresols, quaternary ammonium compounds (QACs), and chlorhexidine. *Pseudomonas* species are particularly implicated in these cases, as they present a wide metabolic diversity, using a range of compounds as carbon sources for growth; however, the levels of tolerance tend to be within the normal inhibitory and sometimes bactericidal range observed with pseudomonads, with higher concentrations of the biocide generally being effective against these isolates. Many of these strains are beneficial, as they are used for the biodegradation of toxic compounds within the environment. Degradation of cresols and phenols as carbon sources has been demonstrated in strains of *P. putida* and *Pseudomonas pickettii,* due to the presence of various metabolic enzymes, like dehydrogenases and hydroxylases. Similarly, inactivation of formaldehyde has been reported with *P. aeruginosa*, *P. putida*, and *Pseudomonas syringae* and is mediated by the production of glutathione-dependent formaldehyde dehydrogenases. Various formaldehyde dehydrogenases and transketolases are involved in the metabolism of formaldehyde in methanotrophs, like *Methylococcus*. The degradation of formaldehyde by *E. coli* has been studied in some detail; glutathione reacts with formaldehyde to form hydroxymethylglutathione, which is then oxidized by the dehydrogenase to *S*-formylglutathione and subsequently metabolized by the cell. Similar alcohol dehydrogenases in *E. coli* and yeasts facilitate the conversion between alcohols and aldehydes; for example, ethanol is oxidized by a dehydrogenase to form acetaldehyde, which is rapidly converted into acetyl-coenzyme A for use by the cell. Other enzymes are directly involved in neutralizing biocides in a cellular response to their presence. Various oxidases and reductases have been identified in bacterial tolerance of toxic metals, including arsenate reductase, mercuric reductase, and copper oxidases (see section 8.3.6). Others are catalases and peroxidases, which degrade hydrogen peroxide (see section 8.3.3). Glutathione reductase plays an important role in the reduction of oxidized glutathione (formed on reaction with an oxidant) to form reduced glutathione. Reduced glutathione is an example of a chemical antioxidant that may afford some tolerance at low levels of oxidizing agents by direct oxidant neutralization and by reversing disulfide bond formation in proteins. Other enzymes (like DNA gyrases) are involved in increasing the tolerance by bacteria of heat damage and (like endonucleases, exonucleases, and proteases) repairing biocidal damage to the cell.

8.3.6 Intrinsic Resistance to Heavy Metals

Metal ions play important roles in many cellular functions, including roles in the macromolecular structure, as cofactors in enzymatic reactions, and as cellular catalysts. Relatively low concentrations are required for these essential roles, while increased cellular concentrations have toxic effects, as exemplified by their use as biocides (see section 3.12). The most widely utilized biocides are copper and silver, but intrinsic mechanisms of resistance to various heavy metals in *Bacteria* and *Archaea* have been described. These are considered in more detail, as they represent typical mechanisms of intrinsic (and, in some cases, acquired) resistance to biocides and other antimicrobials. Many of these mechanisms developed to allow microorganisms to survive under restrictive concentrations of heavy metals. However, further investigation of the potentials of these mechanisms to induce cross-resistance to other antimicrobial agents is required.

Five intrinsic mechanisms of heavy-metal tolerance have been described (Fig. 8.9), and examples of each are considered below.

The first mechanism is exclusion from the cell. This can be due to the effects of various surface structures, including the cell wall structure

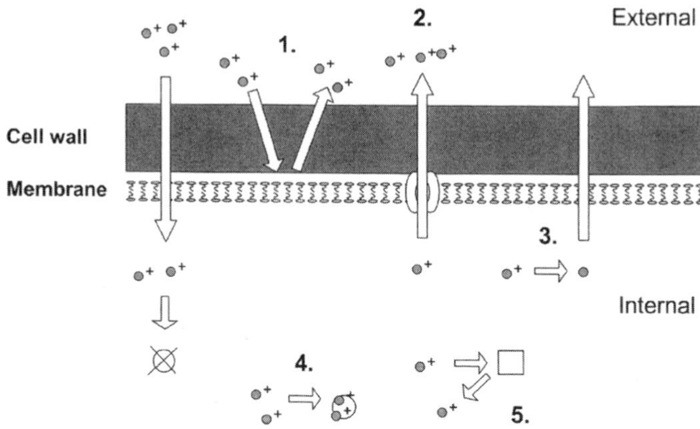

FIGURE 8.9 Intrinsic mechanisms of microbial resistance to heavy metals. The heavy-metal ions can pass through the cell wall and membrane with a subsequent intracellular increase in concentration and inhibitory or biocidal effects (shown on the far left). Mechanisms of resistance are exclusion, due to the presence of various surface structures or more subtle changes in the porin or pump specificity to allow the uptake of essential but not biocidal ions (1); active efflux out of the cell, against a concentration gradient (2); enzymatic conversion of the ion to a different form, which can be released from the cell (3); sequestration, in which macromolecules can absorb the biocide, reducing the available concentration (4); and changes in the structure of the target molecule, reducing its susceptibility to biocidal action (5).

and the presence of capsules, slime layers, or S-layers (see section 8.3.7) that can entrap the metal ions or repel their penetration. More subtle mechanisms have been described for arsenic uptake. Arsenate ions (As^{5+}) can permeate into the periplasmic space or, in gram-negative bacteria, are actively transported into the cell across the outer membrane by the same protein transport mechanism as for phosphate influx. In *E. coli*, the outer membrane porin PhoE mediates this mechanism. Similar transport is mediated across the cell membrane by two mechanisms: the transmembrane Pit protein, which transports both phosphate and arsenate, and the Pst system, which demonstrates greater specificity for phosphate and exclusion of As^{5+}. The Pst system is an inner-membrane ATPase-coupled uptake system induced during phosphate starvation, which demonstrates a link between starvation responses and increased metal resistance. It should also be noted that specific mutations within the Pit gene could also allow greater specificity for phosphates over arsenic as a mechanism of acquired resistance (see section 8.7).

Efflux plays an important role in intrinsic and acquired resistance to heavy-metal ions. In another example of arsenic tolerance in *E. coli*, the chromosomally encoded ArsB protein is a transmembrane efflux pump (ABC type) (see section 8.3.4), using energy to transport arsenic ions against a concentration gradient. In some bacteria, but also described in archaea and yeasts, ArsB-like proteins are coupled with an ATPase (ArsA) that uses ATP hydrolysis as a source of energy for transport; ArsA-associated operons are commonly found to be acquired (plasmid-encoded) mechanisms of resistance. Other acquired mechanisms have been described in bacteria and archaea for a variety of toxic metals, including silver (Ag^{+}), copper (Cu^{2+}), mercury (Hg^{2+}), and lead (Pb^{2+}). As for arsenic efflux, these include PMF- and ATP-driven mechanisms (see section 8.3.4). Specificity of various ATP-driven pump families has been reported for monovalent (e.g., Cu^+ and Ag^+) and divalent (e.g., Hg^{2+}, Zn^{2+}, and Pb^{2+}) ions.

The next mechanism (Fig. 8.9, mechanism 3), involves enzymatic conversion (reduction) of the toxic ion, followed by active or passive expulsion from the cell. Arsenic may be present in two ionic forms, As^{5+} (arsenate) and As^{3+} (arsenite). Arsenate demonstrates intracellular toxicity similar to that of other heavy metals (see section 7.4.5), including As^{5+} replacing phosphate in various metabolic processes, the affinity of As^{3+} for protein thiol groups (thereby disrupting protein structures), and promoting the formation of DNA-DNA and DNA-protein cross-links. ArsC is an arsenate reductase expressed in *E. coli* in response to increased levels of arsenic. The *ars* operon encodes three proteins, ArsC, ArsB (the efflux pump), and ArsR, a regulator protein that controls expression of the operon. ArsC reduces As^{5+} to As^{3+}, which can then be pumped from the cell. This enzyme is also associated with the ArsA-based plasmid-encoded operons described above. Similar arsenate reductases have been described as metal tolerance mechanisms in yeast (*Saccharomyces*) and algae. The reduction of the pentavalent ion to the trivalent ion may seem unusual, considering that As^{3+} is more toxic to the cell than As^{5+}; this appears to be due to the greater specificity for arsenite efflux from the cell. In other cases, including *Pseudomonas* strains and the acidophilic archaea of the genus *Thiomonas,* arsenate oxidases that convert As^{3+} to As^{5+} as a tolerance mechanism have been described; these cases represent interesting mechanisms of bioremediation of environmental arsenic contamination. Further examples of enzymatic conversion have been described for mercury resistance, with the chromosomal or plasmid-mediated expression of mercuric reductases. In this case, ionic mercury (Hg^{2+}) is reduced by the enzyme to its elemental form (Hg), which then volatilizes from the cell. Other enzymes (hydrolases) also play roles in the tolerance of toxic mercuric compounds, causing the hydrolysis and release of the Hg^{2+}, which can then be neutralized.

Two other mechanisms of toxic-metal resistance, which can also be intrinsic or acquired, have been described. Sequestration involves the binding of the metal (known as metallochaperones), thereby reducing access to key intracellular targets. This may simply be due to nonspecific interaction with external proteins or other macromolecules to reduce penetration through the cell wall and/or membrane or by a more specific mechanism. A particular example has been described for copper resistance, including the expression of intracellular, periplasmic, and extracellular copper-binding proteins. CutC is a chromosomally encoded cytoplasmic protein in *E. coli* which appears to bind and transport copper to efflux-associated proteins, although the exact mechanisms of action remain to be elucidated. A similar protein (CopZ) in *Enterococcus* also has a metallochaperone function associated with CopB, an ATPase-associated efflux pump. Similarly, the *P. syringae* plasmid-encoded CopA and CopC are periplasmic proteins that bind Cu^+ and Cu^{2+} to reduce influx into the cytoplasm and proposed transport to the outer membrane efflux pump, CopB; Cu^+ is particularly toxic to the cell, and oxidase activity to the less toxic Cu^{2+} ion has been associated with CopC/CopA in *Pseudomonas* and the periplasmic CueO oxidase in *E. coli*. Finally, particularly in extremophiles (see sections 8.3.9 and 8.3.10), various intracellular proteins that are less sensitive to the effects of toxic metals have been identified. For example, mercury specifically interferes with cellular oxidase systems; in *Thiobacillus* strains, cytochrome *c* oxidases have been shown to be less sensitive to mercury, although the exact mechanism is unknown.

Overall, these resistance mechanisms allow the cell to survive in the presence of inhibitory or microbicidal concentrations of toxic metals. The most efficient appear to be gram-negative bacteria (e.g., *E. coli* can survive up to 4 mM As^{3+} and 1 mM Cu^{2+}) and *Archaea*, including *Acidiphilium* and *Thiobacillus* (up to 30 mM As^{3+} and 10 mM Cu^{2+}).

TABLE 8.6 Protective cell surface structures external to the bacterial cell wall

Structure	Constituents	Examples
S-layer	Protein, glyco-protein	*Bacteria (Bacillus, Geobacillus, Aeromonas)* and *Archaea (Halobacterium)*
Capsule	Polysaccharide, protein	*Bacillus, Acinetobacter, E. coli, Streptococcus, Pseudomonas, Staphylococcus*
Slime layer	Polysaccharide, protein	*Myxococcus, Azotobacter, Staphylococcus, Streptococcus*

8.3.7 Capsule and Slime Layer Formation and S-Layers

In addition to the protective cell wall structure on the external surfaces of bacteria, some bacteria also produce materials on the outside of the cell wall (see section 1.3.4.1). They include S (surface)-layers, capsules, and slime layers (Table 8.6).

Capsules and slime layers are also referred to as glycocalyx structures and generally consist of insoluble polysaccharide materials present on the cell surface. A bacterial capsule is a well-defined layer of polysaccharide that is tightly associated with the cell wall. In some cases, the capsule may also be protein based. In contrast, slime layers are much thinner and easily deformed or removed layers of partially soluble material. A major function of these layers is protection from drying, bacterial viruses, immune systems, and adverse environmental conditions. The exact composition of the glycocalyx varies depending on the bacterial species and its environment, although the main components are polysaccharides. The polysaccharide may consist of a single-sugar polymer or more complex polymers of different sugars. These polysaccharides include the streptococcal dextran capsule, which is enzymatically generated from glucose and allows *Streptococcus mutans* to effectively bind to the surfaces of teeth, while other glycan polysaccharides allow the binding of *Staphylococcus epidermidis* strains to inanimate surfaces. Many proteins and other components, like lipids, are often associated with the glycocalyx. Only in rare cases is the capsule found to be primarily composed of protein, with notable examples being the poly-D-glutamic acid capsule of *Bacillus anthracis* and the polypeptide slime on *S. epidermidis*; in the case of *B. anthracis*, the genes required for capsule formation are actually plasmid based.

The extent to which the presence of a capsule or slime layer contributes to bacterial tolerance of biocides is unknown, but at a minimum it can present a barrier to biocide penetration. An example is the increased resistance to chlorine reported for *Vibrio cholerae*, which expresses an amorphous exopolysaccharide causing cell aggregation ("rugose" morphology) without any loss in pathogenicity.

In nature, *Staphylococcus aureus* may exist as mucoid strains, with the cells surrounded by a slime layer. In a comparison of mucoid and nonmucoid cells, the mucoid cells demonstrated greater resistance to chloroxylenol, QACs, and chlorhexidine but little or no difference with phenols or chlorinated phenols; removal of the slime by washing the cells rendered them sensitive. However, in other investigations with *S. aureus*, no increase in tolerance was observed between capsular and noncapsular strains. A disinfectant-tolerant *Klebsiella* strain has also been linked to the expression of a mucoid capsule. Capsule formation is believed to play an important role in the unique and varied intrinsic tolerance of *Pseudomonas* strains for various biocides, which is further considered in relation to the resistance of microorganisms in biofilms below (see section 8.3.8). Overall, the capsule or slime has a protective role, either as a physical barrier to disinfectant penetration or as a loose layer reacting with or absorbing the biocide molecules. Variations in results are related to greater penetration of some biocides (e.g., phenolics) than others (QACs) and the nature of the capsule or slime, including the specific bacterial strain, stage of growth, and types and extents of polysaccharides or other materials present. It should also be noted that the capsule affords protection to a microorganism by attachment to a surface, which can indirectly protect the target cell. The development of a capsule may also be considered the initial step in the development of a biofilm, which affords greater resistance to the effects of biocides (see section 8.3.8).

S-layers are found in gram-positive and gram-negative bacteria, as well as many *Archaea*. They consist of protein or glycoprotein in a regular crystalline array. The functions of the S-layer are similar to those described for capsules. The specific contribution of the S-layer to biocide tolerance is not known, although in some cases, the S-layer provides resistance to changes in pH, to some enzymes, and to other environmental stresses, suggesting that further protection from biocide damage may be afforded.

8.3.8 Biofilm Development

Vegetative microorganisms, like bacteria and fungi, are often considered planktonic, or "free-growing," cells, but this is certainly not the case in their natural environments, where they associate, multiply, and survive on surfaces or at surface interfaces. Microbial growth may more accurately be considered "biofilms," which are defined as communities of microorganisms (either single or multiple species) developed on or associated with surfaces (Fig. 8.10). These surfaces include solid inanimate surfaces, foods, soft tissues, and any liquid-air or liquid-liquid interfaces. Biofilms can consist of monocultures or mixed cultures either actively growing (like bacteria and fungi) or associated with the community (including viruses and protozoa). Bacterial (gram-positive and gram-negative) and fungal (particularly yeast) biofilms have been described in some detail, and some of the more prevalent microorganisms associ-

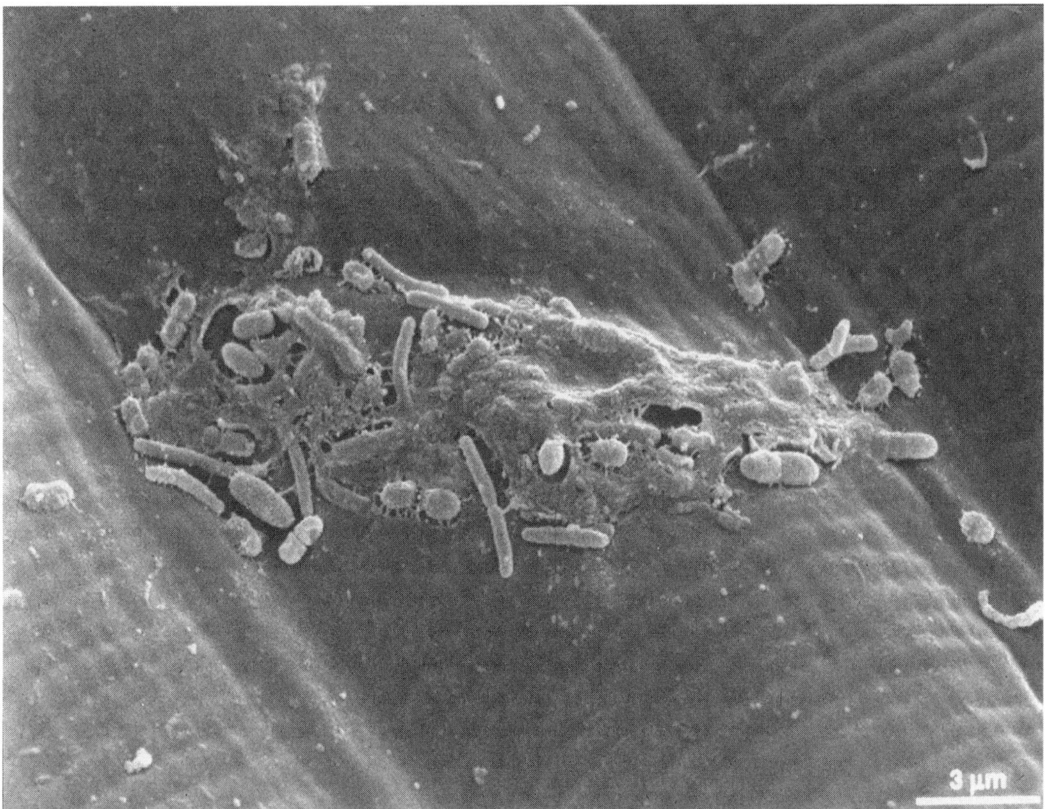

FIGURE 8.10 A *P. aeruginosa* biofilm on a surface. Individual rod-shaped bacteria can be seen developed in a polysaccharide matrix. © William Fett and Peter Cooke (USDA Agricultural Research Service). Courtesy of Peter Cooke and Paul Pierlott (USDA Agricultural Research Service).

TABLE 8.7 Typical bacteria and fungi associated with biofilm formation

Microorganism(s)	Associated biofilms
S. mutans, Streptococcus sobrinus	Cause tooth plaque and periodontal disease; consist of layers of bacteria and polysaccharide growing on the teeth, which can cause damage to the teeth and gums over time; one of the first types of biofilms to be described
P. aeruginosa and other pseudomonads, including *B. cepacia*	Most prevalent biofilms associated with water surfaces/systems, including water pipes, washing machines, and water circulation systems; often associated with industrial biofouling (including corrosion and clogging) and nosocomial infections (related to devices like implants, washer-disinfectors, and contaminated water lines). *P. aeruginosa* also forms biofilms in the lungs of patients with cystic fibrosis, leading to persistent infections.
L. pneumophila	Legionnaires' disease associated with contaminated aerosolized moisture from air and heat/cooling water distribution systems
S. aureus, S. epidermidis	Skin and device-related infections
M. fortuitum, M. chelonae	Biofouling and water-borne infections or "pseudo" infections (e.g., misdiagnosed as pathogenic mycobacteria)
Propionibacterium acnes	Often considered the cause of acne, a persistent skin infection, particularly in young adults
Deinococcus geothermalis	Biofouling of paper machines, impairing operation and causing product defects
C. albicans	Most prevalent fungal biofilms; has been reported in device-related infections and root canal or endodontic infections

ated with problematic biofilms are shown in Table 8.7.

Biofilms are important for several reasons, notably due to their association with biocorrosion, biofouling, and reduced water quality and their acting as foci for the contamination of products such as foods, devices, waterlines, and manufactured drugs. The control of biofilm development and proliferation is therefore an important clinical and industrial challenge. In other cases, biofilms may be beneficial, for example, in the intestine, where various associated microorganisms play protective (preventing the invasion of pathogenic organisms) and nutritional (producing some amino acids and vitamins) roles.

The formation of a biofilm may be considered to go through a series of stages (Fig. 8.11). The initial step is the association of the microorganism with the surface (adsorption). Individual bacteria have been found to use a variety of mechanisms to aid in preliminary attachment to a surface, including electrostatic attraction, physical forces (such as van der Waals forces), fimbriae, pili, and surface capsules or slime layers (see section 8.3.7). The presence of carbohydrate or other organic molecules on a given surface, which is known as "conditioning," can provide sites for adhesion and may enhance these mechanisms. In some bacteria, an initial reversible attachment to the surface is observed, which develops into a more permanent adsorption, for example, due to production of and affinity with capsules. The adsorbed cells begin to multiply and produce various extracellular polymeric materials, particularly various polysaccharides of mannose, glucose, *N*-acetylglucosamine, and other sugars. The associated polysaccharide assists in maintaining the cells in close contact and acts to trap nutrients from the environment, allowing cell metabolism and division. As the biofilm continues to develop, the individual cells within the community are at various stages of growth and metabolism in response to their environment. For example, facultative bacteria require less oxygen and fewer nutrients, which are available in the depths of the biofilm with cells growing anaerobically in comparison to the surface layers, where cells grow aerobically. These stresses surrounding the cell are sensed by the microorganism, causing the initiation of the various

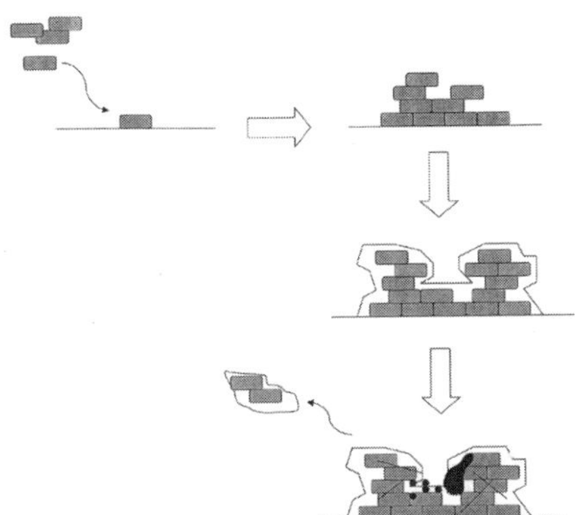

FIGURE 8.11 The development of a biofilm. Initial attachment (adsorption) of a microorganism may be reversible or permanent, leading to profileration and extracellular-polysaccharide production. This matrix develops over time, allowing the entrapment of nutrients and other microorganisms, which can also proliferate to produce a mature biofilm. Sections of the biofilm can slough off over time, bind to other surfaces, and subsequently develop further biofilms.

responses described in section 8.3.3. There is also some evidence of complex interactions between cells; for example, "quorum sensing" as a response to population density within a bacterial community has been described in *S. aureus* and *P. aeruginosa*. The extracellular matrix development plays an important role in the protection of the cells from various environmental challenges, including penetration by and contact with biocides and biocidal processes. In most cases, the matrix is predominantly composed of polysaccharide and water, with various other associated proteins (including enzymes) and organic and inorganic materials that are excreted from the cells or trapped from the environment. This also acts as a trap for various other microorganisms (including bacteria, fungi, viruses, protozoa, and algae), many of which also proliferate within the matrix. Therefore, the mature biofilm can vary considerably depending on the environment, but clearly, it will be a complex and cooperative interaction. Sections of the biofilm can also slough off, with subsequent binding to other surfaces and further biofilm formation (Fig. 8.11).

Biofilms present a significant challenge to disinfection and sterilization processes, as well as to the activities of other chemical antimicrobial agents. Several factors can account for the reduced sensitivity of bacteria and other microorganisms within a biofilm (Table 8.8).

Probably the major factor in biofilm resistance is reduced access to the cells within the biofilm. It is known that binding to a surface alone affords some protection, as planktonic cells are more sensitive to the effects of biocides than those on a surface (see section 1.4.2.2); this may be partially due to the surface itself interfering with the biocide or to bacteria being shielded from these effects within various microscopic imperfections at the surface. More significantly, the biofilm consists of cells at various depths within the thick polysaccharide matrix that the biocide needs to penetrate to elicit its effects. The biocide attacks the various

TABLE 8.8 Biofilms and microbial response to antimicrobial agents

Mechanism of resistance associated with biofilms	Comment
Exclusion or reduced access of biocide to underlying cell	Depends on (i) nature of biocide or biocidal process, (ii) nature of surface, (iii) binding capacity and reaction of glycocalyx to biocide, and (iv) rate of growth of biofilm relative to diffusion rate of biocide
Sensitivity of individual cell	Associated with (i) stress responses, (ii) growth rate/phase, and (iii) metabolic activity
Increased production of degradative enzymes and other neutralizing agents	Enzymes decrease the available concentration of some biocides. Neutralizing agents can include organic and inorganic materials.
Increased genetic exchange between or mutations within cells	Close interaction between cells may enhance exchange of genetic and associated acquired tolerance of biocides.

polysaccharides and proteins of the biofilm, as they are often themselves key targets, and this reduces the actual concentration available for action against the microorganism. Organic and inorganic components of the biofilm also directly neutralize the activities of biocides. An example is the presence of enzymes, like peroxidases and catalases, that reduce the attacking concentration of biocides such as hydrogen peroxide (see section 8.3.3). The direct chemical interaction between the disinfectant and the biofilm itself is also important. Cross-linking agents (like aldehydes) may allow the formation of polymeric surface barriers that can inhibit penetration of the biocide to bacteria deeper within the biofilm; in contrast, other biocides (like peracetic acid and other oxidizing agents) may allow degradation of the biofilm structure and its removal from the surface and therefore greater penetration. As penetration can be reduced within a biofilm, many of the other intrinsic resistance mechanisms may play greater roles in protecting the cell at lower concentrations of the biocide. These include the various responses to environmental stress (see section 8.3.3), a decreased growth rate (see section 8.3.1), and allowing the cells time to develop into their respective dormant stages (see section 8.3.11). Bacteria in different parts of a biofilm have been shown to experience different nutrient environments, so that their physiological properties are affected. Slowly growing bacteria are known to be less sensitive than more actively metabolizing cells. Similarly, the presence of biocides can induce cells to increase the production of polysaccharide and other agents as defense mechanisms.

In most cases, bacteria removed from a biofilm, isolated, and recultured under laboratory conditions are generally no more resistant than the original planktonic cells of that species; however, it has been suggested that under biofilm growth conditions, the microorganism can mutate or acquire extrinsic genetic material to allow greater resistance to biocides and antibiotics (as acquired resistance mechanisms) (see section 8.7). These mechanisms can be retained by the bacteria on subculturing. For this reason, it is often suggested (particularly in industrial applications) that periodic rotation of different disinfectant types may be more efficient for microbial control, e.g., routine biocidal treatment with frequent temperature disinfection or rotation of biocidal treatments with different modes of action. There is mixed evidence on the advantages of such practices.

Biofilms are a constant challenge to control in manufacturing, commercial, health care, and food-processing facilities (Table 8.7). Several instances of the contamination of antiseptic or disinfectant solutions by bacteria are known, although when subcultured, the bacteria appear to be rapidly sensitive to the preparations. Examples are the prolonged survival of *Serratia marcescens* in 2% chlorhexidine solutions and of *Burkholderia cepacia* in chlorhexidine and contamination of iodophor antiseptics with *Pseudomonas*. All of these cases were attributed to the embedding of these organisms within thick biofilm matrices that adhered to the walls of storage containers or were associated with other interfaces within a formulated product, thereby allowing the bacteria to survive. In the *Pseudomonas* investigation, the source of the biofilm was found to be the interior surfaces of polyvinyl chloride pipes used during the manufacture of providone-iodine antiseptics. Pseudomonads and other gram-negative bacteria are often cited as causes of industrial water pipe contamination, which over time can lead to the corrosion of surfaces and cross-contamination of various manufactured products. Filters are particularly sensitive to biofilm proliferation, as by their nature, they trap various microorganisms and nutrients, allowing their proliferation over time. In some extreme cases, bacteria have been shown to be capable of "growing through" the filter, allowing downstream contamination; theoretically, this may be due to gradual damage to the filter by chemicals or the biofilm itself, reducing its retentive capabilities. For this reason, the integrity of filters should be periodically verified and they should be frequently disinfected (by biocides or heat) during use (see section 2.5). A further example of biofilm contamination is with *Legionella pneumophila*, which is often found in hospital and commercial water distribution systems and cooling towers. Chlorination, in combination with continuous heating (60°C) of incoming water, is usually the most appropriate disinfection measure; however, because of biofilm production, the contaminating organisms are often less susceptible to this treatment than expected. Incidences of biofilm contamination of various medical devices, particularly indwelling devices, have been well described. Indwelling devices, including contact lenses (on the eyes), intravenous or urinary catheters, and various prosthetic devices, are placed in or on the body for a variety of applications. Many of these devices are provided sterile but can become contaminated by contact with the skin (from the patient during insertion or handling) or with other surfaces or by aerosolization. Contamination can lead to overgrowth, biofilm formation, and protection of the microorganisms from the host's immune system. Contamination and biofilm formation on devices with gram-positive bacteria (*Staphylococcus* and *Enterococcus* spp.), gram-negative bacteria (*Escherichia* and *Pseudomonas* spp.), and fungal (*Candida* spp.) pathogens have been reported. These biofilms invariably resist the antimicrobial effects of integrated or applied biocides and antibiotics used to control bacterial growth; further, the release of high concentrations of endotoxins from gram-negative bacterial biofilms can also lead to further complications and, potentially, death. A further consideration is multiple-use surgical or investigational devices, which require reprocessing (cleaning, disinfection, and/or sterilization) between uses. Recent advances in noninvasive procedures (including minimally invasive surgery and flexible-endoscope interventions) offer significant advantages but pose cleaning and disinfection challenges. Many of these devices are designed with lumens (to allow access during surgery), which can be difficult to clean and disinfect, and can be made of heat-sensitive materials (e.g, flexible endoscopes). Biofilm or pseudobiofilm contamination is often cited as a cause of infections related to these devices, primarily due to inadequate reprocessing and/or recontamination following reprocessing. Inadequate reprocessing can be due to the device design restricting penetration of cleaning and disinfection processes or inadequate removal or disinfection of patient material, allowing subsequent overgrowth of microorganisms. Nosocomial outbreaks due to a variety of microorganisms, like *P. aeruginosa, Mycobacterium chelonae, Mycobacterium tuberculosis,* human immunodeficiency virus, and hepatitis C virus, underscore the importance of biofilm formation in the contamination of flexible fiberoptic scopes. These outbreaks were associated with inadequate cleaning of endoscopes, which compromised subsequent disinfection with high-level disinfectants and allowed bacterial overgrowth. The use of cross-linking agents, like glutaraldehyde, can cause a buildup of insoluble residues and associated microorganisms on scopes and in automated reprocessing machines. Recontamination is a particular concern due to rinsing of devices with water after chemical disinfection. Biofilm formation within the reprocessing machine or in the incoming water lines can recontaminate the device and allow biofilm development during subsequent storage.

The optimum treatment against biofilms is a continuous process that includes an antimicrobial component and physical disruption, with removal of the extracellular matrix. For this reason, liquid oxidizing agents are used, due to their structure-disrupting mode of action (see section 7.4.2). Chlorine, as sodium hypochlorite, is particularly used for this purpose, but at much higher concentrations than those required for normal biocidal activity. Similar effects have been shown for other oxidizing agents, including ozone, chlorine dioxide, and peracetic acid, although the activities of these biocides can be dramatically influenced by various formulation effects. Nonoxidizing agents that are often recommended include the QACs, due to their surfactant, physical removal, and cleaning activities. Other biocides are less attractive due to their modes of action. Examples are aldehydes and heat, which can allow entrapment of viable bacteria within the biofilm and, by fixing material on a surface, provide enhanced sites for bacterial attachment. Despite this, successful biofilm control depends on the physical and chemical properties of the biocide, its formulation, and the field of application; for example, glutaraldehyde has been used for biofilm control in the oil industry. In the pharmaceutical industry, where the quality of water is maintained at a high standard (e.g., water-for-injection), the water is kept at high temperatures (generally ≥80°C), which significantly decreases (if it does not remove) the risk of bacterial and fungal survival and proliferation within these systems. Other physical methods, like nonionizing radiation (particularly UV treatment), reduce or remove microbial contamination within the water stream only at the site of application, allowing biofilm growth up- or downstream of the light source. Overall, the frequent use of antimicrobial processes is only one consideration in the control of biofilms. Other control mechanisms include the integration or generation of biocides and/or antibiotics on surfaces to prevent or reduce attachment, the use of materials with reduced surface attachment properties (e.g., as claimed for Teflon), nutrient restriction, and design of water systems (e.g., ensuring that there is no standing water or inaccessible areas, like dead legs or crevices).

8.3.9 Bacteria with Extreme Intrinsic Resistance

Many of the intrinsic mechanisms of resistance discussed above allow some survival of bacteria under various adverse conditions, although in most cases, the bacterial cells are still considered relatively sensitive to biocides at typical concentrations and/or under typical conditions. There are a number of notable exceptions that demonstrate more extreme intrinsic resistance to various adverse conditions. Examples of these are given in Table 8.9.

The extremophiles, including thermophiles (which grow under different temperature extremes) and acidophiles (which grow in acidic environments) are considered in section 8.3.10. They have been isolated from various extreme environments, although it should be noted that these bacteria have unique growth requirements that allow them to grow under what we may consider "extreme" conditions (e.g., high or low temperature and high or low pH). These conditions are often required for their normal growth and survival. Unlike the extremophiles, some bacterial species (including *Geobacillus, Bacillus*, and *Clostridium*) optimally grow under conditions similar to those for many other bacteria; however, under adverse conditions, they develop into dormant spores, which are protected from the environment until suitable conditions are available for normal vegetative growth. These spores demonstrate tremendous intrinsic resistance to physical and chemical disinfection and sterilization processes and are discussed in detail, along with other dormancy mechanisms, in section 8.3.11.

Deinococcus species have dramatic intrinsic resistance to radiation (including ionizing and

TABLE 8.9 Examples of known extreme resistance to biocides and biocidal processes

Bacteria	Resistance	Mechanisms of resistance
Thermophiles, including *Thermococcus* and *Pyrococcus*	Heat and salt conditions	Multiple, including unique cell wall structures, heat-resistant proteins and lipids/lipid membranes, and protein/DNA protective/repair mechanisms
Acidophiles, including *Thiobacillus* and *Thermoplasma*	Acids and heat (some)	Multiple, including unique cell wall structures and active efflux and exclusion methods
Bacterial endospores, including *Geobacillus* and *Clostridium*	Heat, biocides (including gases and liquids), radiation, desiccation	Dormant-spore production with various intrinsic resistance mechanisms
Deinococcus	Radiation, oxidizing agents, and desiccation	Multiple, including efficient repair mechanisms and unique cell wall structure

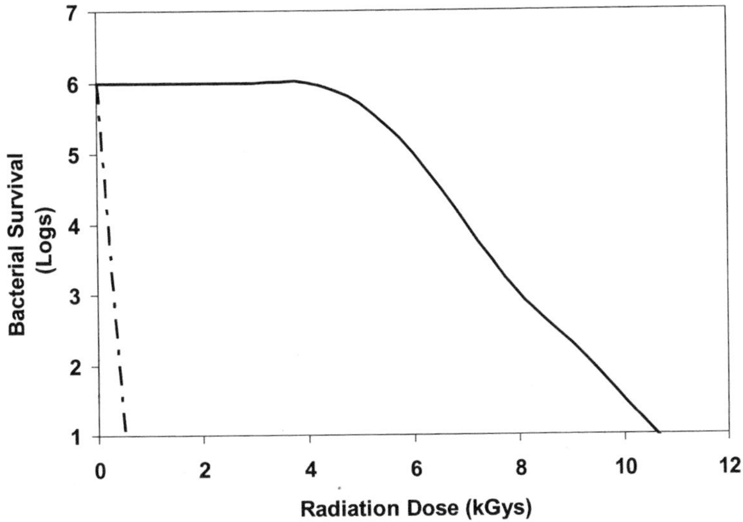

FIGURE 8.12 An example of *D. radiodurans* survival of radiation. The survival of *D. radiodurans* (solid line) is compared to that of a typical radiation-sensitive bacterial strain (dotted line) when exposed to increasing doses of γ-irradiation (measured in kilograys) (see section 5.4).

nonionizing radiation) (see section 2.4), even in comparison to bacterial spores (Fig. 8.12). *Deinococcus radiodurans* was first identified in canned meat products that had been irradiated. The microorganisms were subsequently found to survive typical disinfection and sterilization doses of γ-irradiation, even up to 5- to 20-kGy doses. These results were considered unusual, since *D. radiodurans* and other deinococcal isolates were shown to be nonsporulating, gram-positive, nonmobile, aerobic bacteria (Fig. 8.13). Further radiation-resistant strains, classified as *Deinobacter* species, were similar to *Deinococcus* but were found to be gram-negative bacteria.

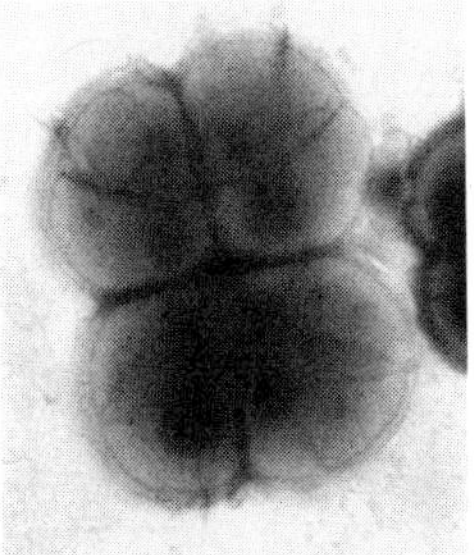

FIGURE 8.13 Micrograph of *D. radiodurans* cells in a typical tetrad formation.

These bacteria are widely distributed in the environment and have been isolated from soil and dust and in association with nuclear waste.

In addition to radiation resistance, strains have also been shown to be resistant to oxidative damage (e.g., the effects of oxidizing agents) and dehydration. In these cases, damage to bacterial DNA is considered to be a major part of the modes of action of the agents. One of the key mechanisms of resistance in *Deinococcus* is efficient DNA repair activity. Although many bacteria and fungi have been shown to tolerate minor DNA damage by the induction of response mechanisms (like the SOS response [see section 8.3.3]), *Deinococcus* species are capable of tolerating a significantly greater extent of DNA strand breakage (in the case of ionizing radiation) and the presence of other photoproducts (like thymine and other base dimers on exposure to UV light) (see section 7.4.4). Similar to other bacterial stress responses, various repair mechanisms are induced (mediated by a RecA homologue [see section 8.3.3]), including increased DNA repair and recombination, DNA replication, cell wall metabolism, and other increases in metabolic functions. Multiple

DNA lesions are efficiently repaired within 12 to 24 h following radiation exposure by two major processes: single-strand annealing and homologous recombination. During recombination, the RecA protein facilitates the repair of double-strand DNA breaks by cutting out a section of the molecule and replacing it with a similar section of DNA. This procedure is further enhanced in radiation-resistant strains by the presence of multiple (sometimes 4 to 10) copies of the bacterial genome; alignment of these copies allows the efficient recovery of a viable genome. Other significant defense mechanisms have been identified. *D. radiodurans* has a typical red colony color due to the presence of carotenoid pigments that act as free-radical scavengers and can protect the cell from hydroxyl radicals, which are formed on contact with various oxidizing agents. In addition, high levels of defense enzymes, like catalase and superoxide dismutase, confer some protection against biocides, like ozone and hydrogen peroxide (see section 8.3.3). Finally, the deinococcal cell wall structure is considered unique among gram-positive bacteria (see section 1.3.4.1). The cell wall has unusual thickness (50 to 60 nm) and consists of a substantial inner layer of peptidoglycan, an outer membrane, and an external S-layer, which itself varies in thickness. The peptidoglycan structure is similar to that of other gram-positive bacteria but has the amino acid ornithine instead of diaminopimelic acid in the various peptide cross-linkages. The outer membrane is a lipid bilayer but does not contain LPS, as in gram-negative bacteria; overall differences in phospholipid and fatty acid profiles have also been reported, which may also contribute to the intrinsic resistance. Although less studied, strains of *Deinobacter* appear to have a cell wall structure similar to that of *Deinococcus* but stain gram negative, presumably due to a thinner peptidoglycan layer.

8.3.10 Extremophiles

Microorganisms are found in a number of diverse environments and vary considerably in their growth requirements. Research into various "extremophiles" has identified unique and multiple intrinsic mechanisms of resistance or tolerance of extreme conditions. The term "extremophilic" is taken from the original Greek word *philein*, "to love," and can be further subdivided into descriptive groups based on the major requirement(s) for growth: temperature, pH, water or salt concentration, and oxygen. For example, thermophiles (or "thermophilic microorganisms") can survive at high temperatures (with many archaea described as hyperthermophiles, which multiply under even more extreme temperature conditions), while their opposites, psychrophiles, grow in cold environments, halophiles survive extreme salt conditions, and acido- or alkaliphiles are found in low- or high-pH environments. It should be noted that these growth conditions are generally not "extreme" for the actual microorganism and in many cases are actually required for growth. For example the hyperthermophilic *Pyrolobus fumarii* cannot grow at temperatures lower than 85°C.

The optimum temperatures for microbial growth have been found to vary considerably, particularly with fungi, bacteria, and archaea. The organisms can be grouped into three temperature ranges: psychrophiles (which grow optimally at low temperatures), mesophiles (which grow within an ambient- or mid-temperature range), and thermophiles (which grow preferably at high temperatures) (Fig. 8.14).

Within the mesophilic group, many bacteria and fungi can tolerate lower or higher temperatures within a given range but show slower metabolism at lower temperatures and specific protective responses, like the heat shock response (see section 8.3.3), at higher temperatures. These varied responses allow some protection and survival for the cells under less-than-optimal temperature conditions. The psychrophiles and thermophiles are dramatically different in that they have modified microbial structures and processes that allow them to thrive under cold or hot growth conditions. Overall, the mechanisms of heat and cold tolerance are similar yet distinct. In particular, they include specific protein-enzyme and lipid structures that are more tolerant of specific

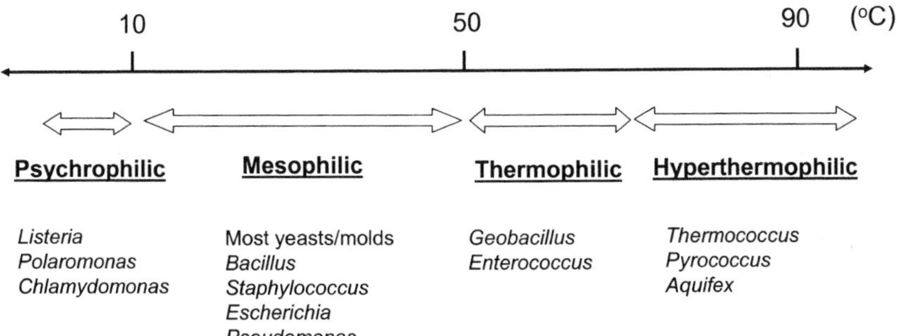

FIGURE 8.14 Microbial growth and optimum temperature conditions. Examples of various vegetative microorganisms are shown, although the sensitivities of specific species to heat vary. *Geobacillus* spores may be considered hyperthermophilic but are dormant (see section 8.3.11).

growth conditions. Mesophilic enzymes have significantly less activity at lower temperatures and are denatured at higher temperatures (see section 7.4.4). In psychrophiles, many of the key metabolic enzymes and structural proteins show a greater proportion of α-helix secondary structure and increased polar (hydrophilic) amino acids (with decreased hydrophobic residues), which appear to allow proteins greater flexibility at lower temperatures; however, the exact contributions of protein primary and secondary structures to cold tolerance are not known. A further difference is the increased occurrence of unsaturated fatty acids, particularly in the cell membrane, which provide greater fluidity than typical saturated fatty acids at lower temperatures. There is also a higher concentration of polyunsaturated long-chain lipids in the cytoplasm. The opposite effects are observed in thermophiles. Proteins are found to have greater heat stability due to increased chemical (ionic) bonds between amino acid residues in their secondary and tertiary structures and to some minor changes in primary structure (e.g., a lower proportion of glycine residues), which resist unfolding. A further difference is the presence of various proteins or other molecules that protect the proteins from heat inactivation; they include chaperones (which are discussed under heat shock responses in section 8.3.3) and sugars, like diglycerol phosphate and manosylglycerate. There are also many repair or protective mechanisms to reduce the effects of heat on DNA, including DNA gyrases that increase the supercoiling and DNA-binding proteins. In contrast to the lipids prevalent in psychrophiles, thermophiles have a larger proportion of saturated fatty acids, which allow greater membrane stability and resistance to phospholipid bilayer separation. In some hyperthermophiles among the *Archaea*, heat-resistant membrane lipids include monolayers of long-chain fatty acids that are more resistant to disruption; many thermophilic archaea are also acidophiles, growing at low pH ranges (pH 1 to 5).

Microorganisms can also be separated on the basis of their pH requirements or tolerance (Fig. 8.15). The concentration of hydrogen ions (H^+) in solution is expressed as pH, which is a logarithmic scale ranging from acidic through neutral to basic, or alkaline, conditions. Microorganisms have been isolated at the extremes of this range, from acidophiles that can tolerate low-pH conditions to alkaliphiles that prefer high-pH conditions. It should be noted that although these extreme pHs can be tolerated and even required for growth, cells have developed mechanisms to maintain the internal cytoplasm close to neutral pH, allowing the various metabolic functions. This is primarily maintained by efficient membrane-associated efflux pumps that pump hydrogen ions in either direction across the membrane to maintain internal neutral conditions (see section 8.3.4). Acidophiles, which generally survive at pH

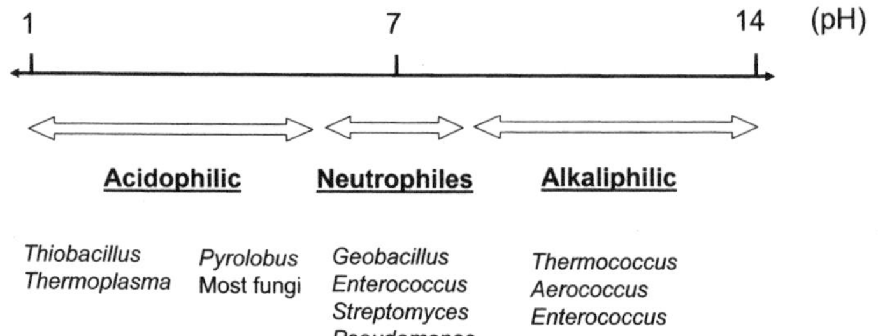

FIGURE 8.15 Microbial growth and optimum pH conditions. Examples of various microorganisms are shown, although the sensitivities of specific species to pH vary.

levels less than 5, pump H^+ ions out of the cell at a constant high rate to maintain internal pH levels between 6.5 and 7. The internal pH levels in alkaliphiles are generally within the pH 7 to 8 range and are maintained by pumping H^+ into the cytoplasm. A well-studied acid-tolerant bacterium is *Helicobacter pylori*, which can survive in the stomach (pH ~1 to 2) and is the causative agent of peptic ulcers. *H. pylori* is actually a neutrophilic organism, but a variety of acid-tolerating mechanisms have been identified. An interesting mechanism was identified in studies of dependence on the presence of urea for growth at pH <4. Urea is transported into the gram-negative periplasm under acidic conditions, where the presence of a urease causes the formation of NH_3, allowing neutralization of the periplasm, the generation of a PMF, and active efflux of H^+ from the cell. Further, an exclusion mechanism involving specific inner and outer membrane proteins of *H. pylori* that reduce the overall proton permeability of the cell has been described. Many acidophiles also present tolerance to various toxic heavy metals, which can be due to an intrinsic (see section 8.3.6) and/or acquired (see section 8.7) resistance mechanism.

Similar effects have been described in the tolerance of varying salt concentrations by some microorganisms; an example of tolerances to sodium chloride (NaCl) is shown in Fig. 8.16. The concentration of salt surrounding a microorganism affects its survival due to the diffusion of water into or out of the cell. Water is required for metabolism, but an increase in cytoplasmic water content can lead to cell lysis, and equally, a loss of water can lead to loss of cell viability. The diffusion of water naturally occurs from an area of low solute (or salt) concentration to a high concentration in a process known as osmosis. These effects have been studied to some extent in bacteria and fungi, with some isolates (known as nonhalophilic) growing under high-water-activity (or low-solute) conditions and others (halophiles) requiring much lower water (and therefore higher solute) activity for growth. In some cases, extreme halophiles that require a concentration of >10% NaCl have been described, including the *Halobacterium* archaea. A wide range of organisms also grow within an intermediate salt range and are known as halotolerant; for example, *Vibrio* species can survive in seawater (~3% salt) (Fig. 8.16).

Various adaptations in *Bacteria* and *Archaea* that allow them to survive osmotic effects have been described. Intracellular water loss in bacteria can be controlled by increasing the cytoplasmic salt (or solute) concentration to inhibit the loss of intracellular water, which effectively reduces the osmotic effect. This is achieved by a combination of the activity of influx pumps (to pump inorganic ions, like K^+, into the cell) and by the synthesis of intracellular organic solutes, which are compatible with metabolic processes (including glycerol, glutamate, and amino acids). An example has been described in *S. aureus* strains, which can grow in up to ~7.5% NaCl by increasing the internal concentration of proline (an amino acid) as a solute. Other mechanisms have been studied in extreme halophiles. Cytoplasmic proteins have high levels of acidic amino acids, with much lower levels of basic and hydrophobic residues; these pro-

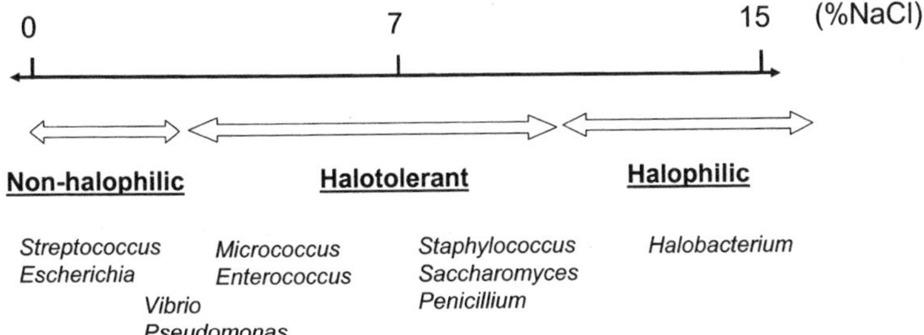

FIGURE 8.16 Microbial growth and optimum salt conditions. Examples of various microorganisms are given, although the sensitivities of specific species to salt concentrations vary.

teins appear to be less sensitive to high concentrations of salts. Exclusion is also a key mechanism. *Halobacterium* spp. and other halophiles among the *Archaea* have unique cell wall structures in comparison to bacteria. They include thick polysaccharide or protein or glycoprotein cell walls (instead of the bacterial peptidoglycan) and paracrystalline S-layers (see section 8.3.7), which appear to assist in preventing water loss to the environment. *Halobacterium*, in particular, has a predominantly glycoprotein-based cell wall (also with a high proportion of acidic amino acids), which is further stabilized by the presence of a high concentration of Na^+.

Another example of microbial survival under extreme conditions is different oxygen requirements. Microorganisms can be classified based on their requirements for oxygen for growth. Aerobic organisms require oxygen at the typical concentrations in air (~21%), while anaerobic organisms require the absence of oxygen for growth. Within these extremes are bacteria that specifically require reduced oxygen levels (<20%, microaerophilic) or that can grow under aerobic and anaerobic conditions (facultative) and those anaerobes that can tolerate the presence of oxygen but do not use it (aerotolerant anaerobes). These requirements reflect differences in metabolic activity. Aerobes metabolize by using oxygen in aerobic respiration, while anaerobes metabolize by fermentation, or anerobic respiration. In some cases, for example, with *Clostridium*, the presence of oxygen can lead to cell death that may be linked to the lack of protective response mechanisms against active oxygen species in these bacteria (see sections 8.3.4 and 8.3.5). With the exception that strict anaerobes may be more sensitive to the effects of peroxgyens and other forms of oxygen, the various oxygen requirements for growth do not appear to affect sensitivity to biocides.

8.3.11 Dormancy

Bacteria display a variety of adaptive processes that allow them to survive limiting environmental conditions, including the presence of biocides and restricted nutrient availability. In some cases, they become dormant, with very low levels of metabolism; examples are pathogenic *Mycobacterium* species, which can remain dormant within the body, and *Vibrio* species, which can remain dormant in water. The dormant forms may be less sensitive to various biocides due to lower metabolic rates, but overall, they have not been particularly investigated. The most dramatic dormant adaptation is displayed by certain gram-positive bacteria known generally as the gram-positive endospore-forming rods and cocci (see section 1.3.4.1). Examples of bacteria in this group include *Geobacillus, Bacillus*, and *Clostridium* spp., with examples given in Table 8.10; they are widely isolated from various environments, and many are known pathogens (primarily due to the production of toxins) (see section 1.3.7).

These bacteria undergo a remarkable change in their normal vegetative growth processes in response to environmental stress to produce dormant and resilient forms of themselves,

TABLE 8.10 Spore-forming bacteria and their significance

Bacterium	Significance
Geobacillus	Aerobic, gram-positive rods; thermophilic; previously defined under the genus *Bacillus*
G. stearothermophilus	Regarded as the microorganism most resistant to steam and other sterilization processes; used to test the efficacies of these processes, for example, in biological indicators
Bacillus	Aerobic, gram-positive rods; generally mesophilic; diverse species; common environmental contaminants
B. anthracis	Has been used as a bioterrorism agent; causative agent in anthrax, a disease of animals and humans
B. atrophaeus	Regarded as the microorganism most resistant to ethylene oxide and other sterilization processes; therefore, used to test the efficacy of these processes, for example, in biological indicators; formerly known as *B. subtilis* var. *niger*
B. cereus	Causative agent of food poisoning
Clostridium	Anaerobic, gram-positive rods
C. difficile	A common cause of institution-related diarrhea
C. perfringens	Used as a test organism to verify the sporicidal efficacies of biocides in the United States; also a known wound contaminant
C. tetani	Causative agent of tetanus; linked to deep-wound infections
C. botulinum	Causative agent of botulism, a food poisoning disease

known as bacterial spores or "endospores." They are referred to as endospores because they are developed within the "mother" cell in a process known as sporulation (Fig. 8.17).

The sporulation process has been particularly well studied in *Bacillus subtilis* and involves a coordinated adaptation in the transcription and translation machinery of a cell to become dedicated to the development of an endospore. The resulting endospores are invariably the most resistant of all types of bacteria, if not all microorganisms, to antiseptics, disinfectants, and sterilants. For this reason, they are used in the development and routine monitoring of

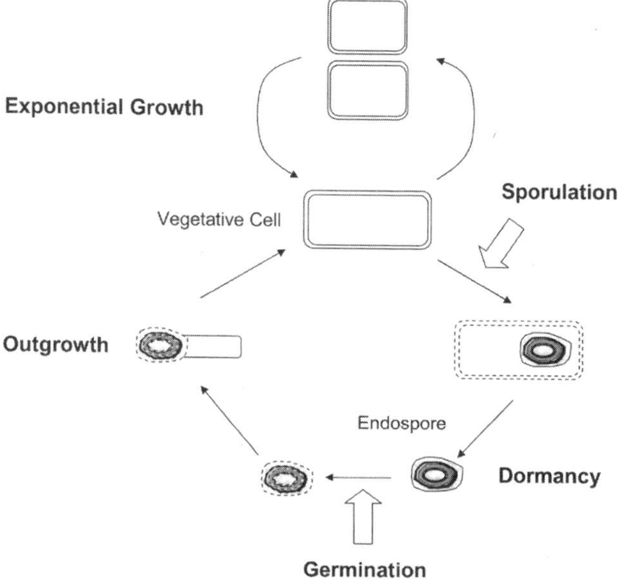

FIGURE 8.17 The basic life cycle of gram-positive endospore-forming rods. The vegetative growth of the bacteria is limited due to the reduction of essential nutrients (for example, carbon or nitrogen sources) or other environmental factors, causing the initiation of the sporulation cascade, death of the mother cell, and release of the dormant spore. Under the right environmental conditions, conducive to bacterial growth, the spore becomes activated, germinates, and grows out to produce a viable vegetative bacterial cell, which resumes metabolism and multiplication.

TABLE 8.11 Sporistatic and sporicidal concentrations of liquid biocides[a]

Biocide	Concn (mg/liter)	
	Sporistatic	Sporicidal
Benzalkonium chloride	5	—[b]
Chlorhexidine	1	—
Ethanol	700	—
Sodium hypochlorite	1	100
Phenol	500	—
Hydrogen peroxide	500	50,000
Peracetic acid	10	100
Glutaraldehyde	50	10,000
Formaldehyde	500	20,000

[a]Concentrations are approximate and vary depending on the bacterial-endospore type and test conditions. All biocides were tested as suspensions in water.

[b]—, little or no sporicidal activity has been reported at maximum solubility, but this can vary depending on the endospores tested.

various sterilization processes (see section 1.4.2.3). Many biocides are bacteriostatic or even bactericidal at low concentrations for nonsporulating bacteria, including the vegetative forms of *Bacillus* and *Clostridium* species, but high concentrations and/or temperatures with longer contact times are necessary to achieve a sporicidal effect (e.g., with oxidizing agents, aldehydes, and steam) (Table 8.11).

In contrast, even high concentrations of alcohol, phenolics, QACs, and chlorhexidine lack any appreciable sporicidal effect, although in some cases, effects may be achieved when these compounds are used at elevated temperatures or in synergy with other biocides. Endospores, depending on the species, also show varying abilities to survive high temperatures (particularly the thermophilic *Geobacillus* species) and drying, or desiccation; they can therefore survive in the environment for up to many years, depending on the genus, species, and environmental conditions. In spite of this, under the right environmental conditions for growth, including temperature and presence of nutrients, the spore can become activated and germinate (Fig. 8.17). The germination process is quite rapid and irreversible and is the first indication of the dormant spore resuming metabolism. During this stage, the protective spore coats are broken, with release of the spore core contents and breakdown of proteins intrinsic and unique to the spore core (the small acid-soluble spore proteins [SASPs] [see below]). The germinated spores then move on to a further regeneration stage, known as outgrowth. During this stage, water is reabsorbed into the spore and the normal cellular processes (including protein, lipid, carbohydrate, and nucleic acid synthesis and their respective activities) resume, allowing the regeneration of a vegetative cell and normal growth and proliferation.

A closer understanding of endospore structure is of interest in understanding their resilience in the environment and intrinsic resistance to biocides. A so-called "typical" endospore has a complex structure in comparison to the parent vegetative cell, consisting of an inner spore core that is surrounded by protective spore layers (Fig. 8.18).

The innermost part of the endospore is the spore core (or "protoplast"), which, similar to the mother cell cytoplasm, contains the essential components for viability but differs substantially in its constituents (Table 8.12).

The core, in particular, contains DNA, some RNAs, acidic proteins, and metal ions but demonstrates little or no metabolic activity. The first major difference is the degree of hydration. A typical endospore contains ≤30% of the normal water concentration in the vegetative cell. This limits any macromolecular activity but also acts as a barrier to the penetration of liquids and gases, as well as being a poor conductor of heat, thereby protecting the nucleic acid from damage. The spore core contents are further protected by the presence of dipicolinic acid (DPA), which is associated with a high concentration of calcium ions, overall comprising approximately 10% of the dry weight of the endospore. The Ca-DPA (calcium dipicolinate) appears to protect the spore core from heat and chemicals by stabilization of the bacterial DNA. In addition to calcium, other metals that may also play roles in the protection of the nucleic acid, including potassium, manganese, and phosphorus, are present in the spore core.

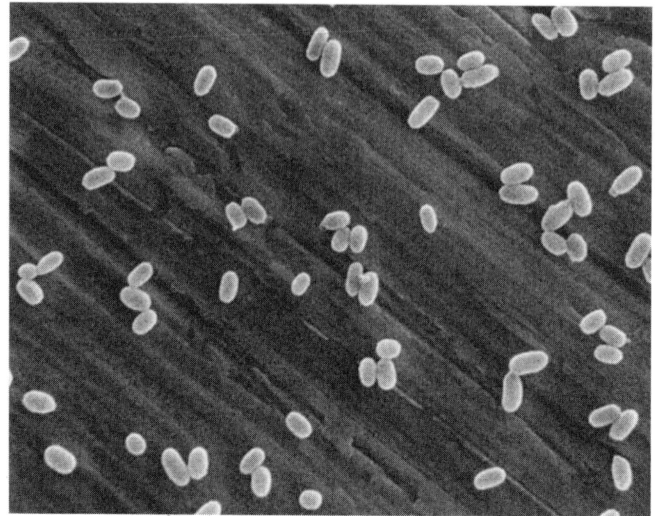

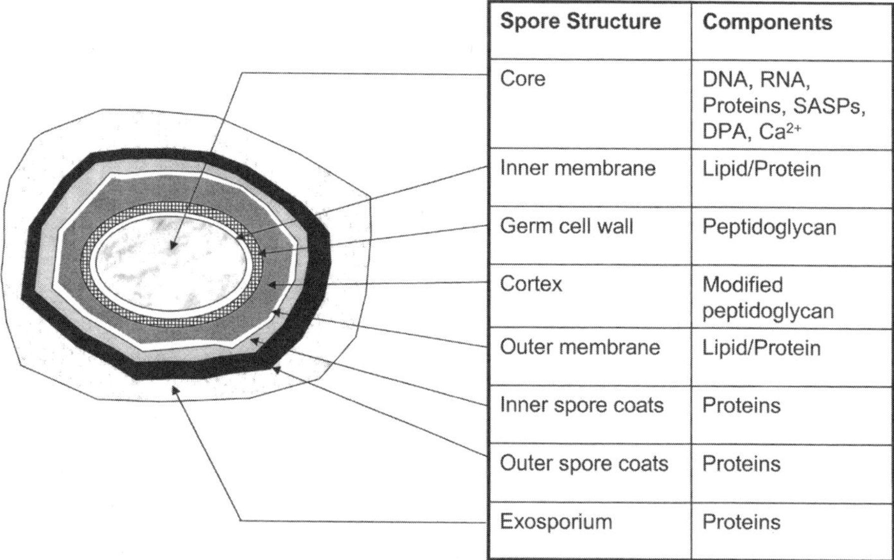

Spore Structure	Components
Core	DNA, RNA, Proteins, SASPs, DPA, Ca^{2+}
Inner membrane	Lipid/Protein
Germ cell wall	Peptidoglycan
Cortex	Modified peptidoglycan
Outer membrane	Lipid/Protein
Inner spore coats	Proteins
Outer spore coats	Proteins
Exosporium	Proteins

FIGURE 8.18 Typical bacterial-endospore structure. An actual micrograph of endospores on a surface is shown, with a representation of the various spore layers shown below (not to scale). The shapes of the spores vary, depending on the bacterial genus and species.

The protein component is predominantly SASPs, which are produced during the sporulation process and used as an energy or nutrient source during the germination of the spore. They appear to protect the viability of the spore by tightly binding to the bacterial DNA and preventing biocides or other environmental damage to the nucleic acid. Spores lacking SASPs are more sensitive to oxidizing agents and radiation methods.

In addition to the protective mechanisms described above, the spore core is further protected from the environment by a series of spore layers, including lipid and protein membranes, cell wall-type layers, cortex, and spore coats (Fig. 8.18). The inner and outer mem-

TABLE 8.12 Structures, components, and activities of endospores and their vegetative cells

Characteristic	Value	
	Endospore	Vegetative cell
Internal pH	~6	~7
Heat resistance	High; some strains can survive at >100°C	Low, although some thermophiles grow optimally at ~55°C
Chemical resistance	High	Low, with the exception of some extremophiles
Structure	Various protective layers surrounding an inner spore core	Typical gram-positive cell wall structure
Water content (%)	<30	~80
Calcium level	High	Low
Macromolecular synthesis	None	Active
Dipicolinic acid	Present	Absent
ASP	Present	Absent
Typical life span	Years in some cases	Days, depending on environment

branes are similar to (and derived from) the mother cell membrane, consisting of a bilipid membrane and integrated proteins. During the development of the spore, they further differentiate in their structures and functions in comparison to the cell membrane. The cortex is actually similar in structure to the gram-positive cell wall peptidoglycan; an inner germ cell wall consisting of peptidoglycan may be present, but the majority of the cortex consists of a specific muramic lactam (i.e., a structure similar to peptidoglycan but with the addition of muramic lactam-*N*-acetylglutamic linkages) that demonstrates greater rigidity and resistance to biocide penetration. The cortex also appears to play a role in regulating the observed water content of the inner core. The inner and outer spore coats comprise a major part of the overall spore content. These structures consist largely of protein, with an alkali-soluble fraction made up of acidic polypeptides that is found in the inner coat and an alkali-resistant fraction associated with the presence of disulfide-rich bonds in the outer coat. Finally, where present, the exosporium provides a further penetration challenge to biocides and predominantly consists of proteins. Overall, the observed layers vary from species to species; for example, the exosporium coat is present only in the spores of some species, while others are more simply surrounded by just one spore coat layer. These aspects, especially the roles of the spore coat(s) and cortex, are all relevant to the mechanism(s) of resistance presented by bacterial spores to biocides and biocidal processes.

As mentioned above, the endospore structure is developed in a sequential and controlled manner over approximately 8 h (Fig. 8.19). The sporulation process has been particularly well studied in *B. subtilis* as a primitive yet instructive and complex example of how cells are capable of differentiating during their life cycles. The control of the transcriptional and translational machinery of the cell is coordinated by a series of RNA polymerase-associated sigma factors that specifically direct the translation of genes, and therefore the production of proteins, away from normal housekeeping functions to those required for the development of the spore. The overall process has been defined as a series of seven integrated yet definitive stages, called stages I to VII (Fig. 8.19).

During this process, the vegetative cell (stage 0) undergoes a series of morphological changes that culminate in the release of a mature spore (stage VII). A cell undergoing the first stages of sporulation demonstrates a change from normal binary fission to asymmetric cell division (stages

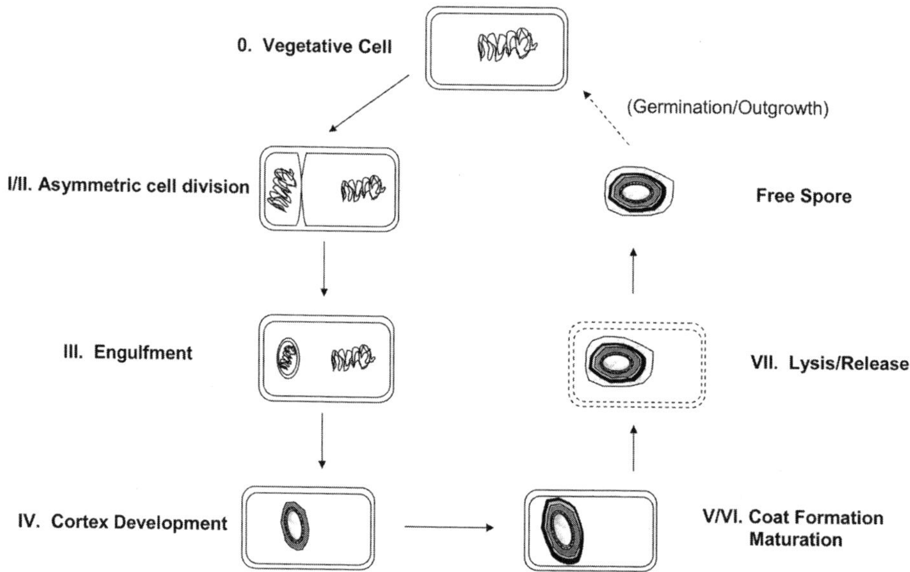

FIGURE 8.19 A representation of a typical sporulation process, with the key stages identified.

I and II), followed by engulfment of the forespore (stage III). The forespore then develops the cortex (stage IV) and spore coats (stages V and VI), in parallel with dehydration of the spore core and accumulation of calcium, DPA, and the SASPs. The final stages demonstrate further maturation of the spore structure and lysis of the mother cell to release the mature endospore. Studies with a normal *B. atrophaeus* strain (particularly strain 168) and various sporulation (Spo^-) mutants that develop only to a certain stage in the cascade have been used to understand the genetic and biochemical nature of each stage and to study at which stage biocide resistance is observed. In particular, stages IV to VII (cortex development, maturation, and release) have been identified as the most important stages in the development of resistance. Resistance has been found to depend on the nature of the biocide and has been defined as being either an early, intermediate, late, or very late event. Useful markers for monitoring these phases of resistance are toluene (resistance to which is an early event), heat (intermediate), and lysozyme (an enzyme effective against the normal bacterial cell wall peptidoglycan, to which spores become resistant late in sporulation). From these studies (Fig. 8.20), the order of development of resistance was found to be toluene (marker), formaldehyde, sodium lauryl sulfate, phenol, cresols, chlorhexidine gluconate, QACs (like cetylpyridinium chloride), moist heat (marker), sodium dichloroisocyanurate, sodium hypochlorite, lysozyme (marker), and glutaraldehyde.

Other techniques have also been useful in understanding mechanisms of spore resistance. They include removing the spore coat and cortex, using a "step-down" technique to achieve highly synchronous sporulation (so that cellular changes can be accurately monitored), adding a biocide at the commencement of sporulation and determining how far the process can proceed, and examining the role of SASPs.

The various layers of the spore can be removed, using chemical and enzymatic treatments, to study their roles in resistance. Forms without spore coats can be produced by treatment of spores under alkaline conditions with urea, dithiothreitol, and sodium lauryl sulfate, while further treatment with the enzyme lysozyme can be used to remove the inner cortex. These studies have shown that both the spore coats and the cortex play roles in con-

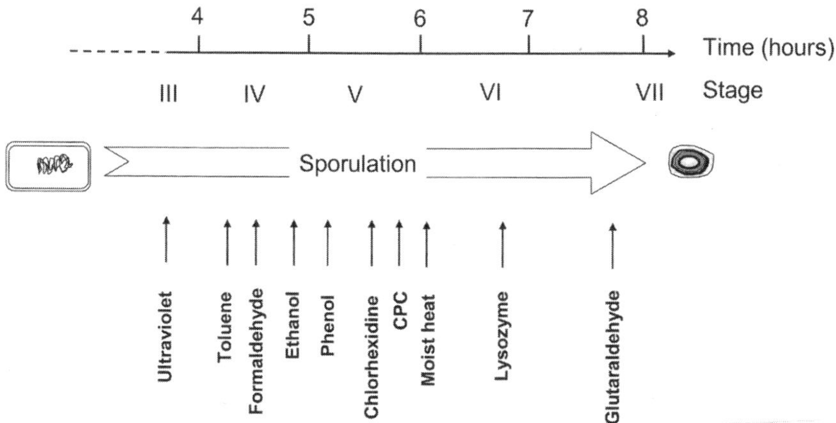

FIGURE 8.20 The development of resistance of bacterial endospores to biocides and biocidal processes. The various defined stages of sporulation are given from stage III (engulfment of the forespore) to stage VII (release of the mature spore), as shown in Fig. 8.19. The point at which the developing spore demonstrates resistance to each biocide or biocidal process is indicated.

ferring resistance, where the sensitivity of the spore increases as the various layers are removed. The initial development and maturity of the cortex are implicated in the development of resistance to phenolics, chlorhexidine, and QACs; this resistance is further enhanced in developing spores by the initiation of spore coat synthesis.

Development of resistance during sporulation to formaldehyde was found to be an early event, but it depended on the concentration (1 to 5% [vol/vol]) of formaldehyde employed. This appears to be at odds with the extremely late development of resistance to the dialdehyde glutaraldehyde. As glutaraldehyde and the monoaldehyde formaldehyde contain an aldehyde group(s) and are alkylating agents (see section 7.4.3), it would be plausible to assume that they have similar modes of sporicidal action, even though the dialdehyde is a more powerful alkylating agent. If this is true, then it could also be assumed that spores would exhibit the same resistance mechanisms against these disinfectants. In aqueous solution, formaldehyde forms a glycol in equilibrium; thus, formaldehyde could well be acting poorly as an alcohol-type disinfectant rather than an aldehyde. Alkaline glutaraldehyde does not readily form glycols in aqueous solution. Resistance to formaldehyde, then, may be more linked to cortex maturation and resistance to glutaraldehyde to coat formation.

As spores develop resistance to biocides during sporulation, they also lose resistance as they germinate and outgrow to reinitiate normal metabolism and growth (Fig. 8.21).

The activation of the endospore is a key stage in dedicating the spore to develop into a vegetative cell. Activation alone allows the spore to be more sensitive to heat and other biocides, like phenolics and normally sporistatic concentrations of aldehydes. Further biocide access and damage to the inner spore membrane and spore core following germination clearly play roles in inhibiting further outgrowth of the spore; during germination, the protective barriers of the spore coats are lost and the integrity of the cortex and spore core is broken, as indicated by the release of core constituents. As the outgrowth stage proceeds, biocides demonstrate their typical bacteriostatic and bactericidal activities, as observed in vegetative cells. It is interesting to note that biocide-treated spores may remain viable but be difficult to revive. Heat shock and culture conditions have been cited as improving the efficiency of revival of endospores. In contrast, the revival of disinfectant-treated spores has been little

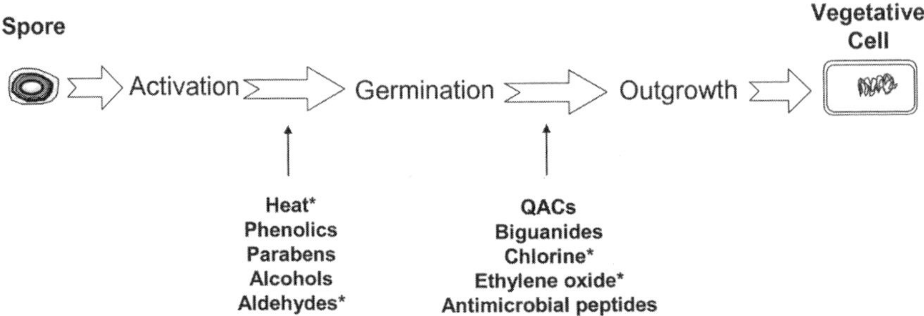

FIGURE 8.21 Loss of resistance to various biocides and heat during bacterial-endospore germination and outgrowth. Various biocides inhibit the activation of endospores (sporistatic) and are bactericidal to vegetative cells. Others (marked by asterisks) are also sporicidal at higher concentrations and temperatures and longer exposure times. Biocides at low concentrations and temperatures have also been shown to specifically inhibit germination or outgrowth following activation of the spore.

studied. Experiments designed to distinguish between germination and outgrowth in the revival process have demonstrated that sodium hydroxide-induced revival increases the potential for germination. Some reports have suggested that *B. atrophaeus* and *Geobacillus stearothermophilus* spores treated with formaldehyde or glutaraldehyde could be revived following a subsequent heat shock process, but not with chlorine or iodine treatment. It is likely that this is not related to an intrinsic resistance of the endospore but may be related to the test method or mode of action of the biocide. Inadequate neutralization of the biocide during laboratory investigations inhibits the activation and germination of the endospore, even at low concentrations. It can also be suggested that the mode of action of aldehydes, where lack of penetration of the aldehydes allows viable spores to be trapped in a cross-linked matrix, inhibits the germination of the spore but that the spore can be released and allowed to germinate following disruption by heat shock or other methods. This has been shown to be the case in a different situation with the use of aldehydes to treat viruses in vaccine preparations, where insufficient contact with the virus suspension allowed viable virus to survive normal virucidal treatment (see section 8.8).

In addition to the bacterial species listed in Table 8.10, some actinomycetes also produce spores (exospores). Actinomycetes are true bacteria that grow in long branched filaments similar to those of fungi. They are prokaryotes in that they lack mitochrondria and a nuclear membrane (see section 1.3.4). They can be further classified into aerobic and anaerobic species. Aerobic species include the mycolic-acid-containing species (like *Nocardia* and *Corynebacterium*), which are nonsporulating, and those without mycolic acids, which form exospores (including *Streptomyces*). Facultative and anaerobic species, including *Actinomyces*, are also spore-forming bacteria; actinomycetes themselves can be mesophilic or thermophilic. The growth of *Streptomyces* has been well studied due to the various developments identified during a typical life cycle (Fig. 8.22). These include antibiotic synthesis, stress responses, and morphological differentiation; similar to bacteria, the coordinated control of these developments is primarily due to transcriptional control of various operons by specific sigma factors (>65 have been identified) in response to environmental stresses.

Under the right environmental conditions for growth, *Streptomyces* species initially grow as surface (or subsurface) hyphal groups. Over time, the cells differentiate (by the coordination of a specific set of genes) to form aerial hyphae and, subsequently, exospores. During spore development in response to nutrient depletion,

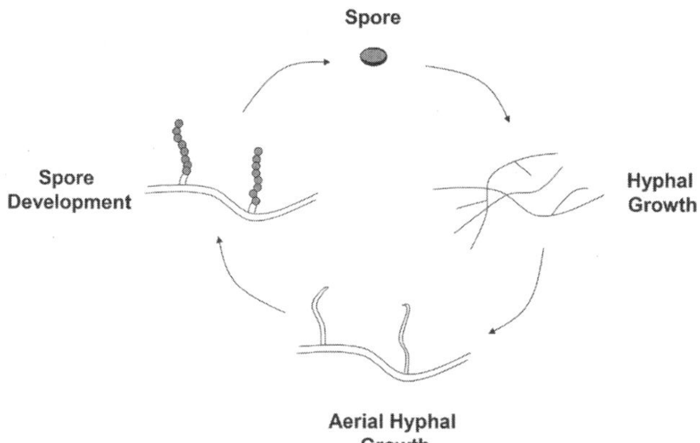

FIGURE 8.22 Typical life cycle of *Streptomyces*. A desiccated spore, under the right environmental conditions, will germinate and initiate hyphal growth. Under conditions of environmental stress and/or nutrient limitation, aerial hyphae develop in parallel with the production of secondary metabolites, including antibiotics and hydrolytic enzymes, to assist in survival. The aerial filaments separate by simple cross-wall division to form prespore compartments and to develop desiccated spores, which are released into the environment.

the aerial hyphae form initial prespore compartments (by cross-wall divisions of the filamentous growth), followed by spore development with observed wall thickening (containing glycogen and trehalose), production of a spore pigment, and spore desiccation. Different strains demonstrate various arrangements of spores, which have been used for classification. The purpose of sporulation is similar to that of bacterial endospores: the survival of cells under extreme nutrient depletion and harsh environmental conditions, although exospores are significantly less resistant to biocides and biocidal processes. Exospores are resistant to drying, surviving for extended periods, which actually aids in their dispersal; however, they are easily destroyed by heat, chemical, and radiation processes. Overall, the resistance of exospores to biocides has not been considered significant, although further investigations are warranted.

8.3.12 Revival Mechanisms

Biocidal processes are applied in different situations and in many cases may not be sufficient for the complete inactivation of various target microorganisms. Many of these situations have been described, including limited accessibility of the biocide through cell wall or other cell surface structures (see section 8.2), bacterial-endospore development (see section 8.3.11), and microorganisms within biofilms (see section 8.3.8). In many of these cases, damage to the target microorganisms may occur but may not be sufficient to render them nonviable (Fig. 8.23).

Biocidal damage may be tolerated by the microorganism and in some cases repaired to allow subsequent growth. These "revival" mechanisms can contribute to intrinsic resistance to biocides or biocidal processes, as they

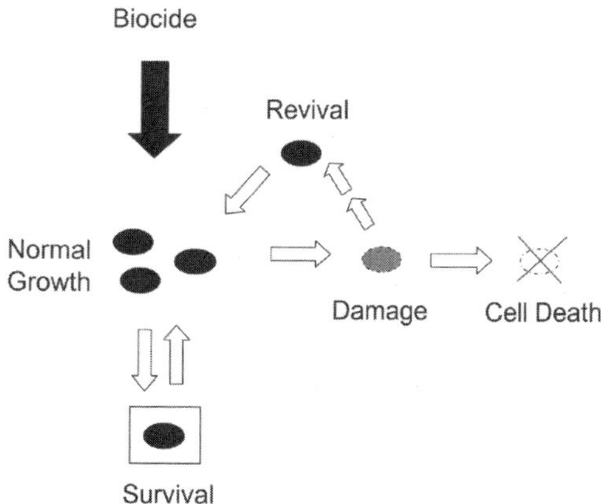

FIGURE 8.23 The revival of microorganisms after biocidal treatment. On exposure, microorganisms may survive due to lack of contact or intrinsic resistance to the biocide. In other cases, the damaged microorganisms can be revived by active repair mechanisms and undergo subsequent growth or infectivity. Damaged microorganisms may therefore be initially uncultivable by normal laboratory methods but remain viable. Biocidal effects may also be sufficient to render the microorganism nonviable (cell death or loss of infectivity).

TABLE 8.13 Examples of revival mechanisms that have been described following biocidal exposure

Revival mechanism	Comments
Cell wall/membrane regeneration	Described in fungi and bacteria, including known mechanisms of enterococcal resistance to antibiotics and in alcohol resistance in yeast and bacteria
Nucleic acid repair	Identified in all prokaryotes and eukaryotes in response to DNA damage by radiation; extremely efficient in some bacteria, like *Deinococcus* (see section 8.3.9)
Heat shock response	Repair of damage to various cellular components in bacteria and fungi, including DNA repair mechanisms and macromolecular regeneration (see section 8.3.3)
Growth medium factors	Described in the recovery of endospores and in the revival of some vegetative bacteria after heat, radiation, and chemical treatments
Viral reassociation or cooperation	Multiplicity reactivation in bacteriophages and other viruses, e.g., herpes simplex virus (demonstrated only under laboratory conditions)

allow microorganisms to recover over time. They are also important to consider in the evaluation of the efficacies of disinfection or sterilization processes (see section 1.4.2), as injured microorganisms (particularly bacterial spores) may not initially grow on or in recovery media at the same rate as untreated cultures but can demonstrate growth over a longer period or under the right environmental conditions.

Various examples of revival mechanisms have been described (Table 8.13).

Revival mechanisms have been particularly studied in the recovery of bacterial endospores from moist-heat treatment, but also following the application of radiation, dry-heat, and chemical sporicidal methods. Studies have shown that the recovery of spores following these treatments can be increased by various growth medium factors and conditions. These include the composition of the recovery medium, pH, temperature, and incubation time. This was first described in the recovery of *Clostridium botulinum* spores, which were found to be more fastidious than untreated spores, requiring various medium supplements to support their recovery. This was subsequently found to be common to all bacterial spore formers. Examples are the increased recovery of *B. atrophaeus* spores in media supplemented with amino acids (glycine, threonine, or homoserine) and with sodium bicarbonate (a known germination stimulant) for *Clostridium* spores. The incubation temperature is a further consideration. In one respect, the recovery of endospores and vegetative cells (including those of *E. coli* and *S. aureus*) has been shown to be greater when they are incubated at temperatures below the known optimal temperature for the untreated bacterial culture. For example, in some studies with *G. stearothermophilus* spores, greater survival was observed when cultures were grown at 45 to 50°C instead of the normal optimal temperature of ~55°C. In other reports, the heat shock of various heat- and chemically treated spores at 70 to 80°C for a number of minutes was also shown to increase recovery. It is not known why these treatments aid in spore revival, but in the case of lower growth temperatures, it may be associated with a lower initial metabolic rate to allow efficient repair of any damage. An alternative explanation of some of these findings has been proposed for aldehyde-treated spores. Increased revival by treatment with hydroxides (NaOH and KOH) and in some cases by heat shock has been shown with glutaraldehyde- and formaldehyde-treated spores, but not with spores treated with iodine, chlorine, or hydrogen peroxide. Considering the cross-linking mode of action of aldehydes (see section 7.4.3), it has been proposed that recovery may not be due to any true specific repair mechanism(s) but to the release of viable spores that are protected within cross-linked masses of spores or debris. During exposure to aldehydes, it is possible that viable spores become trapped within these forms and are not released for growth until physical or chemical disruption occurs. Similar explanations may be considered for the recovery of heat-, chemical-, or radiation-treated endospores. These mechanisms of revival have not been studied with fungal spores or other dormant microbial forms, which are generally less resistant than bacterial spores.

Exposure to sublethal concentrations of biocides damages bacteria and fungi but also activates various stress responses (see section 8.3.3). These stress responses include repair mechanisms that allow injured cells to recover from biocide damage. Radiation, particularly UV, damage repair mechanisms have been described in some detail and have been identified in most prokaryotes and eukaryotes. Although these mechanisms are normally present in cells, they have been shown to be upregulated in response to DNA damage, e.g., during the SOS response in *E. coli* (see section 8.3.3). Two major repair mechanisms have been identified: excision repair and photoreactivation. Excision repair involves the removal of various DNA photoproducts (including pyrimidine dimers) that are formed on exposure to radiation by incisions on either side of the lesion and removal and replacement of the DNA sequence. The mechanisms of repair are similar in prokaryotes and eukaryotes but involve different enzymes. Photoreactivation (which requires light for repair) involves the repair of dimers via photolyase enzymes. The repair of DNA lesions affords some recovery of exposed cells, depending on the extent of damage, although it should be remembered that radiation methods cause damage to other macromolecules in addition to DNA. A further mechanism of revival, which has been observed in bacteria and fungi, concerns the regeneration of the cell wall and membrane. As these structures are the front line in any biocide attack, a significant amount of damage can be observed even at sublethal concentrations of biocides. The ability to regenerate damaged cell walls has been shown in the generation of bacterial protoplasts (cell wall-deficient forms) under laboratory conditions, and protoplasts have been found to be very sensitive to various biocides but subsequently increase their tolerance on redevelopment of the cell wall.

As viruses are nonmetabolizing, they are not expected to express mechanisms of active repair of biocidal damage. Despite this, radiation-damaged DNA viruses (e.g., herpes simplex viruses and bacteriophages) have been shown to be repaired by host cell mechanisms following infection. Further studies have found that suspensions of damaged or disintegrated viruses or viral components can cooperate in a phenomenon known as "multiplicity reactivation" to allow the infection of cells; this appears to occur at a high concentration of virus under laboratory conditions, and its environmental or clinical significance is unknown.

8.4 INTRINSIC RESISTANCE OF MYCOBACTERIA

Mycobacteria are well known to demonstrate resistance to biocides that is roughly intermediate between those of other nonsporulating bacteria and bacterial spores. There is no evidence that enzymatic degradation of harmful molecules takes place. The most likely mechanism for the high resistance of mycobacteria is associated with their complex cell walls, which provide an effective barrier to the entry of these agents. To date, plasmid- or transposon-mediated resistance to biocides has not been demonstrated in mycobacteria.

The mycobacterial cell wall (Fig. 8.24) is a highly hydrophobic structure with a mycoylarabinogalactan-peptidoglycan skeleton.

The peptidoglycan is covalently linked to the polysaccharide copolymer (arabinogalactan) made up of arabinose and galactose esterified to mycolic acids (see section 1.3.4.1). Also present are complex lipids, LPSs, and proteins, including those that form porin channels through which hydrophilic molecules can diffuse into the cell. Similar cell wall structures exist in all the mycobacterial species examined to date. The cell wall composition of a particular species is also influenced by its environmental niche. Pathogenic bacteria, such as *Mycobacterium tuberculosis*, exist in a relatively nutrient-rich environment, whereas saprophytic mycobacteria living in soil or water are exposed to natural

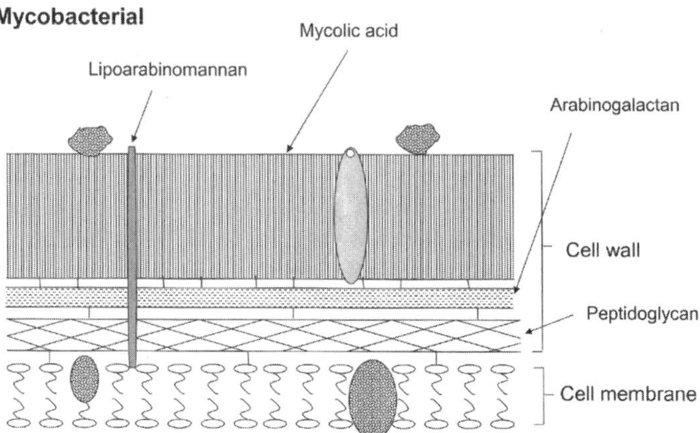

FIGURE 8.24 A representation of the mycobacterial cell wall structure.

antibiotics and tend to be more intrinsically resistant to these drugs.

Biocides that exhibit mycobacterial activity include phenolics, peracetic acid, hydrogen peroxide, alcohols, and aldehydes. By contrast, other well-known bactericidal agents, such as chlorhexidine and QACs, are mycobacteriostatic even when employed at high concentrations. However, their activities can be substantially increased by formulation effects. Thus, a number of QAC-based products claim to have mycobacterial activity. It has been proposed that the resistance of mycobacteria to QACs is related to the lipid content of the cell wall. In support of this contention, *Mycobacterium phlei*, with low total cell lipid content, was found to be more sensitive to QACs than *M. tuberculosis*, which has a higher lipid content. It was also noted that the resistances of various species of mycobacteria were related to the contents of lipid material in their walls. It is now known that, because of the highly hydrophobic nature of the cell wall, hydrophilic-type biocides in their own right are generally unable to penetrate the mycobacterial cell wall in sufficiently high concentrations to produce a lethal effect. However, low concentrations of biocides such as chlorhexidine must presumably traverse this permeability barrier, because their MICs are on the same order as those for nonmycobacterial strains, such as *S. aureus*, although *Mycobacterium avium-Mycobacterium intracellulare* is particularly tolerant. The other component(s) of the mycobacterial cell wall that contributes to high biocide resistance is largely unknown, although some information is available. Inhibitors of cell wall synthesis increase the susceptibility of *M. avium* to drugs; inhibition of glycolipids, arabinogalactan, and mycolic acid biosynthesis also enhances drug susceptibility. Treatment of this organism with *m*-fluoro-DL-phenylalanine, which inhibits glycolipid synthesis, produces significant alterations in the outer cell wall layers. Ethambutol, an antibiotic inhibitor of arabinogalactan and phospholipid synthesis, also disorganizes these layers. In addition, ethambutol induces the formation of dead cells without the dissolution of peptidoglycan ("ghost" cells). Methyl-4-(2-octadecylcyclopropen-1-yl) butanoate is a structural analogue of a key precursor in mycolic acid synthesis. Thus, effects of methyl-4-(2-octadecylcyclopropen-1-yl) on mycolic acid synthesis and of *m*-fluoro-DL-phenylalanine and ethambutol on outer-wall biosynthetic processes leading to changes in cell wall architecture appear to be responsible for increasing the intracellular concentrations of chemotherapeutic drugs. These findings support the concept of the overall cell wall structure acting as a permeability barrier to various drugs. Fewer specific studies have been done of the mechanisms involved in the resistance of mycobacteria to biocides. However, the activities of chlorhexidine and of a QAC, cetylpyridinium chloride, against *M. avium* and *M. tuberculosis* can be potentiated in the presence of ethambutol. From these data, it may be inferred that arabinogalactan is another cell wall component that acts as a permeability barrier to chlorhexidine and QACs.

One species of mycobacteria that is a cause for concern is *M. chelonae*, since the organism is sometimes isolated from endoscopes, washer-disinfectors, and dialysis water. One such (presumably mutant) strain was not killed even after a 60-min exposure to 2% alkaline glutaraldehyde; in contrast, a reference (wild-type) strain showed a 5-log-unit reduction after a contact time of 10 min. These glutaraldehyde-resistant *M. chelonae* strains demonstrated a slightly increased tolerance to peracetic acid but not to sodium dichloroisocyanurate or to a phenolic. Other workers have also observed above-average resistance of *M. chelonae* to glutaraldehyde and formaldehyde but not to peracetic acid; an additional aldehyde used for low-temperature disinfection, orthophthaldehyde (OPA), was also found to be less effective against these strains, but more effective than glutaraldehyde over time. The reasons for this high glutaraldehyde resistance are unknown but appear to be related to changes in cell wall structure and may in part be due to reduced uptake of glutaraldehyde by these *M. chelonae* strains (see section 8.7.2). *M. chelonae* is also known to adhere strongly to smooth surfaces, which may render cells within a biofilm less susceptible to disinfectants and increase the potential development of tolerance by mutation at sublethal concentrations of biocides.

8.5 INTRINSIC RESISTANCE OF OTHER GRAM-POSITIVE BACTERIA

The cell wall of staphylococci has been studied in some detail; it is composed essentially of peptidoglycan and teichoic acid (Fig. 8.25). Neither of these appears to act as an effective barrier to the entry of various biocides. Since substances of high molecular weight can readily traverse the cell walls of staphylococci and vegetative *Bacillus* spp., this possibly explains the sensitivity of these organisms to many antibacterial agents, including QACs and chlorhexidine. However, the plasticity of the bacterial cell wall is a well-known phenomenon. The growth rate and any growth-limiting nutrient will affect the physiological state of the cells. Under such circumstances, the thickness and degree of cross-linking of peptidoglycan are likely to be modified, and hence, cellular sensitivities to various biocides may be altered. For example, the sensitivity of *Bacillus megaterium* cells to chlorhexidine and 2-phenoxyethanol is altered when changes in growth rate and nutrient limitation are made in actively multiplying cultures. However, lysozyme-induced protoplasts of these cells remained sensitive to, and were lysed by, these membrane-active agents. So-called "fattened" cells of *S. aureus* that are produced by repeated subculturing in glycerol-containing media also showed changes in their surface structure and were found to be more resistant to alkyl phenolics and some antibiotics, like benzylpenicillin; subculture of these cells in routine culture media resulted in rever-

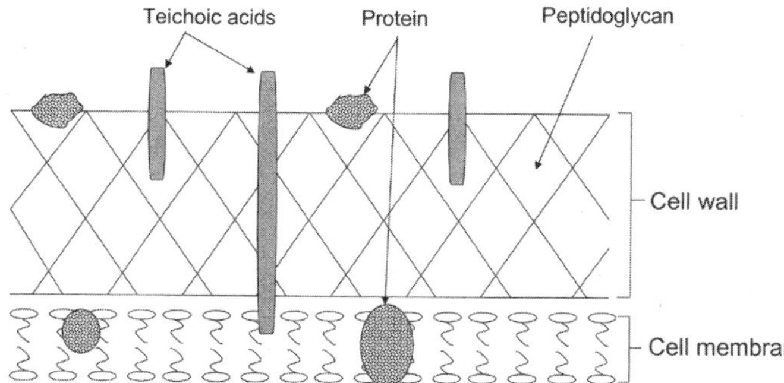

FIGURE 8.25 A representation of a typical gram-positive bacterial cell wall structure.

sion to biocide sensitivity. Thus, the cell wall in whole cells appears to be responsible for their modified response to biocides.

Antibiotic-resistant gram-positive bacteria, particularly methicillin-resistant *S. aureus* (MRSA) and vancomycin-resistant *Enterococcus*, are significant concerns in hospitals and other health care facilities. Some reports have suggested that these strains may also have increased tolerance of various antiseptic biocides, particularly triclosan and chlorhexidine (see section 4.6.2). Efflux as a mechanism of acquired tolerance of biocides like chlorhexidine and QACs in staphylococci has been shown to be linked to antibiotic resistance in MRSA strains (see section 8.7); however, the actual MICs of these biocides have been found to vary considerably in *S. aureus* environmental and clinical isolates. For example, chlorhexidine MICs range from ~0.2 to 20 mg/liter independently of the presence of methicillin resistance (Table 8.14). There is currently no standard method of determining biocide MICs, and therefore, reports in the literature can vary greatly. The exact mechanisms of resistance in these strains have not been studied and may be due to various intrinsic factors rather than acquired by mutation or plasmid or transposon acquisition (see section 8.7). Further, no significant differences have been observed in the bactericidal concentrations of biocides (Table 8.14) or in the bactericidal activities of antiseptic products under in-use conditions. There is no evidence to date that vancomycin-resistant enterococci or enterococci with high-level resistance to aminoglycoside antibiotics are more resistant to biocides than are antibiotic-sensitive enterococcal strains. However, enterococci are generally less sensitive to biocides than staphylococci, and differences in inhibitory and bactericidal concentrations have also been found among enterococcal species.

Various other intrinsic mechanisms of biocide tolerance have been described in gram-positive bacteria. The development of bacterial endospores in gram-positive bacteria, like *Bacillus* and *Clostridium*, is clearly an important mechanism (see section 8.3.11). Various staphylococci, including *S. aureus* strains, are mucoid and are surrounded by polysaccharide-rich capsules or slime layers (see section 8.3.7). Nonmucoid strains are generally inactivated more rapidly than mucoid strains by some biocides, including QACs and chlorhexidine, but not significantly by others, like phenolics (depending on their concentrations). Removal of the capsule or slime layer has been found to render the cell more sensitive, confirming that these layers play important protective roles either as a direct barrier to prevent penetration into the cell or by absorbing or inactivating the biocide.

8.6 INTRINSIC RESISTANCE OF GRAM-NEGATIVE BACTERIA

Gram-negative bacteria are generally more resistant to biocides than are nonsporulating, nonmycobacterial gram-positive bacteria. Examples of MICs for gram-positive and gram-negative organisms are provided in Table 8.15.

Based on these data, there is a marked difference between the sensitivities of *S. aureus* and *E. coli* to QACs (benzalkonium, benzethonium, and cetrimide), hexachlorophene, diamidines, and triclosan but little difference in chlorhexidine susceptibilities. *P. aeruginosa* is considerably

TABLE 8.14 Ranges of MICs and MBCs of chlorhexidine and triclosan against *S. aureus* and *Enterococcus* sp. isolates

Strain	MIC (mg/liter)		MBC (mg/liter)	
	Chlorhexidine	Triclosan	Chlorhexidine	Triclosan
S. aureus[a]	0.2–20	0.05–2	20–30	12–20
Enterococcus[b]	1–15	10–15	75	15–20

[a]Including methicillin-sensitive and MRSA isolates.

[b]Including vancomycin-sensitive and -resistant isolates of *E. faecium* and *E. faecalis*.

TABLE 8.15 MICs of various biocides (determined in test media) for gram-positive and gram-negative bacteria

Chemical agent	MIC (mg/liter) for:		
	S. aureus	*E. coli*	*P. aeruginosa*
Benzalkonium chloride	0.5	50	250
Cetrimide	4	16	64–128
Chlorhexidine	0.2–20	1	5–60
o-Phenylphenol	100	500	1,000
Propamine isothionate	2	64	256
Dibromopropamidine isothionate	1	4	32
Triclosan	0.05–2	5	>300

more resistant to all of these agents, including chlorhexidine; other gram-negative bacteria, like *Proteus* species, also possess above-average resistance to cationic agents, such as chlorhexidine and QACs.

The outer membrane of gram-negative bacteria acts as a barrier that limits the entry of many chemically unrelated types of antibacterial agents (Fig. 8.26).

This conclusion is based upon the differences in observed biocide sensitivities between gram-positive and gram-negative bacteria, but also on studies with outer-membrane mutants of *E. coli*, *Salmonella enterica* serovar Typhimurium, and *P. aeruginosa*. In wild-type gram-negative bacteria, intact LPS molecules (see section 1.3.7) (Fig. 8.26) are a major component of the outer membrane. Low-molecular-weight hydrophilic molecules can readily pass through the outer membrane porins into the cells, but hydrophobic molecules are required to diffuse across the outer-membrane bilayer. Outer membranes are known to prevent the access of hydrophobic molecules (including antibiotics and biocides) to the periplasm, presumably due to the LPS molecules providing a highly ordered, limited-fluidity structure on the cell surface. In gram-negative deep-rough mutants, the outer-membrane structure is quite distinct, essentially lacking the O-specific side chain and most of the core polysaccharide of LPS molecules, which are replaced with phospholipid patches. These mutants, with increased surface hydrophobicity, tend to be hypersensitive to hydrophobic antibiotics and biocides, which are normally more effectively excluded from wild-type strains. Some of the possible transport mechanisms for biocides into gram-negative bacteria are listed in Table 8.16.

In addition to these hydrophilic and hydrophobic entry pathways, a third pathway has been proposed for cationic agents, such as

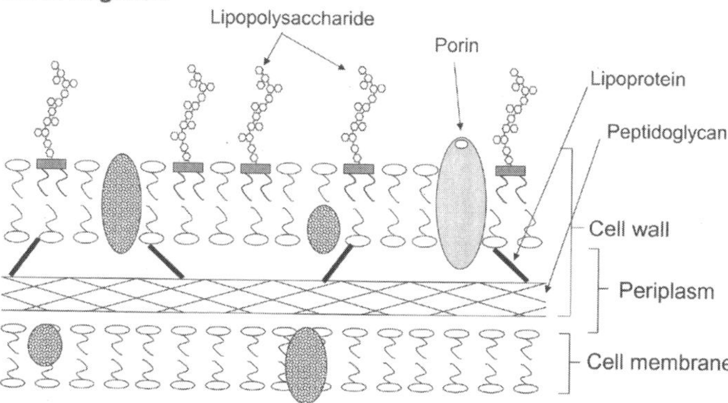

FIGURE 8.26 A representation of a typical gram-negative bacterial cell wall structure.

TABLE 8.16 Possible transport mechanisms of some biocides into gram-negative bacteria

Biocide	Passage across OM[a]	Passage across IM[a]
Chlorhexidine	Self-promoted uptake due to OM damage	IM is a major target site; damage to IM enables biocide to enter cytoplasm, where further interactions occur.
QACs	OM may present an important barrier. Self-promoted uptake, due to OM damage.	IM is a major target site; damage to IM enables biocide to enter cytoplasm, where further interaction occurs.
Phenolics	Hydrophobic pathway (activity increases as hydrophobicity of phenolic increases)	IM is a major target site, but high phenolic concentrations have been shown to coagulate cytoplasmic constituents, suggesting penetration.

[a]OM, outer membrane; IM, inner membrane.

QACs, biguanides, and diamidines. It is claimed that these agents damage the outer membrane, thereby promoting their own uptake. Polycations have been found to disorganize the outer membrane of *E. coli*. It must be added, however, that the QACs and diamidines are considerably less active against wild-type than against deep-rough strains, whereas chlorhexidine has the same order of activity (MIC increase, ~2- to 3-fold) against both types of *E. coli* strains. However, *S. enterica* serovar Typhimurium outer-membrane mutants are more sensitive to chlorhexidine than is the wild-type strain. External damage to allow greater penetration of biocides can also be expected for other types, including oxidizing agents.

Gram-negative bacteria that show a high level of resistance to many biocides include *P. aeruginosa*, *B. cepacia*, *Proteus* spp., and *Providencia stuartii*. The outer membrane of *P. aeruginosa* is responsible for its high resistance; in comparison with other organisms, there are notable differences in LPS composition and in the cation content of the outer membrane. The high Mg^{2+} content aids in producing strong LPS-LPS links; furthermore, because of their small size, the porins may not permit general diffusion. *B. cepacia* has often been shown to be considerably more resistant in the environment than in artificial culture media; the high content of phosphate-linked arabinose in its LPS decreases the affinity of the outer membrane for polymyxin antibiotics and other cationic and polycationic molecules. *Pseudomonas stutzeri*, in contrast, is normally highly sensitive to many biocides, which implies that such agents have little difficulty in crossing the outer layers of the cells of the organism. Members of the genus *Proteus* are invariably insensitive to chlorhexidine. Some strains that are highly resistant to chlorhexidine, QACs, EDTA, and diamidines have been isolated from clinical sources. The presence of a less acidic type of outer-membrane LPS could be a contributing factor in its intrinsic resistance. A particularly troublesome member of the genus *Providencia* is *P. stuartii*. Like *Proteus* species, *P. stuartii* strains have been isolated from urinary tract infections and are intrinsically resistant to different types of biocides, including chlorhexidine and QACs. Strains of *P. stuartii* that showed low-level, intermediate, and high-level resistances to chlorhexidine formed the basis of a series of studies of the resistance mechanism(s). Gross differences in the compositions of the outer layers of these strains were not detected, although it was concluded that subtle changes in the structural arrangement of the cell wall could be responsible for their resistance.

The peptidoglycan content of gram-negative bacteria has not been considered a potential barrier to the entry of biocides; this appears likely, as the overall peptidoglycan contents of these organisms are much less than in gram-positive bacteria, which are inherently more sensitive to biocides. Nevertheless, there have been instances where gram-negative bacteria grown in subinhibitory concentrations of penicillin (which targets peptidoglycan synthesis) have been found to have deficient permeability barriers. Furthermore, penicillin-induced spheroplasts and lysozyme-EDTA-Tris "protoplasts" of gram-negative bacteria are also rapidly lysed by membrane-active agents, such as chlorhexidine. It is conceivable that the destabilized nature of both the outer and inner membranes in the absence of peptidoglycan and loss of cell wall integrity are responsible for increased susceptibility to biocides.

The possibility exists that the cytoplasmic (inner) membrane could be a further mechanism of intrinsic resistance. This membrane is composed of a phospholipid-protein mosaic and would be expected to prevent passive diffusion of hydrophilic molecules. It is also known that changes in the membrane lipid composition affect sensitivity to ethanol in some bacteria. Various other factors have been implicated in the intrinsic resistance of gram-negative bacteria to biocides, including chlorhexidine degradation in *S. marcescens, P. aeruginosa*, and *Alcaligenes (Achromobacter) xylosoxidans* and biofilm development. Planktonic cultures grown under conditions of nutrient limitation or reduced growth rates have cells with altered sensitivity to biocides, probably as a consequence of modifications in their outer membranes and other stress responses (see sections 8.3.1 and 8.3.3).

8.7 ACQUIRED BACTERIAL RESISTANCE MECHANISMS

8.7.1 Introduction

Microorganisms demonstrate intrinsic variability in their responses to the range of biocides or biocidal processes. For example, alcohols are rapidly bactericidal, fungicidal, and virucidal but demonstrate little or no effect on bacterial spores (see section 3.5). Similarly, gram-positive bacteria and enveloped viruses are particularly sensitive to QACs, which have less activity against gram-negative bacteria, fungi, and mycobacteria (see section 3.16). Biocides that are more restrictive include the anilides and diamidines, although even these toxic compounds still display broad antibacterial and microstatic activities (see sections 3.6.and 3.9). In contrast, many antibiotics or other chemotherapeutic drugs demonstrate much narrower spectra of activity (see section 7.2). Antibiotics are generally effective only against bacteria, due to the presence of specific targets and the lack of these targets in other microorganisms. With the β-lactam antibiotic penicillin, for example, the mode of action is specific to peptidoglycan biosynthesis (Fig. 8.27).

Penicillin specifically binds to and inhibits the penicillin-binding proteins (PBPs), which are associated with the cytoplasmic membrane and specifically involved in the building and cross-linking of peptidoglycan. Most gram-positive bacteria are sensitive to penicillin, which generally has less activity against gram-negative bacteria, despite the presence of peptidoglycan and PBPs. The overall therapeutic effect of penicillin is to restrict the growth of sensitive bacteria at relatively low concentrations of the antibiotic by preventing cell wall biosynthesis. Intrinsic bacterial resistance to penicillin is primarily due to decreased uptake of the antibiotic and/or the presence of enzymes (β-lactamases) that degrade it. These mechanisms of resistance are not dissimilar to those described for various biocides (see section 8.3); however, it is clear that penicillin will not be effective against microorganisms that do not contain peptidoglycan, like fungi and

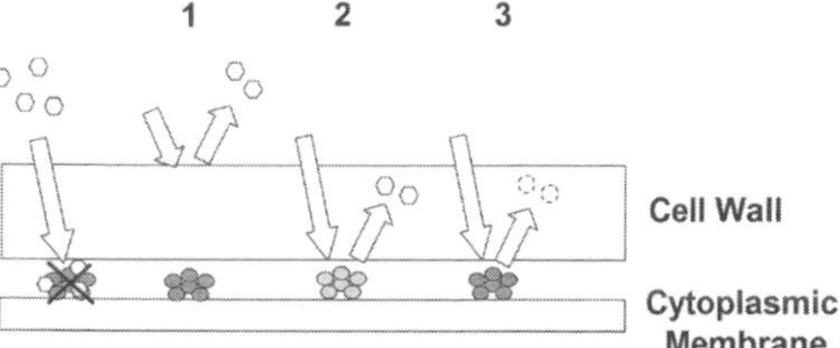

FIGURE 8.27 The primary mechanisms of action of penicillin and of bacterial resistance to it. The antibiotic penetrates through the cell wall to the cytoplasmic-membrane-associated PBPs and disrupts their role in the synthesis of the cell wall peptidoglycan (shown on the left). The first mechanism of resistance (1) is exclusion from the cell, which can be intrinsic or acquired. In the second (2), the target PBPs have mutated to become less sensitive to penicillin binding. The third (3) is the presence (naturally induced or otherwise acquired) of β-lactamases, which hydrolyze the antibiotic.

viruses. In addition, with the widespread use of penicillin, various bacterial acquired resistance mechanisms have been identified and investigated. These have arisen due to various mutations and the acquisition of genetic material in the form of plasmids or transposons.

Mutations are inherited changes in the nucleotide sequences of nucleic acids that can result in altered structures and functions within a microorganism. In the case of penicillin, an important example of the effects of genetic mutations is the direct modification of the structures of the PBPs, changing their affinities for the antibiotic. In these cases, specific mutations in the PBP gene lead to specific changes in the primary amino acid sequence of the protein, and subsequently, to adopting a secondary structure that is nonsusceptible to penicillin. Other mutational effects include the loss of proteins (including the outer-membrane porin proteins in gram-negative bacteria, thereby restricting access to the inner cell membrane and the location of the PBPs) and the overexpression of proteins due to the loss of transcriptional control. Examples of protein overexpression are the PBPs (sequestering the effect of the antibiotic) and β-lactamases (demonstrating greater degradation of the antibiotic [Fig. 8.27]).

Plasmids and transposons are transmissible genetic elements that can be transferred between bacteria. They have been studied primarily in bacteria but have been identified in archaea and in eukaryotes. Plasmids are extrachromosomal DNA molecules that replicate independently within the cell and are separate from the chromosomal DNA, although in some cases, a plasmid can insert (or integrate) into the chromosome (so-called episomes). Plasmids have been found to encode various functions, including replication, virulence determinants, degradative enzymes (e.g., against toluene and salicylic acid), and other mechanisms of resistance to antibiotics and biocides. They can be transferred between cells by three basic mechanisms: transformation, conjugation, and transduction. Transformation involves the ability of the cell to naturally take up plasmids from the environment (e.g., during competence in *Bacillus* or otherwise induced). Conjugation involves direct cell-to-cell contact, and this ability is actually encoded by the plasmid itself. Finally, transduction involves the transfer of the plasmid or genetic material by virus (or, in the case of bacteria, bacteriophage) transfer. Transposons are similar to plasmids, as they are also mobile genetic (DNA) sequences, but they are not capable of autonomous replication. Transposons are capable of inserting ("transposing") into the host chromosome or plasmids, replicating as part of those genetic elements. Similar to plasmids, transposons contain various sequences that encode essential functions (e.g., enzymes involved in the transposition process), as well as antibiotic and biocide resistance mechanisms. Mechanisms of resistance to antibiotics are encoded and can be transferred between bacteria on plasmids and transposons. Using the example of the β-lactams, β-lactamases (Fig. 8.27) are plasmid or transposon encoded and can be transferred between bacteria to confer penicillin resistance. Examples of other acquired mechanisms of resistance to antimicrobial drugs are given in Table 8.17.

Acquired mechanisms of biocide resistance have also been described and are discussed in detail below. Some of these biocide resistance mechanisms may also demonstrate increased resistance to antibiotics. However, it is important to note that "biocide resistance" as a term can often be misused and needs to be interpreted with some prudence. This is particularly true with MIC analysis, which determines the level of a drug that inhibits the growth of the microorganism. Unlike antibiotics, "resistance" or a significant increase in the MIC of a biocide does not necessarily correlate with therapeutic or functional failure. An increase in an antibiotic MIC may have significant clinical consequences, often indicating that the target organism is simply unaffected by its antimicrobial action. This is also true if the change in MIC is sufficient to allow the survival of the microorganism at typical therapeutic concentrations that cannot be further increased due to toxicological concerns. Increased biocide MICs due to acquired mechanisms have also

TABLE 8.17 Acquired mechanisms of resistance to antimicrobial drugs

Antimicrobial agent	Resistance	Example(s)
Antibacterials		
Sulfonamides	Chromosomal	Mutations in dihydropteroate synthetase with lower affinity for the antibiotic
	Plasmid	Expression of antibiotic-resistant synthetases
Rifampin	Chromosomal	Mutations in target β-subunit of bacterial RNA polymerase, which are less sensitive to the antibiotic
Aminoglycosides	Chromosomal	Mutations in the sequence of ribosomal proteins and loss of the antibiotic-binding site
	Plasmid or transposon	Expression of enzymes that modify the antibiotic, e.g., acetyltransferases
Tetracyclines	Chromosomal	Mutational loss of outer membrane proteins and reduced penetration of the antibiotic
	Plasmid or transposon	Expression of efflux proteins
β-Lactams	Chromosomal	Mutational changes in the structures of target penicillin-binding proteins and less affinity for the antibiotic Mutational loss of outer membrane proteins and less penetration of the antibiotic
	Chromosomal, plasmid, or transposon	β-Lactamase expression, which degrades the antibiotic
Antivirals		
Viral polymerase inhibitors, including reverse transcriptases (e.g., zidovudine) and DNA polymerases	Nucleic acid	Single or multiple mutations in the polymerase structure with less affinity for the antiviral
Protease inhibitors (e.g., saquinavir)	Nucleic acid	Single or multiple mutations in the polymerase structure with less affinity for the antiviral
Antifungals		
Flucytosine	Chromosomal	Loss or mutation of enzymes involved in the uptake, metabolism, or incorporation of the drug into RNA
Polyenes, e.g., amphotericin	Chromosomal	Membrane alterations (e.g., reduced content of ergosterol)
Azoles, e.g., ketoconazole	Chromosomal	Cell membrane changes; increased expression of efflux pumps; mutations in target enzymes in ergosterol synthesis (e.g., demethylases)

been reported and in some cases misinterpreted as indicating "resistance." It is important that issues, including the pleiotropic actions of most biocides, bactericidal activity, concentrations used in products, direct product application, and formulation effects, be considered in evaluating the clinical implications of these reports.

8.7.2 Mutational Resistance

A mutation is a change in the genetic material (i.e., DNA or, in some viruses, RNA) that results in a change in the nucleotide sequence of the nucleic acid. Mutations can occur due to a variety of reasons and in many cases have no effect on the respective genes and their functions within the cell or virus. However, in other cases, a mutation can occur which allows the microorganism to survive various environmental challenges and to pass on this beneficial change to its descendants. Mutations can range from small spontaneous changes in the nucleotide sequence to rather large deletions of sections of the nucleic acid. Chromosomal mutations leading to antibiotic resistance have been recognized and studied in some detail. These investigations have allowed a greater understanding of the modes of action of antibiotics and have identified a variety of mechanisms by which bacteria can circumvent the antibacterial activities of antibiotics. Examples of these mutations are specific protein targets that are no longer affected by the presence of the antibiotic and various other regulatory proteins or sequences that change the expression of target proteins, allowing the bacteria to overcome the inhibitory or lethal effects. In contrast, fewer studies have been made to determine whether mutation confers resistance to biocides; however, specific examples have been described demonstrating mechanisms similar to and distinct from those of antibiotics.

Many attempts have been made to induce bacterial tolerance of biocides under laboratory conditions. This can be investigated by growing the microorganism at subinhibitory and/or inhibitory concentrations of the biocide over time. In some cases, stable mutants have been identified; however, more often, these mutants are unstable and revert to normal sensitivity following removal of the biocide. One of the first reported examples was the identification of *S. marcescens* mutants that allowed growth in the presence of a QAC at 100 to 1,000 times the MIC for the wild type (or sensitive parent) strain. The wild-type strain was normally inhibited at ~100 mg of the QAC/liter, in comparison to the resistant strains at up to 100,000 mg/liter; however, it should be noted that some practical problems are associated with QACs and other, similar biocides, like chlorhexidine, in that they precipitate (due to limited aqueous solubility) in liquid culture media, which can be mistaken for bacterial growth (due to observed turbidity). Similarly, these and other biocides also interact with agar components to give inaccurate MIC determinations. Despite this, these strains clearly had higher-than-normal resistance to the biocide. The exact mechanism of resistance was not identified, but the resistant strains were reported to have different surface characteristics, presumably due to increased or altered lipid content on the cell surface. Although it can be speculated that the resistance mechanism may have been due to a developmental response to reduce the penetration of the biocide into the cell, the more likely conclusion was that these strains had mutated to become more resistant. The QAC-resistant strains were unstable, reverting to QAC sensitivity when cultured in the absence of the biocide. Despite subsequent reports of many unstable biocide-tolerant bacteria, a number of exceptions have been investigated, which suggests the need for further studies of the induction of biocide resistance by mutation.

Triclosan is a bisphenol widely used in antiseptic formulations, including surgical scrubs, antimicrobial soaps, and deodorants (see section 4.6). It demonstrates potent activity against gram-positive bacteria, like staphylococci, but is less active against most gram-negative organisms, probably by virtue of a permeability barrier (see section 8.6). The mechanisms of action of and resistance to triclosan have been the focus of recent research, particularly due to the isolation of various stable triclosan mutants in bacteria. Gram-positive (e.g., *Staphylococcus*) and gram-negative (e.g., *Escherichia* and *Pseudomonas*) bacterial mutants can be developed by serial passage in subinhibitory and inhibitory concentrations of triclosan. In contrast to the unstable *S. marcescens* mutants discussed above, stable mutational changes as a mechanism of triclosan resistance were first reported in *E. coli*, due to changes in the fatty acid composition of the cell wall. The *E. coli* mutants were developed under laboratory conditions, exhibiting a 10-fold-greater triclosan MIC than a wild-type strain, but only in the presence of divalent ions. Analysis of these strains showed no significant differences in total envelope protein profiles but did show significant differences in envelope fatty acids. Specifically, a prominent $C_{14:1}$ fatty acid was absent in the resistant strain, along with minor differences in other fatty acid species. It was proposed that in these mutants the divalent ions and fatty acids may adsorb triclosan and limit its permeability to its site of action. The effect of triclosan on the phospholipid membrane has been investigated in bacteria; studies have shown that the hydrophobic biocide can integrate into the upper region of the membrane via its hydroxyl group, which causes membrane disruption and loss of various functions (including catabolic and anabolic processes) and integrity. Overall, changes in the structures of membrane-associated lipids may decrease these interactions. Minor changes in fatty acid profiles were also found in stable triclosan-tolerant gram-positive (*S. aureus*) isolates, which had elevated triclosan MICs but not MBCs; again, the mechanism(s) of resistance was not further investigated. More recent investigations have identified at least four different mechanisms of resistance due to mutations, many of which have also been shown with other biocides: decreased uptake (as described above), increased efflux, chromosomal mutations (leading to decreased sensitivity of key target proteins), and overproduction of target proteins (Fig. 8.28).

In addition to the lipid changes observed in *E. coli* mutants, downregulation or mutation in outer-membrane proteins (porins) responsible for the influx of compounds into gram-negative bacteria has been shown to affect the MIC of triclosan. An example is mutations in the *ompF* porin gene in *E. coli* or those due to the overproduction of a protein regulator (MarA) that downregulates the expression of the protein. In section 8.3.4, efflux was discussed as a mechanism of intrinsic tolerance of some biocides and antibiotics. Mutations in the expression or control of these efflux systems have been shown to increase or decrease the sensitivities of biocides. The predominant efflux system in *E. coli* is the AcrAB-TolC proteins, which play roles in the survival of the bacteria in the gut due to the export of toxic fatty acids and bile salts. The efflux system is typical of the RND family (see section 8.3.4), consisting of the inner membrane antiporter efflux protein AcrB (driven by energy from the PMF), the periplasm-associated AcrA, and the outer-membrane factor TolC. The systems have been associated with the active efflux of triclosan from the cell, but also include other biocides, like antimicrobial dyes (e.g., crystal violet), detergents (like sodium dodecyl sulfate [SDS]), organic solvents (like *n*-hexane), acriflavine, QACs, chlorhexidine, and pine oil. Mutations that cause the loss of expression of these efflux proteins lead to the loss of this intrinsic mechanism of tolerance; equally, mutations that allow the overproduction of the proteins have been shown to allow some (although in many cases slight) increase in biocide tolerance. Overproduction was due to mutations associated with transcriptional control of efflux protein expression. The expression of the AcrAB-TolC system is under various levels of control within the cell. AcrR is a protein repressor that negatively controls the expression of the AcrAB genes by binding to a DNA sequence (known as an operator) and preventing their transcription. Mutations in *acrR* (leading to loss of the protein or changes preventing its binding) or within the operator sequence that AcrR binds to have been shown to cause overproduction of the efflux system. Similarly, MarA is a positive regulator of AcrAB and TolC, which, when present, also allow increased expression of efflux activity. MarA is a key regulator protein in *E. coli, Salmonella*, and other gram-negative bacteria

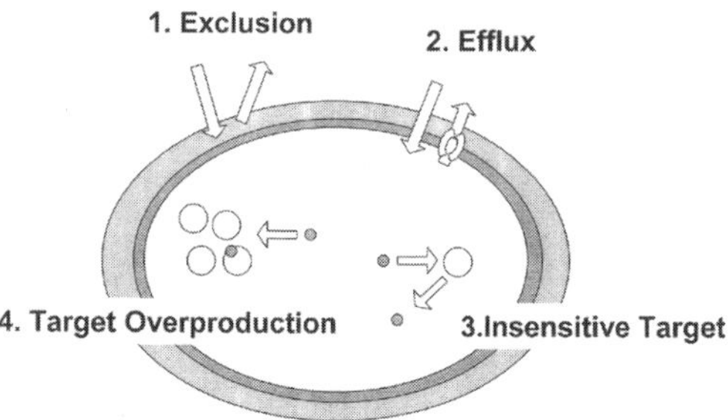

FIGURE 8.28 The modes of bacterial tolerance of triclosan due to acquired mutations. Exclusion (1) may be due to loss of outer membrane porin proteins (reduced influx) or changes in the outer or inner membrane lipid structure. Efflux mechanisms (2) include overproduction of cell membrane- or wall-associated efflux pumps due to the mutation of regulator proteins. Enoyl reductases have been shown to be specific targets for triclosan in the inhibition of fatty acid biosynthesis, with mutations identified with less affinity for these enzymes (3). Finally, the overproduction of enoyl reductases or other proteins provides greater tolerance of the biocide (4).

that is activated under stressful environmental conditions, leading to responses that allow increased tolerance of oxidative stress, organic solvents, antibiotics, and some biocides. It itself is under negative control by a repressor, MarR. As with the AcrR repressor, removal of this control allows the constitutive expression of MarA and increased expression of the efflux system. Further, MarA downregulates the outer membrane porin OmpF, which also causes a decrease in the influx of various biocides, including triclosan (discussed above as an exclusion mechanism). Overexpression of MarA was found to allow a two- to threefold increase in triclosan tolerance, as well as slight increases in pine oil tolerance. Mutations or overexpression of other associated control proteins (including SoxA and RobS) also affect the levels of AcrAB-TolC expressed in the cell, although these mechanisms of resistance are less well understood. Other similarly chromosomally encoded efflux systems have been identified in *E. coli* (e.g., the EmrAB system), as well as in other bacteria, like *Haemophilus influenzae, Neisseria gonorrhoeae, Vibrio parahaemolyticus*, and *Pseudomonas.* It should be noted that differences in the overall spectra and extents of biocides and antibiotics that are effluxed vary. Studies of the intrinsic or mutation-acquired tolerances of biocides are limited in comparison to those of antibiotics, although effects similar to those observed in *E. coli* are expected. Various RND efflux pumps have been identified in *P. aeruginosa*, with various antibiotic and biocidal resistance patterns (Table 8.18) (see section 8.3.4).

The Mex systems are similar to AbrAB-TolC. For example, overexpression of MexAB-OprM has been reported due to mutations associated with the NfxB regulatory protein, which performs a function similar to that of AbrR in *E. coli.* In these cases, increased tolerance of triclosan has been reported. Similarly, overexpression of MexEF-OprN, MexCD-OprJ, and MexJK-OprM has also been shown to allow increased tolerance of triclosan. These mechanisms may play important roles in the cumulative resistance mechanisms described in *Pseudomonas* biofilms (see section 8.3.8), although many of the mutations have not been stable. Interestingly, this is not the case in the overexpression of MexXY-OprM; indeed, limited cross-resistance has been reported with the heavy-metal-associated resistance of CzrAB-OpmN (Table 8.18). The overexpression of other cell wall-associated proteins has been implicated in biocide resistance in *Pseudomonas*, for example, the outer membrane protein OmpR, although the exact reasons for this are unknown. Overall, the increase in efflux of triclosan and other antimicrobials allows the survival of the cell around typical MICs of the biocide but has not been shown to be significant in survival at typical bactericidal concentrations. Of greater importance may be the observed cross-resistance to various antibiotics, like tetracycline and fluoroquinolones. It is interesting that *E. coli* mutants with pine oil- or triclosan-induced tolerance (due to overexpression of MarA and therefore increased efflux activity) were also found to have low-level increases in antibiotic (e.g., ampicillin and tetracycline) MICs; however, if tolerance was similarly induced with the antibiotic tetracycline, much higher levels of cross-resistance

TABLE 8.18 Examples of RND efflux pumps associated with biocide resistance in *P. aeruginosa* due to overproduction

Efflux system	Antibiotic resistance	Biocide resistance
MexAB-OprM	β-Lactams, tetracycline, fluoroquinolones	Triclosan, SDS
MexXY-OprM	Fluoroquinolones	Unknown
MexCD-OprJ	β-Lactams, tetracycline, fluoroquinolones	Triclosan, crystal violet, acriflavine
MexEF-OprN	Fluoroquinolones	Triclosan
MexJK-OprM	Tetracycline	Triclosan
CzrAB-OpmN	Unknown	Cadmium, zinc

were observed. It may well be that efflux-mediated mechanisms allow the survival of bacteria under restrictive environmental conditions and therefore provide time to further adapt by intrinsic or acquired resistance mechanisms. The clinical significance of these results is unclear and deserves further investigation.

Although triclosan appears to have multiple mechanisms of action, it is clear that a key bacterial target is intracellular enoyl (acyl carrier protein) reductases (see section 3.15); these enzymes are also specifically targeted by another bisphenol, hexachlorophene. Enoyl reductases are involved in type II fatty acid synthetic processes. Type II fatty acid synthase systems in bacteria use a dissociated group of enzymes (in contrast to mammalian type I synthases, which use a multienzymatic polypeptide complex) for the synthesis of fatty acids; this involves the cyclic addition of two carbon units to a growing fatty acid chain. Enoyl reductases catalyze the last stage in this elongation cycle, which is dependent on the presence of the cofactor NADH or NADPH. Both biocides, as well as some antibiotics, like isoniazid and the diazoborines, specifically bind to the substrate target site on the enzyme to selectively inhibit its activity (see section 3.15). Specific binding of triclosan to FabI-like enoyl reductases has been observed in gram-positive (*S. aureus, Mycobacterium smegmatis*, and *M. tuberculosis*) and gram-negative (*E. coli, P. aeruginosa*, and *H. influenzae*) bacteria. Triclosan preferably binds noncovalently to the enzyme and its respective cofactor, mimicking the enzyme's natural substrate. It should be noted that not all enoyl reductases are intrinsically sensitive to triclosan. In the case of *E. coli*, FabI is believed to be the only enoyl reductase that is sensitive to triclosan; hence, low concentrations of triclosan have the ability to inhibit wild-type *E. coli* strains; in contrast, the structurally different FabK enoyl reductase in *Streptococcus pneumoniae* has been found to be intrinsically resistant to triclosan binding. In other bacteria, including *P. aeruginosa, B. atrophaeus, S. aureus, M. tuberculosis*, and *Enterococcus faecalis*, homologues of both enoyl reductase types have been identified, suggesting that both triclosan-resistant and -sensitive forms are expressed. In these cases, triclosan tolerance is due to the various intrinsic mechanisms; for example, in *P. aeruginosa*, resistance is due to the presence of an effective outer-membrane permeability barrier and efficient efflux systems. The most studied triclosan-sensitive enoyl reductases have been *E. coli* FabI and its homologue, InhA, in *M. smegmatis*. Specific genetic mutations producing amino acid changes within the active site of the enzyme have been shown to dramatically reduce the affinity for triclosan. FabI mutations were first identified in vitro by passaging wild-type *E. coli* strains through increasing concentrations of triclosan. Triclosan-tolerant strains were found to rapidly develop and could grow at significantly higher MICs, from approximately 1 to >75 μg/liter, depending on the specific mutation. The *M. smegmatis* enoyl reductase (InhA) was found to develop cross-resistance with triclosan to the antimycobacterial antibiotic isoniazid; isoniazid had previously been shown to target fatty acid biosynthesis, particularly that of InhA, in mycobacteria, and resistance to the antibiotic could develop due to similar mutations.

A further mechanism of resistance to triclosan has been found to be due to the overproduction of enzymes. *E. coli* mutants (with MICs in the range of 25 to 50 mg/liter) have been described which did not show any mutations in the DNA sequence of *fabI* but did show overproduction of the FabI protein. Hyperexpression of FabI in *S. aureus* mutants has also been reported to cause an increase in triclosan resistance. The exact mechanism of resistance has not been reported in these strains. In a further mode of resistance to triclosan, distinct *E. coli* mutants have been identified that had no mutations associated with the enoyl reductase but appeared to overexpress glucosamine-6-phosphate aminotransferase, which is involved in biosynthesis of various amino sugar-containing macromolecules. In both cases, these mutants also showed increased resistance to triclosan in *E. coli*, but not to other biocides, including hexachlorophene or antibiotics. Overproduction of target proteins may allow cellular processes to proceed due to sequestration of the available biocide. Further reports on the mode of action of triclosan have shown direct inhibition of other enzymes, including various transferases, in vitro, suggesting that other mutations may contribute to triclosan resistance.

The triclosan MIC for wild-type laboratory *E. coli* strains is quite low (typically between 0.1 and 2 μg/liter), but the MBC is actually quite high (50 to 75 μg/liter); in all cases of triclosan resistance investigated, although significant changes in MICs could be developed, no changes in MBCs were found, suggesting that triclosan has multiple targets of action. In some cases, triclosan resistance has been shown to be >75 mg/liter, but it should be noted that triclosan is soluble in water or growth media only up to ~75 μg/liter, above which it precipitates. In an interesting link to decreased penetration as a mechanism of resistance, many of these triclosan-tolerant *E. coli* strains lose their resistant phenotypes when cultured in the presence of EDTA; EDTA is a permeabilizing agent that may allow greater penetration of triclosan to the inner cell membrane and cytoplasm.

Many mutational studies have also focused on chlorhexidine. Chlorhexidine is a bisbiguanide widely used in antiseptics (see sections 3.8 and 4.6). It also demonstrates broad-spectrum bacteriostatic and bactericidal activities, particularly against gram-positive bacteria. Increased tolerance of chlorhexidine has been induced in some organisms but has not been successful in others. In studies with the gram-negative bacteria *Proteus mirabilis* and *S. marcescens*, mutants have been developed under laboratory conditions that have up to 128 and 258 times higher initial chlorhexidine MICs, respectively; however, it was not possible to develop resistance to chlorhexidine in *S. enterica* serovar Enteritidis. The mutants appeared to be stable in *S. marcescens* but not in *P. mirabilis*. Some of the chlorhexidine-tolerant strains were also shown to be cross-tolerant of a QAC, benzalkonium chloride, suggesting similar mechanisms of resistance. Analysis of these strains did not show any obvious changes in their biochemical properties or in their virulence in mice. More recent studies demonstrated the development of stable chlorhexidine resistance in *P. stutzeri*; these strains showed various levels of increased tolerance of QACs, triclosan, and some antibiotics, probably by a nonspecific alteration of the cell envelope or, particularly, the outer membrane. Despite extensive experimentation using a variety of procedures, many investigators have been unable to develop stable chlorhexidine resistance in *E. coli*, *Staphylococcus*, and *Enterococcus*.

Clinical reports of chlorhexidine tolerance include the adaptation and growth of *S. marcescens* that also had cross-resistance to a QAC in contact lens disinfectants containing chlorhexidine. In contrast to mutations leading to increased tolerance of chlorhexidine, other mutations have been shown to cause hypersensitivity to the biocide. Examples are a series of outer-membrane *E. coli* and *P. aeruginosa* mutants, including outer-membrane protein and LPS strains, which are more sensitive to chlorhexidine, and QACs, confirming the importance of the outer-membrane structure in the intrinsic resistance of gram-negative bacteria to biocides (see section 8.6).

Other examples of mutations leading to increased sensitivity to biocides are given in Table 8.19. A number of studies have investigated the resistance mechanisms of bacterial spores. In studies with sodium hypochlorite and chlorine dioxide, no difference in biocide sensitivity was observed in spore mutants lacking the various acid-soluble spore proteins. However, mutations in proteins required for the assembly of the various spore coats (see section 8.3.11) produced spores that were hypersensitive, confirming the exclusion of these active agents from the spore core by the spore coats as a major mechanism of intrinsic resistance to these oxidizing agents. Other spore mutants that lack DPA appeared to have increased water contents, with a subsequent decrease in resistance to moist heat, hydrogen peroxide, iodophors, and formaldehyde; no effects were observed on resistance to dry heat and glutaraldehyde, but the mutants did demonstrate increased resistance to UV light. It can be speculated that as mutations

TABLE 8.19 Examples of mutations causing increased sensitivity to biocides

Bacteria	Biocide sensitivity	Mechanism
E. coli, *P. aeruginosa*	Chlorhexidine, some QACs	Mutants lacking key outer membrane proteins or LPS
P. putida	Peracetic acid	Catalase mutants
B. subtilis spores	Sodium hypochlorite, chlorine dioxide	Loss of spore coat structure/assembly
	Moist heat, hydrogen peroxide, iodophors, formaldehyde	Lack of dipicolinic acid
Acinetobacter calcoaceticus, *P. putida*, and *G. stearothermophilus*	Phenol and phenolics	Mutants lacking enzymes responsible for phenol degradation, including phenol hydroxylases and catechol dioxygenases
Gram-negative and gram-positive bacteria, including *Pseudomonas*, *Acinobacter*, *Bacillus*, and *Thiobacillus*	Mercury	Loss of mercuric reductase activity[a]

[a]Can be plasmid, transposon, or chromosomally mediated.

that lead to the loss of enzymatic mechanisms of intrinsic tolerance of biocides (like mercuric ion reductases and catalases and peroxidases, as discussed in section 8.3.5), adaptations of mutations leading to overexpression of these enzymes may be expected to allow some increase in tolerance of the respective biocides.

Efflux as a mechanism of acquired biocide resistance has been the focus of more recent investigations, as highlighted for triclosan resistance above. This was first proposed as a mechanism of resistance in proflavine (an acridine)-resistant bacteria, where the cells had an increased ability to expel the bound dye. More recent studies of triclosan and other biocides have demonstrated the significance of efflux in resistance of bacteria and cross-resistance to antibiotics. MDR is a particularly serious problem in enteric and other gram-negative bacteria. MDR is a term employed to describe resistance mechanisms by genes that comprise part of the normal cell genome. These genes are activated by induction or mutation caused by some types of stress, and because they are distributed ubiquitously, genetic transfer is not considered a high risk. Although such systems are most important in the context of antibiotic resistance, several examples of MDR systems in which an operon or gene is associated with changes in biocide susceptibility have been described, including the following:

- Mutations at an *acr* locus in the Acr system render *E. coli* more sensitive to hydrophobic antibiotics, dyes, and detergents.
- The *robA* gene is responsible for overexpression in *E. coli* of the RobA protein, which confers multiple antibiotic and heavy-metal resistances (interestingly, Ag^+ may be pumped out).
- The MarA protein controls a set of genes (*mar* and *soxRS* regulons) that confer resistance, not only to several antibiotics, but also to superoxide-generating agents.

Low concentrations of pine oil (used as a disinfectant and containing pinene and terpineol as the major biocides) (see section 3.10) allowed the selection of *E. coli* mutants that overexpressed MarA and demonstrated low levels of cross-resistance to antibiotics. Deletion of the *mar* or *acrAB* locus (the latter encodes a PMF-dependent efflux pump) increased susceptibility to pine oil; deletion of *acrAB*, but not of *mar*, increased the susceptibility of *E. coli* to chloroxylenol and to a QAC. In addition, the *E. coli* MdfA (multidrug transporter) protein confers greater tolerance of both antibiotics and a QAC (benzalkonium). The significance of these and other MDR systems in bacterial susceptibility to biocides needs to be studied further, particularly the issue of cross-resistance with antibiotics. At present, it is difficult to translate these laboratory findings to actual clinical use, and some studies have demonstrated that antibiotic-resistant bacteria are not significantly more resistant to the lethal (or bactericidal) effects of disinfectants than are antibiotic-sensitive strains.

The adaptation of *P. aeruginosa* to QACs and other biocides is a well-known phenomenon, but in most cases, this is due to a physiological adaptation rather than to specific mutations. In many of these reports, the actual mechanisms of tolerance have not been identified. Chloroxylenol-resistant strains of *P. aeruginosa* were isolated by repeated exposure in media containing gradually increasing concentrations of the phenolic, but resistance was also unstable. Resistance to amphoteric surfactants has also been observed, and interestingly, cross-resistance to chlorhexidine was noted. This may suggest that the mechanism(s) of such resistance is nonspecific and that it involves cellular changes that modify the responses of organisms to unrelated biocidal agents. Outer-membrane modification is an obvious factor and has indeed been found with QAC-resistant and amphoteric-resistant *P. aeruginosa* and with chlorhexidine-resistant *S. marcescens*. Such changes involve fatty acid profiles and, perhaps more importantly, outer-membrane proteins. Evidence for this was shown in the analysis of *Pseudomonas fluorescens* isolates that had increased tolerance of QACs, which could be reduced when EDTA was present with the QAC; similar results have been found with laboratory-generated *E. coli* mutants with increased MICs of triclosan (as discussed above). EDTA has long been known to produce changes in the outer membranes of gram-negative bacteria, especially pseudomonads. *E. coli* mutants with increased resistance to triclosan and some solvents have shown specific changes in their cell membrane lipid contents; in the case of solvent resistance, a decrease in the ratio of the phospholipids (phosphatidylethanolamine-phosphatidylglycerol-cardiolipin, with the last being more anionic) in the cell membrane was observed, suggesting exclusion as the mechanism of resistance. Thus, it appears that, again, the development of resistance can be associated with changes in the cell membrane or envelope, limiting uptake of biocides.

One of the most significant reports of mutation as a mechanism of resistance to a biocide concerned the isolation and analysis of glutaraldehyde-resistant mycobacteria. Water is a common source of atypical mycobacteria, which include the "rapidly growing" species, like *Mycobacterium fortuitum*, *Mycobacterium abscessus*, and *M. chelonae* (in relation to the other "slowly growing" mycobacteria, like *M. tuberculosis*). It was noted that *M. chelonae* strains had been isolated from flexible endoscopes and washer-disinfectors used to reprocess such temperature-sensitive medical devices. These microorganisms have been linked to nosocomial infections and "pseudoinfections," the latter due to misdiagnosis of these strains as pathogens, such as *M. tuberculosis* and *M. avium*. The identification of these isolates was initially speculated to be due to the development of biofilms over time within the machines and devices, which became intrinsically resistant to the 1 to 2% glutaraldehyde formulations that are widely used for low-temperature disinfection (see section 3.4). The isolation and investigation of a number of these *M. chelonae* strains found that they not only showed increased MICs of glutaraldehyde, but also were dramatically resistant to the biocidal effects of glutaraldehyde products (Fig. 8.29).

A range of glutaraldehyde-based products (normally effective concentrations between 0.5 and 2.5% glutaraldehyde) have been shown to be ineffective against these mutant strains. Testing with other aldehydes showed mixed results; 10% succine dialdehyde-formaldehyde showed little or no change in resistance, while 0.55% OPA was effective, but at a lower rate than observed with wild-type *M. chelonae* strains (Fig. 8.29). Little or no difference in tolerance was observed with other biocides, including 70% ethanol, peracetic acid, and hydrogen peroxide; however, in some cases, changes in MICs and MBCs that may be formulation (or product) specific have been reported. The nature of glutaraldehyde resistance in these strains has been investigated and was found to be related to cell wall or surface changes. The mutant

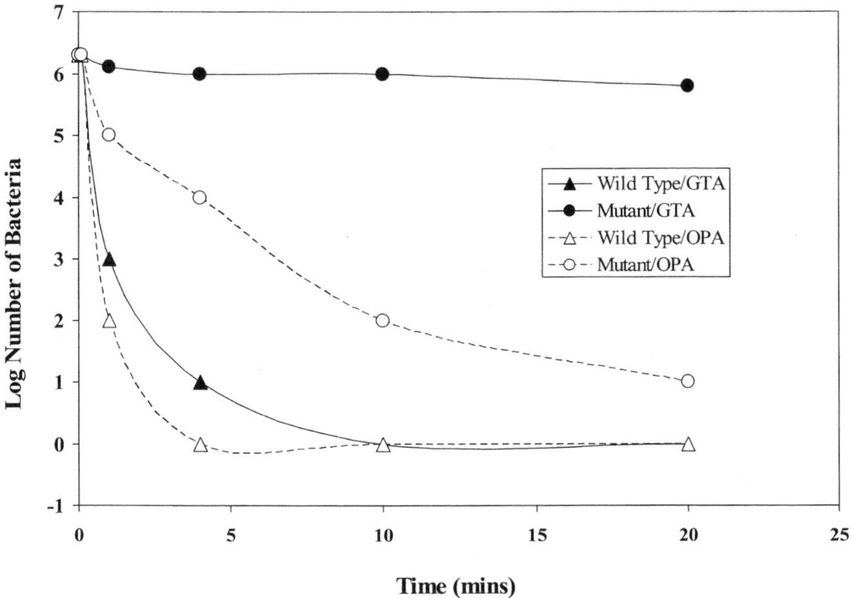

FIGURE 8.29 Demonstration of the resistance of *M. chelonae* glutaraldehyde-resistant strains. The aldehyde antimicrobial activity of a wild-type glutaraldehyde-sensitive strain of *M. chelonae* was compared to that of a glutaraldehyde-resistant strain. Glutaraldehyde (2%) demonstrated little or no effect against the resistant strain; another aldehyde (0.55% OPA) demonstrated efficacy but required a longer exposure time than for the wild-type strain.

colonies appeared to be physically drier and waxier than those of the wild-type strains and were found to have greater hydrophobicity. Cell wall analysis found no differences in the extractable fatty acids or mycolic acids (although there could be differences in the proportions of these lipids), but there was an obvious change in the monosaccharide contents of the cell wall polysaccharides arabinogalactan and arabinomannan. The exact mutation(s) in these strains has not been identified, but changes in the polysaccharide structure appear to decrease the cell wall permeability. A slight increase in the MIC was observed with some antimycobacterial antibiotics (notably rifampin and ethambutol), but not others (isoniazid). It is interesting that these strains remained somewhat sensitive to other aldehydes, including OPA, presumably due to greater penetration of the aldehydes into the cell wall (see section 7.4.3). Following these reports, subsequent isolation and testing of *M. chelonae* and *Mycobacterium gordonae* strains from washer-disinfectors that used glutaraldehyde have found a prevalence of glutaraldehyde-resistant strains (up to 50% of isolates); in one study, efflux pumps were confirmed not to be involved as a resistance mechanism. It has also been demonstrated that some strains have increased tolerance of 70% ethanol in comparison to other mycobacteria. Overall, the mechanism of resistance in these strains appears to be due to exclusion of the biocide from the cell or inaccessibility of key cell wall targets.

It is generally accepted that environmental isolates of bacteria are invariably less sensitive to biocides than are laboratory strains. Although it is thought that in many cases this is primarily due to physiological adaptation of bacteria within their respective environments (see section 8.3), various challenges in these situations may also play an important role in the mutational adaptation of the isolates. These mutations may directly affect key biocide targets within cells or otherwise provide the cell with greater resistance to the biocide. In addition, other subtle mutations or adaptations can afford further benefits to allow the bacteria to survive in the presence of biocides. For example, subinhibitory antibiotic concentrations have been speculated to cause subtle changes in the bacterial outer structure, thereby stimulating cell-to-cell contact and other responses or survival mechanisms; whether residual concentrations of biocides in clinical or industrial situations can produce the same subtle effects remains to be tested, although some studies have suggested such adaptations.

8.7.3 Plasmids and Transmissible Elements

Initial investigations into plasmid- and/or transposon-mediated resistance to biocides identified certain specific examples of plasmid-mediated resistance in bacteria to heavy metals, like silver, other metal ions, and organomercurials. Despite this, unlike many reports of antibiotic resistance in bacteria, plasmids and transposons were not generally considered responsible for the elevated levels of biocide resistance associated with certain species or strains. Further investigations, however, have shown numerous cases linking the presence of plasmids in bacteria with increased tolerance of chlorhexidine, QACs, and triclosan, as well as of diamidines, acridines, and other dyes, such as ethidium bromide. In many cases, the exact mechanisms are unknown and may be linked indirectly to other plasmid determinants, which indirectly lead to changes in the cell membrane or cell wall. Despite this, specific examples of plasmid-encoded tolerance of various biocides by degradation and efflux have been identified and investigated (Table 8.20).

Plasmid-encoded resistance to biocides has been extensively investigated with mercurials (both inorganic and organic), silver compounds, and other cations and anions. Mercurials have been less used in recent years as disinfectants, but inorganic salts (e.g., $HgCl_2$) and organomercurial compounds (e.g., merbromin and thiomersal) are still employed as preservatives in some types of industrial products (see section 3.12). Mercury resistance in bacteria can be intrinsic (chromosomally encoded) in some cases, including strains of *Pseudomonas* and *Thiobacillus*, but is more often described as being acquired through plasmids or transposons (Table 8.21).

These plasmids and transposons are particularly widespread within gram-negative bacteria, although a number of chromosome-associated (e.g., in *Bacillus*) and plasmid-based (e.g., *S. aureus* pI258) mechanisms in gram-positive bacteria have been described. They can be transferred between bacteria by conjugation, transduction, and transformation (as discussed in

TABLE 8.20 Identified and possible mechanisms of plasmid-encoded resistance to biocides

Biocide	Mechanism
Chlorhexidine	Inactivation: chromosomally mediated; not yet found to be plasmid mediated Efflux in *S. aureus* and other staphylococci Decreased uptake
QACs	Efflux in *S. aureus* and other staphylococci Decreased uptake
Silver compounds	Efflux in *Salmonella*
Formaldehyde	Inactivation by formaldehyde dehydrogenase Cell surface alterations (outer membrane proteins)
Acridines[a]	Efflux in *S. aureus* and *S. epidermidis*
Diamidines	Efflux in *S. aureus* and *S. epidermidis*
Crystal violet[a]	Efflux in *S. aureus* and *S. epidermidis*
Mercurials[b]	Inactivation (reductases, lyases)
Ethidium bromide	Efflux in *S. aureus* and *S. epidermidis*.

[a]Now rarely used for antiseptic or disinfectant purposes (see section 3.7).
[b]Organomercurials are still used as preservatives, e.g., in paints (see section 3.12).

TABLE 8.21 Examples of acquired (plasmid or transposon) resistance to mercury in bacteria

Bacterium	Plasmid or transposon[a]
P. fluorescens	pMER327
P. putida	Group G and H plasmids, Tn*5041D*
Xanthomonas spp.	Tn*5053*
E. coli	pR100, pNR1, Tn*5057*
Acinetobacter spp.	pKLH102, pKLH104, pKLH1
S. marcescens	pDI1358
S. aureus	pI258

[a]Plasmids are generally designated pXXX (p for plasmid) and transposons TnXXX (Tn for transposon).

section 8.7.1). Mercury itself is an antimicrobial metal (see section 3.12). It is a particularly potent intracellular toxin, binding to the sulfhydryl groups of proteins and enzymes. The mechanisms of mercury tolerance have been particularly well studied due to their potential use for bioremediation of mercury-contaminated wastewater. As described in section 8.3.6, the mechanism of resistance is based on the expression of mercuric reductases, irrespective of whether it is intrinsic or acquired, which causes the enzymatic conversion of the mercury ion (Hg^{2+}) to mercury vapor (Hg^0), which then vaporizes from the cell. Mercuric reductases are encoded by *merA* genes that demonstrate significant similarities in their respective amino acid sequences, suggesting a common original source, with the exception of the gram-positive reductases, which appear to be more distinct and diverse. In some cases, the plasmids can also carry antibiotic resistance genes; for example, inorganic (Hg^{2+}) and organomercury resistance is a common property of clinical isolates of *S. aureus* containing plasmids that also express penicillinases (which break down penicillin). MerA is expressed from an operon that is also relatively conserved within gram-negative bacteria (Fig. 8.30).

Expression of the various genes involved in mercury resistance is inducible in the presence of mercury, under the control of the MerR activator-repressor protein, which allows the expression of the resistance proteins in the presence of Hg^{2+} and their repression in its absence. The mechanisms involved in the neutralization of mercury are summarized in Fig. 8.31.

In gram-negative bacteria, Hg^{2+} binds to the periplasmically encoded MerP protein that transfers the toxic ions to the cytoplasmic membrane protein MerT and from there to the cytoplasmic MerA enzyme. MerA is an NADPH-dependent flavoprotein that causes the reduction of Hg^{2+} to Hg^0; due to the high vapor pressure of Hg^0, it rapidly volatilizes out of the cell. In some plasmids, an additional

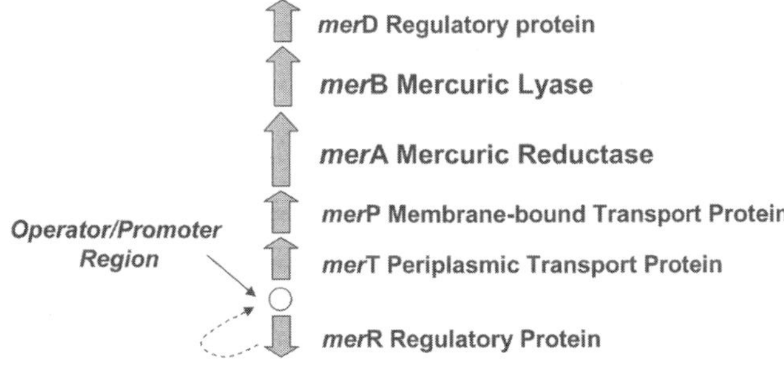

FIGURE 8.30 The simplified structure of a typical mercury resistance operon in gram-negative bacteria. The numbers, types, and control of expression of proteins from the operon can vary from isolate to isolate. In all cases, a mercuric reductase (MerA) is expressed; however, only broad-spectrum plasmids and transposons are found to have MerB homologues (which are enzymes that hydrolyze organomercurial compounds to release the mercuric ion for subsequent reduction). The other proteins expressed are involved in mercury transport and control of the expression of the operon.

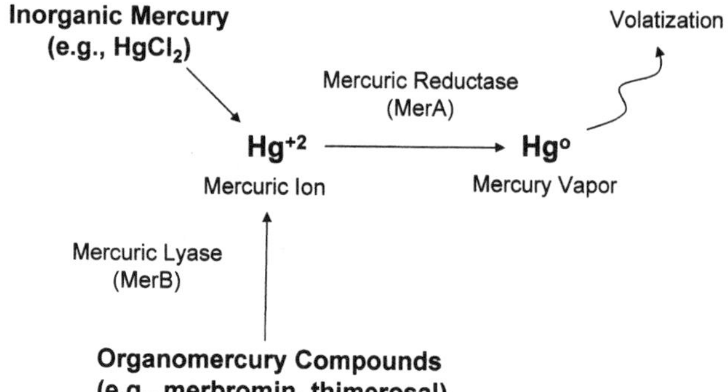

FIGURE 8.31 Mechanisms of resistance to mercury.

enzyme, MerB, which is an organomercuric lyase, is also expressed; this enzyme catalyzes the separation of Hg^{2+} from various organomercury compounds (like phenylmercury), thereby allowing further resistance to these compounds. Plasmids and transposons that confer resistance to mercurials may therefore be further considered as either (i) "narrow spectrum," specifying resistance to Hg^{2+} and to some organomercurials (like merbromin), or (ii) "broad spectrum," with resistance to narrow-spectrum compounds and to additional organomercurials. In the case of narrow-spectrum elements, the resistance may be simply due to exclusion from the cell, suggesting that other resistance mechanisms may also be present.

Unlike mercury, silver and copper are still widely employed as biocides (see section 3.12). In both cases, plasmid-mediated resistance in bacteria has been described (Table 8.22). Plasmid-encoded resistance to silver in *Salmonella, Pseudomonas, Serratia, Klebsiella, Enterobacter,* and *Citrobacter* species has been described. Resistance to silver was a significant concern in the treatment of wounds with silver nitrate and silver sufadiazine. In the investigation of particular *Enterobacter cloacae* wound infections, resistance to therapeutic concentrations of silver appeared to be associated with the presence of a plasmid, although in other cases, the resistance mechanism was thought to be chromosomally encoded. The mechanisms of resistance have yet to be elucidated in these cases, but they appear to be associated with decreased silver accumulation. At least two main mechanisms, efflux systems (e.g., silver efflux proteins encoded by *Salmonella* plasmids) and sequestering of the metal ions (e.g., *P. syringae* Cop proteins expressed from pPT23D for copper sequestration) have been identified, although other mechanisms remain to be elucidated.

TABLE 8.22 Examples of plasmid-mediated resistance to silver and copper in bacteria

Bacterium	Resistance	Mechanism
E. coli	Copper	Chromosomal and plasmid-mediated resistances described. An example is the plasmid pRI1004, which carries the *pco* genes (e.g, for the proteins PcoE and PcoC), which are known to detoxify copper in the periplasm, but by an unknown mechanism.
Klebsiella pneumoniae	Copper, silver	pLVPK expresses periplasmic proteins that are thought to sequester copper and silver ions.
Salmonella spp.	Silver	Plasmids encoding P-type ATPase and cation/protein antiporter efflux proteins
P. syringae	Copper	Plasmids (e.g., pPT23D) encoding Cop extracellular and periplasmic proteins that sequester copper ions

TABLE 8.23 Plasmid-mediated resistance to various toxic metals in bacteria

Bacterium	Plasmid or transposon	Resistance	Mechanism
Gram-positive			
S. aureus	pI258	Cadmium, zinc	Efflux-ATPase (CadA)
		Arsenic	Efflux-antiporter (ArsB)
	pII147	Cadmium	Membrane-associated sequestration
Staphylococcus xylosus	pSX267	Arsenic	Efflux-membrane potential (ArsB)
Gram-negative			
R. eutropha	pMOL28, pMOL30	Cadmium, zinc, copper, mercury, chromium, nickel	Efflux systems, e.g., the Czc system on pMOL30 for copper, cadmium, and zinc and the Cnr system on pMOL28 for copper and nickel; other, still unknown mechanisms exist.
Listeria monocytogenes	pLm74, Tn*5422*	Cadmium	Efflux similar to pI258 in *S. aureus* but specific to cadmium (CadAC); also encoded on a transposon but found to be plasmid rather than chromosome associated
E. coli	pR773	Arsenic	Efflux-ATPase (ArsAB)

Plasmid-encoded resistances to a variety of toxic metals, including arsenic, cadmium, lead, and zinc, have also been described (Table 8.23), although in many cases, the exact mechanisms of resistance are unknown.

Many of these systems have also been investigated for potential use in the bioremediation of metal contamination in various industrial applications. Examples are the plasmid-encoded arsenic resistance mechanisms in *E. coli* (pR773) and *S. aureus* (pI258), which encode arsenic efflux systems. In the *E. coli* plasmid pR773, resistance is mediated by the expression of the *arsRDABC* operon. When arsenate enters the cytoplasm, it is first reduced (by ArsC) to arsenite and then pumped out of the cell by the arsenite-specific ArsAB ATPase efflux system. The expression of the *ars* operon is controlled by the two regulator proteins ArsR and ArsD. ArsR has been shown to repress the transcription of the operon, which is relieved in the presence of arsenite. The *S. aureus* mechanism is similar yet distinct; the simpler operon *arsRBC* encodes an efflux protein, which is driven by energy from the membrane potential, with action similar to that of the ArsR and ArsC proteins in *E. coli*. Further examples are strains of *Ralstonia eutropha* (previously known as *Alcaligenes eutrophus*), which have a remarkable capability to survive in the presence of a variety of toxic metals. They appear to have multiple resistance mechanisms that include those encoded by the bacterial chromosome, by transposons, and by two megaplasmids (or large plasmids) (pMOL28 and pMOL30). Both plasmids encode efflux pumps that have specificity for various metals (Table 8.23) but are also known to encode other, as yet unspecified mechanisms of resistance. As with copper and silver, multiple acquired resistance mechanisms have been proposed, including (i) efflux; (ii) the expression of cell surface proteins that bind the metal ions; (iii) metal-detoxifying proteins expressed in the cytoplasm, including those in bacteria, yeasts, and fungi, like metallothioneins and other metal-binding proteins; and (iv) specific mutations or overexpression of key target enzymes or other proteins. A number of these resistance mechanisms have also been found in yeasts (see section 8.10).

Occasional studies have examined the possible roles of plasmids in the resistance of gram-negative bacteria to other biocides. Plasmid RP1 (which encodes resistance to the antibiotics carbenicillin, tetracycline, and neomycin-kanamycin) did not significantly alter the resistance of *P. aeruginosa* to QACs, chlorhexidine, iodine, or chlorinated phenols, although an increased resistance to hexachlorophene was observed. This compound has a much greater effect on gram-positive than on gram-negative bacteria, so it is difficult to assess the significance of this finding. Transformation of this plasmid into *E. coli* or *P. aeruginosa* did not increase sensitivity to a range of biocides tested. Strains of *P. stuartii* have been reported to be highly tolerant of mercury, cationic disinfectants (such as chlorhexidine and QACs), and various antibiotics. As yet, no evidence has been presented to show that there is a plasmid-linked association between antibiotic and biocide resistances in these organisms, pseudomonads, or *Proteus* species, although it has been speculated. High levels of biocide tolerance have been reported in other hospital and industrial isolates, although no clear-cut role for plasmid-specified resistance has emerged. High levels of tolerance of chlorhexidine and QACs may be intrinsic or may have resulted from mutations due to low-level yet constant exposure in the environment. It has been proposed that the extensive use of these cationic agents could be responsible for the selection of biocide- and antibiotic-resistant strains; however, there is little evidence to support this conclusion. Studies with these biocides demonstrated that it was difficult to transfer chlorhexidine or QAC resistance under normal conditions and that plasmid-mediated resistance to these chemicals in gram-negative bacteria was an unlikely event. By contrast, plasmid pR124 alters the OmpF outer-membrane porin protein in *E. coli*, and cells containing this plasmid are more resistant to at least one QAC (cetrimide) and to other agents. Changes in the presence, structure, or proportion of various cell envelope porins or LPS in gram-negative bacteria may indirectly allow increased or decreased sensitivity to biocides by altering biocide penetration (as discussed in section 8.6).

Bacterial mechanisms of resistance to formaldehyde and industrial biocides can be plasmid encoded in gram-negative bacteria. Alterations in the cell surface (outer-membrane proteins) and formaldehyde dehydrogenase (see section 8.3.5) are considered to be responsible. Formaldehyde resistance plasmids in *S. marcescens* and *E. coli* have been reported to change the expression of some outer-membrane proteins and therefore cell surface hydrophobicity. The various membrane proteins were found to be identical; however, the expression of a number of proteins appeared to be reduced in the plasmid-containing strains. Other reports of formaldehyde resistance in gram-negative bacteria have also shown changes in the composition and structure of the outer membrane, which were also cross-resistant to glutaraldehyde and independent of the expression of formaldehyde dehydrogenase. Toluene resistance in pseudomonads due to degradation by oxygenase-catalyzed hydroxylation has been shown to be chromosome and plasmid encoded. The plasmids include the *Pseudomonas* TOL plasmids for toluene resistance and the TOM (for toluene *ortho*-monooxygenase) plasmid, which encodes enzymes for toluene and phenol degradation in *B. cepacia*. In both cases, they allow phenols and/or toluene to be used as single sources of carbon and energy. The TOM pathway is a three-component enzyme system consisting of a hydroxylase, an oxidoreductase, and a protein involved in the electron transfer between these enzymes. Its significance as a mechanism of resistance to phenol- and cresol-based disinfectants or preserved products is not known.

MRSA strains are a major cause of sepsis in hospitals throughout the world, although not all strains have increased virulence. Many can be referred to as "epidemic" strains because of the ease with which they have been shown to spread or transfer between patients. Individuals who are at particular risk are those who are debilitated or immunocompromised or have open wounds. MRSA strains demonstrate marked resistance to various antibiotics, including methicillin, penicillin, and gentamicin, that can be chromosomally and/or plasmid encoded. The analysis of plasmids from these

TABLE 8.24 Examples of *qac* genes and susceptibilities of *S. aureus* strains to biocides

qac gene[a]	MIC ratio[b]						
	PF	CHG	Pt	Pi	CTAB	BZK	CPC
A	>16	2.5	>16	>16	4	>3	>4
B	8	1	>4	2	2	>3	>2
C	1	1	1	1	6	>3	>4
D	1	1	1	1	6	>3	>4
MIC (μg/ml)	40	0.8	<50	50	1	<2	<1

[a]*qac* genes are also known as nucleic acid binding (NAB) compound resistance genes, as many of the biocides have a mode of action related to nucleic acid binding.

[b]For comparison, the ratios shown are the MICs for strains of *S. aureus* carrying the various *qac* genes divided by the MIC for a strain carrying no gene or plasmid. The actual MIC of the sensitive strain that did not carry the gene or plasmid in shown in the last row. PF, proflavine; CHG, chlorhexidine diacetate; Pt, pentamidine isothionate; Pi, propamidine isothionate; CTAB, cetyltrimethylammonium bromide; BZK, benzalkonium chloride; CPC, cetylpyridinium chloride.

strains found that *S. aureus* and coagulase-negative staphylococci (like *S. epidermidis*) can have one or more plasmids, which can vary in size and copy number. These plasmids have been subdivided into three different types:

1. Large, β-lactamase–heavy-metal resistance plasmids, which carry transposons (e.g., Tn*552*) that confer penicillin resistance (penicillinase expression) and also tolerance of heavy metals (including mercury and arsensic, as discussed for the plasmid pI258 above)

2. The pSK41 family of conjugative plasmids

3. The pSK1 plasmid family, which can confer increased tolerance of aminoglycoside antibiotics (including kanamycin and gentamycin), as well as cross-tolerance of various cationic biocides

Based on MICs, *S. aureus* strains carrying these plasmids (with various *qac* genes) were found to have less sensitivity to the inhibitory effects on biocides, including QACs, chlorhexidine, and diamidines, together with intercalating dyes, like ethidium bromide and acridines (Table 8.24). No decrease in the susceptibilities of antibiotic-resistant strains to phenolics (phenol, cresol, and chlorocresol), povidone-iodine, or tested preservatives (parabens) were shown. These plasmids have been the focus of research to identify the genetic aspects of plasmid-mediated biocide resistance mechanisms. In clinical strains of *S. aureus*, these mechanisms have been found to be encoded by at least four separate multidrug (efflux) resistance determinants that are widely distributed (Table 8.25).

These determinants were all found to encode efflux proteins driven by energy from the PMF (see section 8.3.4) and have been described as two gene families (*qacA*/*qacB* and *qacC*/*qacD*) that show sequence similarities. The *qacA*/*qacB* family of genes (Table 8.25) encodes proton-

TABLE 8.25 *qac* genes and resistance to QACs and other biocides

Multidrug resistance determinant[a]	Gene location	Resistance encoded[b]
qacA	pSK1 family of multiresistant plasmids; also, β-lactamase and heavy-metal resistance families	QACs, CHX, diamidines, acridines, EB
qacB	β-Lactamase and heavy-metal resistance plasmids	QACs, acridines, EB
qacC[c]	Small plasmids (<3 kb) or large conjugative plasmids	Some QACs, EB
qacD (or *smr*)[c]	Large (50-kb) conjugative, multiresistance plasmids	Some QACs, EB

[a]Other *qac* genes have also been described, including *qacG*, *qacH*, and *qacJ*, most of which are similar to the QacC gene.

[b]CHX, chlorhexidine salts; EB, ethidium bromide.

[c]These genes have identical target sites and show restriction site homology.

dependent export proteins (of the MFS SMR subtypes) (see section 8.2.4) that develop significant homology to other energy-dependent transporters, such as the tetracycline transporters found in various strains of tetracycline-resistant bacteria. QacA and QacB were among the first bacterial multidrug-resistant transporters identified. The *qacA* gene is present predominantly on the pSK1 family of multiresistance plasmids but is also likely to be present on the chromosomes of clinical *S. aureus* strains as an integrated family plasmid or part thereof. pSK1 is a 28.4-kb plasmid that can also carry the transposon Tn*4001* (which confers resistance to the aminoglycosides gentamicin, kanamycin, and tobramycin) and may also carry a gene that confers resistance to trimethoprim. Efflux of >30 different toxic substances has been described, including cationic and lipophilic biocidal compounds, with transcription of *qacA* under the control of the QacR repressor, which is relieved in the presence of QacA substrates. The *qacB* gene is detected on large heavy-metal resistance plasmids, like pSK23, but despite similarities to *qacA*, it appears to have a narrow range of biocide efflux activity (more specific to intercalating dyes, like ethidium bromide and QACs). The *qacC* and *qacD* genes (e.g., on pSK89 and pSK41) have identical phenotypes and sequence homologies; the *qacC* gene may have evolved from *qacD* (also known as *smr*). They also encode SMR-type PMF-dependent efflux proteins (see section 8.3.4).

pSK41 (Fig. 8.32) is a 46.4-kb conjugative plasmid that is a typical example of the evolution of plasmids in staphylococci. The plasmid consists of multiple resistance mechanisms on a single plasmid that have evolved from the insertion of transposons and the integration of other plasmids. The transposon Tn*4001* confers aminoglycoside resistance, neomycin and bleomycin antibiotic resistance is conferred by genes provided by the integration of a plasmid (pUB110), and the *smr/qacD* gene encodes a QAC efflux pump. Other members of the pSK41 family of plasmids can also confer trimethoprim resistance. Other genes carried on pSK41 are those required for the conjugation of the plasmid from one strain to another (*tra* genes).

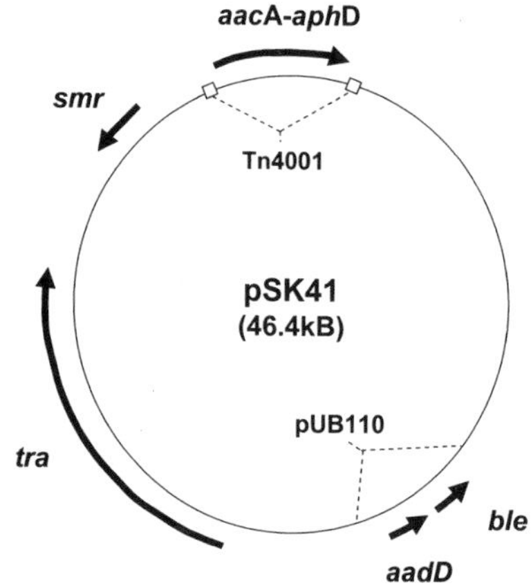

FIGURE 8.32 pSK41, an example of a multidrug resistance plasmid in staphylococci (not drawn to scale). pSK41 is a 46.4-kb plasmid carrying various genes for its transfer by conjugation (*tra*), resistance to antibiotics (gentamycin, tobramycin, and kanamycin by *aacA-aphD*, neomycin by *aadD*, and bleomycin by *ble*), and a biocide efflux pump (*smr*). The plasmid contains sequences from a transposon (Tn*4001*) and an integrated plasmid (pUB110).

In addition to Qac efflux pumps from clinical isolates, other efflux pumps similar to QacC-SMR have been identified in strains isolated in the food industry (QacG and QacH), as well as from *S. aureus* strains isolated from animals (e.g., QacJ). Overall, plasmid-encoded resistance determinants are considered widespread among *S. aureus* strains and have caused some concern over their demonstrated relationship to increased MICs of biocides (like chlorhexidine and benzalkonium chloride, often used in antiseptics and disinfectants) and β-lactam antibiotics. QacA, QacB, and QacC homologues have also been identified in *S. epidermidis* (e.g., on pST6) and other coagulase-negative staphylococci. Other gram-positive bacteria have also been found to have similar efflux pumps. For example, *Lactococcus lactis* strains have been identified with efflux pumps driven by both proton pumps (LmrP) and ATP hydrolysis (QacA), although the spectrum of biocides pumped out appeared to be restricted to certain intercalating dyes, like ethidium bromide, which are not generally used as biocides.

Plasmid-mediated efflux pumps are therefore important mechanisms of resistance to many antibiotics, metals, and cationic biocides, such as QACs, chlorhexidine, diamidines, and acridines, as well as to dyes, like ethidium bromide. Recombinant *S. aureus* plasmids transferred into *E. coli* are responsible for conferring increased MICs of similar cationic agents on the gram-negative organism. For example, a plasmid-borne ethidium bromide resistance determinant from *S. aureus* cloned into *E. coli* encoded resistance to ethidium bromide and to QACs, which are expelled from the cells. A similar efflux system was also found to be present in *Enterococcus hirae*. The plasmid-encoded efflux pump Smr (previously known as QacD or Ebr) has been identified in antibiotic-sensitive and -resistant strains of *S. aureus*, coagulase-negative staphylococci, and *Enterococcus* strains. Strains with increased tolerance of biocides appear to have identical nucleotide sequences of *smr* but are proposed to have an increase in the copy number of the gene or the plasmid, as the usual function of Smr could be to remove toxic substances from normal cells of staphylococci and enterococci. Based on DNA homology, it has also been proposed that *qacA* and related genes carrying resistance determinants evolved from preexisting genes responsible for normal cellular transport systems and that the biocide resistance genes evolved prior to the introduction and use of topical antimicrobial products and other antiseptics and disinfectants. In the case of antibiotics, the presence of a specific resistance mechanism frequently contributes to the long-term selection of resistant variants under in vivo conditions. Whether low-level resistance to cationic antiseptics, e.g., chlorhexidine and QACs, can also provide a selective advantage to staphylococci carrying *qac* genes remains to be elucidated.

To date, there is little or no evidence of plasmid-associated resistance to biocides in other gram-positive bacteria, despite some attempts to investigate them. Antibiotic-resistant corynebacteria have been implicated in human infections, especially in the immunocompromised. "Group JK" coryneforms (e.g., *Corynebacterium jeikeium*) were found to be more tolerant than other coryneforms of cationic disinfectants, ethidium bromide, and hexachlorophene, but studies with plasmid-containing and plasmid-cured derivatives produced no evidence of plasmid-associated resistance. Similarly, *Enterococcus faecium* strains showing high-level resistance to vancomycin, gentamicin, or both antibiotics are not more resistant to chlorhexidine or other investigated biocides. Further, despite the extensive dental use of chlorhexidine as an oral antiseptic, strains of *S. mutans* remain sensitive.

Transformation involves the ability of the cell to naturally take up plasmids or other genetic material from the environment (e.g., in the gram-positive bacteria *Bacillus* and *Streptococcus*). Transformation has not been described as a natural mechanism of acquisition of biocide tolerance genes, but it may occur. Under experimental conditions, chlorhexidine-tolerant strains of *Streptococcus sanguis* were isolated, and the DNA was extracted and directly mixed with chlorhexidine-sensitive strains. Subsequent recovery at normally inhibitory concentrations of chlorhexidine allowed the isolation of tolerant transformants, with resistance profiles similar to those of the original mutants. The nature of resistance in these strains was not identified, and further investigations are warranted to verify transformation as a mechanism of biocide resistance exchange.

It is of some interest that the transfer of genetic material by conjugation, transformation, or tranduction can be inhibited by the presence of biocides. Subinhibitory concentrations of biocides, like chlorhexidine, povidone-iodine, phenols, and QACs, have been shown to reduce the conjugation of plasmids between gram-positive and gram-negative bacteria. Similar results have been reported for phage transduction.

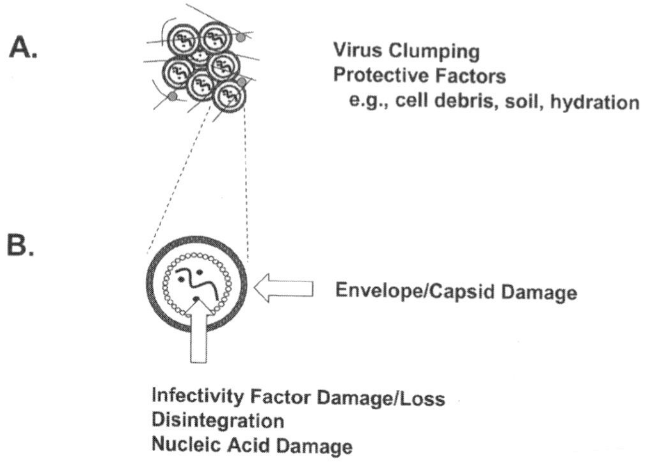

A.

Virus Clumping
Protective Factors
e.g., cell debris, soil, hydration

B.

Envelope/Capsid Damage

Infectivity Factor Damage/Loss
Disintegration
Nucleic Acid Damage

FIGURE 8.33 Mechanisms of viral resistance to biocides. The typical structure of an enveloped virus is shown as an example (see section 1.3.5). Resistance can be due to indirect factors, like viral clumping and the presence of soils (A), or directly to the structure of the virus particles (B), such as the presence of an envelope and lack of damage to the nucleic acid.

8.8 MECHANISMS OF VIRAL RESISTANCE

Viruses are nonmetabolizing and dependent on host cells for their survival and multiplication (see section 1.3.5). Therefore, the mechanisms of resistance of viruses to biocides have been shown to be directly related to the virus structure. Other associated yet indirect factors have been shown to provide some protection against virucidal agents (Fig. 8.33).

Like other microorganisms, viruses are normally associated with various extraneous materials, including cell debris, proteins, carbohydrates, lipids, and various inorganic salts. The presence of these materials affects the activity and penetration of the biocide to the individual viral particles, providing a protective mechanism of resistance. These materials are often directly associated with viruses, as they require host cells for multiplication and can be found within or closely associated with cells or cellular debris. This mechanism is an important consideration for the safe disinfection of viruses associated with various organic and inorganic materials, including body fluids, like blood, serum, and saliva. The presence of these materials also aids the virus to survive on surfaces for extended periods, presumably by preventing drying; this is particularly true of the enveloped viruses, which generally do not survive long on surfaces but can survive for a number of days in the presence of soil (as observed with hepatitis B virus in blood). In contrast, some nonenveloped viruses, including poxvirus and poliovirus, can survive for up to a number of years. Although viruses cannot form true biofilms (see section 8.3.8), some studies with polioviruses in water have shown that they have affinity for and can accumulate within biofilms as an indirect mechanism of resistance to biocides.

A further indirect mechanism involves viral aggregation, or clumping. Viral clumping has been implicated in various outbreaks of viral disease. A notable example has been studied with the preparation of polio vaccines. Polio vaccines are produced from either live attenuated ("less virulent") strains or as inactivated poliovirus (IPV or enhanced IPV) preparations. IPV vaccines were first introduced during the 1950s by the treatment of live, infectious poliovirus preparations with formaldehyde (typically mixed at 37% for up to 12 days). The surface structure of the virus is directly affected by formaldehyde, dramatically reducing its infectious nature; however, the virus particles retain most of their immunogenic properties and therefore their potential as a vaccine. In the investigation of an outbreak of poliovirus associated with IPV preparations, it was found that viral clumping allowed the protection of individual virus particles from contact with formaldehyde; these preparations subsequently retained their infectivity when introduced into sensitive hosts. Various techniques are now used to ensure adequate contact with the biocide, including prefiltering of virus pools through 0.2-μm filters to remove viral aggregates prior to inactivation. The direct effects of formaldehyde on the surface structure of the virus are unknown but are believed to be due to cross-linking of the capsid proteins. Studies with poliovirus and the similarly nonenveloped foot-and-mouth disease virus have found that formaldehyde-treated preparations become more resistant to acid pH (at which they normally disintegrate) and are difficult to extract the viral nucleic acid (RNA) from. It is not known if the viral RNA was directly affected by formaldehyde, and it seems likely that both of these effects are due to cross-linking of the viral capsid to produce a more rigid structure. A further example of viral persistence against biocides by clumping has been described with outbreaks of Norwalk virus in drinking water and tolerance of chlorination. Laboratory investigations of the virucidal effects of peracetic acid on enteroviruses and rotaviruses showed a biphasic survival curve, which may also be interpreted as evidence of a more sensitive population of viruses that are rapidly killed by the biocide and a more resistant population of viral aggregates that require a longer time for penetration.

After penetration of the biocide through any extraneous material to the virus particles, the major viral targets are the viral envelope (when present), the capsid, and the viral genome. The viral envelope is characteristic of the enveloped viruses (see section 1.3.5) and contains various lipids and proteins typical of a cell membrane. This envelope may be considered to offer some protection to the inner viral core against initial biocide damage; however, viral envelopes play an important role in the infectivity of the virus, and damage to the envelope can therefore dramatically reduce the ability to infect cells. Enveloped viruses are actually less resistant to biocides than nonenveloped viruses. The presence or absence of an envelope was the basis of an original classification of viruses proposed in the 1960s based on their relative susceptibilities to disinfectants and their chemical natures. This classification was based on whether the viruses were "lipophilic" in nature because they possessed a lipid envelope (e.g., herpes simplex virus and human immunodeficiency virus) or "hydrophilic" because they did not (e.g., poliovirus and parvovirus). Lipid-enveloped viruses were found to be sensitive to lipophilic-type biocides, such as 2-phenylphenol, cationic surfactants (QACs), chlorhexidine, and isopropanol, as well as to solvents, like ether and chloroform. The initial classification was further refined into three groups (Table 8.26): A, lipid-containing (enveloped) viruses; B, small, non-lipid-containing (nonenveloped) viruses; and C, a group of some larger non-lipid-containing viruses with moderate resistance to some bio-

TABLE 8.26 Viral classification and response to biocides[a]

Viral group	Lipid envelope[b]	Examples of viruses	Effects of disinfectants[c]	
			Lipophilic	Broad spectrum
A	+	Herpes simplex virus, human immunodeficiency virus, Newcastle disease virus, rabies virus, influenza virus	S	S
B	–	Nonlipid picornaviruses (poliovirus, coxsackievirus, echovirus), parvoviruses	R	S
C	–	Other larger nonlipid viruses (adenovirus, reovirus)	R	S

[a]This is often referred to as the Klein and Deforest classification.

[b]Present (+) or absent (−).

[c]Lipophilic disinfectants include QACs and chlorhexidine. S, sensitive; R, resistant.

cides. In general, larger viruses are more sensitive to biocides than smaller viruses, although this varies, depending on the virus family, type, and strain. Adenovirus serovars, for example, have been found to vary in their intrinsic tolerance to disinfectants, presumably due to differences in their capsid proteins. Disinfectants were also classified into two groups, broad-spectrum disinfectants that inactivated all viruses and lipophilic disinfectants that failed to inactivate small, non-lipid-containing viruses, like picornaviruses and parvoviruses. These classifications are still used today as the basis for testing and verifying the virucidal efficacies of disinfectants in the United States and other countries; indicator viruses of each type, poliovirus (small, nonenveloped), adenovirus (large, nonenveloped), and herpes simplex virus (enveloped), are used to establish the virucidal activity of the disinfectant under the recommended conditions of use.

The viral capsid is proteinaceous in nature. Therefore, biocides that disrupt the structures and functions of these proteins (including glutaraldehyde, hypochlorite, ethylene oxide [ETO], and hydrogen peroxide) have broad-spectrum virucidal activities. This is presumably due to the loss of infectivity associated with damage to the capsid in the case of the nonenveloped viruses. Chlorine dioxide or iodine treatment of polioviruses has been shown to interact directly with the capsid proteins, leading to their disintegration and release of the viral RNA. Separation of the nucleic acid was proposed to be important for total viral inactivation; however, chlorine dioxide alone was also shown to damage the viral RNA and prevent subsequent viral replication in the host cell. Other virucidal effects include damage to or loss of capsid-associated proteins that are required for viral infectivity (e.g., reverse transcriptase is carried by retroviruses and is required for release into the cell with the nucleic acid for replication). It is important to note that the destruction of the viral capsid can result in the release of a potentially infectious nucleic acid and that viral inactivation may not be complete unless it is accompanied by damage to or destruction of the viral nucleic acid. Viruses are either RNA or DNA based and can be single stranded or double stranded. The infectivity of poliovirus RNA genomes and the effects of biocides have been particularly well studied. Poliovirus RNA retains its infectivity when isolated from the viral capsid. The nucleic acid is less infectious than the whole virus, but in some studies, similar infectivities could not be shown with other RNA viruses, like hepatitis A virus and feline calicivirus. Free nucleic acids are more sensitive to biocides with known activity against RNA or DNA (see chapter 7). The effects of radiation treatment, for example, with UV, is dose dependent, with lower doses directly affecting the nucleic acid and forming photoproducts (like dimers) typical of their modes of action (see section 7.4.4). Higher doses of UV also affect the structures and functions of capsid and other associated proteins. Oxidizing agents, like chlorine and peracetic acid, cause viral disintegration, with specific effects on viral proteins, lipids, and nucleic acids. Polioviruses are relatively sensitive to the effects of heat, with loss of capsid structure observed at 45 to 55°C; the effects of heat can vary, depending on the virus and capsid type, with parvoviruses, for example, demonstrating greater resistance to heat than other viruses. These effects are related to the secondary and tertiary structures of the capsid proteins, with varying degrees of protein denaturation (see section 7.4.4). Clearly, at higher temperatures, general denaturation of macromolecules (including nucleic acids) leads to a general loss of viral structure and infectivity.

The specific effects on viral nucleic acids are important in consideration of viroid disinfection. Viroids are naked, infectious, single-stranded RNA molecules but are relatively stable in structure and have been reported to be easily transmitted between plants. Their inactivation has not been studied in any detail, and they were originally considered to be relatively sensitive to hard-surface disinfectants; however, some studies have found that viroids were not affected by some detergents (including QACs) and phenolics. It may be expected that biocides that target nucleic acids would be effective against viroids, but further testing is required to establish the sensitivity of viroids to disinfectants.

Unfortunately, the penetration of various biocides into different types of viruses and their interaction with viral components has been little studied. Some insights into these effects have been provided by investigations with bacteriophages (see section 1.3.5). Bacteriophages (or phages) are bacterial viruses and have been proposed as potential surrogates for assessing the virucidal activities of disinfectants due to their relative resistance in comparison to eukaryotic viruses. Morphological changes in the structure of the *P. aeruginosa* phage F116 on exposure to biocides have been studied under electron microscopy. Various effects were noted, including changes in the head and tail structures, leading to loss of phage infectivity and release of head DNA, which were dependent on the biocide concentration and exposure time. These effects were particularly observed with biocides that disrupt protein structure, including phenol, alcohol, peracetic acid, and glutaraldehyde; in contrast, chlorhexidine had little effect on phage structure and infectivity. Some studies have found that phage preparations have varying tolerances of the effects of sodium hypochlorite, with more resistant fractions being isolated at increased concentrations of available chlorine. These effects did not seem to be due to phage aggregation or obvious morphological differences in their structures. It is likely that this is due to differences in the intrinsic structures of the various phage proteins and their sensitivities to biocides.

Overall, there are many conflicting reports on the actions of and resistance to biocides on different virus types. This is primarily due to the different test systems used to study virus inactivation. An important example is virus preparation, where viral suspensions are generally associated with cellular debris and attempts to prepare purified fractions can lead to loss of infectivity. Other variables are the specific virus strain, the cell culture method, and the disinfectant tested, as well as the neutralization method used (see section 1.4.2). Liquid biocide formulation can play an important role in virucidal activity. For example, clumping has already been discussed as a mechanism of viral resistance to disinfection. As cross-linking biocides can trap viruses within clumps, the effects of various detergents or some biocides can cause their dispersion, but not necessarily their inactivation. Further, some reports have suggested that the structural integrity of a virus could be altered by an agent that reacted with viral capsids to cause an increase in viral permeability to other biocides. An interesting phenomenon described for bacteriophages and other viruses is referred to as "multiplicity reactivation," which has been observed under laboratory conditions. It is envisaged that the viral particles are damaged due to the various effects of the biocide to render them noninfectious but that complementary reconstruction of infectious particles can occur by reassociation of various virus components. In the case of UV- or alkylating-agent-treated double-stranded DNA viruses (like herpes simplex virus), this may be due to various virus components cooperating to allow virus infectivity or by damaged DNA sections being repaired within the host cell.

It seems unlikely that viruses with acquired resistance to biocides will be described, but they have shown the ability to become resistant to various antiviral agents by genetic changes in specific viral targets. A proposed mechanism is the development of key capsid proteins with increased resistance to the effects of biocides and biocidal processes by secondary or tertiary structural changes. With this is mind, there remains the possibility of viral adaptation to new environmental conditions. A number of reports have suggested that this can occur. Laboratory poliovirus preparations with increased tolerance of chlorine inactivation were selected by gradual passage through increasing sublethal concentrations of chlorine, and a similar development was described with *Pseudomonas* bacteriophages. In these cases, the mechanism of resistance was not identified. Clearly, much remains to be learned about the mechanisms of viral inactivation by, and viral resistance to, biocides.

8.9 MECHANISMS OF PRION RESISTANCE

The transmissible spongiform encephalopathies form a group of fatal neurological diseases of humans and other animals. Transmissible spongiform encephalopathies are caused by prions, abnormal proteinaceous agents that appear to contain no agent-specific nucleic acid (see section 1.3.6). An abnormal protease-resistant form (PrP^{res}) of a normal host protein is implicated in the pathological process, although other factors have been proposed to be involved.

Prions are considered highly resistant to most physical and chemical agents, with even greater resistance than bacterial spores in some cases (Table 8.27).

It is important to note that crude preparations (brain homogenates from infected animals) have been used to investigate the efficacies of various biocides and biocidal processes against prions. The presence of extraneous materials (particularly a high concentration of lipid associated with brain tissue) could, at least to some extent, mask the true efficacies of these processes against the infectious agent. For disinfection of these crude extracts, there is currently no known decontamination procedure that can guarantee the complete absence of infectivity in prion-infected tissues. The most effective process is boiling (or superheating under pressure) of the tissues in concentrated solutions of sodium hydroxide (1 to 2 N), which over time can totally dissolve any proteins present. In contrast, prions can survive harsh acid treatment. Formaldehyde, unbuffered glutaraldehyde (acidic pH), and ETO have little effect on infectivity, although chlorine-releasing agents (especially hypochlorites), sodium hydroxide, some phenols, and guanidine thiocyanate are more effective. Lower concentrations of hydroxides (NaOH and KOH) and hypochlorides have been shown to be effective against surface prion contamination, in combination with surfactants and other formulation effects. Extended steam sterilization is effective, although hydration of the prion-infected material appears to be important for optimal inactivation of prions. Further research is required on developing formulations and processes against prions, including the use of oxidizing agents, like gaseous hydrogen peroxide, which has shown effectiveness.

Prions are hydrophobic proteins and have been shown to have affinity for surfaces, including metals and plastics. In most surface disinfection recommendations for use against prions, cleaning is considered a key step to remove most of the contamination prior to chemical or heat inactivation of the prions. However, certain cleaning formulations have been shown to increase the intrinsic resistance of prions (or

TABLE 8.27 Effects of various disinfection and sterilization methods on prions

Effective	Partial or possible effectiveness[b]	Ineffective
Steam sterilization (121°C for ≥1 h)[a]	Hydrogen peroxide (particularly gaseous peroxide)	Formaldehyde
1–2 N NaOH ≥ 1 h	Peracetic acid (in formulation at ≥50°C)	Glutaraldehyde
Steam sterilization (132–136°C for ≥18 min)[a]	Ozone	Alcohols
≥2% available chlorine for ≥1 h[a]	Plasma	Radiation
Incineration[a]		Dry heat
Some phenolics		Ethylene oxide
Some alkaline cleaners (pH ≥12)		Acids
Prolonged boiling in SDS or 1 N NaOH		Phenolics
4 M guanidinium hydrochloride (≥1 h)		QACs
Prolonged protease digestion[a]		

[a]Some reports have shown incomplete inactivation.

[b]The effectiveness of these methods has not been fully confirmed.

prion-contaminated materials) by an unknown mechanism. This has also been observed in treatment with some biocides, including formaldehyde, presumably due to protein fixation. Although prions are considered resistant to proteases (hence their designation PrP, for "protease-resistant protein"), various proteases, including proteinase K and keratinases, have been shown to degrade prions over time, depending on their concentrations and the exposure conditions.

The proposed mechanisms of prion resistance are summarized in Fig. 8.34.

Prions aggregate to form protein particles (or fibrils) within various tissues but are predominantly observed within brain tissue. These particles are hydrophobic and are associated with various cellular materials present within the contaminated tissue; for example, brain tissue contains a high concentration of lipid materials. These effects create a penetration challenge for the biocidal process. Various biocides and biocidal processes have been shown to be ineffective against prions. With the information presently available, it is difficult to explain the extremely high resistance of prions, save to comment that the PrP is abnormally stable against degradative processes. In the case of radiation, the mechanism of resistance is proposed as evidence for the lack of any nucleic acid associated with prion infectivity; however, the effects of various radiation sources have not been studied in any detail, and radiation can damage other macromolecules, including proteins (see section 7.4.4). Biocides that have a cross-linking or fixing mode of action, including alcohols and alde-

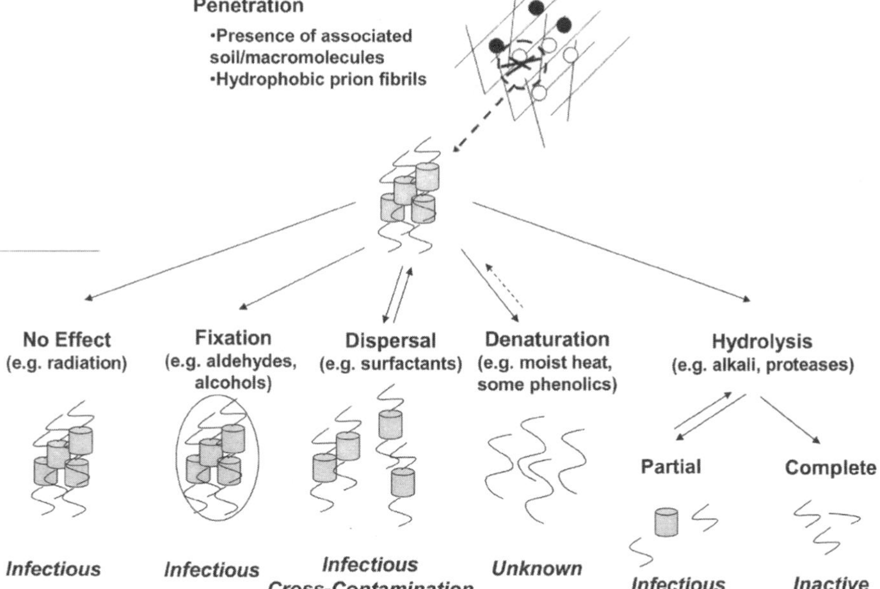

FIGURE 8.34 Mechanisms of resistance of prions to biocides and modes of action of biocides against prions. Prions (hydrophobic protein fibrils) are present in associated macromolecules (including lipids, carbohydrates, and proteins), through which the biocidal process must penetrate. Following penetration, ineffective processes are those that have no effect on proteins, that fix proteins, or that cause prion protein dispersal (potentially leading to cross-contamination). Biocidal processes that denature and/or hydrolyze (or degrade) proteins have been shown to be effective against prions; however, with denaturation alone, renaturation of the protein could occur to produce the reassociated infectious protein form. Further, protein hydrolysis may be partial or complete. In some cases, partial hydrolysis of the protein is ineffective, because smaller components of the protein retain an infectious nature.

hydes, have also been shown to be ineffective against prions, presumably due to a lack of any degradative effect on the target protein but actual cross-linking with other associated extraneous materials. Biocides or biocidal processes that denature or cause the fragmentation of proteins have been shown to be effective against prions. Moist heat and certain phenolic formulations are proposed to inactivate prions by denaturation. It has been speculated that renaturation of the denatured protein could occur under some conditions, although this has not been observed. Biocides, like sodium hypochlorite, sodium hydroxide, and hydrogen peroxide at high concentrations, appear to cause fragmentation or other structural changes to prions, rendering them noninfectious. It is still possible (but considered unlikely) that other, as yet unidentified factors are involved in prion infectivity and need to be similarly degraded to ensure complete inactivation.

8.10 MECHANISMS OF FUNGAL RESISTANCE

In comparison with bacteria, very little is known about the ways in which fungi can circumvent the actions of biocides and biocidal processes. As with bacteria, two general mechanisms of resistance can be identified: intrinsic resistance, a natural property or development of the organism during normal growth, and acquired resistance, with examples of both identified or proposed (Table 8.28).

Filamentous fungi (molds) grow by cell division but do not separate, instead forming long lines and branches of cells, known as hyphae, which develop further to form a mass known as a mycelium (plural, mycelia). As mycelial growth enters stationary phase, a variety of fruiting bodies or other structures, which contain spores, develop. Fungal spores are found in a variety of shapes and sizes and can be asexual and/or sexual. A variety of unicellular fungi grow similarly to bacteria, for example, yeasts; they also produce spores. The vegetative forms of fungi (yeasts and molds) are generally found to be more resistant to biocides than most nonsporulating bacteria (Table 8.29). It is tempting to speculate that the cell wall composition in fungi (see section 1.3.3.2) confers a high level of intrinsic resistance on these organisms. Vegetative molds are also generally more resistant than yeasts (Table 8.30).

The various types of fungal spores also present a wide variety of sensitivities to biocides. Fungal spores are more resistant than vegetative fungi but considerably less resistant than bacterial endospores.

The overall tolerance of fungi for biocides is most likely due to various mechanisms of intrinsic resistance. The predominantly polysaccharide-based (glycan) cell wall presents a protective barrier to reduce or exclude the entry of an antimicrobial agent. The cell wall structures of fungi are varied and differ from those of bacteria (see section 1.3.3.2). A typical fungal cell wall consists of fibrils of chitin or

TABLE 8.28 Possible mechanisms of fungal resistance to biocides

Type of resistance	Possible mechanism	Example(s)
Intrinsic	Sporulation	Phenolics, QACs, desiccation, radiation, UV, ETO
	Hyphal clumping	UV, ETO
	Exclusion	Chlorhexidine
	Enzymatic inactivation	Formaldehyde
	Phenotypic adaptation	Ethanol
	Efflux	Not demonstrated[a]
Acquired	Mutation	Some preservatives
	Inducible efflux	Some preservatives[a]
	Plasmid-mediated responses	Not demonstrated

[a]Efflux is known to be one mechanism of fungal resistance to antifungal drugs.

TABLE 8.29 Comparison of the relative resistances of bacteria and fungi to biocides

Antimicrobial agent	pH	Concn (% [wt/vol])	*D* value (min)[a]				
			Aspergillus niger	*C. albicans*	*E. coli*	*P. aeruginosa*	*S. aureus*
Phenol	5.1	0.5	20	13.5	0.94	<0.1	0.66
	6.1	0.5	32.4	18.9	1.72	0.17	1.9
Benzalkonium	5.1	0.001	—[b]	9.66	0.06	3.01	3.12
chloride	6.1	0.002	—	5.5	<0.1	0.05	0.67

[a]The *D* values were estimated at 20°C on exposure to phenol and benzalkonium chloride. The *D* value is defined as the time required to kill 1 log unit (or 90%) of the microbial population under the stated tested conditions.

[b]—, no inactivation; fungistatic effect only.

cellulose embedded within a matrix of various cross-linked glycans and associated proteins and lipids. These structures are considered effective barriers against the penetration of biocides. The cell walls of some yeasts have been described in detail, although less is known about the specific structures of other fungi (Table 8.31). In general, mold cell walls predominantly consist of glucans, also with specific linked outer cell wall glucans and inner polysaccharides, like chitin-cellulose and/or proteins. Further, the various structures are known to be dynamic, with the compositions and proportions of components varying in response to different nutritional and environmental factors, not dissimilar to the various phenotypic changes observed in bacteria (see section 8.3.1). For example, during the stationary phase of fungal growth, various adaptations of metabolism and structure are observed, the most obvious being the formation of aerial mycelia and spores. An example of phenotypic adaptation to antifungals has been described in *Aspergillus*, where an accumulation of cell membrane ergosterol may be partially responsible for increased tolerance of azoles and may also be expected to increase tolerance of certain biocides that target the cell membrane. A further example of this has been described with yeasts grown under different conditions and having variable levels of sensitivity to ethanol. Cells with linoleic-acid-enriched plasma membranes appeared to be slightly more tolerant of ethanol than cells with enriched oleic acid, from which it has been inferred that a more fluid membrane enhances ethanol resistance. The roles of various fungal cell membrane sterols in the activity and penetration of biocides are not known. Further, active response mechanisms have been described in yeasts that salvage and repair damage to the cell wall, which may provide some protection to the cell at subfungicidal concentrations of biocides. Overall, the impact of phenotypic changes during the normal growth of fungi has not been studied in detail for variations in biocide sensitivity.

The role of the cell envelope or wall in intrinsic resistance is primarily due to exclusion from the cell. Of the various fungi tested, strains

TABLE 8.30 Fungicidal concentrations of biocides for yeasts and molds

Antimicrobial agent	Fungicidal concn (μg/ml)		
	Yeast (*C. albicans*)	Mold	
		Penicillium chrysogenum	*Aspergillus niger*
QACs			
Benzalkonium chloride	10	~100–200	~100–200
Cetrimide/CTAB[a]	25	100	250
Chlorhexidine	20–40	400	200

[a]CTAB, cetyltrimethylammonium bromide.

TABLE 8.31 Various cell wall structures of fungi

Species	Presence of cell wall component[a]			
	β-Glucans	α-Glucans	Mannoproteins	Chitin
S. cerevisiae	+ (~50–60%)	–	+ (~40%)	+ (~2%)
C. albicans	+ (~40–60%)	–	+ (~40%)	+ (~2%)
C. neoformans	+ (~15%)	+ (~35%)	+	+
Aspergillus fumigatus	+ (~80%)	+	+ (~3%)	+
Histoplasma capsulatum	+	+	?	?

[a]+, present; –, absent.

of *Aspergillus* are generally considered to be the most resistant to biocides and biocidal processes. This may be due to the higher proportion of linked β-glucans in the cell wall, but it is also clear that hyphal clumping (preventing biocide penetration) and the production of spores (ascospores [see below]) also play roles in the intrinsic resistance of these and other fungi. A particular example of this has been described with isolates of *Pyronema domesticum* and their intrinsic resistance to ETO. ETO is a broad-spectrum biocide that is widely used in the low-temperature sterilization of devices (see section 6.2). Isolates of *P. domesticum* have been found to survive typical ETO sterilization processes associated with various devices using cotton (e.g., in sponges and gauzes), particularly from China. Other *Pyronema* strains have been identified in cotton from the United States. Studies of these strains showed that they were sensitive to steam sterilization but exhibited significantly increased tolerance of radiation (E beams and γ-irradiation). In the case of ETO, resistance has been described as being up to 10 times higher than those typically described for *B. atrophaeus* spores, which are considered the most resistant to ETO. *P. domesticum* organisms are ascomycete molds that appear to have two significant mechanisms of tolerance for ETO. Typical of ascomycetes, they produce asexual spores (known as ascospores [see below]) within bodies known as apothecia. Further, they also produce hardened (or desiccated) clumps of fungal hyphae known as sclerotia, which appear to be dormant and can also include asexual spores (a more detailed discussion of the various types of spores found in fungi is provided below). The desiccated nature of the sclerotia is presumed to reduce the penetration of ETO, which requires humidity for activity (see section 6.2). Interestingly, the ascospores themselves appear to present greater resistance to radiation than the sclerotia, although they are not considered as resistant as *Bacillus pumilus* spores, which are used to monitor the efficacy of radiation sterilization (see section 5.4).

The cell wall structures of yeasts are similar to yet distinct from those of molds, with differences in the glucans and linked proteins identified. Although various yeast cell wall mutants have been described, their respective sensitivities to biocides have not been investigated. Overall, the yeast cell wall appears relatively flexible, which allows a cell to be dimorphic, changing from single-celled to hyphal growth. In some limited studies of chlorhexidine susceptibility in the yeast *Saccharomyces cerevisiae*, the penetration of the biocide was inhibited by the cell wall glucan, the wall thickness, and the relative porosity (Table 8.32).

These findings can provide a tentative picture of the cellular factors that modify the response of *S. cerevisiae* to chlorhexidine. Cell wall-free cells (protoplasts) of *S. cerevisiae* have been prepared with glucuronidase in the presence of β-mercaptoethanol and were found to be readily lysed by chlorhexidine concentrations well below those effective against "normal" (whole) cells. Furthermore, the culture age influences the response of *S. cerevisiae* to chlorhexidine; cells walls are much less sensitive at stationary phase than those in the logarithmic growth phase, and the uptake of chlorhexidine was much less during stationary phase.

TABLE 8.32 Parameters affecting the response of *S. cerevisiae* to chlorhexidine

Parameter	Role in susceptibility of cells to CHG[a]
Cell wall composition	
Mannan	No role found
Glucan	Possible significance; at lower concentrations and with cell wall-free forms, CHG can cause cell lysis.
Cell wall thickness	Increases in cells of older cultures; expected reduced CHG uptake
Relative porosity	Decreases in cells of older cultures; expected reduced CHG uptake
Plasma membrane	Seems to be as sensitive as bacterial membrane, but alterations in lipids/proteins could change CHG susceptibility

[a]CHG, chlorhexidine.

Studies with the antifungal antibiotic amphotericin B demonstrated a phenotypic increase in resistance of *Candida albicans* as the organisms entered the stationary growth phase, which was attributed to cell wall changes involving tighter cross-linking. These reports suggest that a similar increase in biocide resistance may occur, but this has not been investigated in any detail.

The porosity of the yeast cell wall is affected by its chemical composition, with the wall acting as a barrier to or modulator of the entry and exit of various agents. Assays have been developed to study the porosity of the yeast cell under normal growth conditions, including the uptake of fluorescein isothiocyanate-labeled dextrans and the periplasmic enzyme invertase or polycation-induced leakage of UV-absorbing compounds as indicators of yeast cell wall porosity. Studies using these assays have found that the relative porosity of cells decreases with increasing culture age. As the age of the *S. cerevisiae* culture increased, there was a significant increase in the cell wall thickness. In parallel, biocide permeability was reduced as the culture aged, as indicated by the uptake of radiolabeled chlorhexidine. Mannan mutants of *S. cerevisiae* showed an order of sensitivity to chlorhexidine similar to that of the parent strain, suggesting that mannan did not play a significant role in cell wall tolerance of biocides. The yeast wall mannoprotein consists of two fractions, SDS-soluble mannoproteins and SDS-insoluble, glucanase-soluble ones: the latter limit cell wall porosity. Thus, glucan and possibly some mannoproteins play key roles in determining the uptake, and hence activity, of chlorhexidine in *S. cerevisiae*. *C. albicans* is less sensitive and takes up less chlorhexidine, but studies with that organism and with molds are few.

A limited number of fungi have been shown to produce capsules, or capsule-like structures, external to the cell wall that can present a further intrinsic barrier to biocide penetration. They include species of *Tremella, Trichosporon*, and *Sporothrix*, but the best studied is the *Cryptococcus neoformans* capsule (Fig. 8.35).

C. neoformans is an opportunistic human pathogen, particularly in immunocompromised patients. This blastidomycete fungus presents

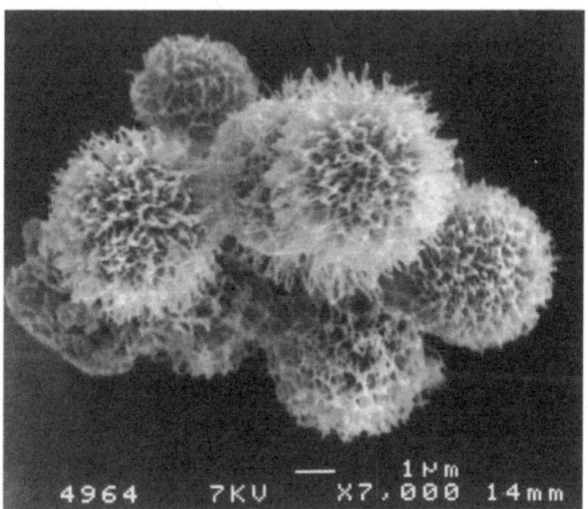

FIGURE 8.35 Scanning electron micrograph of an encapsulated *C. neoformans* strain. The capsule appears as a loose fibrillar network in encapsulated strains. Reprinted from A. Casadevall and J. R. Perfect, *Cryptococcus neoformans* (ASM Press, Washington, D.C., 1998), with permission. Micrograph originally supplied by Wendy Cleare (Albert Einstein College of Medicine, Bronx, N.Y.).

various intrinsic mechanisms of resistance to biocides, including capsule formation on vegetative cells; the production of asexual fruiting bodies, which consist of desiccated clumps of cells; and the sexual production of spores (basidiospores). The last two mechanisms develop upon nutrient starvation, suggesting stress response mechanisms similar to those of bacteria (see section 8.3.3). Vegetative cells produce an exopolysaccharide capsule, which is tightly associated with the cell wall and plays an important role in the pathogenic nature of the microorganism in evading the immune response to infection and in persistence. The capsule consists of two major polysaccharides: glucuronoxylomannan and galactoxylomannan. Approximately 90% of the capsule consists of glucuronoxylomannan, which is a mannose polymer with various sugar side chains; galactoxylomannan, which is a similar galactose polymer, is a much smaller component (~5%). Various other associated polysaccharides and proteins have also been described. Capsule formation is induced during asexual budding and by changing growth conditions, suggesting a protection mechanism similar to that described for bacteria as a stationary-phase phenomenon (see section 8.3.1). Capsule synthesis is mediated by the *CAP* and *CAS* genes; various mutants that lack capsules or capsule components have been isolated, and they are more sensitive to some biocides at typical inhibitory or fungicidal concentrations. The relative tolerances of capsulated and noncapsulated cells have not been studied in any detail. As with bacteria, the presence of a capsule allows greater affinity for surfaces. In studies with clinical isolates of *C. albicans*, *C. neoformans*, and *Rhodotorula rubra* of the activities of various biocides (including iodine, chlorhexidine, hydrogen peroxide, alcohol, and sodium hypochlorite) and UV radiation, dramatic differences in susceptibility were observed between planktonic and surface-bound cells (possibly in biofilms).

Fungi, particularly molds, grow within tangled webs of individual hyphae and as part of a larger mass of mycelia forming a mat-like structure (Fig. 8.36); this provides a penetration challenge to various biocidal processes. An example has been described with UV radiation (see section 2.4), against which fungi demonstrate high resistance, presumably due to lack of penetration into the mycelium structure. At the level of individual hyphae, it should be noted that some studies have suggested that the hyphae of "lower" fungi are more sensitive to biocides than those of "higher" fungi due to the presence of septation (or separation between cells) in the latter. The septa may provide some protection to neighboring cells in the presence of a biocide, although these effects are considered minor. In addition, the cells at the ends of hyphae are actively dividing ("apical growth"), with other cells in a more dormant form. It is also expected, although it has not been investigated in any detail, that actively growing and multiplying cells are more sensitive to biocides than the dormant cells, suggesting that within a given fungal mycelium cells display various levels of tolerance of antimicrobials.

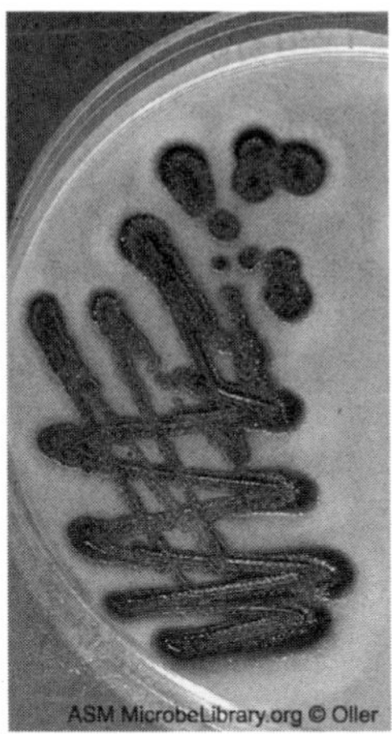

FIGURE 8.36 Typical growth of a fungus on a medium surface. Shown are 7-day-old *Aureobasidium pullulans* colonies grown on Ueda medium at 28°C in a humid environment. Courtesy of Anna Oller (Central Missouri State University).

Various fungi have been associated with biofilm formation. Biofilms are communities of microorganisms that are attached to surfaces and can include various microorganisms, such as bacteria, protozoa, and fungi (see section 8.3.8). Various molds and yeasts have been described as being biofilm formers by binding to surfaces and proliferating within a protective exopolymeric structure. They include *Aspergillus, Candida, Rhodotorula, Cladosporium*, and *Cryptococcus*. They have been identified in water system biofilms, as well as on implantable or indwelling devices. *C. albicans* biofilm development is a particular concern on implantable devices and has been shown to be highly resistant to antimicrobial agents. In addition, various fungi can become associated with bacterial biofilms, along with debris, but can subsequently proliferate and cooperate within the biofilm. This also offers them protection against the effects of biocides, similar to bacteria.

The typical life cycle for a fungus is shown in Fig. 8.37. In most cases, fungi reproduce by both sexual and asexual reproduction. Asexual reproduction can be simple budding or binary fission in yeast (where one cell produces a bud to form another cell) but can also be simple fragmentation of the fungal hyphae, allowing the fragment to disperse and multiply. However, the most common form of asexual reproduction is by the production of asexual spores in response to various environmental factors, including nutrient limitations.

Fungi can be classified based on their microscopic morphology, including the presence of septation between individual cells within the hyphal structure and the types of spores or spore-forming ("fruiting") bodies developed. The various types of fungal asexual and sexual spores are shown in Fig. 8.38 and classified in Table 8.33. Genetically, asexual spores are produced by mitosis and sexual spores are produced by the fusion of the protoplasts and nuclei of two cells, followed by meiosis.

Similar to some bacteria, fungi form spores in response to various environmental stimuli, including nutrient restrictions, competition, and low concentrations of fungistatic or fungicidal biocides. Spores, therefore, have two major

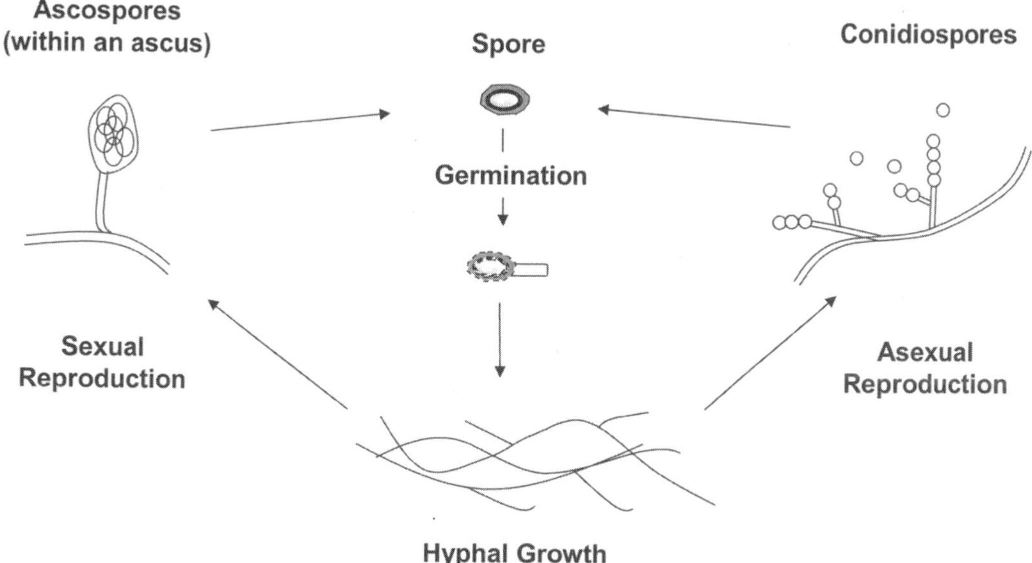

FIGURE 8.37 Fungal life cycle (ascomycota). The life cycle shown is typical of ascomycota, such as *Neurospora*. In the case of the yeast ascomycetes, including *Saccharomyces*, the single cells reproduce asexually by binary fission or budding and sexually by two cells uniting, leading to the development of ascospores. Similar asexual and sexual spores are formed in other fungi, although in some cases, only asexual conidiospores have been described (Table 8.33).

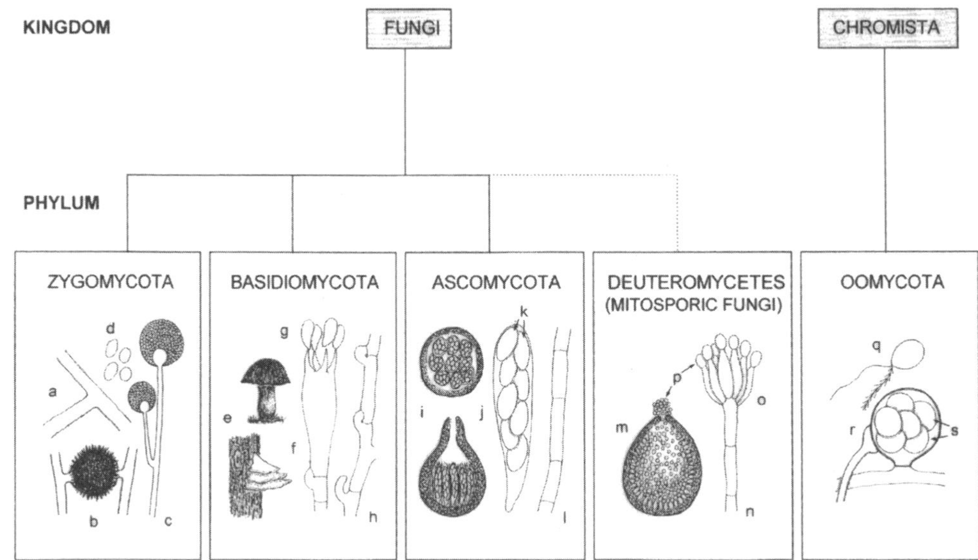

FIGURE 8.38 Examples of various types of fungal spores and spore-bearing structures. Zygomycota: a, aseptate hypha; b, zygospore; c, sporangiophore (with spores within sporangia); d, sporangiospores. Basidiomycota: e, basidiomata; f, basidium; g, naked basidiospores; h, hypha with clamp connections. Ascomycota: i, ascomata; j, ascus-containing spores; k, ascospores; l, septate hypha. Deuteromycetes: m, pycnidium; n, conidiophore; o, conidiogenous cells; p, conidia. Oomycota: q, zoospore (motile); r, gametangia; s, oospores. Reprinted from J. Guarro et al., *Clin. Microbiol. Rev.* **12:**454–500, 1999, with permission.

fundamental functions: survival and dispersal. The main types of asexual spores are conidia and sporangiospores. Conidia are developed from specialized aerial hyphae known as conidiophores that bud spores, and they are borne naked on the hyphal structure. In contrast, sporangiospores are formed within fruiting bodies known as sporangia, which are also mounted on specialized hyphae (sporangiophores). Asexual spores develop by nutrient accumulation within a specific vegetative cell, where they swell, convert available nutrients into lipid or carbohydrate reserves, and develop a specialized external spore wall. In some cases, sporangiospores are considered more tolerant of biocides than conidia, as they develop a double

TABLE 8.33 Examples of spores produced by fungi

Group[a]	Examples	Septation[b]	Asexual spores	Sexual spores
Low				
Zygomycota	*Rhizopus, Mucor*	–	Sporangiospores	Zygospores
Oomycota	*Phythophthora, Pythium*	–	Zoospores	Oospores
High				
Ascomycota	*Saccharomyces, Aspergillus, Candida, Neurospora*	+	Conidia (conidiospores)	Ascospores
Basidiomycota	*Cryptococcus*, mushrooms, puffballs	+	Uncommon	Basidiospores
Deuteromycota ("imperfect" fungi)	*Thermomyces, Nattrassia*	+	Conidiospores	–

[a]The classification of fungi often shows discrepancies, but in this case, fungi can be classified into a "low" class, whose members do not have true septa between individual cells, and a "high" class, whose members are septate, as well as by the types of spores they produce.

[b]+, present; –, absent.

spore wall rather than the single conidial spore wall. The different types of sexual spores also develop within specialized structures (including oospores, zygospores, and ascospores, the last within an ascus) (Fig. 8.38) or naked on specialized hyphae (basidiospores). There are various mechanisms of sexual-spore development which generally involve the development and maturation of a spore wall around a cell nucleus and cytoplasm. In development within a fruiting body, like an ascus, the spores can be further protected from attack by various materials that surround and support the spore within these structures. A further class of fungi, the deuteromycota, or "imperfect" fungi, do not (or are not known to) produce sexual spores.

The various molecular structures of fungal spores have not been described in detail. In general, they are surrounded by a rigid wall of various thicknesses, primarily composed of polysaccharides but also containing proteins, lipids, and pigments. The spore wall is distinct in structure from the normal vegetative-cell wall, being less fibrous and more multilayered. Internally, they contain nutrient reserves (carbohydrates and fats) and have low water content (as low as 1% of that normally found in vegetative mycelia) and low metabolic activity. The thickness of the spore wall appears to be related to the extent of dormancy. Some spores (generally asexual spores, like conidia and sporangiospores) have thin walls and low nutrient reserves and can be easily disseminated and germinate rapidly under suitable conditions. These spores also contain typical vegetative-cell organelles and are actively metabolizing, but at a much lower rate. Some asexual zoospores are motile due to the expression of flagella. In contrast, other spores develop thicker cell walls and higher nutrient reserves, which are more suitable for survival under adverse conditions. Fungal spores are generally more resistant than vegetative fungal cells or hyphae, but not to the same extent as bacterial spores. Sexual spores are particularly more resistant to being dried or heated and to some biocides. Typically, most fungal vegetative forms and spores are heat sensitive at 50 to 60°C. Despite this, some fungi that produce ascospores with a higher resistance to heat than normally observed for fungi have been isolated. They include heat-resistant species of *Byssochlamys, Talaromyces*, and *Eurotrium*. They have been identified as frequent contaminants in thermally processed foods (particularly fruit juices) and have been implicated in food spoilage. Pasteurization (see section 2.2) is a heat disinfection process generally applied to solid or liquid foods to reduce the risk of the presence of pathogens and/or food spoilage organisms. It is widely used for the treatment of milk and milk products, beer, and juices to extend shelf life. A typical pasteurization process can range from 63 to 66°C for ≥30 min and 71 to 72°C for ≥15 to 16 s. Many of these strains survive these processes and require higher temperatures for fungicidal effects (in the 80 to 95°C range). The mode of resistance is unknown but is clearly related to the structure of the ascospores. As described above in the case of *Pyronema*, ascospores and related structures with higher resistance to other biocidal processes, like radiation and ETO, have been identified. It is expected that the nature of the resistance of these spores is due to both protection within masses of hyphae and the intrinsic resistance of the developed spores, including having desiccated protoplasm and multiple spore wall layers. Studies with *Aspergillus* have shown that conidia and vegetative cells are relatively sensitive to QAC and alcohols, with ascospores demonstrating greater tolerance. The overall resistance of the ascospores also increased with age and varied from species to species. The level of desiccation of *Aspergillus* ascospores has been linked with intrinsic resistance to ETO and most likely other gaseous biocides.

The germination of fungal spores is similar to that described for bacterial endospores (see section 8.3.11). It includes actual germination of the spore, water uptake with an increase in spore size, and development of a germ tube, which grows into a vegetative cell or actively growing hyphae. The initiation of germination has been shown to vary in different spore types. In some cases, there are factors that prevent the germination of the spore and that need to be relieved. These include inhibitory factors within the spore (for example, spore phosphate levels) or, in the case of *Microsporium* spores, an external protein layer that must be degraded by an intrinsic spore enzyme before germination can proceed. Other germination mechanisms are similar to those of endospores, with the spore sensing the environment for the presence of nutrients and water or the absence of inhibiting factors, including biocides. These mechanisms play roles in the survival of fungi at fungistatic concentrations of biocides.

As in bacteria, heavy-metal resistance in *C. albicans* and, to a lesser extent, *S. cerevisiae* has been described. Two major mechanisms of resistance have been described in eukaryotes: the expression of metal-binding proteins (e.g., metallothioneins) and efflux mechanisms. In the case of *C. albicans*, both mechanisms have been described in response to toxic levels of copper. They include the expression of copper metallothioneins, which bind copper via thiol groups of exposed cysteine residues within the protein (e.g., CUP1), and copper efflux by P-type ATPases (e.g., CRP1 and CRD1p, with the latter extruding both copper and silver ions). The difference in tolerance between *C. albicans* and *S. cerevisiae* has been proposed to be due to the lack of copper efflux in *S. cerevisiae*, where both strains examined produced metallothioneins. Overall, there is little evidence of efflux as a mechanism of biocide tolerance in fungi. In some yeasts, the extrusion of formic acid has been described as giving a greater level of tolerance to formaldehyde. Efflux mechanisms that are expressed early in biofilm development have been described in *C. albicans*; they have been linked to antifungal (azole) resistance and include two different types of efflux mechanisms, ABC and MFS pumps (see section 8.3.4). The significance of these pumps in the tolerance of biocides remains to be investigated.

Similarly, there is little evidence of acquired resistance by mutation (except to some preservatives) or by plasmid-mediated mechanisms. The mutational loss of a cytoplasmic membrane pump in *S. cerevisiae* was shown to cause an increase in resistance to QACs, like benzalkonium chloride; this pump was involved in the transport of leucine into the cell, suggesting a similar mechanism of transport and tolerance due to exclusion from the cell cytoplasm. *Schizosaccharomyces* mutants with stable tolerance of various heavy metals have been isolated. Resistance linked to plasmid acquisition has not been studied, but increased tolerance of various antifungal agents has been artificially produced under laboratory conditions; the significance of these results in the environment of biocidal resistance is not known. Overall, it may be expected that mechanisms of acquired biocide tolerance similar to those described in bacteria remain to be identified in yeasts and molds.

Various enzymes that are involved in the degradation and metabolism of formaldehyde in fungi and other eukaryotes have been identified. These mechanisms can be a particular concern in the use of formaldehyde or formaldehyde-releasing agents as preservatives (see section 3.4). They include glutathione-dependent formaldehyde dehydrogenases and alcohol dehydrogenases in *Candida* and *Saccharomyces* species. The expression of these enzymes can be considered an intrinsic mechanism of resistance similar to those described in bacteria (8.3.5). A further example is the expression of formate oxidase in *Aspergillus* species, which can grow and metabolize in the presence of up to 0.45% formaldehyde. In addition to intrinsic expression of the enzymes, associated acquired mechanisms have also been described. *Saccharomyces* mutants that have increased sensitivity to formaldehyde due to the loss of enzyme activity and increased tolerance due to overexpression of the associated enzyme(s) have been described. Similar hypersensitive yeast mutants have been described with alkylating agents, like ETO. Some strains of yeast have also been reported to produce catalase and cytochrome *c* peroxidases that degrade hydrogen peroxide.

Overall, relatively few rigorous studies have been done to understand intrinsic and extrinsic mechanisms of resistance to biocides in yeasts and molds. As vegetative microorganisms, various fungi have demonstrated mechanisms of resistance similar to those described in more detail in bacteria, including cell wall structures, stationary-phase phenomena, biofilm development, degradative-enzyme production, and sporulation. Less is known about acquired mechanisms of resistance, but it may be expected that similar mechanisms remain to be identified and further described in fungi.

8.11 MECHANISMS OF RESISTANCE IN OTHER EUKARYOTIC MICROORGANISMS

The helminths (generally known as "worms") are a diverse group of multicellular eukaryotic microorganisms (see section 1.3.3). They can be further subclassified into the nematodes (roundworms) and flatworms (including trematodes and cestodes). Although many helminths are pathogenic and are frequently identified, their responses to various biocides and biocidal processes have not been studied in any detail. Many are described as important animal pathogens that can be difficult to control environmentally, and others are often associated with contaminated water and indicative of poor sanitation conditions. The adult worms and larval forms vary in their shapes and sizes, with the adults protected externally by a rigid proteinaceous cuticle; these forms are relatively sensitive to exposure conditions outside their respective hosts, including to the presence of biocides. A greater consideration is the production of dormant eggs or cysts (Fig. 8.39), which demonstrate marked resistance to biocides, during their respective life cycles.

The structure of *Ascaris* eggs has been investigated in some detail, as it is a frequent contaminant of wastewater. They consist of an inner core (oocyte), which is enclosed within a lipid membrane and surrounded by three main layers: an inner layer of lipoprotein, middle layers of the polysaccharide chitin, and an external proteinaceous layer. Other helminth eggs are morphologically similar but vary in their shapes (generally oval), sizes (ranging from ~30 to 150 μm in length), and the chemical constituents of various egg layers. Helminth eggs are generally found in water at low concentrations but have a low infectious dose and can survive typical bac-

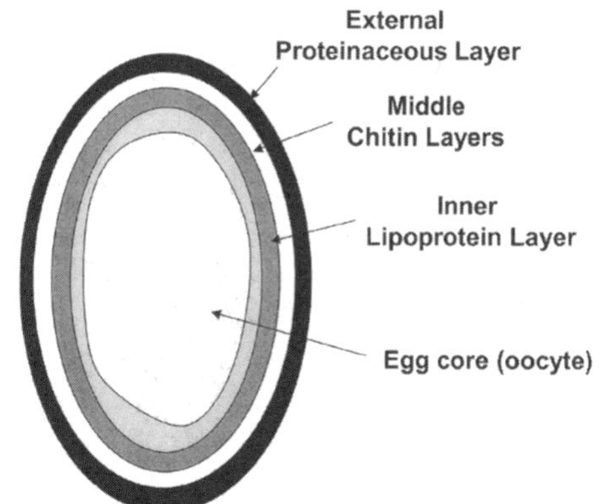

FIGURE 8.39 Representation of the structure of a helminth (*Ascaris*) egg.

tericidal concentrations of chlorine and ozone; studies of the effects of other biocides have been limited, but efficacy has been observed with oxidizing agents. The biocidal resistance of helminth eggs is presumably due to reduced uptake of chemical biocides through the various egg layers to the sensitive core. Further, helminth eggs also demonstrate tolerance of radiation (UV disinfection) and heat, although temperatures of >70°C have been found to be effective over time. Chlorine, ozone, UV radiation, and heat have all been shown to be effective in a dose-dependent manner, requiring high concentrations or temperatures or long exposure times to be efficient in comparison to those tested and used to control levels of bacteria and viruses in water. Ozone treatment appears to cause the disintegration of the various shell walls and loss of viability. In some cases, strong acids or alkali are also used, which are believed to hydrolyze the egg layers. Overall, the multiple-layered structure of helminth eggs is the main intrinsic mechanism of resistance to biocides and biocidal processes. Other resistance determinants, including acquired mechanisms, have not been described, although they are possible, considering the development of resistance to specific antihelminthic drugs.

Algae are also often associated with poor or nutrient-rich water conditions (see section 1.3.3.3). They are a diverse group of single-celled eukaryotes that can grow as free-living cells or as associated filaments. Some algae are known to be pathogens of fish and humans, including *Gonyaulax* and *Pfiesteria*. Similar to those of fungi, their cell wall structures vary significantly and include different polysaccharides, like cellulose and chitin, but in some cases (like *Euglena*) they lack a cell wall. In limited investigations, algae have been found to be relatively sensitive to most biocides that are used for water disinfection, including chlorine, chlorine dioxide, ozone, bromine, and UV radiation. The most widely used biocides for control of algae (generally algistatic rather than algicidal applications) are copper compounds, including copper sulfate, QACs, chlorine, bromochlorodimethyl hydantoin, and hydrogen peroxide. They are used to reduce algal growth in pools, water baths, tanks, and other water applications. Since many algae can grow as associated filaments, their close association within a biofilm either on or in water or associated with a surface can provide a mechanism for limited resistance to biocidal activity. Algae can be associated with bacterial biofilms, but they have also been found to produce extracellular polysaccharides, which can protect the cells within an algal biofilm. There is some evidence to suggest that algae have active stress responses similar to those of bacteria (see section 8.3.3) that allow greater tolerance of sublethal concentrations of biocides. Increased resistance to copper and other heavy metals has also been described. Algae are capable of accumulating heavy metals; physiological adaptations to the presence of copper include thickening of cell walls (when present) and an increase in the presence of vacuoles, which contain copper precipitates. In some strains, the presence of heavy metals also causes an increase in the presence of lipid and starch deposits within the cell. Active efflux as a mechanism of biocide resistance and cadmium tolerance in *Euglena* has been described; other algae have shown evidence of heavy-metal efflux, which is activated on exposure to the biocide. The extent of cross-resistance to other biocides has not been investigated. In addition to physiological adaptations, there is also evidence of acquired mechanisms of biocide tolerance in algae. Stable *Chlamydomonas reinhardtii* mutants with increased tolerance of heavy metals were developed in the laboratory. In some of the mutants, tolerance was restricted to increased concentrations of cadmium, but other mutants were cross-resistant to cadmium, copper, hydrogen peroxide, and UV light. Although the exact mechanism of resistance was not identified, it was proposed to be due to a specific chromosomal mutation event and to be associated with a change in the stress response. There are many reports of the isolation of copper-tolerant algal strains following exposure to sublethal concentrations of copper; in some cases, these mutant strains appeared to be smaller than the parent strains and had reduced metabolic activity. Finally, algae reproduce both asexually (by mitosis) and sexually (by the production of zygospores or zoospores). In the case of *Chlamydomonas*, sexual reproduction leads to the formation of a zygote, which then excretes a thick wall to form a zygospore. Similar to other sporulation processes, sexual reproduction is initiated under unfavorable environmental conditions. The zygospore consists of food (starch and lipid) reserves surrounded by the multilayered wall and is a resistant, dormant structure. Many zygospore developmental (maturation) mutants have been identified and are under investigation. The intrinsic tolerance of zygospores or other algal spores for biocides has not been studied but is clearly an important intrinsic mechanism of resistance to drying, lack of nutrients, and other environmental stresses.

Protozoa are also single-celled eukaryotes, but they do not contain a true cell wall (see section 1.3.3.4). Their vegetative forms (including trophozoites and sporozoites) do not present a significant challenge to most biocides at low-level concentrations. The modes of action of the various biocides and biocidal processes are not considered to be different from those described in bacteria. For example, chlorhexidine and other biguanides have been shown to primarily affect the structure and function of the plasma membrane, as observed by electron microscopy analysis of treated protozoa. Various intrinsic mechanisms of resistance that are similar to those identified in bacteria and fungi have been described in these forms, but they have not been well described. Vegetative forms survive various hostile environments, including the presence of host resistance mechanisms, like the production of superoxide ions and hydroxyl radicals. One intrinsic mechanism that has been discovered in *Leishmania* is the production of superoxide dismutase, which neutralizes superoxide ions (see section 8.3.5). This may be part of an overall stress response, as found in *Acanthamoeba castellanii* trophozoites, with the expression of various shock proteins on exposure to heat, oxidizing agents, and pH changes; the exact functions of these proteins have not been defined but are likely to be similar to those described in bacteria. They may include DNA repair mechanisms, which have been found in UV-irradiated *Cryptosporidium* species. Other physiological adaptations are the overproduction of surface glycoproteins or other proteins or carbohydrates, which may act to sequester the presence of the biocide, and alterations in protozoal permeability. Efflux and/or decreased-influx mechanisms have also been described and have been implicated in antiprotozoal drug (e.g., chloroquine) resistance. MDR ABC efflux pumps have been identified in *Plasmodium falciparum* and may also provide increased tolerance of biocides, as described in bacteria (see section 8.3.4). Many protozoa grow and multiply within host cells, including *Plasmodium* in hepatocytes and red blood cells and *Leishmania* in white blood cells; the intracellular locations of these protozoa may provide a protective mechanism against the effects of biocides. Further, various protozoa (including *A. castellanii*) have been associated with bacterial biofilms and become an integral part of the biofilm community. As an interesting note, *Legionella* strains and other bacteria have been found to survive within *Acanthamoeba* (including during the development of cysts and remaining viable within them, as discussed below) and subsequently within biofilms, providing them protection from biocides.

Acquired mechanisms of resistance have not been identified or investigated in any detail in protozoa, but it may be expected that various mutations could develop to increase tolerance of biocides. An example is the demonstration that triclosan inhibits protozoa like *Plasmodium*, *Toxoplasma*, and *Babesia* by interacting with enoyl acyl carrier protein reductases involved in fatty acid synthesis and similar to specific targets identified in bacteria (see section 8.7.2); it is likely, considering identified mutations that provide resistance to antiprotozoal drugs, that mechanisms for tolerance of triclosan similar to those described in bacteria may also occur in protozoa.

Similar to helminths, protozoa can produce dormant forms during their life cycles, such as cysts or oocysts (see section 1.3.3.4). Intestinal protozoa, such as *Cryptosporidium*, *Entamoeba*, and *Giardia*, are all potentially pathogenic to humans and animals and produce resistant, transmissible cysts (or oocysts for *Cryptosporidium*) that can be transmitted via water or contaminated surfaces. Although the intrinsic resistances of various types of oocysts and cysts vary, these dormant protozoal forms are considered more resistant to biocides than viruses, vegetative bacteria, and fungi but less resistant than *Ascaris* eggs and bacterial spores. *Giardia* cysts and *Cryptosporidium* oocysts have been isolated from chlorinated water and have been implicated in disease outbreaks due to inadequate disinfection. *Cryptosporidium parvum* is an obligate intracellular pathogen that can cause severe gastrointestinal disease, particularly in immunocompromised individuals. In response to environmental stress, it develops oocysts, which consist of a double layer of a protein-lipid-carbohydrate matrix that is produced within the oocyst itself during maturation (Fig. 8.40). *C. parvum* oocysts are considered the most resistant to chemical disinfection in comparison to other protozoal cysts, like those of *Giardia lamblia*. Of the biocides widely used for water disinfection, oxidizing agents, like ozone and hydrogen peroxide, are considered the most effective protozoal cysticides, followed by chlorine dioxide, iodine, and free chlorine, all of which are more effective than the chloramines. The thicknesses of *Cryptosporidium* oocyst walls

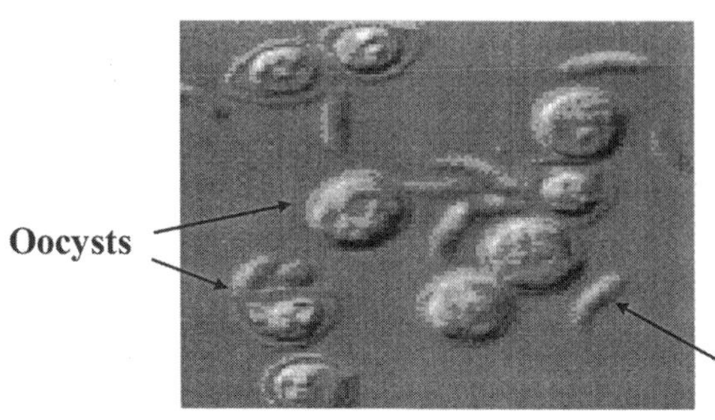

FIGURE 8.40 *C. parvum* oocysts and sporozoites.

vary, and thinner-walled oocysts are considered less resistant to biocides and other environmental factors than the thicker-walled types. In studies with various surface sterilization and disinfection methods, steam, ETO, and hydrogen peroxide gas-plasma sterilization processes were confirmed to be effective against *C. parvum* oocysts. Liquid hydrogen peroxide formulations (at 6 to 7.5%) were also effective, but oocysts have been described as being resistant to normal, in-use concentrations of peracetic acid, sodium hypochlorite, phenolics, QAC, iodophores, glutaraldehyde, and OPA-based disinfectants. As with other microorganisms, the presence of soils limited the activities of the disinfectants due to reduced penetration. Peracetic acid-based formulations were effective at higher exposure temperatures (>40°C), but oocysts were also found to be relatively sensitive to temperatures in the 50 to 60°C range, thus presenting little resistance to heat in comparison to chemical biocides. Oocysts were also inactivated by UV radiation, freeze-thaw cycles, and desiccation, unlike bacterial spores. The mechanisms of chemical biocide resistance are unknown, but it is reasonable to assume that cysts, similar to spores, take up fewer disinfectant molecules from solution than do vegetative forms. In some studies, resistance appeared to be primarily due to the protein components of the cyst wall layers.

The cysts of the amoeba *A. castellanii* have also been studied in some detail (Fig. 8.41). They are significantly more resistant than vegetative trophozoites (Table 8.34).

Some recent studies have compared the responses of cysts and trophozoites of *A. castellanii* to disinfectants employed in contact lens solutions and followed the development of resistance during encystation and the loss of resistance during excystation. Similar to the development of bacterial spores (see section 8.3.11), as *A. castellanii* trophozoites developed and matured into cysts, resistance to various bio-

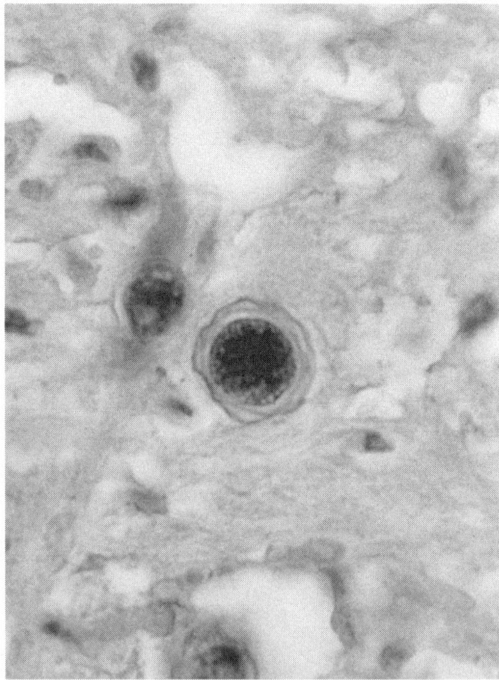

FIGURE 8.41 An *Acanthamoeba* cyst. Reprinted with permission of the U.S. Armed Forces Institute of Pathology.

TABLE 8.34 Minimum amoebicidal concentrations for *Acanthamoeba* trophozoites and cysts

Biocide	Minimum amoebicidal concn (mg/liter)	
	Trophozoites	Cysts
Chlorine	2	>50
Peracetic acid	15	150
BNPD[a]	250	>5,000
BKC[b]	60	>5,000

[a]BNPD, bromonitropropanediol, a bromine-releasing agent.
[b]BKC, benzalkonium chloride, a QAC.

cides could be detected; earlier in development, tolerance of hydrochloric acid was observed, followed by benzalkonium chloride, hydrogen peroxide, and moist heat, with resistance to chlorhexidine observed later. The lethal effects of chlorhexidine and of a polymeric biguanide were found to be time and concentration dependent, and mature cysts were clearly more resistant than preencysted trophozoites or post-excysted cysts. The cyst wall structure appeared to act as a barrier to the uptake of these agents, presenting a classical type of intrinsic resistance mechanism. The multilayered walls of *A. castellanii* cysts develop around the inner cyst core, which is surrounded by a cell membrane, with the initial deposition of inner cellulose-based wall layers and subsequent maturation of external proteinaceous wall coats. The development of the inner cellulose-based layers appears to play a major role in resistance to biocides, although the outer protein layers seem to present a greater barrier to biocide penetration. *Acanthamoeba* is capable of forming biofilms on surfaces, such as contact lenses. Although protozoal biofilms have yet to be studied extensively in terms of their response to disinfectants, it is apparent that they could play a significant part in modulating the effects of chemical agents.

FURTHER READING

Baron, H., J. Safar, D. Groth, S. J. DeArmond, and S. B. Prusiner. 2001. Prions, p. 659–674. *In* S. S. Block (ed.). *Disinfection, Sterilization, and Preservation*, 5th ed. Lippincott Williams & Wilkins, Philadelphia, Pa.

Block, S. S. 2001. *Disinfection, Sterilization, and Preservation*, 5th ed. Lippincott Williams & Wilkins, Philadelphia, Pa.

Brown, N. L., A. P. Morby, and N. J. Robinson (ed.). 2003. Interactions of bacteria with metals. *FEMS Microbiol. Rev.* **27:**129–447.

Cabiscol, E., J. Tamarit, and J. Ros. 2000. Oxidative stress in bacteria and protein damage by reactive oxygen species. *Int. Microbiol.* **3:**3–8.

Denyer, S. P., and W. B. Hugo. 1991. *Mechanisms of Action of Chemical Biocides.* Blackwell Scientific, Cambridge, Mass.

Donlan, R. M., and J. W. Costerton. 2002. Biofilms: survival mechanisms of clinically relevant microorganisms. *Clin. Microbiol. Rev.* **15:**167–193.

Fields, P. A. 2001. Protein function at thermal extremes: balancing stability and flexibility. *Comp. Biochem. Physiol. A* **129:**417–431.

Fraise, A. P., P. A. Lambert, and J.-Y. Maillard. 2004. *Russell, Hugo & Ayliffe's Principles and Practice of Disinfection, Preservation & Sterilization*, 4th ed. Blackwell Science Ltd., Malden, Mass.

Gilbert, P., and A. J. McBain. 2003. Potential impact of increased use of biocides in consumer products on prevalence of antibiotic resistance. *Clin. Microbiol. Rev.* **16:**189–208.

Grkovic, S., M. H. Brown, and R. A. Skurray. 2002. Regulation of bacterial drug export systems. *Microbiol. Mol. Biol. Rev.* **66:**671–701.

Guarro, J., J. Gene, and A. M. Stchigel. 1999. Developments in fungal taxonomy. *Clin. Microbiol. Rev.* **12:**454–500.

Lappin-Scott, H. M., and J. W. Costerton. 2003. *Microbial Biofilms.* Cambridge University Press, Cambridge, England.

Madigan, M. T., J. M. Martinko, and J. Parker. 2003. *Brock Biology of Microorganisms*, 10th ed. Pearson Education, Upper Saddle River, N.J.

Maillard, J.-Y., and A. D. Russell. 1997. Viricidal activity and mechanisms of action of biocides. *Sci. Progr.* **80:**287–315.

Makarova, K. S., L. Aravind, Y. I. Wolf, R. L. Tatusov, K. W. Minton, E. V. Koonin, and M. J. Daly. 2001. Genome of the extremely radiation-resistant bacterium *Deinococcus radiodurans* viewed from the perspective of comparative genomics. *Microbiol. Mol. Biol. Rev.* **65:**44–79.

McDonnell, G., and A. D. Russell. 1999. Antiseptics and disinfectants: activity, action and resistance. *Clin. Microbiol. Rev.* **12:**147–179.

Paulsen, I. T., and K. Lewis. 2002. *Microbial Multidrug Efflux.* Horizon Press, Norwich, United Kingdom.

Poole, K. 2005. Efflux-mediated antimicrobial resistance. *J. Antimicrob. Chemother.* **56:**20–51.

Rothschild, L. J., and R. L. Mancinelli. 2001. Life in extreme environments. *Nature* **409:** 1092–1101.

Russell, A. D. 1982. *The Destruction of Bacterial Spores.* Academic Press, London, United Kingdom.

Russell, A. D. 1990. Bacterial spores and chemical sporicidal agents. *Clin. Microbiol. Rev.* **3:**99–119.

Russell, A. D. 1997. Plasmids and bacterial resistance to biocides. *J. Appl. Microbiol.* **82:**155–165.

Russell, A. D. 2003. Similarities and differences in the responses of microorganisms to biocides. *J. Antimicrob. Chemother.* **52:**750–763.

Russell, A. D., and I. Chopra. 1996. *Understanding Antibacterial Action and Resistance*, 2nd ed. Ellis Horwood, Hemel Hempstead, England.

Russell, A. D., J. R. Furr, and J.-Y. Maillard. 1997. Microbial susceptibility and resistance to biocides. *ASM News* **63:**481–487.

Russell, A. D., W. B. Hugo, and G. A. J. Ayliffe. 1992. *Principles and Practice of Disinfection, Preservation & Sterilization*, 2nd ed. Blackwell Science, Cambridge, Mass.

Schweizer, H. P. 2001. Triclosan: a widely used biocide and its link to antibiotics. *FEMS Microbiol. Lett.* **202:**1–7.

Springthorpe, V. S., and S. A. Satter. 1990. Chemical disinfection of virus-contaminated surfaces. *Crit. Rev. Environ. Contam.* **20:**169–229.

INDEX